Handbook of Violence Risk Assessment and Treatment

Joel T. Andrade, MSW, LICSW, is a licensed independent clinical social worker in Massachusetts. He received his Master's degree in social work from the Boston College Graduate School of Social Work where he is currently a PhD candidate. Andrade's dissertation focuses on psychosocial precursors of psychopathy in adult psychiatric patients.

For 11 years, Andrade worked at Bridgewater State Hospital, which is the only maximum-security forensic hospital in Massachusetts. While there, he was the admission coordinator, director of the intensive treatment unit, and clinical risk assessment coordinator. At Bridgewater State Hospital he evaluated and treated hundreds of individuals that require "strict security" under Massachusetts General Law. He testified as an expert witness in the area of violence risk assessment and risk management of violent offenders, and conducted violence risk assessment evaluations of forensic patients being considered for transfer to less secure settings.

Andrade currently works as a clinical operations specialist for MHM Services, Inc., the leading national specialist in providing mental health programming and services to correctional systems, including state prisons and local jails. In this capacity, he writes clinical program guidelines for mental health treatment within correctional facilities, consults with staff nationwide regarding violence risk assessment, and ongoing risk management of violent offenders, and provides clinical consultation for individual cases and when implementing treatment programs within correctional facilities in several states.

He has presented at numerous national and international conferences in the areas of: violence risk assessment, treatment, and risk management of violent offenders; self-injurious behavior in correctional facilities; behavior management within correctional facilities; psychopathy in juvenile and adult populations; psychopathy as a risk factor for violence; evaluation and treatment of adult and juvenile sex offenders; and psychopathy among sex offenders. He has also published in peer-reviewed journals, and is a reviewer for several peer-reviewed journals.

Handbook of Violence Risk Assessment and Treatment

New Approaches for Mental Health Professionals

JOEL T. ANDRADE, MSW, LICSW

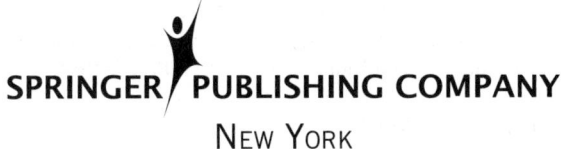

SPRINGER PUBLISHING COMPANY

NEW YORK

Copyright © 2009 Springer Publishing Company, LLC

All rights reserved.

No part of this publication may be reproduced, stored in a retrieval system, or transmitted in any form or by any means, electronic, mechanical, photocopying, recording, or otherwise, without the prior permission of the publisher or authorization through payment of the appropriate fees to the Copyright Clearance Center, Inc., 222 Rosewood Drive, Danvers, MA 01923, 978-750-8400, fax 978-646-8600, info@copyright.com or on the web at www.copyright.com

Springer Publishing Company, LLC
11 West 42nd Street
New York, NY 10036
www.springerpub.com

Acquisitions Editor: Jennifer Perillo
Production Manager: Julia Rosen
Cover Design: David Levy
Composition: Apex CoVantage, LLC

E-Book ISBN: 978-0-8261-9904-1

09 10 11 / 5 4 3 2 1

The author and the publisher of this work have made every effort to use sources believed to be reliable to provide information that is accurate and compatible with the standards generally accepted at the time of publication. Because medical science is continually advancing, our knowledge base continues to expand. Therefore, as new information becomes available, changes in procedures become necessary. We recommend that the reader always consult current research and specific institutional policies before performing any clinical procedure.

The author and publisher shall not be liable for any special, consequential, or exemplary damages resulting, in whole or in part, from readers' use of, or reliance on, the information contained in this book. The publisher has no responsibility for the persistence or accuracy of URLs for external or third-party Internet Web sites referred to in this publication and does not guarantee that any content on such Web sites is, or will remain, accurate or appropriate.

Library of Congress Cataloging-in-Publication Data

Handbook of violence risk assessment and treatment : new approaches for mental health professionals / Joel T. Andrade.
    p. ; cm.
  Includes bibliographical references and index.
  ISBN 978-0-8261-9903-4 (alk. paper)
  1. Forensic psychiatry—Handbooks, manuals, etc. 2. Violence—Forecasting—Handbooks, manuals, etc. I. Andrade, Joel T.
    [DNLM: 1. Forensic Psychiatry—methods. 2. Adolescent. 3. Risk Assessment. 4. Violence. W 740 H2369 2009]
  RA1151.H27 2009
  614'.15—dc22   2008050928

Printed in the United States of America by Bang Printing.

—To my wife, Susanne
You are my constant source of support and inspiration

—To the victims of violence
So we are able to prevent future victims

Contents

Contributors xi
Foreword xv
Preface xix
Acknowledgments xxiii

PART I: ADULT VIOLENCE 1

1 Violence Risk Assessment and Risk Management: A Historical Overview and Clinical Application 3
   Joel T. Andrade, Katherine O'Neill, and Robert B. Diener

2 Violence Risk Assessment Evaluation: Practices and Procedures 41
   Michael H. Fogel

3 The Utility of Dynamic and Static Factors in Risk Assessment, Prediction, and Treatment 83
   Stephen C. P. Wong, Mark E. Olver, and Keira C. Stockdale

4 Contextualizing Women's Violence: Gender-Responsive Assessment and Treatment 121
   Judith S. Willison and Yvonne L. Lutter

5 Intimate Partner Violence 157
   Gretchen E. Ely and Chris Flaherty

6 Sex Offender–Specific Treatment: Historical Foundations, Current Challenges, and Contemporary Approaches 179
   Laurie L. Guidry

7 Keeping Vigil: Neuropsychiatry in the Forensic Setting   221
Joseph H. Baskin

8 Psychopathy: Assessment, Treatment, and Risk Management   241
Joel T. Andrade

9 Treatment and Management of Violence and Criminal Risk Among Mentally Ill Offenders   291
José B. Ashford, Katherine O. Sternbach, and Maureen F. Balaam

10 Treating the Morally Objectionable   311
James Knoll IV

PART II: YOUTH VIOLENCE   347

11 Youth Violence: Prevalence, Etiology, and Treatment   349
Frank DiCataldo, Matt C. Zaitchik, and Kate Provencher

12 Risk/Needs Tools for Antisocial Behavior and Violence Among Youthful Populations   377
Gina M. Vincent, Anna M. Terry, and Shannon M. Maney

13 Reducing Risk for Violence and Aggression in Youth   425
Craig S. Schwalbe

14 Contextualizing Girls' Violence: Assessment and Treatment Decisions   449
Judith A. Ryder, Cindy Gordon, and Jessica Bulger

15 Identifying and Responding to Criminogenic Risk and Mental Health Treatment Needs of Crossover Youth   495
Denise C. Herz, Sharon Harada, Gregory Lecklitner, Michael Rauso, and Joseph P. Ryan

16 Understanding Complexity in Sexually Abusive Youth   529
Phil Rich

17 Juvenile Stalking: An Overview of Assessment and
Management Issues   561
R. Gregg Dwyer and Deborah L. Laufersweiler-Dwyer

18 Applying Skills Directed Therapy to Aggressive Children   573
Tammie Ronen and Michael Rosenbaum

19 Ecological and Evidence-Based Family Intervention
for Juvenile Justice Practitioners   601
Susan B. Stern, Jeanine A. Webber, and Leena K. Augimeri

Index   639

Contributors

José B. Ashford, MSW, PhD, LICSW
Professor and Associate Director
School of Social Work
Arizona State University
Director of the Office of Forensic Social Work
Affiliate Professor of Criminology and Criminal Justice and Justice and Social Inquiry

Leena K. Augimeri, PhD
Director, Centre for Children Committing Offences & Program Development
Child Development Institute
Toronto, Canada
Adjunct Assistant Professor and Sessional Lecturer
University of Toronto

Maureen F. Balaam, MS, MFT
Private psychotherapy practice and consultation services
Monterey, CA

Joseph H. Baskin, MD
Forensic Psychiatrist
Assistant Clinical Professor
The Ohio State University Department of Psychiatry
Columbus, OH

Jessica Bulger, LICSW
Senior Clinical Director
Germaine Lawrence, Inc.
Arlington, MA

Frank DiCataldo, PhD
Forensic Psychologist
Assistant Professor of Psychology
Roger Williams University
Bristol, RI
Clinical Director
Forensic Evaluation Service
Northeast Family Institute–Massachusetts
Danvers, MA

Robert B. Diener, MD
Medical Director of Bridgewater State Hospital
MHM Services, Inc.
Bridgewater, MA

R. Gregg Dwyer, MD, EdD
Assistant Professor and Director
Sexual Behaviors Evaluation, Research and Treatment Clinic and Laboratory
Department of Neuropsychiatry and Behavioral Science
University of South Carolina School of Medicine
Columbia, SC

Gretchen E. Ely, PhD
Assistant Professor
University of Kentucky College of Social Work
Lexington, KY

Chris Flaherty, PhD
Assistant Professor
University of Kentucky, College of Social Work
Lexington, KY

Michael H. Fogel, PsyD, ABPP
Chair, Department of Forensic Psychology
The Chicago School of Professional Psychology
Chicago, IL

Cindy Gordon, MSW, LICSW
Director of Juvenile Services
Forensic Health Services Inc.
Braintree, MA

Laurie L. Guidry, PsyD
Clinical Psychologist
Director, Mentally Ill/Problematic Sexual Behavior Program
Massachusetts Department of Mental Health
President, Massachusetts Association for the Treatment of Sexual Abusers
Boston, MA

Sharon Harada, BA
Bureau Chief, Juvenile Field Services
County of Los Angeles Probation Department
Los Angeles, CA

Denise C. Herz, PhD
Professor in the School of Criminal Justice and Criminalistics
California State University–Los Angeles
Los Angeles, CA

James Knoll IV, MD
Director of Forensic Psychiatry
Associate Professor of Psychiatry
SUNY Upstate Medical University
Syracuse, NY

Deborah L. Laufersweiler-Dwyer, PhD
Professor, Department of Criminal Justice
University of Arkansas at Little Rock
Little Rock, AR

Gregory Lecklitner, PhD
Mental Health Clinical District Chief
Los Angeles County Department of Mental Health
Los Angeles, CA

Yvonne L. Lutter, PsyD
Clinical Director
Forensic Health Services of MHM
New Mexico Women's Correctional Facility
Grants, NM

Shannon M. Maney, MA, MA
Department of Psychiatry
University of Massachusetts Medical School
Worcester, MA

Mark E. Olver, PhD
Assistant Professor
Department of Psychology
University of Saskatchewan
Saskatoon, Saskatchewan, Canada

Katherine O'Neill, MSW, LICSW
Director of a Maximum-Security Unit at Bridgewater State Hospital
MHM Services Inc.
Bridgewater, MA

Kate Provencher, MA
Doctoral Student
Massachusetts School of Professional Psychology
Boston, MA

Michael Rauso, PsyD, MFT
Los Angeles County Department of Children and Family Services
Los Angeles, CA

Contributors   **xiii**

Phil Rich, EdD, LICSW
Clinical Director
Stetson School Inc.
Barre, MA

Tammie Ronen, PhD
Social Worker,
  Full Professor
The Bob Shapell School of
  Social Work
Tel-Aviv University
Tel-Aviv, Israel

Michael Rosenbaum, PhD
Clinical Psychology, Full
  Professor
Department of Psychology
Tel-Aviv University
Tel-Aviv, Israel

Joseph P. Ryan, MSW, PhD
Assistant Professor and Faculty
  Fellow
Children and Family Research
  Center
School of Social Work
University of Illinois at
  Urbana-Champaign
Champaign, IL

Judith A. Ryder, PhD
Criminal Justice
Assistant Professor, Sociology and
  Anthropology Department
St. John's University
Queens, NY

Craig S. Schwalbe, MSW, PhD
Assistant Professor
Columbia University School of
  Social Work
New York, NY

Susan B. Stern, PhD
Associate Professor
Factor-Inwentash Faculty of
  Social Work
University of Toronto
Toronto, ON, Canada

Katherine O. Sternbach, MEd, MBA
Principal and Senior
  Consultant
Mercer Government Human
  Services Consulting
San Francisco, CA

Keira C. Stockdale, PhD
Clinical Associate, Young
  Offender Team
Mental Health and Addiction
  Services
Saskatoon Health Region
Saskatoon, Saskatchewan,
  Canada

Anna M. Terry, MA
Doctoral Student
Massachusetts School of
  Professional Psychology
Boston, MA

Gina M. Vincent, PhD
Assistant Professor
Center for Mental Health
  Services Research
Department of Psychiatry
University of Massachusetts
  Medical School
Worcester, MA

Jeanine A. Webber, MSW, RSW
PhD Candidate
  (University of Toronto)
Factor-Inwentash Faculty of
  Social Work
University of Toronto
Program Coordinator & Professor,
  Community and Justice
  Services Program
Humber Institute for
  Technology and Advanced
  Learning
Toronto, ON, Canada

Judith S. Willison, MSW, LICSW
Director of Operations
Forensic Health Services
Braintree, MA

Stephen C. P. Wong, PhD
Professor, Personality Disorder
  Institute
University of Nottingham
Visiting Professor
Department of Forensic Mental
  Health Science, Institute of
  Psychiatry
King's College,
  University of London
Adjunct Professor
Department of Psychology
University of Saskatchewan

Matt C. Zaitchik, PhD, ABPP
Associate Professor of Psychology
Roger Williams University
Bristol, RI

Foreword

It has been fascinating to watch the growth of scientific and clinical knowledge about violence risk assessment and management during the past 35 years. Until the 1970s, the practice of identifying the violence potential of persons with mental disorders received little research attention. In the ensuing three decades, however, research has provided a wealth of scientific and clinical knowledge about the best ways to estimate violence potential in clinical populations.

Chapter 1 of this volume provides a key to how this happened. Violence risk assessment is driven by two imperatives, whose icons are two of the most important mental health law cases of the 1970s. One was the *Tarasoff* case, which held that a mental health professional must do something to protect others if they are at risk of serious harm by the professional's patient. The other was *O'Connor v. Donaldson*, which held that doctors could not simply lock up patients against their will for treatment purposes unless they also presented a risk of harm to others or to themselves.

Tarasoff was intended to protect society from patients' potential violence, and *O'Connor v. Donaldson* was intended to protect patients from society's potential impulse to lock them up unfairly. This conflict between the state's interests in avoiding violence and the individual's right to be protected from unwarranted state intervention was a classic product of the mid-twentieth-century civil rights movement in U.S. law. And it put a spotlight on the importance of identifying violence risk, which was essential for a just conclusion when such conflicts arose.

Requiring that one protect endangered people from patients' violence, or allowing for patients' hospitalization due to dangerousness, necessarily required that someone must identify whether a patient's condition required either of these things. Mental health professionals, of course, were perceived as the most likely persons to have the expertise to predict violence among patients with mental illnesses. Yet, ironically,

Tarasoff and *O'Connor* arose at the very same time that research was revealing the dismal quality of clinicians' predictions about their patients' harm to others. How could society or patients be legally protected when no one could claim to be able to make a valid assessment of the likelihood of patients' future violent behavior?

Thus began an extraordinary scientific effort to identify ways to improve estimates of future violence among patients with mental disorders, as well as among offenders with violence histories. What ensued was the rise of what has become one of the most prolific areas of research in the history of forensic psychology and psychiatry. The foundation for this enterprise was laid by several large-scale research efforts in the 1990s (described in Chapter 1) that discovered actuarial and standardized, structured clinical methods that could create at least reasonably valid estimates of the likelihood of future violence.

By the beginning of our present decade, research had turned to translating the findings of the 1990s into methods that clinicians could use in everyday practice. Practical tools were developed to structure clinicians' evaluations of risk of violence. And variations on the methods were developed and tested for use with many special populations, including sex offenders, youth, and women.

Researchers also came to recognize that the ultimate goal of violence risk assessment was not only identifying risk, but also reducing it. Thus assessment methods were modified to offer not only risk estimates, but also indicators of the best ways to reduce the risk of patients' future violence through treatment and clinical management of the factors that increased the risk. This involved the dynamic notion that a patient's assessed risk level was not simply a static characteristic of the patient. It was something that could be altered—for example, by altering the factors in a patient's environment that increased the risk. Thus an assessment of risk—if it identified such risk factors—could in itself reduce the risk, rather than simply giving the patient a risk-level label.

The requirements for mental health practitioners in this area are far different from the days when *Tarasoff* and *O'Connor* issued the challenge to violence risk assessment. Clinicians of that era could not be expected to do much more than use their clinical intuition when judging their patients' violence potential. Today, however, using unstructured clinical speculation to assess risk of violence is incompetent practice and, in some cases, unethical practice. The practice standards of all mental health professionals hold them responsible for using the best evidence-based practices that our research has developed and translated for their use over the past three decades.

And that is what this book prepares clinicians to do. The authors of these chapters have distilled the field's efforts to translate our best research into best practices for estimating our patients' likelihood of harm to others. They have written not just for those who work in forensic settings, but for all mental health professionals who work with a wide range of populations in a variety of clinical circumstances. Their perspectives cross all disciplinary lines, consistent with their own professional training in social work, psychology and psychiatry. Most of these authors themselves are practitioners who experience every day the demands of real-world clinical and forensic settings, and who are champions for the use of practical methods that have been informed by rigorous empirical research. As such, they are more than authors. They are role models for the practitioners whom they seek to assist in developing empirically-based clinical practice. Hear them, and dedicate yourself to the ideals they represent.

Thomas Grisso
University of Massachusetts Medical School

Preface

In 2006, there were 1,417,745 violent crimes reported in the United States. Of these, 17,034 were crimes resulting in the death of a victim; 92,455 were forcible rapes; and 860,853 were aggravated assaults (U.S. Department of Justice, Federal Bureau of Investigation, 2006). Statistics such as these increase the public's concern for being victimized by violent offenders and raise the concern of policy makers (Lowry, Nio, & Leitner, 2003). Highly publicized cases of extreme violence perpetrated by individuals with a history of criminal activity have led to the widespread perception that violent offenders will continue their violent behavior despite intervention. As a result, public policy has increased sanctions in the form of confinement, often without increasing rehabilitative services. The result is a significant increase in incarcerated individuals that require mental health services and ongoing management. In 1956, 550,000 individuals were treated within state psychiatric hospitals in the United States. This has declined 90% over a 40-year period; in 1996, 61,700 individuals were treated within these psychiatric facilities. During this same time period, the number of incarcerated offenders presenting with mental health needs increased dramatically. As a result, correctional facilities have become the leading provider of mental health services in the United States (American Psychiatric Association, 2004).

Ninety-seven percent of all incarcerated individuals will eventually reintegrate into society at a rate of 650,000 per year (Council of State Governments, 2005). Those released from prisons and jails are frequently at the same level of risk for future violence as when they were initially incarcerated. Forensic practitioners are often called on to assess the risk such offenders pose to the general public. As such, these practitioners are frequently caught between public perception, policy makers, and the criminal justice system.

During the past 30 years great strides have been made in the area of violence risk assessment, treatment, and risk management. The empirical literature of the 1970s focused on the "prediction" of violence. However, this research evolved from attempting to "predict" violence to quantitatively assessing factors that increase an individual's risk for future violence. The current research literature is asking more specific questions regarding the assessment and management of risk. Typical questions now being asked of practitioners and in the literature include: How can we manage an individual's risk for future violence? and How can we intervene in a way to decrease this individual's risk for future violence? The ability to conduct violence risk assessment evaluations that inform decision making and ongoing risk management is a necessary skill for forensic practitioners. These questions have typically been asked of those working in forensic or correctional settings, but are now asked of civil psychiatric, school-based, and outpatient practitioners. To answer such questions requires astute clinical skill as well as a comprehensive grasp of the relevant research literature.

The goal of this volume is to provide practitioners with the knowledge base necessary to conduct violence risk assessments and to synthesize clinical and research data into comprehensive reports and oral testimony. There are hundreds of articles and book chapters dedicated to violence risk assessment, but far fewer address the treatment and risk management of individuals who engage in violent behavior. This volume is dedicated to both. Assessment is an ongoing process that requires practitioners to determine the current level of risk and intervene so as to prevent future violence. Therefore, included in each practitioner's opinion regarding an individual's level of risk for future violence, a well-formulated and comprehensive risk management plan is also necessary. To that end, each chapter in this volume addresses the issue of treatment and risk management. This task is large and requires a wealth of information from various disciplines including social work, psychology, psychiatry, sociology, and criminology, all of which are represented in this volume. All chapters are authored by leading experts in their respective fields who were asked to take what is known from the empirical research literature and apply it to clinical practice. Authors were also encouraged to consider difficult cases that often require intensive intervention and collaboration between treatment providers.

Research findings and treatment interventions germane to adult populations are often not applicable to juvenile and youthful populations, and vice versa. Forensic practitioners often work with clientele of all ages, so this volume is divided into two sections, one focusing on violence in adult populations and the other dedicated to violence among youthful populations. This book will provide practitioners with knowledge of the developmental course of aggressive behavior throughout the life cycle, as well as appropriate risk assessment techniques and ongoing risk management strategies based on the individual's developmental level.

Each section begins with chapters devoted to reviewing what is known about violence risk assessment in general, the etiology of violent behavior, and analysis of the relevant research literature (chapters 1–3 and 11–13). The following chapters in each section are dedicated to special populations of concern to practitioners. The adult section addresses female offenders (chapter 4), intimate partner violence (chapter 5), sexual offenders (chapter 6), neurological issues (chapter 7), and psychopathic offenders (chapter 8). The youth section addresses aggression in girls and young women (chapter 14), crossover youth (chapter 15), sexually abusive youth (chapter 16), and juvenile stalking (17).

Finally, each section concludes with two chapters dedicated to specialized treatment interventions. For adults, chapter 9 focuses on the treatment of mentally ill offenders and chapter 10 discusses the difficulties in treating the morally objectionable. For youth, chapter 18 examines skills-directed therapy and chapter 19 reviews family interventions.

Clinical examples are used throughout this volume to illustrate the process of conducting violence risk assessments, the tools used in these evaluations, and how information is translated into an overall assessment and guide for future risk management.

This book is multifaceted in order to address the needs of practitioners from various fields including social work, psychology, psychiatry, and students in these disciplines. Practitioners involved in all phases of intervention, from initial assessment to long-term treatment and risk management, will use this volume to inform their clinical practice. This book was also designed for officials—such as judges, lawyers, correctional officials, probation officers, and public policy makers—who make decisions in cases where risk for future violence is an issue. These groups will gain invaluable insights into the current state-of-the-art of violence risk assessment and risk management of violent individuals. While this volume will be useful to these diverse groups, the goal is to provide practitioners with an understanding of the current risk assessment, treatment, and risk management research literature and how to apply empirical findings to forensic practice.

Because our understanding of violence is growing rapidly, it is the responsibility of practitioners to remain current with best practices specific to the population they serve. This volume will do so for those involved in decision making in the areas of risk assessment, treatment, and risk management of violent individuals. It is also my hope that this volume will contribute to the prevention of future violence by providing practitioners and other decision makers with the appropriate tools necessary to ensure evidence-based assessment and methods of intervention.

REFERENCES

American Psychiatric Association. (2004). *Mental illness and the criminal justice system: Redirecting resources toward treatment, not containment.* Arlington, VA: Author.

Council of State Governments. (2005, January). *Report of the Re-Entry Policy Council: Charting the safe and successful return of prisoners to the community.* New York: Author.

Lowry, D. T., Nio, T.C.J., & Leitner, D. W. (2003). Setting the public fear agenda: A longitudinal analysis of network TV crime reporting, public perceptions of crime, and FBI crime statistics. *Journal of Communication, 53*(1), 61–73.

U.S. Department of Justice, Federal Bureau of Investigation. (2006). *Uniform crime reports for the United States.* Washington, DC: Author.

Acknowledgments

First, many thanks to the 40 distinguished authors who worked diligently on this project. Your chapters stand alone as individual contributions to the evidence-based literature on violence risk assessment, treatment, and risk management. Together these chapters make up a comprehensive volume addressing the current state-of-the-art in these areas.

This work would not have been possible without the support of the incredible group of individuals at Springer Publishing. Special thanks to Jennifer Perillo, senior acquisitions editor, who helped cultivate this volume from its earliest stages and kept it on track throughout this process. Your understanding and guidance is very much appreciated.

Several academic mentors and professional colleagues sparked my interest in forensic practice as a master's student, and sustained this interest through their support, scholarly discussions, and ongoing friendships. I would like especially to thank Thomas O'Hare, Thomas Walsh, Elaine Pinderhughes, Karen Kayser, Ce Shen, Richard Rowland, Gina Vincent, and Ira Packer.

I also would like to thank the team of forensic practitioners, correctional officers, and nurses at Bridgewater State Hospital who I worked with and learned so much from over the years. Each day was a learning experience that required the application of what is known from empirical research to actual practice. It is my hope that this book is a tribute to your dedication to prevent violence through proper assessment and intervention. In particular I would like to thank Paul Caratazzola for his encouragement, sense of humor, and for sharing his wealth of knowledge with me over the years. I would also like to thank the clinical and correctional administration at Bridgewater State Hospital for their support, especially Robert Diener, Susan Lantagne, Rhonda Cantelli, Kenneth Nelson, Karin Bergeron, Susan Skea, and many more. I would also like to thank the Clinical Operations Team and others at MHM Services, Inc. for leading the way in ensuring the delivery of evidenced-based mental health services within correctional facilities. Special thanks to Jane Haddad, Sharen Barboza, John Wilson, Hal Smith, Richard Bennett, and Sandra Lasater.

A very special thanks to my family for their lifelong support, encouragement, and for sacrificing our time together as I worked on this project. Thank you Mom, Dad, and Jason. Finally, to my wife, Susanne, who always responded to my requests to review a paragraph, a section, or an entire chapter no matter how late into the night. Without your love, patience, and unending encouragement this would not have been possible.

Adult Violence

PART I

1

Violence Risk Assessment and Risk Management: A Historical Overview and Clinical Application

JOEL T. ANDRADE, KATHERINE O'NEILL, AND ROBERT B. DIENER

Forensic practitioners are increasingly asked to conduct assessments and evaluations for criminal justice systems, such as adult and juvenile courts, parole and probation departments, and correctional facilities, as well as for child protective services agencies, school departments, community mental health centers, and more. Although a variety of questions may be asked of the practitioner, this chapter will focus on those related to violence risk assessment. A typical question posed to the forensic practitioner is: Does this individual pose a risk to society at large, and, if so, what is the nature of that risk? As our ability to conduct violence risk assessment evaluations has improved, additional, often more difficult, questions usually follow, such as: What treatment interventions or strategies will decrease this individual's risk? and How will we know when this individual can safely reintegrate into society?

Such questions are difficult to answer but are at the heart of forensic practice. To answer such questions requires both astute clinical skill as well as a comprehensive grasp of the empirical research literature. The goal of this chapter is to provide a historical overview of the violence risk

---

The authors would like to thank Paul Caratazzola, MSW, LICSW, for his helpful comments and suggestions on an earlier draft of this chapter.

assessment literature and to detail the clinical application of a violence risk assessment evaluation.

To that end, this chapter will begin with a brief discussion of the diverse types of violence risk assessment evaluations conducted by forensic practitioners. Next, two court cases that call for mental health professionals to conduct such assessments will be reviewed. This will be followed by a discussion of what is now referred to as the three generations of risk assessment literature. Risk assessment tools that are a product of this research will be examined. Next, individual risk factors found to correlate with future violence will be reviewed. Guidelines for the specification of risk assessment, treatment and risk management, and risk communication will also be presented. Finally, a forensic case will illustrate how violence risk assessment evaluations are practically conducted by the forensic practitioner.

WHAT IS VIOLENCE RISK ASSESSMENT?

The phrase *violence risk assessment* may have various meanings to forensic practitioners, depending on the setting in which they practice including correctional facilities, forensic hospitals, and civil psychiatric facilities. The following paragraphs provide a brief overview of the different types of violence risk assessment evaluations conducted in such settings.

In correctional settings, prison officials often request a violence risk assessment as part of assigning offenders to various levels of security. Individuals who are at high risk for violence are placed in maximum-security facilities, while those at lower risk are placed in medium- or minimum-security facilities. Also, in such settings, parole considerations often rely on the recommendations made by clinical staff responsible for evaluating an offender.

In a forensic psychiatric setting, the practitioner is most likely asked to consider an individual's short- and long-term risk for violence and to recommend treatment strategies to mitigate such risk. Forensic practitioners are asked to assess the distal (long-term) risk an individual poses to society in the context of the need for continued hospitalization. This differs from situations in which the practitioner is asked to assess the proximal or short-term risk. The latter evaluation guides decisions around internal placement, including seclusion or segregation.

Practitioners working in civil psychiatric settings are relied upon to determine the potential risk for violence an individual poses prior to release to the community. In this context, it is incumbent upon the clinician to consider the type of outcome behavior that is being assessed. Such factors to be examined could include violent behavior, general criminal behavior, sexual violence, risk for suicide, and treatment noncompliance.

This list illustrates the range of potential risk assessments conducted by forensic practitioners. The type of assessment, variables to be considered, and the level of potential risk vary widely among these evaluations.

Regardless of the setting, to prepare a comprehensive evaluation, the practitioner must be an authority in two areas: (1) the patient's developmental, psychiatric, criminal, and violence history and (2) the research literature in the area of violence risk assessment and risk management. A forensic practitioner's understanding of the research literature must be specific both to the question being asked as well to the specific risk and protective factors with which an individual presents.

Preliminary Questions to Be Addressed

Prior to conducting any violence risk assessment, forensic practitioners must understand the parameters of the evaluation they are being asked to conduct. To determine whether such an assessment is appropriate, the following questions must be answered:

1. **Am I qualified to conduct such an assessment?**
   Qualifications to conduct violence risk assessment evaluations vary depending on jurisdiction and local laws. However, even in cases when a practitioner meets statutory requirements, advanced knowledge of the subject area is required. A practitioner with experience in conducting violence risk assessments may deem that a particular case does not fall into his or her area of expertise depending on the nature of the case. Practitioners must be familiar with the research literature in the area in which they are conducting an evaluation. Thorough attention to this issue is critical.
2. **What is the specific question to be addressed?**
   In many cases, this may appear obvious, but, in the process of conducting the evaluation, the specific question often becomes unclear. It is the practitioner's responsibility to clarify the specific question being asked with the referring agency (e.g., criminal court, parole board, detention facility, school department, etc.).

3. What are the parameters of the assessment and are all possible outcomes clearly defined prior to beginning the evaluation? To answer this question, the practitioner must determine with the authority requesting the risk assessment which recommendations can and cannot be fulfilled. For example, if conducting an assessment of an individual who is serving a sentence in a correctional facility, a recommendation of release to the community would not be possible.

Legal Precedent: The Need for Practitioners to Conduct Risk Assessments

This section reviews two major legal decisions that led to an increased need for practitioners to add the assessment of risk for violence to their clinical repertoire. Although the facts of each case and the topics they address are different, the outcomes support the same conclusion—mental health practitioners need to be able to assess an individual's risk for violence. This brief review is intended to place our understanding of violence risk assessment into a historical context, not to fully explore the legal aspects of these cases.

The first case is that of *Tarasoff v. Regents of the University of California,* 1974. This case involves a clinician's "duty to warn" an identified potential victim of the risk of potential violence and a "duty to protect" an identified potential victim. The second case is *O'Connor v. Donaldson,* 1975, which resulted in the requirement that clinicians who hospitalize an individual must demonstrate that the individual is at imminent risk to him- or herself or others due to mental illness. These two landmark cases illustrate the need for practitioners to understand the violence risk assessment literature with sufficient fluency to provide an opinion regarding an individual's risk for future violence.

Tarasoff v. Regents of the University of California

In 1974, the Supreme Court of California ruled that mental health professionals are required by law to warn identified potential victims who are at risk of being harmed. Based on the facts of this case, the court concluded, "When a doctor or a psychotherapist, in the exercise of his professional skill and knowledge, determines, or should determine, that a warning is essential to avert danger arising from the medical or psychological condition of his patient, he incurs a legal obligation to give that warning." This ruling came in response to the murder of a young college student by the client of an outpatient therapist.

In 1968, Prosenjit Poddar was a 25-year-old student in a master's degree program at the University of California, Berkley (Quinn, 1984). Poddar, originally from Bengal, India, became romantically interested in a 19-year-old woman named Tatiana Tarasoff. The couple attended a New Year's Eve party and exchanged a kiss. Poddar's intention to pursue a relationship was later rejected by Tarasoff. Subsequently, Poddar became depressed and began to receive counseling at the Cowell Memorial Hospital, which was affiliated with the University of California, Berkeley (VandeCreek & Knapp, 1989). Poddar was initially diagnosed with paranoid schizophrenia, prescribed a neuroleptic medication, and referred for psychotherapy on an outpatient basis (Slovenko, 1988). Over the course of therapy, Poddar disclosed his obsession with Tarasoff, expressing fantasies of harming and potentially killing her. During this time, Tarasoff was vacationing in Brazil. Upon her return, Poddar arrived at her residence with a pellet gun and demanded to see her. When Tarasoff declined to see him, he shot her with the pellet gun. Tarasoff fled from the house, but Poddar eventually caught her and stabbed her to death with a kitchen knife. Poddar then went into her home and called the police (Schwartz, 1985).

The events of this case raised three critical questions: (1) Does the mental health practitioner have the ability to assess risk of potential violence? (2) If so, is it the responsibility of the practitioner to warn the potential victim? and (3) Does the public's safety supersede the client's right to confidentiality? Based on the facts of the *Tarasoff* case, the court opined that mental health professionals do have a duty to warn potential victims of violence and that public safety supersedes the practitioner's responsibility to maintain confidentiality (see Simone & Fulero, 2005, and Kachigian & Felthous, 2004, for a thorough review of the *Tarasoff* case).

O'Connor v. Donaldson

The second case highlights the requirements for involuntary commitment of an individual to a psychiatric facility. Kenneth Donaldson, a 34-year-old husband and father, experienced his first psychotic break and subsequent hospitalization in 1943. While hospitalized at Marcy State Hospital in Florida, he was successfully treated with electric convulsive therapy, recompensated, and was released. Some years later, in 1956, he was committed to Florida's Chattahoochee State Hospital after developing delusions that he was being poisoned. He remained hospitalized for 15 years on the basis that he was mentally ill, uncooperative with treatment, and lacked sufficient insight into his condition. Donaldson persistently petitioned the courts for his release throughout his hospitalization on the basis that he was not dangerous to himself or others, and that, because he was being detained involuntarily, hospital staff were denying him his right to liberty.

In examining the facts of the case, the court concluded the following: "A finding of 'mental illness' alone cannot justify a State's locking a person up against his will and keeping him indefinitely in simple custodial confinement" (*O'Connor v. Donaldson*, 1975). The ruling emphasized an individual's civil rights and declared it unconstitutional to hospitalize an individual involuntarily solely on the basis of mental illness. The court further ruled that, in order to commit an individual against his or her will, the individual must be deemed to be at imminent risk of harm to him- or herself or others. From this point forward, involuntary hospitalization was driven by violence and/or suicide risk secondary to mental illness and not by the mere presence of mental illness.

This brief overview of these two landmark cases illustrates the need for clinicians—particularly forensic clinicians—to be able to conduct evaluations that address an individual's risk for future violence. The following sections will review the violence risk assessment research literature.

VIOLENCE RISK ASSESSMENT RESEARCH

The belief that individuals who suffer from major mental illness are at greater risk to act out violently is long-standing. Historically, research has been both slow to validate these socially held beliefs and unable to draw correlations between mental illness and violence. In fact, what is now referred to as the first generation of research regarding violence and mental illness asserted that there was no connection between the two (Monahan, 1981). The following discussion describes the transition from the first to the third generation of this research, which is not only relevant for historical purposes, but useful as an aid to understanding current practices in conducting risk assessments.

The First Generation of Risk Assessment Research

The first generation of risk assessment research was concerned with *predicting* violent behavior in psychiatric samples. At the time, there were limited risk assessment measures, and the overall literature was sparse. Mental health professionals were charged with the difficult task of predicting which psychiatric patients would become violent in the future and attempting to prevent such violence through continued inpatient hospitalization with very limited tools. These assessments relied heavily on unsubstantiated clinical/forensic judgment based on the practitioner's clinical/forensic experience.

Research at the time found a significant rate of overprediction (false positive predictions; Steadman & Cocozza, 1974). Such findings led a task force of the American Psychiatric Association (1974) to conclude that "the state of the art regarding predictions of violence is very unsatisfactory. The ability of psychiatrists or any other professionals to reliably predict future violence is unproved." Due to the paucity of research literature, the ability of clinicians to successfully predict when an individual would be violent remained a significant problem. In his often cited book on the subject, John Monahan (1981) concluded,

> Outcome studies of clinical prediction with adult populations underscore the importance of past violence as a predictor of future violence, yet lead to the conclusion that psychiatrists and psychologists are accurate in no more than one out of three predictions of violent behavior. (p. 92)

However, the research literature at the time had four main methodological flaws that confounded findings. First, research used heterogeneous clinical samples without a comparison or control group. Such research has very limited external validity, meaning that results cannot be applied to a population different from the one studied. Second, there was very little data regarding the base rate of violent behavior in the general population. Therefore, comparisons made between mentally ill samples could not be made with the general population with any degree of certainty. Third, the criterion for violence used in studies was typically conviction for violent behavior. Due to issues inherent in the criminal justice system, such as difficulty in gaining convictions and the effect of plea bargaining, the conviction rate for violent offenses is much lower than the level of actual violence. Therefore, conviction is a poor outcome measure for violence. Finally, because this area of study was in its infancy, very few studies used standardized measures between studies.

Rather, studies in the first generation of risk assessment literature often used subjective measures of risk, such as a clinician's opinion.

A major contribution to the advancement of this literature was an epidemiological study of violent behavior in the general population (Swanson, Holzer, Ganju, & Jono, 1990). This study was the first to establish the base rate of violent behavior in the general population by collecting data on over 10,000 randomly selected individuals residing in the community (both mentally ill and non–mentally ill). The catchment areas used were Baltimore, MD, Raleigh-Durham, NC, and Los Angeles, CA. The findings indicate that those with affective disorders were 3 times as likely to be violent, those with schizophrenia or schizophreniform disorder were 4 times as likely to be violent, those with alcohol abuse or dependence were 12 times more likely to be violent, and those with other drug abuse or dependence were 17 times more likely to be violent. When counting the number of diagnostic categories into which each individual fell, a near linear relation was found between the number of diagnoses and violent behavior, meaning the more diagnoses an individual had, the more likely he or she was to engage in violent behavior. For example, the rate of violence for those with no diagnosis was 2.05%. The rate for those with one diagnosis was 6.81%, two diagnoses 17.51%, and three or more diagnoses 22.36% (Swanson et al., 1990).

Initially, this area of research was referred to as the "prediction of violence," but it has since become known as violence risk assessment. The shift in terminology reflects a more accurate understanding of clinical capabilities. Clinicians assess the level of risk an individual poses by examining whether certain risk factors that increase the likelihood of violent behavior are present as opposed to "predicting" violent behavior (Grisso & Tomkins, 1996).

This research literature further progressed to ask which specific psychiatric symptoms are most statistically predictive of violent behavior (i.e., which symptoms place individuals at increased risk for violent behavior). A study comparing psychiatric patients with community controls found that psychotic symptoms were the only set of variables examined that accounted for differences between these two groups (Link, Andrews, & Cullen, 1992).

A later study found that a specific cluster of psychotic symptoms substantially increased the risk for violence (Link & Stueve, 1994). These symptoms were referred to as threat/control-override symptoms. As the label indicates, individuals who experience these symptoms feel as though they are being threatened in some way or that their internal capacity to control their thoughts and/or behavior has been overridden by some external force. This study noted, "the threat/control override scale remains a significant predictor even when other psychotic symptoms are held constant" (p. 153). This scale included 13 items from the Psychiatric Epidemiology Research Interview (Dohrenwend, Shrout, Egri, & Mendelsohn, 1980), three of which are classified as threat/control-override symptoms.

Swanson, Borum, Swartz, and Monahan (1996) examined the relation between threat/control-override symptoms and violence. Subjects in this study who experienced these symptoms were twice as likely to report engaging in violent behavior when compared with individuals who experience other types of psychotic symptoms. Subjects who experienced threat-control/override symptoms were five times as likely to report violence when compared to individuals with no major mental illness. Those who experienced threat-control/override symptoms combined with substance use (drugs and/or alcohol) were 8 to 10 times as likely to report engaging in violent behavior when compared to individuals with no major mental illness (Swanson, Borum, Swartz, & Monahan, 1996).

Perhaps the single most important contribution of the first generation of research is our understanding of base rates. Base rates refer to the frequency with which an event occurs in the natural environment. Without knowledge of the base rate for violence, the literature struggled to show any relation between individual risk factors, such as mental illness, and violence. Let's suppose that of 1,000 individuals, 100 become violent. In this case, the base rate of violence is 10%. Therefore, the prediction that no individual in this group will become violent would be correct 90% of the time. Alternatively, the prediction that all individuals in this group will be violent in the future would be correct only 10% of the time. To successfully predict the 10% who will become violent requires the identification of risk factors that are highly predictive of violence. Because it is very difficult to predict an event that rarely occurs, our understanding of base rates led researchers to study populations with higher rates of violence, such as criminal offenders, as opposed to groups with low rates of violence, such as civil psychiatric patients.

The Second Generation of Risk Assessment Research

Based on knowledge gleaned from the first generation of research, the second generation focused on identifying specific risk factors that increase the likelihood that an individual will engage in violent behavior in the future. The literature began to focus on actuarial assessments of historical/static factors to assess an individual's risk for future violence. In their 1996 article, Monahan and Steadman compared this methodology to that of meteorology. The most salient commonality between the actuarial risk assessment methodology and meteorology is the collection of large amounts of data points to determine which are most predictive of a certain outcome. For example, information gathered by a meteorologist, such as temperature, barometric pressure, and time of year, is combined to produce a statistical prediction for the chance of rain on a given day. The prediction is based on the combination of these variables and resultant precipitation in the past. Because such meteorological data have been collected for decades, the accuracy of the prediction is increased. Similarly, in the area of violence risk assessment, findings from studies that collect large amounts of data on factors that increase an individual's risk for violence increases the predictive accuracy of individualized assessments (Borum, 1996; Douglas & Webster, 1999; Serin & Amos, 1995).

The second generation of research examined specific risk factors for future violence. As a result, actuarial tools have been developed that assign numeric value to particular risk factors. A total score on such a measure provides the forensic clinician with a percentile rank or predictive number for a specific individual.

The VRAG

The most widely researched actuarial assessment tool in the violence risk assessment literature is the Violence Risk Appraisal Guide (VRAG; Harris, Rice, & Quinsey, 1993). The VRAG was normed on a sample of 618 mentally disordered offenders from a maximum-security psychiatric institution in Ontario, Canada. Over 40 variables found to retrospectively correlate with violent recidivism were examined. Statistical analysis of the data resulted in 12 items that were most statistically predictive of violence, 9 of which were positively predictive of violence and 3 that were negatively predictive of violence.

The following nine items were positively predictive of violence:

1. A high score on the Psychopathy Checklist–Revised (PCL-R; Hare, 1991, 2003) (the PCL-R will be discussed in more detail later in this chapter)
2. Elementary school maladjustment

3. DSM diagnosis of any personality disorder
4. Young age at index offense
5. Separation from parents before age 16
6. Failure on prior conditional release
7. History of nonviolent offenses
8. Never being married
9. History of alcohol abuse

The following three variables were negatively predictive of violence:

10. DSM diagnosis of schizophrenia
11. Victim injury at index offense
12. Female victim at index offense

These 12 variables were found to be significantly correlated with violent recidivism in this sample ($r=0.459$; Harris et al., 1993). Each item has a weighted score, and the final score is the sum of all individual item scores. Based on the VRAG final score, an individual is placed into one of nine categories, one through nine. The higher the category, the higher the risk of future violence. Each category indicates a probability of violent recidivism based on 7 and 10 years post release from incarceration follow-up studies. For example, an individual in category 5 has a 35% chance of violent recidivism within 7 years and a 48% chance of violent recidivism within 10 years (Quinsey, Harris, Rice, & Cormier, 2006). In a prospective replication study with 347 male forensic patients, 11% of the patients who scored in category 2 on the VRAG were later found to commit a new violent act. Also, 42% of the patients in category 5, 70% of patients in category 7, and 100% of the patients in category 9 committed a new violent act (Harris, Rice, & Cormier, 2002).

Studies found actuarial tools to be more accurate estimates of risk than unsubstantiated clinical judgment (Borum, 1996; Douglas & Webster, 1999; Serin & Amos, 1995). Some proponents of actuarial methods cautioned against the use of clinical judgment in conducting violence risk assessments. For example, Quinsey, Rice, Harris, and Cormier (1998) asserted,

> what we are advising is not the addition of actuarial methods to existing practice, but rather the complete replacement of existing practice with actuarial methods . . . actuarial methods are too good and clinical judgment too poor to risk contaminating the former with the latter. (p. 171)

Despite the contributions of the second generation of research, there are several compelling criticisms of the actuarial method. First, scores on actuarial assessment tools remain static and do not change with the passage of time. Once an individual is categorized using this method, his or her risk for future violence will not change despite treatment intervention or environmental changes. Second, providing a percentile rating of risk is not necessarily helpful to the authority that requested the risk assessment evaluation. For example, if a criminal court requests a violence risk assessment evaluation as part of a dangerousness hearing to consider whether an individual should be released from a state hospital, and the conclusion is that there is a 35% chance that this individual will become violent within the next 10 years, the court will likely ask the expert to provide a more conclusive opinion. Third, dynamic or changeable factors that may mitigate risk for future violence are not considered by the actuarial method.

The Third Generation of Risk Assessment Research

The third generation of risk assessment literature has moved from actuarial assessment of static risk factors for future violence to the method of structured professional judgment. Structured professional judgment calls for the use of structured assessment tools to guide the forensic practitioner in their assessment. This method works to understand a specific individual and identify whether risk factors are present or absent. Structured professional judgment addresses the problem of using purely static risk factors that will not change with time or intervention.

The HCR-20

The most widely researched assessment tool designed to employ structured professional judgment is the Historical-Clinical-Risk Management-20 (HCR-20; Webster, Douglas, Eaves, & Hart, 1997). The HCR-20 includes 20 items found predictive of violence in the research literature. This structured clinical guide incorporates three areas of risk factors into one tool: *H*istorical factors, *C*linical factors, and *R*isk Management factors. The 10 items that assess the individual's historical/static risk factors include:

1. Previous violence
2. Young age at first violent incident

3. Relationship instability
4. Employment problems
5. Substance use problems
6. Major mental illness
7. Psychopathy
8. Early maladjustment
9. Personality disorder
10. Prior supervision failure

The five clinical items that assess risk factors related to the individual's clinical functioning at the time of the evaluation include:

11. Lack of insight
12. Negative attitudes
13. Active symptoms of major mental illness
14. Impulsivity
15. Unresponsiveness to treatment

The five risk management items that assess anticipated risk factors in the ongoing treatment and risk management of the individual include:

16. Plans lack feasibility
17. Exposure to destabilizers
18. Lack of personal support
19. Noncompliance with remediation attempts
20. Stress

The HCR-20 and other structured professional judgment tools do not provide a specific score as is the case with actuarial tools. Rather, they require the evaluator to determine the risk level of the individual (low, moderate, or high) based on a review of these research-derived risk factors. Research on the HCR-20 finds that such risk ratings add incremental value to the numerical score when the HCR-20 is used as an actuarial tool (de Vogel, de Ruiter, Hildebrand, Bos, & van de Ven, 2004; Douglas, Ogloff, & Hart, 2003).

Comparisons between the VRAG and the HCR-20 consistently find the HCR-20 to be as effective, or more effective, in assessing risk for future violence (Douglas, Yeomans, & Boer, 2005). Because this chapter is dedicated to the clinical applicability of violence risk assessment and not to a research-based discussion of assessment tools, space allows only for a brief discussion of these differences.

Item selection for the VRAG was based strictly on the statistical power of risk factors in the original sample of 618 mentally disordered offenders. Although these 12 items were highly predictive in the original study, replication studies have not shown such accuracy. Alternatively, selection of the 20 items that make up the HCR-20 was based on findings from the violence risk assessment literature across different samples. Clinically useful items found predictive of violence were also included. Therefore, the HCR-20 was designed to be clinically useful in various types of settings.

A recent study comparing the individual items on the VRAG and the HCR-20 found that most of the items on the HCR-20 were related to future violence, while this was not the case for the VRAG (Mills, Kroner, & Hemmati, 2007). Of the 20 items on the HCR-20, 15 (75%) were related to violent recidivism. Of the 12 VRAG items, 5 (42%) were found predictive of violent recidivism. The follow-up time was approximately 4.5 years, and the base rate for violent recidivism in this sample was 35% (Mills et al., 2007).

The MacArthur Violence Risk Assessment Study

The MacArthur Violence Risk Assessment Study was a multisite study designed to assess risk factors for violent behavior in a sample of civil psychiatric patients (Monahan et al., 2001). The goal of the original study was to improve on methodological flaws of earlier research in the area of violence risk assessment. In contrast to previous studies that used reconviction or rearrest for a violence offense as the outcome measure, the MacArthur study used more comprehensive techniques to measure actual violence. The overall sample was made up of psychiatric patients admitted to acute civil inpatient facilities in Pittsburgh, PA, Kansas City, MO, and Worcester, MA.

Inclusion criteria for the sample included the following: (1) subjects were civilly committed to a psychiatric hospital; (2) subjects were between the ages of 18 and 40; (3) subjects were English speaking; (4) subjects were White or Black (the Massachusetts site also included Latino subjects); and (5) subjects had a medical record diagnosis of schizophrenia, schizophreniform, schizoaffective disorder, depression, dysthymia, mania, brief reactive psychosis, delusional disorder, alcohol or other drug abuse or dependence, or a personality disorder. To ensure a consistent distribution of demographic variables, such as age, gender, and race, this study used a stratified random sampling design (Monahan et al., 2001).

Over the course of the study, a total of 12,873 patients were hospitalized across the three study sites. Of these admissions, 7,740 met the inclusion criteria. A total of 1,695 patients were asked to participate in the study. The refusal rate was 20% and additional subjects were lost due to attrition, resulting in a sample of 1,136 subjects.

Three sources of information were used to ascertain the occurrence and details of a violent incident in the community: (1) interviews with the patient, (2) interviews with collateral individuals (i.e., persons named by the patient as someone who would know what was going on in his or her life), and (3) official sources of information (arrest and hospital records). Each patient was interviewed in the hospital by both a research interviewer and a research clinician in order to assess him or her on each of the risk factors. The research interviews collected historical data, while clinical interviews assessed the subject's clinical presentation, particularly the presence of psychiatric symptoms (Monahan et al., 2001). Included in these interviews was the Psychopathy Checklist: Screening Version (PCL:SV; Hart, Cox, & Hare, 1995). The patients and collaterals were interviewed every 10 weeks over a 1-year period to determine whether there were any incidents of aggression or violence.

Over the 1-year follow-up period, 608 violent incidents were recorded. The majority of patients (72%) were not violent during the 1-year follow-up period; whereas 28% of patients were responsible for all violent incidents. Approximately half of all patients who were involved in a violent incident had numerous violent incidents, while half of the violent patients had only one such incident (Monahan et al., 2001).

The MacArthur Violence Risk Assessment Study used 134 potential risk factors for violence and statistically analyzed these variables individually as well as in groups (Monahan et al., 2001). Several risk factors were found to correlate with violence within the first 20 weeks post discharge.

MacArthur Findings

The MacArthur study found that men were more likely than women to be violent, although the difference between these two groups was not large. The types of violence women engaged in were more likely directed toward family, more likely to occur in their own home, and were less likely to result in the need for medical treatment or criminal involvement.

All measures of previous violence (self-report, arrest records, and hospital records) correlated with violence at follow-up. A history of physical abuse correlated with violence at follow-up, as well as having a parent who abused substances or had a criminal history (Monahan et al., 2001). Individuals from economically disadvantaged communities were at increased risk for violence. Black and White subjects from comparably disadvantaged neighborhoods had similar rates of violence at follow-up (Monahan et al., 2001).

Major mental illness, particularly schizophrenia, was associated with a lower rate of violence at follow-up. A diagnosis of a personality disorder was predictive of violence at follow-up. Comorbid mental illness and substance abuse was predictive of violence at follow-up. Delusions in general were not predictive of violence, but a generally "suspicious" attitude toward others correlated with violence at follow-up. Hallucinations in general were not predictive of violence; however, command auditory hallucinations to engage in a violent act increased the subject's risk for violence (Monahan et al., 2001).

The variable with the strongest bivariate correlation with violence in the MacArthur study was psychopathy as measured by the PCL:SV. The antisocial behavior factor (Factor 2) of the PCL:SV was more predictive of violence than the interpersonal and affective factor (Factor 1) or the PCL:SV Total Score. Thinking or daydreaming about harming others correlated with violence at follow-up, particularly persistent violent thoughts. Violence at follow-up was correlated with anger as measured by the Novaco Anger Scale (Monahan et al., 2001).

INDIVIDUAL RISK FACTORS

Now that we have reviewed the three generations of violence risk assessment literature and the most studied risk assessment tools, the following section will detail some of the individual variables most consistently found related to risk for violent behavior.

Demographic Risk Factors

Demographic risk factors related to risk for violent behavior include age, gender, socioeconomic status, education, and employment.

Age has been found to be inversely correlated with violent recidivism in follow-up studies (Bonta, Law, & Hanson, 1998; Gilders,

1997; Hanson & Bussière, 1998; Hirschi & Gottfredson, 1983). In a meta-analysis of predictors of recidivism, which included over 60,000 subjects across 131 studies, young age was a significant predictor of recidivism (Gendreau, Little, & Goggin, 1996). In the epidemiological study of violence in the community, there was a negative linear relationship between age and violent behavior, meaning that, as age increased, incidents of violence decreased (Swanson et al., 1990). For example, for subjects between 18 and 29 years of age, the rate of violence was 7.34%. For those between 20 and 44 years of age, the rate of violence was 3.59%, and for those between 45 and 64, the rate of violence dropped to 1.22% and to below 1% after the age of 65 (Swanson et al., 1990).

In general, men are more likely to engage in violent behavior than women. Women make up 11% of those arrested for violent crimes in the United States, while men make up 89% (Reiss & Roth, 1993). In the epidemiological study, men reported engaging in violent acts more than twice as often as women (Swanson et al., 1990). Despite these findings in criminal populations and the general population, studies of psychiatric patients indicate no difference in the frequency of violent incidents between male and female patients during follow-up periods after release from the hospital (Lidz, Mulvey, & Gardner, 1993). In one study, clinicians' estimates of prediction were better than chance for male patients but not for female patients (Lidz et al., 1993). Such results indicate the general underestimation of female-perpetrated violence in psychiatric patients. Although similar rates of violence are found between male and female psychiatric patients, male patients' violent behavior is more likely to result in injury to the victim (Krakowski & Czobor, 2004).

Socioeconomic status is consistently found to correlate with risk for violence in both psychiatric and community samples. In an epidemiological study, individuals under the age of 45 from the lower socioeconomic group were three times as likely to be violent compared with those from the same age group in the higher socioeconomic group. This increased significantly in younger men (between 18 and 29) from the lower socioeconomic group, as 16% were violent compared with the overall base rate of 2.05% (Swanson et al., 1990). Studies that examine neighborhood context find that individuals living in areas with high concentrations of poverty are at significantly increased risk for violence (Silver, Mulvey, & Monahan, 1999). Studies that find a correlation between race or ethnicity and violence find that, when controlling for socioeconomic status, this correlation disappears (Monahan et al., 2001; Swanson et al., 1990), meaning that race or ethnicity is not correlated with violence when socioeconomic status is taken into account.

Regarding level of education and violence, 80% of incarcerated violent offenders have not completed high school (Monahan, 1993). In studies examining violent recidivism, education level is correlated with violent recidivism (Harris et al., 1993). A meta-analysis examining risk factors for violent recidivism found that lack of education was a strong predictor (Bonta et al., 1998).

Employment problems have been associated with increased risk for general criminal recidivism (Andrews & Bonta, 1995). Unemployment has also been found to increase the risk of violence in mentally disordered offenders (Menzies & Webster, 1995). Overall, "every one percent rise in unemployment increases the mortality rate in this country by two percent, homicides and imprisonment by six percent, and the infant mortality rate by five percent" (Gilligan, 1996, p. 194). In a descriptive analysis of sentenced offenders, 44% of male and 34% of female subjects have a history of unemployment (Singleton, Meltzer, Gatward, Coid, & Deasy, 1998).

Past History of Violence as a Risk Factor

A history of violent behavior is a highly predictive risk factor for future violence regardless of the population being studied (Klassen & O'Connor, 1988; Monahan et al., 2001). Numerous studies find that a history of violence is the best predictor of future violence (Gilders, 1997; Swanson, 1993). In an often-cited follow-up study of forensic patients found criminally insane, historical variables were the most predictive of violent recidivism upon release from the hospital (Cocozza & Steadman, 1974). In this study, the following cluster of historical variables was predictive of violence: a history of juvenile crime, the number of previous arrests, a history of convictions for any type of criminal activity, convictions for violent offenses, and being under the age of 50 (Cocozza & Steadman, 1974). All risk assessment measures assess historical violence, and most analyses of the effectiveness of these measures find that historical items are highly predictive of violent recidivism (Grann, Belfrage, & Tengström, 2000). The HCR-20 has as many historical items as clinical and risk management items combined (Webster et al., 1997).

Although historical violence is one of the most important individual factors included in a violence risk assessment, using an individual's criminal record as the only data point for past violence grossly underestimates actual violence. The MacArthur Violence Risk Assessment Study, which assessed violence using multiple sources, found the vast majority of violent incidents never came to the attention of law enforcement (Monahan et al., 2001). Also, very few violent incidents resulted in arrest or conviction. Therefore, it is important for the forensic practitioner to discuss historical violence with numerous collaterals, because a review of the criminal record is not sufficient. Self-reported violence has been found predictive of future violence (Klassen & O'Connor, 1988; Tardiff, Marzuk, Leon, & Portera, 1997).

Information regarding an individual's history of violence should be ascertained prior to conducting the interview. In cases when this is not possible, the evaluator should interview the individual again when all information regarding historical violence has been collected. Each violent incident requires discussion with the individual to determine common circumstances or situations that may have led to violence. This requires the practitioner to determine the individual's mental state at the time of each violent incident (e.g., psychosis, mania, intoxication, etc.). It is also useful to question family members or others close to the individual regarding their presentation during past incidents of violence.

The assessment of current and historical violent thoughts requires inquiry during the clinical interview. In the MacArthur study, self-reported violent thoughts were predictive of violent behavior over the first 20 weeks after discharge from the hospital (Monahan et al., 2001). The presence of violent thoughts also correlated with measures of psychopathy, anger, and substance abuse. The frequency and content of violent thoughts is important to ascertain and should be asked at numerous times during an interview to determine truthfulness of self-report. In cases when an individual endorses such thoughts or fantasies, the degree of detail or how well formulated these thoughts are should be assessed. Also, the intent to act on these thoughts requires evaluation.

Psychopathy as a Risk Factor

Psychopathy is a clinical construct that has been identified anecdotally for centuries, but not until the validation of the Psychopathy Checklist (Hare, 1991, 2003) and progeny has the construct been reliably measured in the empirical literature.[1] The Psychopathy Checklist–Revised was originally validated among criminal samples (Hare, 1991). The Psychopathy Checklist: Screening Version, which was based on the PCL-R, was normed on civil psychiatric patients as part of the MacArthur Violence Risk Assessment Study.

Research using the PCL-R and PCL:SV show similar results (Hart et al., 1995). Research using the PCL measures indicates that psychopathic individuals are more likely than their nonpsychopathic counterparts to be convicted of violent offenses. A retrospective examination of the criminal histories of a sample of incarcerated individuals found that those diagnosed as psychopathic had significantly more convictions for assault, robbery, fraud, possession of weapons, and escapes from custody (Hare, McPherson, & Forth, 1988). Psychopathic offenders also commit more violent crime than nonpsychopathic offenders (Kosson, Smith, & Newman, 1990). A prospective study of 231 inmates found psychopathic offenders were four times as likely to recidivate violently when compared with their nonpsychopathic counterparts. Sixty-five percent of those above the cutoff score for psychopathy recidivated violently, while 25% of those who scored low on psychopathy did so (Hart, Kropp, & Hare, 1988). In a sample of 169 forensic patients, 77% of those who scored above the cutoff for psychopathy on the PCL-R violently recidivated compared with 21% for those scoring below the cutoff (Harris, Rice, & Cormier, 1991).

Based on this literature, psychopathy as a risk factor for violence is well established. Most research on the PCL-R and PCL:SV finds two distinct factors: Factor 1 measures affective and interpersonal traits, and Factor 2 measures antisocial behavioral traits (for a discussion of alternative factor models, see chapter 8 of this volume). While psychopathy is highly predictive of future violence, the contribution of each of the PCL factors is less clear. This differentiation has important clinical implications in terms of the group that is most at risk for future violence. Most studies that have examined the contribution of each factor report that Factor 2 is more predictive of violence. Among psychiatric inpatients, those with high Factor 2 scores were at increased risk to engage in violent behavior, while Factor 1 scores were not predictive of violent behavior (Heilbrun et al., 1998). A recent meta-analysis examining institutional misconduct among psychopathic and nonpsychopathic individuals found the correlation between aggressive acts was stronger for Factor 2 ($r=0.21$) than for Factor 1 ($r=0.14$) (Walters, 2003).

Although psychopathy measures were not originally designed as risk assessment tools, research consistently finds psychopathy scores to be highly predictive of violence, particularly Factor 2 scores.

SPECIFICATION OF RISK ASSESSMENT

Forensic practitioners are called upon to conduct risk assessments for various types of behavior. Therefore, it is incumbent on forensic practitioners to be familiar with the state-of-the-art assessment schemes and strategies specific to the type of risk assessment evaluations they are asked to conduct. As this field progresses, the specificity of the risk assessment instruments also continues to progress. For example, several assessment tools are currently available to assess risk for sexual violence, including the Sex Offender Risk Appraisal Guide (Quinsey et al., 1998); the Rapid Risk Assessment for Sex Offender Recidivism (Hanson, 1997); the Static-99 (Hanson & Thornton, 1999); and the Sexual Violence Risk-20 (Boer, Hart, Kropp, & Webster, 1997). Forensic practitioners must remain current with the research literature in their specific area of practice. Practitioners must also have an understanding of the various risk assessment tools specifically designed for the population they are assessing.

TREATMENT AND RISK MANAGEMENT

Based on results from violence risk assessment research with both mentally disordered and nondisordered offenders, a model called risk–need–responsivity has proposed useful guidelines for the treatment of violent offenders. Research in the area of correctional treatment finds that treatment interventions that follow these guidelines are more effective than treatments that do not (Andrews & Bonta, 2003; Andrews et al., 1990). The three areas—risk, need, and responsivity—are each made up of certain principles.

- The risk principle calls for an individual's risk level to be matched with intensity of intervention. For example, high-risk offenders should receive the most intensive treatment interventions, followed by their medium-risk and low-risk counterparts.
- The need principle addresses the individual criminogenic needs of the offender. Criminogenic needs are defined as issues directly linked to the commission of violence or other criminal activity and include antisocial attitudes, antisocial peer groups, and a pattern of criminal thinking. Specific interventions aimed at addressing these criminogenic needs that directly relate to recidivism are employed (Andrews, Bonta, & Wormith, 2006).

- The responsivity principle calls for specific characteristics related to the individual's ability to engage in treatment to be addressed. These include cognitive ability, motivation for treatment, and other issues that are not directly related to criminal behavior but may hinder treatment efforts. A lack of motivation to refrain from engaging in criminal activity is a particularly difficult issue to overcome and is common in this population. The presence of psychopathy may also hinder treatment efforts because the psychopathic individual will likely have no interest in changing his or her behavior.

Recent treatment strategies designed for difficult-to-treat populations, such as psychopathic offenders, draws on the risk–need–responsivity literature (Wong & Hare, 2006). The use of such interventions with mentally disordered offenders is supported by findings of similar risk factors for violent recidivism among mentally disordered and nondisordered populations. For example, a meta-analysis examining risk factors for violent recidivism found those that were predictive of violent recidivism in the general offender population were also predictive of violent recidivism in mentally disordered offenders (Bonta et al., 1998).

RISK COMMUNICATION

This chapter has stressed the assessment of risk factors for violent behavior. While an understanding of the research literature and ability to determine which factors increase an individual's risk for violence are of utmost importance, the ability to communicate this risk to the authority requesting the evaluation is equally as critical. The main purpose of a violence risk assessment is to provide useful information to improve decision making, whether clinical or legal. Heilbrun, Dvoskin, Hart, and McNeill (1999) point out:

> The importance of risk assessment is entirely related to the decisions which are in turn influenced by such assessments. These decisions may be legal, such as civil or forensic commitment, or clinical, such as the assignment of an intensive case manager or a change in medication. . . . The only way risk assessors can influence decisions is by effectively communicating their findings to the legal and clinical actors whose decisions they wish to influence. (p. 94)

Table 1.1

COMPONENTS OF RISK ASSESSMENT EVALUATION

The following information should be included in a comprehensive risk assessment evaluation:

1. Demographic/identifying information
2. Sources of information
3. Referral question
4. Notice of limits of confidentiality
5. Historical information
    a. Family history
    b. Developmental history
    c. Educational history
    d. Employment history
    e. Medical history
    f. Psychiatric history
    g. Substance abuse history
    h. Criminal history
    i. Violence history
6. Results of risk assessment measures (HCR-20, PCL-R, PCL:SV, etc.).
7. Current functioning and mental status
8. Clinical formulation and discussion
9. Recommendations

The following section details a forensic case and illustrates how findings from a violence risk assessment evaluation are communicated in the form of a written report. The vignette includes a brief overview of the case, the incorporation of risk assessment tools into a violence risk assessment, and recommendations for the ongoing risk management of this case based on the findings of the evaluation. The entire case will not be presented due to space constraints. Table 1.1 includes all areas that should be included in a complete violence risk assessment evaluation.

CASE VIGNETTE: MR. Z

This case vignette is a conglomeration of clinical data based on the first author's forensic experience. This vignette demonstrates the application of information presented in this chapter to a forensic case, with a focus on risk factors to be considered in a comprehensive violence risk assessment evaluation.

Identifying Information

Mr. Z is a 42-year-old divorced man. He is currently committed to a state hospital secondary to being found not guilty by reason of insanity (NGRI) for breaking and entering, kidnapping, and assault and battery. Mr. Z broke into the home of a family friend and held her and her 4-year-old daughter against their will for 6 hours. During this 6-hour period, Mr. Z was consuming large amounts of alcohol. Mr. Z assaulted the adult victim by slapping her in the face approximately five times. He has been recommitted to the state hospital for the past 8 years on an annual basis.

During the initial criminal responsibility evaluation, Mr. Z reported that he believed the victim was having a sexual relationship with his ex-wife, was supplying her with drugs, and was the reason for their divorce. This incident occurred 1 year after he was divorced. Following Mr. Z's divorce, he lived alone in an apartment for 6 months but was evicted due to not paying his rent. He was homeless for the 6 months prior to the offense.

Risk Assessment Tools

As part of this risk assessment evaluation, two assessment tools were used: the PCL:SV and the HCR-20. These measures and how they relate to Mr. Z's risk for future violence are discussed below. Information gleaned from clinical interviews and record review will be included in this discussion and incorporated into the overall risk assessment.

Psychopathy Checklist: Screening Version

The PCL:SV is a 12-item scale devised to assess psychopathy in civil psychiatric patients. The PCL:SV is a dimensional measure of the degree to which a given individual matches the prototypical psychopath. Items are scored on a 3-point scale: 0=does not apply; 1=item applies to a certain extent; and 2=item applies. Scores range from 0 to 24, and a cut-off score of 18 is used for the diagnosis of psychopathy. Those who score 12 or below are considered nonpsychopathic, and those who score between 13 and 17 show some psychopathic traits. The administration of the PCL:SV entails both a clinical interview and a record review conducted by clinicians trained in its administration. As recommended by the PCL:SV manual, the PCL:SV was scored by two independent raters, and the scores were averaged to increase reliability.

Psychopathy is a clinical construct that accounts for interpersonal, affective, and behavioral characteristics. Interpersonally, individuals that are psychopathic are grandiose, manipulative, and callous. Affectively, psychopathic individuals display shallow emotions; are unable to form long-lasting attachments to others; and lack empathy, guilt, and remorse. Behaviorally, psychopathic individuals are impulsive, sensation seeking, and readily violate social norms. Research finds that individuals who score high on the PCL:SV are at increased risk for future violence and criminal recidivism.

Mr. Z's total score of 11 places him in the 20th percentile among forensic/psychiatric patients and in the 63rd percentile among civil psychiatric patients. The PCL:SV is made up of two factors. Factor 1 is comprised of interpersonal and affective attributes of psychopathy, while Factor 2 is comprised of behavioral traits of psychopathy. Mr. Z's Factor 1 score of 4 places him in the 18th percentile among forensic/psychiatric patients and in the 61st percentile among civil psychiatric patients. His Factor 2 score of 7 places him in the 31st percentile among forensic/psychiatric patients and in the 64th percentile among civil psychiatric patients. Based on the PCL:SV score, Mr. Z does not demonstrate significant character or behavioral traits consistent with psychopathy when compared with a forensic/psychiatric sample; however, his percentile rank when compared with civil psychiatric patients is in the moderate range.

Historical, Clinical, Risk Management-20

The HCR-20 is a structured clinical assessment tool designed to guide clinical judgment when conducting a violence risk assessment. This tool focuses clinical decision making around risk factors found in the research literature to increase an individual's risk for engaging in violent behavior. Unlike actuarial assessment tools that provide a static (unchangeable) score, structured clinical assessment tools guide decision making using both static and dynamic (changeable) risk factors. Historical variables, which remain unchanged and are based on the patient's history, comprise 10 items on the HCR-20. The clinical item section and the risk management section are made up of 5 items per section.

Historical Items

The 10 historical items of the HCR-20 include (1) previous violence, (2) young age at first violent incident, (3) relationship instability, (4) employment problems, (5) substance use problems, (6) major mental illness, (7) psychopathy, (8) early maladjustment, (9) personality disorder, and (10) prior supervision failure. Mr. Z's historical items of concern are discussed here.

Previous violence: Mr. Z's criminal record indicates two convictions for assault and battery and one NGRI finding for breaking and entering, kidnapping, and assault and battery.

- The first assault and battery conviction occurred when he was 21 years old, the second when he was 32, and the NGRI finding when he was 34. Mr. Z was questioned about these incidents, and collateral sources, including his mother, were also interviewed. Mr. Z dropped out of high school at the age of 16. He moved away from home, which he described as an abusive environment. Between the ages of 20 and 21, Mr. Z reports drinking approximately six beers a day. When he was 21, neighbors called the police because Mr. Z was heard yelling in his apartment late into the night, and he would not answer his door. When police officers responded to the disturbance, Mr. Z was yelling, "The end of days is here and I will not let it end without a fight. I know who you are coming to get me. I'm not going out without a fight." Mr. Z became assaultive toward police officers, punching them as they entered his apartment. He was subdued, handcuffed, and transferred to an inpatient psychiatric facility. Mr. Z was later convicted of assault and battery and placed on probation for 1 year.
- Mr. Z's second conviction for assault and battery occurred when he was 32 years of age. He was homeless at the time, not involved in mental health treatment, and was not taking his prescribed medications. Mr. Z was in a bar and began arguing with another patron. The police report indicates that Mr. Z then attempted to leave the bar and was confronted by the bartender for not paying his bill of $24. Mr. Z punched the bartender and left the bar.

The police were called, and Mr. Z was later arrested. He was convicted of assault and battery and sentenced to 6 months at the county jail.

- When Mr. Z was 34, he was charged with breaking and entering, kidnapping, and assault and battery. He was later found NGRI. The NGRI finding will be discussed at length below.

Young age at first violent incident: Mr. Z reports being involved in numerous violent incidents beginning at the age of 14. He stated,

> I started some of the fights and other people started some of them. If I was mad I would just hit someone if I felt like it. I don't do that now, but that's what I did back when I was young. I was in about five or six fights in high school.

Substance abuse problems: Mr. Z has a documented history of substance abuse problems, primarily alcohol. Mr. Z reports abusing marijuana beginning at the age of 13. He reports smoking two joints per day between the ages of 13 and 15. He reports using cocaine approximately "10 times in my life." Mr. Z began abusing alcohol at the age of 12. As an adult, Mr. Z reports drinking alcohol intermittently, at times drinking "up to 15 beers a day, and at other times I've been sober for almost a year at a time." Mr. Z was consuming alcohol at the time of two of the three violent incidents described above.

Mental illness: Mr. Z's clinical presentation is most consistent with a *DSM-IV-TR* diagnosis of schizophrenia, paranoid type. Historically, Mr. Z has presented with the following symptoms: paranoid and grandiose delusional beliefs, command auditory hallucinations instructing him to harm others, and disorganized thought process. Mr. Z has consistently been diagnosed with schizophrenia, paranoid type since the age of 23. He has been hospitalized on eight occasions secondary to paranoid beliefs that others were conspiring against him. All hospital records were reviewed and indicate a discharge diagnosis of schizophrenia, paranoid type.

Personality disorder: Mr. Z meets the *DSM-IV-TR* criteria for antisocial personality disorder. He presents with the following behavioral criteria for this disorder: failure to conform to social norms with respect to lawful behaviors as indicated by repeatedly performing acts that are grounds for arrest; impulsivity or failure to plan ahead; irritability and aggressiveness, as indicated by repeated physical fights or assaults; and consistent irresponsibility, as indicated by repeated failure to sustain consistent employment or honor financial obligations.

Clinical Items

The five clinical items contained in the HCR-20 include (11) lack of insight, (12) negative attitudes, (13) active symptoms of major mental illness, (14) impulsivity, and (15) unresponsiveness to treatment.

Mr. Z has shown significant progress when examining the clinical items on the HCR-20. Mr. Z's insight into his mental illness has improved over the course of his 8-year hospitalization at the state hospital. Upon admission to the state hospital, he denied that his delusional beliefs were due to a mental illness. Currently, he acknowledges suffering from a mental illness that he described as "paranoid schizophrenia." Upon his admission to the state hospital, Mr. Z was frequently involved in physical altercations with other patients. Over the past 2 years, Mr. Z was involved in no such incidents. During the clinical interview, Mr. Z was asked to describe his history of aggression within the hospital. He stated,

> Really, some of the fights I was in when I first got here I really don't remember because I was out of it. I know I would start with people and would just get into fights. Sometimes they were my fault and I hit people, and other times people hit me because I was crazy and being a jerk.

Mr. Z was asked to detail his two convictions for assault and battery and how his mental illness played a role in these incidents. He stated,

> I've been arrested three times for violent stuff. The first two times I got convicted. I did probation the first time and got six months in jail the second time. The third one is this one, and I got an NGRI for it. All three times I wasn't taking medications, and two out of the three I was drinking. When I'm off my meds I get paranoid about people. First I stay to myself and stop talking to my friends and family. Then after a while I don't leave the house. The problem with that is I don't work, and I don't pay rent, and I get evicted. When I'm homeless I usually get worse and really paranoid and eventually I do something that gets me arrested because I feel like people are coming after me, or messing with me.

When asked to describe how his mental illness was related to the offense for which he was later adjudicated NGRI, he stated,

I used to think that my wife was using drugs and having sex with other people and that's why she left me. I thought that [the victim] was the one behind all of it. I wasn't taking my medications at the time and I was drinking almost every day. I thought she was taking my wife to meet other guys. It's embarrassing to say now, but I know it happened because I read the records. I thought they were going to orgies and my wife was having sex with all kinds of people. When I take my medications I don't think crazy things like that. If I stop my medications or start drinking, I would start believing stuff like that again and would probably be violent at some point.

When asked his thoughts about this incident now, Mr. Z stated,

I wish it never happened. I feel really bad about it. I wish I could just apologize for it and it would go away, but it can't because it was scary for her and her child. That's what I feel worst about—that the kid will be screwed up because of what I did when I was crazy.

Risk Management Items

The five risk management items contained in the HCR-20 include (16) plans lack feasibility, (17) exposure to destabilizers, (18) lack of personal support, (19) noncompliance with remediation attempts, and (20) stress. These items provide guidance for the ongoing management of a case. The risk management items of concern for Mr. Z are discussed below, and inform the specific recommendations made at the end of this report.

- *Lack of personal support:* Mr. Z and his treatment team report that he lacks supportive family and friends in the community. He has not had contact with family and reports that he does not know where he would live if he was released to the community. Mr. Z's violent behavior in the past appears to be related to his lack of support. All three violent incidents were in the context of either living alone for extended periods of time without support from mental health professionals or while homeless. Due to Mr. Z's lack of community support at this time, which would assist him during a transition from the state hospital to a community setting, it is recommended that Mr. Z visit and become familiar with staff and other residents of a residential facility prior to discharge from the hospital (see recommendations at the end of this report).

- *Exposure to destabilizers:* Within the custody of the state hospital, Mr. Z has not had access to potentially destabilizing items or situations, such as alcohol or drugs. During a transition to a less secure facility, access to destabilizers will increase. To mitigate this risk, Mr. Z should be observed closely by staff, particularly during the initial phase of his transition to a less-secure facility.
- *Stress:* During a transition to a less-secure facility, patients typically experience increased stress as they become acclimated to their new environment. Mr. Z has been at the state hospital for 8 years, and a transition to a less-secure facility, while clinically indicated, will likely be stressful. Mr. Z will benefit from discussions with the staff from the residential facility where he will be transferred. This will foster a trusting relationship with staff at the residential facility prior to his transition and provide his new treatment staff with a baseline of Mr. Z's level of functioning when he is clinically stable. It is recommended that clinical staff assess his mental status regularly upon transition to determine whether this stress has resulted in increased symptomatology, particularly paranoia.

Conclusions

Based on this review of Mr. Z's case, the administration of risk assessment tools, a clinical interview with Mr. Z, and consultation with his treatment team, it is my opinion that Mr. Z is at low to moderate risk for violence at this time. It is also my recommendation that Mr. Z begin to transition to a community living situation under supervision provided for by a Department of Mental Health community agency.

Mr. Z has made gains in several areas. He has shown an increased understanding that he suffers from a mental illness and how his mental illness and substance abuse is related to his history of violence. Mr. Z has also shown a good understanding of how increased symptoms of his mental illness or abuse of substances would likely result in him becoming violent in the future. He has also shown that he can manage his behavior within a hospital environment. Although it is recommended that Mr. Z begin a transition to the community, this transition should progress slowly to ensure that he builds community ties prior to release from the hospital. The potential harm if this transition occurs too rapidly is that Mr. Z does not form connections with treatment providers, becomes noncompliant with treatment interventions (medications and abstaining from substance use), resulting in the reemergence of paranoid delusional beliefs. If this occurs, then it would be my opinion that Mr. Z is at high risk for violence. However, if treatment providers feel as though Mr. Z has formed meaningful connections, refrains from substance use, participates in ongoing relapse prevention focused on substance abuse, and remains compliant with medications, his risk of harm to others is low to moderate.

Recommendations

The following recommendations are made for Mr. Z's transition from the state hospital to a community living situation under supervision provided for by the Department of Mental Health:

1. It is recommended that the facility where Mr. Z resides has 24-hour staff coverage and the ability to observe medication administration to ensure compliance.
2. Mr. Z should begin meeting with clinical staff from an identified residential facility as soon as possible to afford time for several meetings prior to his transfer. Because Mr. Z lacks outside support from family or friends, which is helpful during such transitions, a lengthy transition over several months is clinically indicated. His only social support system at this time is made up of his treatment providers. The main goal of transitional meetings is to establish Mr. Z's trust in clinical staff from his community placement similar to his current treatment alliances with clinical staff at the state hospital.
3. It is recommended that during these meetings Mr. Z explain his history of violence and how symptoms of his mental illness and substance abuse are related to past violence. This is important because Mr. Z has a difficult time sharing information with new treatment staff. While clinical staff from the state hospital and the community agency are both present, it will afford Mr. Z the safety of sharing important clinical information with new treatment providers.
4. It is recommended that, during clinical meetings between the state hospital treatment team and community agency staff, the topic of Mr. Z's placement be discussed, including the rules of the residential placement and the privilege system. This will alleviate Mr. Z's anxiety regarding what to expect when he arrives at his new residence.

5. It is recommended that Mr. Z visit the residential facility prior to his discharge from the hospital. Visits should occur under the supervision of both hospital staff and staff from the residential facility. Mr. Z should visit the residence on at least three occasions—once in the morning, once in the afternoon, and once in the evening—so he is able to meet staff across shifts and see the routine throughout the day.
6. A psychiatrist with experience working with aggressive patients should be identified prior to Mr. Z's discharge from the state hospital to allow for the psychiatrist to review records and interview Mr. Z. It is recommended that Mr. Z be seen weekly by his psychiatrist over the first 3 months of his transition to a residential facility. This allows for close monitoring of his mental status. In the case that Mr. Z becomes increasingly paranoid, a brief hospitalization is recommended for stabilization.
7. Privileges should initially be limited to supervised community access. When additional privileges are being considered, another formal violence risk assessment is recommended.

DISCUSSION

The assessment of risk for violent behavior is a complicated area and the focus of a significant amount of research over the past 30 years. Forensic practitioners and evaluators are asked to provide opinions regarding the risk of harm an individual poses in a variety of settings. Qualifications to carry out forensic assessments vary depending on jurisdiction and local laws. Even in cases when a practitioner meets statutory requirements, advanced knowledge of the research literature as it pertains to the specific risk assessment being conducted is necessary. It is also essential for forensic practitioners to clearly understand the type of evaluation they are being asked to conduct and to clarify the resources available when making recommendations with the authority requesting the evaluation. The risk assessment literature has progressed sufficiently to the point that forensic practitioners are able to assess risk for violence with greater accuracy and efficiency. Forensic practitioners are required to remain current with this rapidly growing literature, particularly in the specific area in which they practice.

The literature has progressed through three generations of research. The first focused primarily on clinical samples and found difficulty in determining which groups or subgroups of patients were at risk for violence. The second generation examined specific risk factors for violence, resulting in the establishment of actuarial measures. These actuarial measures significantly increased predictive accuracy over subjective clinical opinion. However, these tools focus on historical data and provide a static, unchangeable score and resultant risk level. Once an individual is categorized at a particular risk level, treatment intervention and/or environmental change will not decrease this assigned risk level. The third generation of research focused on structured professional judgment, which uses risk assessment schemes to guide clinical opinion. The most widely researched structured professional judgment guide is the HCR-20 (Webster et al., 1997). Because numerous risk factors have been found to increase an individual's risk for future violence, all should be considered in the course of an evaluation. It is further recommended that structured professional judgment tools, such as the HCR-20 (Webster et al., 1997) be utilized. Such assessment tools compel the forensic practitioner to address empirically derived risk factors found to increase an individual's risk for violence while also individualizing each assessment.

Risk assessment is an ongoing process and is not conducted at one point in time. The ongoing risk management of a forensic case includes the introduction of intervention strategies but also requires ongoing assessment. As additional data become available, this data should be incorporated into the overall risk assessment. The forensic patient's risk level may change over time for a variety of reasons, such as changes in the patient's clinical presentation or new environmental stressors. As new information becomes available over time, this information is also incorporated into the ongoing risk management plan.

Risk assessments should not occur in a vacuum and require collaboration between the practitioner responsible for the violence risk assessment evaluation and other clinicians and collaterals involved in the long-term care and support of the client. The research literature on risk management shows that, to decrease violent recidivism, ongoing management of the case is required. This often begins within inpatient hospitals or correctional facilities, but outpatient oversight is required to ensure successful transitions from detention to the community.

NOTE

1. Chapter 8 of this volume is dedicated to the topic of psychopathy as a risk factor for violence; thus, psychopathy will be discussed only briefly here.

REFERENCES

American Psychiatric Association. (1974). *Task force report on clinical aspects of the violent individual.* Washington, DC: Author.

Andrews, D. A., & Bonta, J. (1995). *The Level of Service Inventory–Revised.* Toronto, Canada: Multi-Health Systems.

Andrews, D. A., & Bonta, J. (2003). *The psychology of criminal conduct* (3rd ed.). Cincinnati, OH: Anderson Publishing.

Andrews, D. A., Bonta, J., & Wormith, S. J. (2006). The recent past and near future of risk and/or need assessment. *Crime and Delinquency, 52,* 7–27.

Andrews, D. A., Zinger, I., Hoge, R. D., Bonta, J., Gendreau, P., & Cullen, F. T. (1990). Does correctional treatment work? A clinically relevant and psychologically informed meta-analysis. *Criminology, 28,* 369–404.

Boer, D. P., Hart, S. D., Kropp, P. R., & Webster, C. D. (1997). *Manual for the Sexual Violence Risk-20 (SVR-20): Professional guidelines for assessing risk of sexual violence.* Vancouver, Canada: British Columbia Institute Against Family Violence.

Bonta, J., Law, M., & Hanson, K. (1998). The prediction of criminal and violent recidivism among mentally disordered offenders: A meta-analysis. *Psychological Bulletin, 123,* 123–142.

Borum, R. (1996). Improving the clinical practice of violence risk assessment: Technology, guidelines, and training. *American Psychologist, 51,* 945–948.

Cocozza, J. J., & Steadman, H. J. (1974). Some refinements in the measurement and prediction of dangerous behavior. *American Journal of Psychiatry, 131,* 1012–1014.

de Vogel, V., de Ruiter, C., Hildebrand, M., Bos, B., & van de Ven, P. (2004). Type of discharge and risk of recidivism measured by the HCR-20: A retrospective study in a Dutch sample of treated forensic psychiatric patients. *International Journal of Forensic Mental Health, 3,* 149–165.

Dohrenwend, B. P., Shrout, P. E., Egri, G., & Mendelsohn, F. S. (1980). Nonspecific psychological distress and other dimensions of psychopathology. *Archives of General Psychiatry, 37,* 1229–1236.

Douglas, K. S., Ogloff, J.R.P., & Hart, S. D. (2003). Evaluation of a model of violence risk assessment among forensic psychiatric patients. *Psychiatric Services, 54,* 1372–1379.

Douglas, K., & Webster, C. (1999). The HCR-20 violence risk assessment scheme: Concurrent validity in a sample of incarcerated offenders. *Criminal Justice and Behavior, 26,* 3–19.

Douglas, K. S., Yeomans, M., & Boer, D. P. (2005). Comparative validity analysis of multiple measures of violence risk in a sample of criminal offenders. *Criminal Justice and Behavior, 32,* 479–510.

Gendreau, P., Little, T., & Goggin, C. (1996). A meta-analysis of the predictors of adult offender recidivism: What works! *Criminology, 34,* 575–607.

Gilders, I. (1997). Violence in the community: A study of violence and aggression in homelessness and mental health day services. *Journal of Community and Applied Social Psychology, 7,* 377–387.

Gilligan, J. (1996). *Violence: Reflections on a national epidemic.* New York: Vintage.

Grann, M., Belfrage, H., & Tengström, A. (2000). Actuarial assessment of risk for violence: Predictive validity of the VRAG and the historical part of the HCR-20. *Criminal Justice and Behavior, 27,* 97–114.

Grisso, T., & Tomkins, A. J. (1996). Communicating violence risk assessments. *American Psychologist, 51,* 928–930.

Hanson, R. K. (1997). *The development of a brief actuarial scale for sexual offense recidivism.* Ottawa, Canada: Department of the Solicitor General.

Hanson, R. K., & Bussière, M. T. (1998). Predicting relapse: A meta-analysis of sexual offender recidivism studies. *Journal of Consulting and Clinical Psychology, 66,* 348–362.

Hanson, R. K., & Thornton, D. (1999). *Static-99: Improving actuarial risk assessments for sex offenders.* Ottawa, Canada: Department of the Solicitor General.

Hare, R. D. (1991). *The Hare Psychopathy Checklist–Revised.* Toronto, Canada: Multi-Health Systems.

Hare, R. D. (2003) *The Hare Psychopathy Checklist–Revised* (2nd ed.). Toronto, Canada: Multi-Health Systems.

Hare, R. D., McPherson, L. M., & Forth, A. E. (1988). Male psychopaths and their criminal careers. *Journal of Consulting and Clinical Psychology, 56*(5), 710–714.

Harris, G. T., Rice, M. E., & Cormier, C. A. (1991). Psychopathy and violent recidivism. *Law and Human Behavior, 15,* 625–637.

Harris, G. T., Rice, M. E., & Cormier, C. A. (2002). Prospective replication of the Violence Risk Appraisal Guide in prediction of violent recidivism among forensic patients. *Law and Human Behavior, 26,* 377–394.

Harris, G. T., Rice, M. E., & Quinsey, V. L. (1993). Violent recidivism of mentally disordered offenders: The development of a statistical prediction instrument. *Criminal Justice and Behavior, 20,* 315–335.

Hart, S., Cox, D., & Hare, R. (1995). *Manual for the Psychopathy Checklist: Screening Version (PCL:SV).* Toronto, Canada: Multi-Health Systems.

Hart, S. D., Kropp, P. R., & Hare, R. D. (1988). Performance of male psychopaths following conditional release from prison. *Journal of Consulting and Clinical Psychology, 56,* 227–232.

Heilbrun, K., Dvoskin, J., Hart, S., & McNiel, D. (1999). Violence risk communication: Implications for research, policy, and practice. *Health, Risk, & Society, 1,* 91–106.

Heilbrun, K., Hart, S. D., Hare, R. D., Gustafson, D., Nunez, C., & White, A. (1998). Inpatient and post-discharge aggression in mentally disordered offenders: The role of psychopathy. *Journal of Interpersonal Violence, 13,* 514–527.

Hirschi, T., & Gottfredson, M. (1983). Age and the explanation of crime. *American Journal of Sociology, 89,* 552–584.

Kachigian, C., & Felthous, A. R. (2004). Court responses to *Tarasoff* statutes. *Journal of the American Academy of Psychiatry and the Law, 32,* 263–273.

Klassen, D., & O'Connor, W. A. (1988). A prospective study of predictors of violence in adult mental health admissions. *Law and Human Behavior, 12,* 143–158.

Kosson, D. S., Smith, S. S., & Newman, J. (1990). Evaluating the construct validity of psychopathy in black and white male inmates: Three preliminary studies. *Journal of Abnormal Psychology, 99,* 250–259.

Krakowski, M., & Czobor, P. (2004). Gender differences in violent behaviors: Relationship to clinical symptoms and psychosocial factors. *American Journal of Psychiatry, 161,* 459–465.

Lidz, C. W., Mulvey, E. P., & Gardner, W. (1993). The accuracy of predictions of violence to others. *Journal of the American Medical Association, 269,* 1007–1011.

Link, B., Andrews, D., & Cullen, F. (1992). The violent and illegal behavior of mental patients reconsidered. *American Sociological Review, 57,* 275–292.

Link, B., & Stueve, A. (1994). Psychotic symptoms and the violent/illegal behavior of mental patients compared to community controls. In J. Monahan & H. Steadman (Eds.), *Violence and mental disorder: Developments in risk assessment* (pp. 137–159). Chicago: University of Chicago Press.

Menzies, R., & Webster, C. D. (1995). Construction and validation of risk assessments in a six-year follow-up of forensic patients: A tridimensional analysis. *Journal of Consulting and Clinical Psychology, 63*(5), 766–778.

Mills, J. F., Kroner, D. G., & Hemmati, T. (2007). The validity of violence risk estimates: An issue in item performance. *Psychological Services, 4,* 1–12.

Monahan, J. (1981). *Predicting violent behavior: An assessment of clinical techniques.* Beverly Hills, CA: Sage.

Monahan, J. (1993). Causes of violence. In U.S. Commission (Ed.), *Drugs and violence in America* (pp. 77–85). Washington, DC: U.S. Government Printing Office.

Monahan, J., & Steadman, H. (1996). Violent storms and violent people: How meteorology can inform risk communication in mental health law. *American Psychologist, 51,* 931–938.

Monahan, J., Steadman, H. J., Silver, E., Appelbaum, P. S., Clark Robbins, P., Mulvey, E. P., et al. (2001). *Rethinking risk assessment: The MacArthur study of mental disorder and violence.* New York: Oxford University Press.

O'Connor v. Donaldson, 422 U.S. 563 (1975).

Quinn, K. M. (1984). The impact of *Tarasoff* on clinical practice. *Behavioral Sciences and the Law, 2*(3), 319–329.

Quinsey, V. L., Harris, G. T., Rice, M. E., Cormier, C. A. (1998). *Violent offenders: Appraising and managing risk.* The Law and Public Policy: Psychology and the Social Sciences series. Washington, DC: American Psychological Association.

Quinsey, V. L., Harris, G. T., Rice, M. E., & Cormier, C. A. (2006). *Violent offenders: Appraising and managing risk* (2nd ed.). The Law and Public Policy: Psychology and the Social Sciences Series. Washington, DC: American Psychological Association.

Reiss, A. J., & Roth, J. A. (Eds.). (1993). *Understanding and preventing violence.* National Academy Report. Washington, DC: National Academy Press.

Schwartz, D. W. (1985). The obligation to assess dangerousness. *New York State Journal of Medicine, 85*(2), 67–68.

Serin, R. C., & Amos, N. L. (1995). The role of psychopathy in the assessment of dangerousness. *International Journal of Law and Psychiatry, 18,* 231–238.

Silver, E., Mulvey, E. P., & Monahan, J. (1999). Assessing violence risk among discharged psychiatric patients: Toward an ecological approach. *Law and Human Behavior, 23,* 237–255.

Simone, S., & Fulero, S. M. (2005). *Tarasoff* and the duty to protect. *Journal of Aggression, Maltreatment & Trauma, 11,* 145–168.

Singleton, N., Meltzer, H., Gatward, R., Coid, J., & Deasy, D. (1998). *Psychiatric morbidity among prisoners.* London: Her Majesty's Stationery Office.

Slovenko, R. (1988). Commentary: The therapist's duty to warn or protect third persons. *Journal of Psychiatry and Law, 16*(1), 139–209.

Steadman, H., & Cocozza. (1974). *Careers of the criminally insane.* Lexington, MA: Lexington Books.

Swanson, J. W. (1993). Alcohol abuse, mental disorder, and violent behavior: An epidemiologic inquiry. *Alcohol Health and Research World, 17,* 123–132.

Swanson, J., Borum, R., Swartz, M., & Monahan, J. (1996). Psychotic symptoms and disorders and the risk of violent behavior in the community. *Criminal Behavior and Mental Health, 6,* 317–338.

Swanson, J., Holzer, C., Ganju, V., & Jono, R. (1990). Violence and psychiatric disorder in the community: Evidence from the epidemiological catchment area surveys. *Hospital and Community Psychiatry, 41,* 761–770.

Tarasoff v. Regents of the University of California, 13 Cal. 3d 117, 529 P.2d 533, 118 Cal. Rptr. 129 (1974).

Tarasoff v. Regents of the University of California, 17 Cal. 3d 425, 551 P.2d 334, 131 Cal Rptr. 14 (1976).

Tardiff, K, Marzuk, P., Leon, A., & Portera, L. (1997). A prospective study of violence by psychiatric patients after hospital discharge. *Psychiatric Services, 48,* 678–681.

VandeCreek, L., & Knapp, S. (1989). Tarasoff *and beyond: Legal and clinical considerations in the treatment of life-endangering patients.* Sarasota, FL: Professional Resource Press.

Walters, G. D. (2003). Predicting institutional adjustment and recidivism with the Psychopathy Checklist factor scores: A meta-analysis. *Law and Human Behavior, 27,* 541–558.

Webster, C. D., Douglas, K. S., Eaves, D., & Hart, S. D. (1997). *HCR-20: Assessing risk for violence* (version 2). Burnaby, Canada: Mental Health, Law, and Policy Institute, Simon Fraser University.

Wong, S., & Hare, R. D. (2006). *Guidelines for a psychopathy treatment program.* Toronto, Canada: Multi-Health Systems.

2
Violence Risk Assessment Evaluation: Practices and Procedures

MICHAEL H. FOGEL

The purpose of this chapter is to highlight contemporary processes and principles associated with violence risk assessment, report writing, and risk communication. The assessment of violence potential permeates the legal system and clinical environments. As a result of the landmark case *Tarasoff v. Regents of the University of California* (1976) and its progeny as well as the efforts of managed health care systems to contain costs and provide treatment in the least restrictive setting, violence risk assessment has become commonplace for mental health practitioners working outside the forensic arena (Borum, 1996; Monahan, 2003). Indeed, Borum (1996) observed:

> The assessment and the management of violence risk are critical issues, not just for psychologists and psychiatrists in forensic settings but for all practicing clinicians. Despite a long-standing controversy about the ability of mental health professionals to predict violence, the courts continue to rely on them for advice on these issues and in many cases have imposed on them a legal duty to take action when they know or should know a patient poses a risk of serious danger to others. (p. 954)

I wish to thank Joel Dvoskin, PhD, ABPP, for his helpful comments on an earlier draft of this chapter.

Regardless of the setting or context in which the risk assessment is performed, it is incumbent on the evaluator to perform a professionally adequate evaluation. In fact, case law illustrates that some jurisdictions are no longer willing to grant experts absolute immunity from civil liability for testimony that is based on a work product that deviates from applicable professional standards (Ewing, 2003; see, e.g., *Levine v. Wiss & Co.*, 1984; *Murphy v. A. A. Mathews*, 1992). Therefore, the issue most relevant to a mental health practitioner conducting a violence risk assessment is not necessarily the accuracy of the assessment (though one should always strive to be accurate), but whether the methods employed were consistent with what a similarly situated reasonable professional would have done (Borum & Verhaagen, 2006; Monahan, 1993). The methodology and guidelines addressed in this chapter are foundational aspects of current good practice standards that should be a component of any violence risk assessment evaluation, report, or communication.

RISK ASSESSMENT DEFINED

The goal of violence risk assessment is the prevention of future violence and the development of management strategies to control or minimize assessed risk; it is not the prediction of dangerousness (Hart, 1998; Otto, 2000; Webster, Hucker, & Bloom, 2002). Grisso and Appelbaum (1992) contend that the phrase "prediction of dangerousness" has "no logical meaning in the context of the behavioral and social sciences" (p. 623). They assert:

> To "predict" is to make a statement about the likelihood of a future event or behavior. *Dangerousness* seems to refer not to an event or behavior, but to a condition that exists as a function of the presence of someone or something perceived as "dangerous." Other definitions are possible; but whatever dangerousness means, it is not a behavior or an event offering a logical criterion for predictive efforts in research or clinical practice. (p. 623, emphasis in original)

The concept of risk is multifaceted. In contrast to dangerousness, which is a static, dichotomous construct that focuses on the person as the determinant of violence potential, risk assessment focuses on the interaction between the person and environmental factors that produce conditions of risk that can change over time (Borum, Swartz, & Swanson, 1996; Otto, 2000). Risk is predominantly viewed as a construct that is contextual (contingent on the situation and circumstance), dynamic (changeable), and continuous (shifting along a continuum of probability) (Borum & Verhaagen, 2006). Furthermore, social scientists have disaggregated risk into its component parts. Five elements of risk appear somewhat consistently across the literature: (1) the nature of the harm (e.g., type of harm, to whom, instrumental/affective); (2) the likelihood that the harm will occur (i.e., probability); (3) the frequency or duration of the harm (e.g., acute or chronic); (4) the severity or seriousness of the harm; and (5) the imminence of the harm (Dvoskin & Heilbrun, 2001; Grisso & Appelbaum, 1992; Hart, 1998; Litwack, Zapf, Groscup, & Hart, 2005; Mulvey & Lidz, 1995). Depending on the purpose of the risk assessment evaluation (i.e., the referral question), some or all of these components will be addressed.

Consequently, it is clear that risk is much more than a dichotomous conclusion that a person will or will not act violently. In fact, most often, it is a judgment that the person poses a substantial risk of physical harm *under certain circumstances* (e.g., stops taking prescribed medications, reengages in substance abuse), which may or may not occur (Litwack et al., 2005). Statutes that require, for example, a "likelihood of serious harm" do not require a finding that the person *will* commit a violent act, but that *sufficient risk* exists to believe that the person might act violently. It is up to society to determine whether the assessed likelihood of future violence warrants a particular legal intervention, given the additional considerations of the nature, frequency, severity, and imminence of the harm (Grisso & Appelbaum, 1992; Monahan & Wexler, 1978). Cohen, Groth, and Siegel (1978) provide:

> It is a perilous, narrow path between the requirements of social order and the expression of individual freedom. To balance order and liberty properly is a sociopolitical, not a clinical, issue, and this must be done by society's courts and legislatures. The clinician should neither be given nor attempt to usurp society's right to determine the risks it is willing to take in resolving the conflict between safety and liberty. (p. 39)

Nevertheless, it is interesting to note that, despite the disaggregation of the construct of risk, the movement away from a binary finding, and the goal of risk assessment being risk management, ultimately mental health practitioners are still making a prediction. Rogers and Shuman (2005) explain that there are three possible temporal frameworks in which forensic evaluations are completed: current, retrospective, and prospective. Violence risk assessment is a prospective evaluation. The objective is to forecast the nature and seriousness of harm an individual may pose within a given time frame, in light of anticipated circumstances (Borum & Verhaagen, 2006). Indeed, Grisso and Appelbaum (1992) suggest, "Statements of risk are no less predictions than statements in dichotomous form; they simply provide additional information concerning the likelihood that others will be right or wrong in drawing their own dichotomous conclusion" (p. 624).

APPROACHING THE ASSESSMENT

In approaching a violence risk assessment evaluation, the legal–empirical–forensic model of forensic practice should be employed. This model underscores the critical elements that establish evaluator competence in forensic practice (Rogers & Shuman, 2005). The *legal* component emphasizes the importance of possessing a fundamental and reasonable level of knowledge and understanding of the laws, rules, and procedures that govern the evaluation or the anticipated role of the evaluation in a legal proceeding. The *empirical* component highlights the special responsibility a forensic mental health professional bears to provide opinions and testimony that are based on adequate scientific foundation and empirically validated methods that are applied reliably to the facts of the case (Committee on Ethical Guidelines for Forensic Psychologists, 1991). And the *forensic* component stresses the idiographic nature of the law, whereby legal interpretation (e.g., case law) and specialized methods (e.g., forensic assessment instruments) are applied to an individual case.

In concert with the legal component of this model, the practitioner must understand the precise reason why the evaluation is being requested (i.e., the referral question). For instance, what behavior on the part of the examinee precipitated the request for the evaluation? Why is there concern that the examinee might be violent? What specific question does the attorney want addressed? What aspect, if any, does the evaluation play in the legal process? What is the relevant statutory law or case law that should be considered in conducting the evaluation? These are questions that will help to identify the legal purpose of the evaluation. It is through this lens that a determination is made as to what information should be contained in the evaluation report, as only that information that directly bears on the legal issue should be included (Committee on Ethical Guidelines for Forensic Psychologists, 1991). Furthermore, identification of the relevant legal issues is critical to ensure an accurate, relevant, credible, and effective risk assessment evaluation (Heilbrun, Marczyk, & DeMatteo, 2002). The threshold for action concerning violence risk depends in part on the consequences of the prediction. It is the legal issue that informs the evaluator how sure she must be of her inferential opinions. That is, a greater degree of uncertainty is permitted when making a referral to an employee assistance program for mental health services than to a state's attorney's office for civil commitment.

The empirical aspect of this model necessitates a systematic approach to the risk assessment evaluation, with emphasis on the reliability and validity of the methodology and decision-making process. Reliability is the consistency or repeatability of a measure. Validity is the accuracy of the measure, or the degree to which the assessment strategy measures what it claims to measure. Inconsistent, unreliable measures virtually guarantee inaccuracy. A systematic, carefully planned, methodical process is more likely to yield reliable and valid findings. Werner, Rose, and Yesavage (1983) assert, "To the extent that predictions are unreliable, they cannot be accurate forecasters of behavior" (p. 815).

Finally, the forensic component of this model highlights the application of the law and scientific principles and practices to a single case. While social scientists prefer to focus on general principles, relationships, and patterns (i.e., to be nomothetic in scope), legal decisions are based on individual cases and the idiosyncratic facts about them (Haney, 1980). The forensic evaluator must possess a firm and accurate understanding of the relevant legal standard and skillfully apply it to the facts of a particular case, utilizing empirically grounded methods and procedures. The reasoning and rationale for conclusions should be explicitly stated and transparent rather than vague and unverifiable and hidden behind the cloak of "clinical judgment" (Rogers & Shuman, 2005).

BIASES AND JUDGMENT ERRORS

The methodology on which the risk assessment is based must be reliable, valid, and consistent with applicable legal standards, such *Frye v. United States* (1923) or *Daubert v. Merrell Dow Pharmaceuticals* (1993). Well-structured and psychologically relevant assessment methodologies can safeguard against potential standard of care challenges and enhance impartiality and comprehensiveness (Weissman & DeBow, 2003).

Furthermore, such methods ensure consistency in information processing and decision making and reduce the operation of individual biases (Hoge, 2002).

Several biases and judgment errors can operate to reduce the accuracy of a forensic evaluation. For instance, confirmatory bias can impact the data that is retrieved and considered, because it is the tendency to seek, use, or selectively remember information that confirms one's beliefs or hypotheses and to disregard or fail to seek information that refutes them (Garb, 1998). The availability heuristic can influence the selection and weighting of predictor variables, because information that is more vivid or salient will be remembered more readily and can lead to the belief that two variables have a greater relationship than actually exists (Borum, Otto, & Golding, 1993; Garb, 1998; Melton, Petrila, Poythress, & Slobogin, 2007). The belief that a relationship between two variables exists when, in reality, the variables are not correlated, correlated to a lesser extent, or correlated in the opposite direction than believed is identified as illusory correlation (Garb, 1998; Melton et al., 2007).

Additional potential sources of error in clinical judgment include the anchoring-and-adjustment heuristic, the utilization of collateral information that is of questionable validity, and the underutilization of base rates. The primacy effect is the tendency to make judgments after collecting relatively little information. Although the judgment may or may not need to be adjusted based on subsequently collected information, anchoring and adjustment is said to occur when different initial impressions yield findings that are biased toward the corresponding start points. That is, estimates are inadequately revised in the face of contradictory information, and the outcome is relative to the anchoring point (also known as anchoring bias) (Borum & Verhaagen, 2006; Garb, 1998).

As detailed below, third-party information is an essential component of a high-quality forensic evaluation. However, merely obtaining additional information does not necessarily improve judgment accuracy. Information that leads to increased validity is said to have incremental validity. Therefore, considering information that is less valid than information that is already possessed can lead to a decrease in accuracy (Borum et al., 1993; Garb, 1998, 2003). For instance, it is better to use only one psychological test that is psychometrically sound and possesses construction and validation samples that closely mirror the examinee than to use a second psychological test that has less empirical support and samples that are unlike the examinee.

In the context of violence risk, the term *base rate* refers to the proportion of a population that engages in a specified type of violent behavior over a specific period of time. Monahan (1981) asserts, "It is clear that *knowledge of the appropriate base rate is the most important single piece of information necessary to make an accurate prediction*" (p. 60, emphasis in original). At least four critical issues must be considered when examining base rate data: (1) the characteristics of the sample population; (2) the manner in which the behavior of interest is defined; (3) the outcome measure (e.g., self-report, agency records, hospitalization, arrest); and (4) the unit of time at risk (e.g., month(s), year(s)). Each of these characteristics affects the utility and applicability of the data to individual cases; therefore, the closer the fit between the examinee and the characteristics underlying the base rate data, the more confidence that can be expressed regarding its applicability (Monahan, 1981). In addition, it is important to note that base rate data represent an average, with each person possessing a different propensity, and associated probability, to commit an act of violence. Consequently, for some, the probability to engage in violence will be higher than the sample base rate, and for others, the probability will be lower than the sample base rate (Prentky & Burgess, 2000).

The antidote to the above biases and judgment errors begins with awareness of these limitations; however, awareness alone is insufficient. Evaluators must be familiar with the research on these limitations, employ systematic data collection and documentation strategies, and seek professional consultation. Professional ethics and evidentiary requirements mandate that the competent forensic evaluator be cognizant of the weaknesses and limitations associated with their assessment methods, procedures, opinions, and recommendations and take reasonable steps to minimize the impact of such weaknesses and sources of error (Borum et al., 1993; Borum & Verhaagen, 2006; Committee on Ethical Guidelines for Forensic Psychologists, 1991).

RISK FACTORS ASSOCIATED WITH VIOLENCE

The empirical component of the above model necessitates a fundamental understanding of the key risk factors associated with an increased risk of violence. A risk factor is a factor that statistically correlates with violence and precedes its occurrence. Statistical association, however, in no way implies causation. Rather, a causal risk factor must be manipulable and, when manipulated, change the likelihood that the outcome will occur (Kraemer et al., 1997; Monahan, 2006). A risk factor is said to be predictive when the observed level of association between the risk factor and the outcome (i.e., violence) exceeds chance or is significantly different from a correlation coefficient (r) of .00, thus indicating that the two variables are independent of one another (Andrews & Bonta, 2006).

Risk factors are either static (fixed) or dynamic (changeable). Static risk factors (e.g., sex, history of violence) identify an individual's absolute or relative level of risk (Otto, 2000), or what Douglas and Skeem (2005) describe as "risk status." These factors have limited utility in the determination of when an individual has substantially reduced their risk or in directing specific treatment or management efforts since, by definition, they cannot change (Douglas & Skeem, 2005; Hanson, 1998; Otto, 2000). Dynamic risk factors (e.g., substance use, psychotic symptomatology) are amenable to change and are associated with an individual's variability in violence potential (Douglas & Skeem, 2005; Otto, 2000). In contrast to static risk factors, these factors facilitate the identification of when an individual may act violently, direct treatment and management efforts, and aid the assessment of when an individual has substantially reduced their risk.

Hanson (1998) further distinguishes stable and acute dynamic risk factors. Stable dynamic factors (e.g., deviant sexual preferences, traits of impulsivity or hostility) have the potential to change but generally only do so gradually over time. Acute dynamic factors (e.g., sexual arousal, intoxication) are states that change rapidly and may immediately precede an act of violence. Douglas and Skeem (2005) describe the propensity of an individual to engage in violence at a particular time, which is determined by the combination of static and dynamic risk factors, as the "risk state."

Before reviewing some of the key risk factors that have the most robust empirical support, it is important to briefly review some of the methodological issues present in their identification and evaluation. A substantial literature identifies a large number of putative risk factors. Indeed, the MacArthur Violence Risk Assessment Study, which assessed community violence in 951 men and women psychiatric patients after hospital discharge and is the largest and most comprehensive study on violence risk assessment to date, tested the predictive association between 134 potential risk factors and violence (Monahan et al., 2001). Several methodological issues potentially impact the applicability of a risk factor to an individual risk assessment evaluation. Specifically, tremendous variability exists across studies concerning the definition and measurement of risk factors and the outcome criterion (i.e., violence), the duration of the follow-up period, and the statistical methods used to evaluate the predictive power (Hart, 1998). Some studies, for instance, use nomenclature associated with the various editions of the *Diagnostic and Statistical Manual of Mental Disorders* (*DSM;* e.g., American Psychiatric Association, 1994), while others use the various editions of the *International Classification of Diseases* (e.g., World Health Organization, 1992). At times, different standardized tests are used to assess the same psychological construct (e.g., empathy, personality disorders). Furthermore, violence is defined in a multitude of ways, varying with regard to severity, degree of contact, and type of act. The measurement of violence is also quite varied across studies in that outcome measures include charges, convictions, self-report, and/or collateral informants. In addition, the duration over which data are collected varies from days, months, years, to several years (Hart, 1998).

In regard to dynamic risk factors, Douglas and Skeem (2005) contend that few studies have investigated whether changes in putative dynamic risk factors affect the likelihood of future violence. Studies investigating such factors at a single time point illustrate the predictive validity of the factor at a given time across individuals. However, minimal evidence is gleaned from this type of study to substantiate the predictive utility of a supposed dynamic risk factor, given that the factor did not have the opportunity to change over time (i.e., there were not multiple time-point evaluations) and the individual's level of risk was not assessed in relation to that change. Additional limitations associated with studies of ostensibly dynamic risk factors include the variation across studies of the criterion measure (i.e., how violence is defined), the lack of consistency across studies concerning what factors are investigated, and the potential error associated with a less-than-valid assessment of the risk factor across studies.

In sum, the above issues underscore the examiner's need to be cognizant of the limitations inherent in the methodology associated with putative risk factors, the reported statistical relationship of the risk factors to violence, and the applicability of risk factors to an individual risk assessment evaluation.

KEY RISK FACTORS

Empirically validated risk factors most consistently related to violent behavior are briefly reviewed. Additional correlates of violence will also be mentioned throughout this chapter. For a comprehensive review of these and other empirically validated risk factors associated with adult violent behavior, see Bonta, Law, and Hanson (1998); Borum et al. (1996); Conroy and Murrie (2007); Monahan (2006); and Monahan et al. (2001); for juvenile violent behavior, see Borum and Verhaagen (2006); and for sexually violent specific behavior, see Hart, Kropp, and Laws (2003); Hanson and Bussière (1998); and Hanson and Morton-Bourgon (2005).

Perhaps the most consistent finding across studies is the predictive utility of past violent behavior or criminal behavior. The probability of future violent behavior and criminal behavior increases with each prior episode, with the risk exceeding 50% among individuals with five or more prior offenses (Borum et al., 1996; Monahan, 1981). In regard to men and women psychiatric patients, Monahan et al. (2001) write, "The strength and consistency of the predictive association between prior violence and criminality and postdischarge violence make obtaining a reliable estimate of past crime and violence a high clinical priority" (p. 47). History of violence is a static risk factor.

Similarly, age at first serious offense or arrest has a strong association with future violence. Specifically, individuals who engage in violence and serious delinquent behavior prior to age 12 are more likely to engage in more chronic and more serious violent acts over the course of their lives (Borum & Verhaagen, 2006; Otto, 2000). In general, however, the association between age and violence is curvilinear. For instance, men have the greatest rate of violence between the ages of 20 and 30, with a sharp decline thereafter (Conroy & Murrie, 2007). Monahan (2006) indicates that the MacArthur Violence Risk Assessment Study found that for discharged men and women psychiatric patients between the ages of 18 and 40, the odds of violence within the first several months after discharge decreased by 20% for every 1-year increase in age. Age at first offense and current age are static risk factors.

In general, violence by men greatly exceeds that by women. However, among psychiatric patients, men and women do not significantly differ in their rate of violent behavior. There are differences, though, concerning the nature and severity of the violence and the context in which it occurs. For instance, violence by men is more likely to result in injury requiring medical attention and to occur after drinking alcohol or using illicit substances. Violence by women is more likely to target family members and to occur in the home (Borum et al., 1996; Monahan et al., 2001). Sex is a static risk factor.

Studies have repeatedly shown a consistent, robust relationship between psychopathy, as measured by the Hare Psychopathy Checklist–Revised, and violence. In comparison to nonpsychopaths, psychopaths commit more violence and more types of violence, and the violence is more likely to be instrumental/predatory, opportunistic, or sadistic (Hart, 1998). Hart (1998) argues that "psychopathy is such a robust and important risk factor for violence that failure to consider it may constitute professional negligence" (p. 133). Psychopathy is distinguished from the *DSM* categorization of antisocial personality disorder. The *DSM* criteria associated with antisocial personality disorder largely focus on delinquent and criminal behavior, whereas critical aspects of psychopathy further include interpersonal and affective functioning (Hemphill & Hart, 2003). So far at least, psychopathy is generally classified as a static risk factor in that treatment programs have shown limited success treating this condition (e.g., Conroy & Murrie, 2007; Otto, 2000; Wong, Gordon, & Gu, 2007).

Substance abuse is another risk factor with substantial empirical support. For instance, Swanson, Holzer, Ganzu, and Jono (1990) found in their analysis of approximately 10,000 community-dwelling individuals who were surveyed in the National Institute of Mental Health's Epidemiologic Catchment Area project that those with a diagnosis of alcohol abuse or dependence were approximately 12 times more likely to have engaged in acts of violence in the 12 months prior to being surveyed than individuals with no psychiatric disorder (i.e., 24.8% versus 2.1%, respectively). Similarly, individuals with a diagnosis of drug abuse or dependence (excluding alcohol and cannabis) were approximately 17 times more likely to have engaged in acts of violence in the 12 months prior to being surveyed than individuals with no psychiatric disorder (i.e., 34.7% versus 2.1%, respectively). Substance abuse or dependence is a stable dynamic risk factor, while substance intoxication is an acute dynamic risk factor.

The explication of the relationship between mental disorder and violence has become clearer over the years with the large and growing body of epidemiological literature on the subject. Summarizing these data, Monahan (2002) writes:

> The data . . . which have only become available since 1990, fairly read, suggest that whether the measure is the prevalence of violence among the disordered or the prevalence of disorder among the violent, whether the sample is people who are selected for treatment as inmates or patients in

institutions or people randomly chosen from the open community, and no matter how many social and demographic factors are statistically taken into account, there appears to be a greater-than-chance relationship between mental disorder and violent behavior. Mental disorder may be a statistically significant risk factor for the occurrence of violence. (p. 108)

In addition, Swanson et al. (1990) found that individuals with schizophrenia were six times more likely to engage in violent behavior than individuals with no diagnosis. Considering only those with a diagnosis of schizophrenia or schizophreniform disorder, and excluding those who met the criteria for substance abuse, affective, or anxiety disorders, the likelihood of violent offending was reduced to four times that of an individual with no diagnosis. However, it is important to consider that approximately 90% of the individuals with a mental disorder in that study were *not* violent. Comparable findings were obtained in the MacArthur Violence Risk Assessment Study (Monahan et al., 2001). Mental disorder is a stable dynamic risk factor, but, as symptoms recur, it becomes an acute dynamic risk factor.

Two symptoms of mental disorder that have been shown to be associated with violence are delusions and hallucinations. Link and Stueve (1994) identify delusional beliefs that result in the affected individuals feeling the threat of personal harm or that their thoughts and/or actions are being controlled by others, thus removing a sense of self-control, as "threat/control-override" (TCO) symptoms. Research has found that TCO symptoms are related to a higher rate of violence (Link & Stueve, 1994; Swanson, Borum, Swartz, & Monahan, 1996). For instance, using data from the above mentioned Epidemiologic Catchment Area project (Swanson et al., 1990), Swanson et al. (1996) found that subjects who reported TCO symptoms were twice as likely to engage in violent behavior as those subjects who reported other psychotic symptoms and five times as likely as those with no diagnosis. However, the MacArthur Violence Risk Assessment Study failed to show an associated increase in violence (Monahan et al., 2001). Nevertheless, they wrote: "These data, of course, should not be taken as evidence that delusions never cause violence. It is clear from clinical experience and from many other studies that they can and do" (p. 77). Moreover, in reporting that most of their subjects who experienced psychotic symptoms did not engage in violent behavior, Link and Stueve (1994) concluded that they view TCO symptoms "only as an 'internal opportunity structure' that makes violence more or less likely, not as an accurate predictor of individual behavior" (p. 156).

As with delusions, it is abundantly clear that auditory hallucinations that command the affected individual to commit violent acts can result in violence. However, it is less clear whether individuals experiencing such command hallucinations are at greater risk for violence than those individuals not experiencing such commands. For instance, on reviewing the literature, Hersh and Borum (1998) reported that compliance with command hallucinations ranged from approximately 39% to 89%. Furthermore, they found that individuals were no more likely to comply with command hallucinations that were violent in nature than with those that were nonviolent. Rather, increased compliance was associated with a hallucinated voice that was familiar and a concurrent delusion that was consistent with or related to the hallucinations. In summarizing their findings regarding the relationship between hallucinations and violence, Monahan et al. (2001) concluded:

> Although command hallucinations per se did not elevate violence risk, if the voices commanded violent acts, the likelihood of their occurrence over the subsequent year was significantly increased. These results should reinforce the tendency toward caution that clinicians have always had when dealing with patients who report voices commanding them to be violent. (p. 80)

Consequently, the assessment of command hallucinations should include exploration of the specific content, tone, and familiarity of the hallucinations as well as any associated delusional beliefs (Conroy & Murrie, 2007).

The combination of a major mental disorder and substance abuse substantially increases an individual's risk for violence. For instance, the MacArthur Violence Risk Assessment Study found that individuals with a major mental disorder but no substance abuse or dependence diagnosis had a 1-year rate of violence of 17.9%. Individuals with a major mental disorder and a co-occurring diagnosis of substance abuse or dependence had a 1-year rate of violence of 31.1%. Incidentally, individuals with a diagnosis of an "other" mental disorder (i.e., primarily individuals with a personality or adjustment disorder) and a co-occurring diagnosis of substance abuse or dependence had a 1-year rate of violence of 43% (Monahan et al., 2001). However, it is notable that even this group of subjects was less than 50% likely to commit an act of violence.

Unfortunately, much less is known about dynamic risk factors. Research regarding the association between these factors and future violence is in its infancy. Douglas and Skeem (2005) identified seven "promising" dynamic risk factors by culling leading risk factors and selecting only those that showed an empirical relationship to violence and possessed empirical evidence that they changed over time. The proposed dynamic risk factors are: impulsiveness, negative affect (i.e., anger and negative mood), psychosis (i.e., delusions and hallucinations), antisocial attitudes, substance abuse, problems in interpersonal relationships, and poor treatment compliance. So far, however, it is unclear in what way these putative dynamic risk factors interact with violence or contribute to its outcome.

Even more conspicuous in its absence is research concerning protective factors, or factors that *reduce* the likelihood of violence. These factors, also either static or dynamic, decrease the risk of violence by buffering the negative effects of risk factors or by independently interrupting the potentially violent behavior (Rogers, 2000). For instance, psychotropic medication may reduce the presence of persecutory delusional beliefs, or a permanent injury may diminish one's physical ability to engage in violent behavior, respectively. Rogers (2000) asserts that attending solely to risk factors without contemplating the effect of protective factors results in "inherently inaccurate" and "implicitly biased" risk assessment evaluations with potentially very serious consequences (p. 598). One cannot presume without empirical support that a protective factor is simply the absence of a specific risk factor. For example, a PCL-R score of less than 30 is not necessarily a protective factor with equal predictive value as a score greater than 30, which is a robust risk factor for violence. In fact, research has shown that low scores on the PCL-R, but not average scores, have operated as a protective factor (Rogers, 2000). To date, there are no well-established protective factors for violence in general; the majority of research conducted has primarily focused on protective factors for children and adolescents (Conroy & Murrie, 2007).

METHODS FOR COMBINING DATA

There are two methods by which decisions are reached about violence risk: clinical assessment (or professional judgment) and actuarial assessment (or actuarial decision making) (Hanson, 1998; Hart et al., 2003; Otto, 2000). Clinical assessment is considered human judgment, with potentially wide discretion as to how assessment data are gathered and contemplated. Actuarial assessment combines predictor variables using a fixed, mechanical method with explicit rules. Most violence risk assessment actuarial schemes utilize a predetermined, numerical weighting system; classification tree models do not. For comprehensive reviews concerning the clinical versus actuarial risk assessment debate, see Grove and Meehl (1996) and Litwack (2001).

There are at least three kinds of clinical assessment methods. The first is unaided clinical judgment (or unstructured professional judgment). Historically, this is the method most commonly used by mental health professionals. It is an unstructured, intuitive decision-making process that can vary considerably across mental health professionals, because the relevance of data and the manner in which data are processed are left to the discretion of the professional. Moreover, there is limited empirical evidence to support the reliability of this approach, and this presumed lack of reliability is considered to limit its validity (Hart et al., 2003; Otto, 2000).

The second clinical method is called anamnestic assessment. In this approach, a detailed investigation is conducted to identify the personal and situational factors associated with an individual's history of violent behavior. Through review of third-party information, direct clinical interview, and perhaps psychological testing, the mental health professional attempts to reveal repetitive themes, or the series of events and circumstances, that led to prior aggressive behavior and thus inform judgments of risk-level and risk management strategies (Hart et al., 2003; Melton et al., 2007; Otto, 2000). Although this method is likely to possess limitations similar to unaided clinical assessment, a potential advantage includes the ability to identify idiographic violent risk factors not found in the empirically derived normative data or approaches based on group design (Conroy & Murrie, 2007; Melton et al., 2007; Otto, 2000).

The third clinical procedure is structured professional judgment (or guided clinical assessment). This method assists decision making in part by providing guidelines, or a structure, to conduct the risk assessment. The set guidelines serve as an aide-mémoire by recommending a set of core risk factors that should be considered in the overall assessment and how they should be gathered. The risk factors are selected based on their demonstrated association with violent behavior. The final decision about violence risk is based on clinical judgment (Hanson, 1998; Hart et al., 2003; Otto, 2000). However, in contrast to unstructured clinical judgment, research has demonstrated greater agreement between raters concerning the presence of risk factors (i.e., interrater reliability) and improved judgment accuracy (i.e., area under the curve values) (Litwack et al., 2005; Melton et al., 2007). The most researched tool for the assessment of violence using the structured professional judgment model of decision making is the HCR-20, which is so named because of its scales and the total number of items it possesses (10 historical items, 5 clinical items, and 5 risk management items; Melton et al., 2007; Webster, Douglas, Eaves, & Hart, 1997). This measure is intended for use with adult offender and psychiatric populations.

There are two kinds of actuarial assessment. The first is simply the use of actuarial risk assessment instruments. This approach generally considers a small number of weighted variables that have been selected on the basis of theory, experience, or a demonstrated association with violent behavior and combines them according to some algorithm to yield a total risk score. Different risk scores are associated with an estimated likelihood of future violence or recidivism within a specific population over some period of time (Hanson, 1998; Hart et al., 2003; Otto, 2000). In some instances, clinical judgment is required to provide data to score an item on an actuarial instrument (e.g., some actuarial measures assign a numerical value to the total score obtained on the Hare Psychopathy Checklist–Revised [Hare PCL-R]).

Research shows that actuarial methods are generally superior to clinical judgment when an algorithmic formula and predictor variables are known, the algorithmic formula has been validated, and the sole purpose of the assessment is the accuracy of the prediction (Dvoskin & Heilbrun, 2001; Grove & Meehl, 1996). However, when any of these three conditions are not met, the strengths associated with actuarial prediction diminish. In addition, the greater the difference between the characteristics of an examinee and the characteristics of the construction and validation samples, the less accurate the actuarial predictive scheme will be for the assessed individual. Furthermore, for an individual who is sufficiently similar to these samples, Monahan (1981) asserts:

> In truth, all one can say in actuarial prediction is that the person whose behavior is being predicted has characteristics X, Y, Z, and that *other* persons who have been studied in the *past*, who have had characteristics X, Y, and Z, have committed violent acts at a certain rate. (p. 98, emphasis in original)

In those instances that the assessed individual is so fundamentally dissimilar to the construction and validation samples of the actuarial measure, Monahan (2003) believes that "one would be hard pressed to castigate the evaluator who took the actuarial estimate as advisory rather than conclusive" (p. 534).

The most researched tool for the assessment of violence using the actuarial method of decision making is the Violence Risk Appraisal Guide (VRAG), which consists of 12 predictor variables, including the Hare PCL-R. This measure was developed on a sample of over 600 violent male offenders who had been housed at a maximum-security hospital in Canada. The outcome measure, or criterion, employed to determine recidivism was any new charge for a violent offense or return to the facility for behavior that would otherwise have resulted in a charge for a violent offense. The VRAG classifies individuals into one of nine risk categories. The instrument is intended for use with adult offender and psychiatric populations (Melton et al., 2007; Monahan, 2006; Quinsey, Harris, Rice, & Cormier, 2006).

Quinsey et al. (2006), the developers of the VRAG, recommend a "pure actuarial" approach to violence risk assessment. They write:

> What we are advising is not the addition of actuarial methods to existing practice, but rather the replacement of existing practice with actuarial methods. . . . Actuarial methods are too good and clinical judgment is too poor to risk contaminating the former with the latter. (p. 197)

An actuarial measure that developed out of the MacArthur Violence Risk Assessment Study is the Classification of Violence Risk (COVR), a software-based assessment tool that employs a multiple iterative classification tree methodology (Monahan et al., 2006). This measure was developed on a sample of over 1,000 patients released from acute civil psychiatric facilities and followed in the community for 20 weeks. Violence was defined as acts of battery that resulted in physical injury, assaultive acts with the use of a weapon, threats made with a weapon in hand, and sexual assaults. Violence was assessed by a review of official police and hospital records, patient self-reports, and the reports of collateral informants, usually family members who knew the patient best in the community. The COVR classifies individuals into one of five levels of risk. Validity studies support its use with adult psychiatric patients in acute facilities in the United States who are soon to be discharged into the community (Monahan, 2006; Monahan et al., 2005, 2006). In contrast to Quinsey et al. (2006), Monahan et al. (2006) maintain that "it is important to keep in mind that the COVR software is useful in informing, but not replacing, clinical decision making regarding risk assessment" (p. 727).

The second actuarial method is the adjusted actuarial approach. In this approach, the results of the actuarial instrument establish the foundation on which additional information not contained in the actuarial formula is considered. At the discretion of the evaluator, the overall prediction is then adjusted or not adjusted. To clarify, the score of the actuarial instrument is not adjusted; rather, the final prediction may be modified in light of the additional information. There is no consensus among clinicians or researchers, however, as to when factors external to the actuarial instrument should be considered (Hanson, 1998; Hart et al., 2003; Otto, 2000). Nevertheless, Monahan (2003) asserts:

> I believe that actuarial instruments . . . are best viewed as "tools" for clinical assessment (cf. Grisso & Appelbaum, 1998)—tools that support, rather than replace, the exercise of clinical judgment. This reliance on clinical judgment, aided by an empirical understanding of risk factors for violence and their interactions, reflects, and in my view should reflect, the standard of care at this juncture in the field's development. (p. 536)

Moreover, Melton et al. (2007) write: "Based upon our reviews of the relevant literatures, we encourage clinicians to adopt an SPJ [structured professional judgment] approach that is based in empirical data (which may include actuarial data)" (p. 309). Finally, Rogers and Shuman (2005) caution that significant consideration must be afforded the psychometric qualities of an assessment tool prior to its utilization. They admonish:

> Risk assessment is rife with poorly validated measures that do not satisfy even the most basic requirements of test development. The goals of justice are stymied by [superficial knowledge] masquerading as science. (p. 299)

INDIVIDUALIZED ASSESSMENT

The *forensic* component of the legal–empirical–forensic model of forensic practice emphasizes the idiographic nature of the law. Goldstein (2003) asserts, "The law exists to regulate human conduct" (p. 4). While nomothetic data provide guidance regarding general principles of human behavior, the complexity and idiosyncratic nature of an individual's behavior requires an individualized assessment to address the various aspects of risk posed by an individual. Although nomothetic data must be the foundation on which the assessment is based, individual characteristics, perceptions, and manifestations of both psychiatric conditions and violent behavior must be thoroughly explored and contemplated. Indeed, Rogers and Shuman (2005) provide:

The accuracy and completeness of future predictions are the most challenging because *they must rely on group data to predict an individual's highly atypical behavior.* By definition, the group data can never capture the complex individual and situational variables that contribute to a particular offender's crime. (p. 378, emphasis in original)

Consequently, review of third-party information and the completion of a comprehensive clinical interview help to achieve this end.

Third-Party Information

Heilbrun, Warren, and Picarello (2003) write, "TPI [third-party information] is one of the most essential components of a high-quality forensic assessment, enhancing the integrity of the process, the impartiality of the evaluator, and the weight given the results by the trier of fact" (p.72). TPI is any data not obtained directly from the examinee. Heilbrun et al. (2003) indicate that there are two primary sources of TPI in forensic assessment: documents and interviews with collateral informants. Documents include personal documents (e.g., victim or witness statements, letters, journals, diaries) and professional documents (e.g., police reports, previous forensic mental health assessment reports, mental health records, presentence investigations, criminal and juvenile history records). Likewise, collateral informants include personal contacts (e.g., spouses or partners, family members, roommates, victims) and professional contacts (e.g., police, correctional facility staff, probation/parole officers, medical and mental health professionals previously involved in the examinee's assessment or care).

Melton et al. (2007) offer three reasons why forensic evaluators are more likely than therapists to rely on TPI: (1) a greater need for accuracy, (2) presumed differences in response style between persons undergoing a therapeutic versus forensic assessment, and (3) greater scrutiny of the evaluator's conclusions. Violence risk assessments are high-stakes evaluations that require navigation of the delicate balance between public safety and individual liberties (Conroy & Murrie, 2007). The quality of a risk assessment is greatly affected by the quality of the information on which it is based. As noted above, information that has poor incremental validity can reduce judgment accuracy. Individuals involved in the legal system have a vested interest in the outcome of the evaluation and therefore operate under a cloud of suspicion insofar as the information shared is not assumed to be reliable. Furthermore, evaluators' conclusions are highly scrutinized by attorneys zealously representing their clients. Consequently, the forensic evaluator must consider the individual merit of the TPI prior to its utilization.

Similarly, it is incumbent on the forensic evaluator to reach an independent conclusion without being overly influenced by the opinions of others. In general, conclusions should be based on the consistency of information or behavior across multiple sources rather than from a single observation. Unless contraindicated, it is reasonable to accept observations by other professionals as accurate. It is *not* recommended, however, that the forensic evaluator accept as accurate other professionals' opinions concerning diagnosis or specific forensic capacities. Such opinions should be documented in the report as collateral information but independently assessed as the forensic evaluator bears the responsibility of drawing her or his own conclusions (Heilbrun et al., 2003).

At the outset of the evaluation, regardless of the referral source (e.g., court order or assessment prior to hospital discharge), collateral documentation should be requested. If at all possible, it is best to review the documentation before completing a comprehensive interview with the examinee. An informed interviewer is able to challenge an examinee's self-report, tailor questions to elicit responses to assess an examinee's response style (e.g., reliable/honest, defensive, uncooperative), provide general memory prompts that might facilitate the recall of events, and possibly possess a better understanding of circumstances that surrounded previous violent behavior. If it is not possible to review collateral data prior to a comprehensive interview with the examinee, it is prudent to conduct a second interview after such time to clarify any inconsistencies. Furthermore, it is also helpful to contact collateral informants, at times, prior to and following the interview with the examinee to verify an examinee's self-report or simply to gather additional information. When possible, it is useful to interview an examinee on more than one occasion to assess functioning over time, to address information that may have come to light following the initial interview, or to follow up on questions that might remain upon review of information gleaned from the initial interview. On some occasions, depending on the referral source, it may be necessary to obtain the examinee's consent prior to requesting collateral documents or contacting collateral informants.

When interviewing collateral informants, most often the examiner should inform the individual of the purpose(s) of the evaluation, the limits of confidentiality and privilege, how the information shared will be used, the voluntary nature of participation, and that unattributed information cannot be used. Exceptions may arise, however, that contraindicate the delivery of this information; for example, when the informant is speaking with the examiner secondary to a court order. Interviews with collateral informants should begin with questions that elicit broad observations, while subsequent questions focus on more specific observations of symptoms and behavior. Questions should not elicit conclusory statements. Finally, if possible, it is best to obtain collateral documents before interviewing collateral informants because such information can provide a context for the interview, help shape questioning, facilitate the recall of events, and clarify any inconsistencies (Heilbrun et al., 2003).

It is notable that some sources of TPI or elements thereof might be challenged as hearsay on the grounds that an out-of-court statement is being offered as evidence to prove the truth of an in-court statement and therefore deemed inadmissible (Heilbrun et al., 2003). Although such exclusions are rare, the issue is generally that the reliability (i.e., accuracy) of the statement cannot be assessed because the declarant of the out-of-court statement is not subject to cross-examination (Melton et al., 2007; see, e.g., *People v. Goldstein,* 2005). However, many states have adopted a version of Federal Rule of Evidence 703 (2007), which provides, in part, "If of a type reasonably relied upon by experts in the particular field in forming opinions or inferences upon the subject, the facts or data need not be admissible in evidence in order for the opinion or inference to be admitted." In instances where the examiner used a source of TPI to form an opinion or inference of the examinee and said source is subsequently adjudged inadmissible, the examiner must determine whether his opinion remains the same in the absence of said information.

Interviewing the Examinee

The *Specialty Guidelines for Forensic Psychologists* (Committee on Ethical Guidelines for Forensic Psychologists, 1991) cautions:

> Forensic psychologists avoid giving written or oral evidence about the psychological characteristics of particular individuals when they have not had an opportunity to conduct an examination of the individual adequate to the scope of the statements, opinions, or conclusions to be issued. Forensic psychologists make every reasonable effort to conduct such examinations. When it is not possible or feasible to do so, they make clear the impact of such limitations on the reliability and validity of their professional products, evidence, or testimony. (p. 663)

The clinical interview, when available and consented to by the examinee, has the potential to provide very rich and useful information. In fact, it can be quite surprising at times the extent to which examinees are willing to discuss the details of their previous behavior and to share their innermost thoughts and fantasies with minimal regard for the potential consequences of the evaluation. In such instances, it is possible that the examinee lost sight of the purpose of the evaluation and perceives the examiner as a therapist rather than a disinterested third party assisting the trier of fact. Consequently, if it seems that the examinee has confused the examiner's role, it is appropriate and ethically responsible to gently remind the examinee about the limits of confidentiality and privilege and the examiner's role in the evaluation process. This is not to say that during the interview an examiner cannot or should not engage in active listening or display empathy. Indeed, Melton et al. (2007) note, "empathic questioning is not coercive and need not be improperly deceptive, as long as the professional makes clear who will get the report" (p. 92).

As highlighted above, the systematic acquisition of data enhances the evaluation process. Borum and Verhaagen (2006) assert that the best practitioners "don't waste time or have to retrace their steps; they don't stare at their word processors and swear during report writing because they forgot to ask about something that was critically important" (p. 80). In an unstructured interview, there are no strict guidelines or an a priori set of questions. The evaluator explores hypotheses generated from the person's elaborations during the course of the interview, and the interview often lacks organization. In contrast, highly structured interviews enlist a rigid set of rules, procedures, and questions from which deviation is not permitted (Craig, 2003). Each interviewing approach has associated strengths and weaknesses. For instance, examiners utilizing an unstructured interview approach do not always ask the requisite questions to obtain the most pertinent data to make an informed decision (Garb, 2005). Conversely, the highly structured interview approach may be overly restrictive and overlook potentially unique aspects of an individual's history of violence and future risk. Consequently, a semi-structured interview approach offers a good balance between the two methods by providing standard questions, optional probes, and the opportunity to use unstructured questions (Rogers, 2001). This approach allows for greater flexibility to explore relevant information, yet a structure within which to operate that enhances reliability across examiners and evaluations.

The basic components of a semistructured interview schedule for violence risk assessment will include questions pertaining to family history, educational history, employment history, medical and psychiatric history, substance use history, child/adolescent/adult antisocial behavior history, relationship history, and, if applicable, psychosexual history. Information from each of these areas may not be incorporated in the evaluation report but should be explored as avenues of potential relevance. Indeed, the report should not contain information that does not bear directly on the legal purpose of the assessment or is not critical as support for the assessment findings (Committee on Ethical Guidelines for Forensic Psychologists, 1991). While standard questions and optional probes facilitate the initial exploration of an individual's behavior, the greatest latitude is often required when carefully reviewing an examinee's history of violent behavior. It is impossible to create a list of standard questions and optional probes to capture the idiosyncratic and heterogeneous nature of violent behavior and the context in which it occurs. Kozol, Boucher, and Garofalo (1972) found that a "meticulous description of the actual assault" is of paramount importance in the assessment of risk for future violence (p. 384). They determined that failure to consider the details in the description of the assault resulted in their most serious errors in assessment. Based on this finding, they asserted, "the description of the aggressor in action [contrasted with the victim's version] is often the most valuable single source of information" (p. 384).

Monahan (1993) offers that the easiest and quickest way to obtain information about an individual's history of violent behavior is to ask him directly and to ask him questions about possible indices of violent behavior, such as arrests or hospitalizations associated with violent behavior. Questions that may be used to assist the screening of an examinee for a history of violent behavior include (Monahan, 1993; Otto, 2000):

- What kinds of things make you angry/mad/frustrated?
- What do you do when you get angry/mad/frustrated?
- What is the most aggressive/destructive/violent thing you have ever done?
- What is the closest you have ever come to being aggressive/destructive/violent?
- Do you ever worry that you might physically hurt someone?

The various terms provided above (e.g., angry, mad, frustrated) highlight the potential influence a single word may have on an examinee's response. An examinee may express the belief that he is rarely "angry," yet describe incidents wherein he was markedly "frustrated" by the actions of others. Although these words are different and may result in distinct behavioral and emotional responses, the purpose of the question is to ascertain the circumstances surrounding the examinee's behavior/behavioral control during highly negative affect-laden states. Consequently, it is important for the examiner to listen closely to the words the examinee uses to describe her feelings and to utilize the same words to ask questions. Active listening can be helpful to ensure the examiner is acquiring an accurate representation of the examinee's self-report. Likewise, it is important for the examiner to carefully attend to the range of nonverbal communication that accompanies the examinee's responses, because negative responses do not necessarily accurately reflect the examinee's history, and behavioral cues may reveal areas that require further inquiry (Borum & Verhaagen, 2006).

With an examinee who is guarded and less than forthright, Borum and Verhaagen (2006) suggest asking the examinee how other people perceive her behavior; for example, "Do your friends or family members ever say that you have trouble controlling your temper?" or "Has your significant other ever expressed concern that you might physically hurt someone?" It can also be extremely helpful to obtain such third-party information directly from the source, but only after any necessary consent is received.

If an examinee has a history of violence, the examiner should conduct a detailed analysis of the examinee's thoughts, feelings, and behavior before, during, and after the violent behavior, or the incidents that almost resulted in violence, to determine whether any patterns associated with the examinee's violent behavior emerge. The examiner should explore the context and setting, or environmental and situational factors, in which the violence occurred; precipitants to the violence; the examinee's mental state at the time of the violence; the nature and severity of the violence; and characteristics of the victims (Borum & Verhaagen, 2006).

In trying to elicit detailed information from the examinee, it is useful for the examiner, at least initially, to assume a position of thoughtful contemplation and inquisitiveness while exploring the examinee's version of events at the most basic level. Rather than accept that the examinee simply "snapped" or "lost it," a slow, deliberate, incremental analysis of the examinee's thoughts, feelings, and behavior before, during, and after the violent or nearly violent behavior will generally reveal otherwise. Indeed, decision points often emerge at which the examinee purposely chose to engage in an action that increased the likelihood of or ultimately resulted in a violent outcome.

Following the examinee's initial review of events or during those instances when the examinee is less than forthright, a more assertive or challenging approach may prove fruitful, especially when executed with the assistance of collateral information. A challenging exchange may also serve to increase the level of irritation and annoyance experienced by the examinee and thus provide the examiner insight into the examinee's frustration tolerance and impulse control (Borum et al., 1996). However, a deliberate escalation of affect should occur only when adequate steps have been taken to ensure the safety of the examinee, the examiner, and any other constituents. Furthermore, the examinee should be very closely monitored during the interaction so that the examiner may quickly de-escalate a potentially violent outburst. In the end, the goal of the interview is for the examiner to have a thorough understanding of the examinee's history of violence in all its variety, including verbal aggression; physical aggression against property, objects, or animals; and physical aggression against persons (Borum & Verhaagen, 2006).

Table 2.1 provides questions that may be used to assist a detailed examination of an examinee's violent behavior. Questions should be asked in a neutral, straightforward manner to avoid response bias; for example, a social desirability bias. To this end, it is recommended that questions regarding the examinee's behavior are framed in the affirmative when the answer may be perceived as socially undesirable or unappealing so that the examinee must deny its occurrence. For instance, in the context of a sex offender risk assessment evaluation, instead of asking "Do you masturbate?" it is better to ask "How often do you masturbate?" In addition, in general, questions should be open-ended (e.g., "Tell me about what happened"), followed by more direct questions that yield specific information. However, it is important that the examiner be mindful not to lead the examinee, though be aware that, on some occasions, it might be inevitable. For instance, rather than asking "You weren't drinking alcohol at the time, were you?" it is better to ask "Were you drinking alcohol at the time?" Yet, if there is concern regarding the perception of the examinee's response, the preferred question may be "How much alcohol were you drinking at the time?" Ultimately, to combat suggestibility, it may prove helpful to review with the examinee his or her initial, uncontaminated version of events and the specific but possibly less impartial account received under detailed inquiry (Heilbrun et al., 2003).

Table 2.1

SUGGESTED INTERVIEW QUESTIONS

- Where and when did the altercation occur?
- Who was the victim/target? Male or female? Approximately how old was the victim/target at the time of the incident? Any relation?
- If applicable, what about the victim made you select him or her? Why did you choose him or her?
- Who was present at the time of the altercation?
- What happened during the altercation?
- What injuries do you believe the victim sustained?
- What injuries did you sustain?
- What types of weapons were involved?
- What did you say to the person before, during, and after the altercation?
- What did the victim say to you before, during, and after the altercation?
- How did you feel before, during, and after the altercation?
- What did you do before, during, and after the altercation?
- How much alcohol did you drink before the altercation? At what point prior to the altercation did you consume alcohol?
- How much (illegal substance/medication) did you use before the altercation? At what point prior to the altercation did you consume (illegal substance/medication)?
- Were you taking any type of medication at the time of the incident? What? Dose? Why were you taking it? How long had you been taking it?
- Did you stop taking any type of medication prior to the incident? What? Dose? Why were you taking it? Why did you stop taking it? How long had you been taking it?
- Were you experiencing any type of perceptual disturbances (e.g., hearing voices, thinking others were out to get you) prior to or during the time of the incident?
- Do you see any pattern or commonalities/similarities across your history of violent behavior?
- Where were you living when the altercation occurred?
- Were you employed when the altercation occurred?

Adapted from "The Violent Patient," by P. Baxter & J. Beck, 1998, in L. E. Lifson & R. I. Simon (Eds.), *The Mental Health Practitioner and the Law: A Comprehensive Handbook* (pp. 153–165). Cambridge, MA: Harvard University Press; "Assessing and Managing Violence Risk in Clinical Practice," by R. Borum, M. Swartz, & J. Swanson, 1996, *Journal of Practical Psychiatry and Behavioral Health, 2*(4), pp. 205–215; "Assessing and Managing Violence Risk in Outpatient Settings," by R. K. Otto, 2000, *Journal of Clinical Psychology, 56*(10), pp. 1239–1262.

Similarly, the examiner should never assume that she understands the examinee's experience or use of a nonspecific term (e.g., "I became *violent*" or "I had *sex* with her") without clarification and confirmation. Each time such a term is used by the examinee, the examiner should ask for a specific explanation or definition. Likewise, the examiner should never assume that he knows the answer to a question before asking it (e.g., "You must have felt very sad" versus "How did that make you feel?"). Finally, questions should avoid unclear, ill-defined language (e.g., "Have you ever been psychotic?" versus "Have you ever believed that people were spying on you?"), though the examiner should be aware that such questions will occur and that subsequent clarification will be needed (e.g., "Have you ever intentionally injured someone or caused them pain?" "What happened?").

RISK APPRAISAL

Notwithstanding brain pathology or mental illness resulting in an exculpatory violent outcome, most often violence is a purposeful choice (Borum & Verhaagen, 2006). It does not "just happen" or occur simply because the person has a history of violent behavior. Indeed, Hart et al. (2003) caution:

> Conceptually, past behavior does not cause future behavior; it is an indication of what a person is capable of doing, given the right circumstances. It is easy to overestimate the utility of past behavior as a predictor of future behavior. If past behavior were such a good predictor, there would be no need for risk assessment. (p. 38)

Violence is an exceedingly complex interaction between neurobiological and social/environmental factors. It is a nonlinear process of cause and effect. Therefore, it is incumbent on the forensic evaluator to consider the myriad reasons that an individual may or may not act violently, the factors that mitigate and aggravate said violence potential, and, when applicable given the referral question and potential legal issue(s), the strategies to manage said violence risk. It is also important to consider moderator and mediating effects on the relationship between predictor and criterion variables (e.g., ethnicity or the administration of psychotropic medication, respectively; Rogers, 2000). Moreover, depending on the purpose of the risk assessment evaluation, some or all of the following five elements should be assessed: the nature of the violence, the likelihood that the violence will occur, the frequency or duration of the violence, the severity of the violence, and the imminence of the violence.

The opinion concerning an individual's violence risk should be empirically based, data driven, and balanced. Base rate data from a sufficiently similar group with a relevant and applicable outcome measure should serve as the foundation on which the initial estimate of violence risk is based. The extent to which the examinee differs from the base rate sample or the assessed type of violence differs from the outcome data, the potentially less useful the base rate value. While true base rates for most types of violence are unknown, the examiner must determine whether and to what extent research-identified base rate values are applicable to the case at hand (Borum et al., 1993; Conroy & Murrie, 2007; Monahan, 1981). To this end, study characteristics to consider include: the sample description, the setting from which the sample was selected, the sample's time at risk, the method of violence detection (e.g., self-report, official record), and the type of violence used as the outcome measure (e.g., battery that resulted in physical injury, verbal threats).

When normative data are unavailable or weakened by, for example, a small sample size or a nonrepresentative sample, one may still cautiously consider base rate values that are most closely related to the case at hand. Using the base rate data as a reasonable starting point, the evaluator then considers the assessment data and any limitations associated with the reference group to determine whether the examinee presents a level of risk that is greater than, equal to, or less than the sample base rate (Borum et al., 1993; Conroy & Murrie, 2007).

Relevant base rate data may also be gleaned from an actuarial measure. For this approach, the base rate of a subgroup of the instrument's construction sample is used as the group to which the examinee is referenced (e.g., individuals who obtained a VRAG score of 0 to +6 had an overall rate of violent recidivism over 7 years of 35%; Conroy & Murrie, 2007; Quinsey et al., 2006). However, it is again recommended that additional assessment data and any limitations of the actuarial instrument are then considered to cautiously determine the examinee's relative risk. Hart (1998) argues that complete reliance on actuarial decision making is unacceptable. He asserts that, because actuarial measures do not consider the case at hand, "failure to exercise discretion by considering the 'totality of the circumstances' means that actuarial assessments may be considered arbitrary and thus a violation of the individual's legal rights" (p. 126).

Modifying an examinee's level of risk relative to the sample base rate may be done through the use of a structured professional judgment tool (e.g., the HCR-20) and/or the consideration of empirically validated risk factors and protective factors associated with violent behavior. Static, or historical, risk factors with proven predictive utility for the type of violence, individual, and context being assessed should anchor such modifications. Consideration should then be afforded empirically based dynamic risk factors, idiographic risk factors, and protective factors. It is also necessary to consider multicultural variables that might moderate said violence risk. For instance, individual belief systems and values have a profound impact on psychological processes and behavior. It is critical to understand and appreciate the worldview and perspectives of the examinee (American Psychological Association, 2003; Tseng, Matthews, & Elwyn, 2004). For example, in a domestic violence context, violence risk may be significantly increased for an examinee who is male, emanates from a culture that practices honor killings, and resides in a location where firearms are readily available. In contrast, violence risk may be greatly reduced for an examinee who is male and emanates from a culture that views violence as a failure to control one's behavior, has a very low incidence of substance abuse, and prevents general citizens from possessing firearms. In sum, it is the complete understanding of the examinee and his or her history of violent or nearly violent behavior in all its variations that illuminates the nature, frequency, severity, imminence, and duration of the risk of violence and provides an overall assessment of the examinee's relative risk.

In his seminal text, Monahan (1981) offered several questions that should be considered by the examiner when assessing an individual's violence risk.

- What are the sources of stress in the person's current environment [e.g., family stressors, peer group stressors, employment stressors]?
- What cognitive and affective factors indicate that the person may be predisposed to cope with stress in a violent manner?
- What cognitive and affective factors indicate that the person may be predisposed to cope with stress in a nonviolent manner?
- How similar are the contexts in which the person has used violent coping mechanisms in the past to the contexts in which the person likely will function in the future?

- In particular, who are the likely victims of the person's violent behavior, and how available are they?
- What means does the person possess to commit violence? (pp. 152–159)

Although it is reasonable to conclude that the more risk factors the examinee possesses, the higher the relative risk, such a simple additive approach should be used cautiously. All factors may not necessarily be of equal importance, and the relationship between risk factors and violence risk may be nonlinear. That is, risk may depend on the specific combination of specific risk factors, not simply the number of risk factors present (Webster et al., 1997). The weight, or authority, given to each variable depends on the case at hand. The evaluator must determine which factors are most important for a particular case (Meloy, 2000; Webster et al., 1997).

Furthermore, it is important to be mindful of the potential over-ascription of weight to unsubstantiated data, such as information obtained during the course of the clinical interview (Webster et al., 1997). Such data should be viewed as a piece of data to be considered in the overall assessment to generate plausible hypotheses that requires validation via other reliable sources of information. Likewise, similar issues sometimes arise concerning allegations of previous violent behavior. For instance, the examinee may have been arrested but not convicted of an alleged violent act. In such cases, the alleged act must be considered in the context of the totality of information known about the examinee to determine whether it is reasonable to conclude that the alleged act actually occurred and, if so, whether it is reasonably consistent with a known, or substantiated, pattern of behavior. The decision about the credibility of the data and the corresponding weight it should be afforded is based on a reasonable degree of professional judgment (Conroy & Murrie, 2007). If the forensic evaluator deems the information to be credible and relies on it to form an opinion or inference about the examinee, the rationale underlying that conclusion must be clearly documented in the report. It is ultimately the trier of fact who contemplates the facts or data underlying the examiner's opinion to determine its admissibility.

REPORT WRITING AND RISK COMMUNICATION

The communication of risk occurs in a variety of contexts and involves individuals with diverse professional backgrounds (e.g., attorneys, judges, members of a jury, parole board members, law enforcement personnel, and mental health professionals). The comprehensiveness (i.e., degree of risk-relevant data concerning the individual's functioning in multiple domains across time), credibility (i.e., data gathered from multiple sources using multiple methods), and clarity (i.e., clear articulation of rationale for opinion) of such communication is fundamental to informed decision making about risk (Hart, 2003). Indeed, Heilbrun, Dvoskin, Hart, and McNiel (1999) assert, "Improper risk communication can render a risk assessment that was otherwise well-conducted completely useless—or even worse than useless, if it gives consumers the wrong impression" (p. 94).

To begin, risk communication should be transparent. The examiner should clearly articulate the referral question, the procedures used, the nature and source of any collateral information, how data were obtained and considered, the results of psychological testing and/or forensic assessment instruments, and the reasoning underlying conclusions and recommendations. In addition, the factual data and descriptive clinical observations should be presented first and separately from any theoretical and inferential formulations. Distinguishing information in this manner allows the recipient to consider the data and inferences independently and to review the logic that links the relevant data to the opinion (Borum & Verhaagen, 2006; Conroy & Murrie, 2007; Heilbrun et al., 2002; Melton et al., 2007).

Transparent risk communication also requires that the examiner clearly communicate the sources of information and attribute said information clearly and accurately. The reader should be able to determine the origin of the data in order to evaluate its relevance to the question at hand and its reliability or consistency and truthfulness (Heilbrun et al., 2002). For instance, potentially self-interested assertions (e.g., Mr. Smith denied a history of substance abuse) should be distinguished from corroborated information (e.g., Mr. Smith's mother, Sherry Smith, reported that Mr. Smith has a significant history of cocaine and heroin abuse). The *Specialty Guidelines for Forensic Psychologists* (SGFP; Committee on Ethical Guidelines for Forensic Psychologists, 1991) emphasize this point: "When a forensic psychologist relies upon data or information gathered by others, the origins of those data are clarified in any professional product" (p. 662). Moreover, the SGFP provide:

> Forensic psychologists, by virtue of their competence and rules of discovery, actively disclose all sources of information obtained in the course of

their professional services; they actively disclose which information from which source was used in formulating a particular written product or oral testimony. (p. 665)

The findings contained in a transparent evaluation report should flow logically from the data and be presented evenhandedly, identifying any limitations or conflicting data associated with the opinion, conclusions, and/or recommendations. For instance, if there were limited collateral data or plausible alternative hypotheses, this information should be addressed candidly (Conroy & Murrie, 2007). Melton et al. (2007) write, "above all, *clinicians should be effective advocates for their data,* whether or not that makes them effective advocates for the party that calls them to court" (p. 578, emphasis in original). In addition, the SGFP underscore the importance of accuracy:

> Forensic psychologists do not, by either commission or omission, participate in a misrepresentation of their evidence, nor do they participate in partisan attempts to avoid, deny, or subvert the presentation of evidence contrary to their own position. (p. 664)

Given the potential consequences and legal implications associated with the results of a violence risk assessment evaluation, it is important for the examiner to communicate her findings in a manner that avoids confusion and guides decision making (Heilbrun et al., 2002). The examiner should strive to educate the audience of the communication and use language that is clear, concise, and free of unnecessary verbiage. Sentences should be short and cogent. When the use of technical terms is unavoidable, they should be carefully defined, and case examples should be employed when possible. Finally, complex aspects of the evaluation that might be difficult to understand should be explained (Conroy & Murrie, 2007; Heilbrun, Dvoskin, et al., 1999). The SGFP provide:

> Forensic psychologists make reasonable efforts to ensure that the products of their services, as well as their own public statements and professional testimony, are communicated in ways that will promote understanding and avoid deception, given the particular characteristics, roles, and abilities of various recipients of the communications. (p. 663)

When addressing the examinee's violence risk, it is best to avoid conclusory statements about whether the examinee is dangerous or will be violent. Instead, contingency statements should be used to explain the interdependent relationship between the examinee, the examinee's environment, and intervention or management strategies (e.g., *if* Mr. Smith remains medication compliant, does not return to licit and illicit substance use, and continues to actively participate in day treatment, *then* the likelihood of a maladaptive outcome is substantially reduced). This approach highlights the contextual, dynamic, and continuous nature of violence risk (Heilbrun et al., 2002; Otto, 2000; Melton et al., 2007).

The description of an examinee's violence risk is also contingent on the circumstances surrounding the evaluation. That is, Heilbrun (1997) argued that there are two legal decision contexts, each of which warrants a different style of risk communication. A prediction-oriented model is operative when postassessment control is not available. This type of communication, in addition to identifying relevant static and dynamic predictor variables, concludes with a statement expressing the likelihood that an examinee will become violent. The format in which the likelihood of violence risk is generally communicated can be verbal or numerical.

A common verbal form for communicating violence risk is categorical (e.g., low, moderate, or high violence risk; Heilbrun, Philipson, Berman, & Warren, 1999). Although verbal labels are viewed as easy to use, the numerical probabilities assigned to these labels are highly variable and dependent on the specific context (e.g., in general use versus an uncommon adverse medical event) (Burkell, 2004). In fact, a study by Kwartner, Lyons, and Boccaccini (2006) suggests that judges assign different probability values of risk to categorical descriptions of risk than clinicians. Incidentally, Heilbrun, Philipson, et al. (1999) found that, of 55 psychiatrists and psychologists surveyed, only one participant reported communicating risk by way of a numerical probability. Some of the reasons cited against the use of numerical figures included the belief that the existing literature or assessment instruments were unable to support that degree of precision.

Because interpretation of verbal labels is variable, such estimates, if possible, should be anchored (with percentages when available) relative to a similarly situated, explicitly referenced comparison group with specific characteristics that the examinee shares (Heilbrun, Dvoskin, et al., 1999; Melton et al., 2007). Furthermore, if appropriate in the context of the referral question, the decision maker may find it useful to outline clear steps for action that correspond to the assigned risk category. For instance, Webster et al. (1997) offer a prescriptive definition associated with such verbal labels:

In general, a judgment of low risk suggests that the individual is not in need of any special intervention or supervision strategies designed to manage violence risk, and that there is no need to monitor the individual closely for changes in risk. A judgment of moderate risk suggests that a risk management plan should be developed for the individual; this plan should include, at the very least, some mechanism for systematic re-assessment of risk. A judgment of high risk suggests that there is an urgent need to develop a risk management plan for the individual, which typically would involve (at a minimum) advising staff, increasing supervision levels, placing the individual on a high-priority list for available treatment resources, and scheduling regular re-assessments. (p. 21)

The likelihood that an event will occur may be expressed numerically in terms of probability or frequency. Probability assigns a percentage of likelihood to whether a specific event will occur (e.g., Mr. Thompson has a 58% likelihood of violence over the next 5 years). Frequency is the number of times an event occurs within a reference group (e.g., of 100 men approximately the same age as Mr. Thompson and with similar risk factors to that of Mr. Thompson, 58 engaged in violence over a period of 3 years). Research has found that probability and frequency representations of likelihood are not equally clear and understandable (e.g., Burkell, 2004). For instance, Slovic, Monahan, and MacGregor (2000) found that a patient was judged to pose a higher risk to commit a harmful act when the likelihood of risk was assessed using a frequency format (e.g., 10 out of 100) versus a comparable probability format (e.g., 10%). Similarly, it was found that communicating a patient's risk in a frequency format (e.g., 2 out of 10) versus a comparable probability format (e.g., 20%) led to a higher perceived level of risk.

Consequently, several authors have suggested employing multiple formats for communicating violence risk (e.g., Kwartner et al., 2006; Monahan, 2003), though Conroy and Murrie (2007) caution that such an approach is not warranted in all instances. Rather, Conroy and Murrie (2007) argue that, for some cases, there may not be relevant base rate data or an actuarial measure available to provide a percentage estimate of risk, a percentage estimate from an actuarial measure accompanied by a categorical label may prove quite sufficient, or adjusting a numerical estimate by using a categorical label and description of compelling idiosyncratic factors to raise or lower risk may be appropriate.

Furthermore, numerical representations of likelihood are not recommended if the likelihood of the occurrence is unknown or vague. By asserting such a numerical representation, the decision maker is unable to consider the alternative without bias, because it is based on the possibly incorrect assumption that the likelihood of the behavior is precisely known (Burkell, 2004). That is, if the assertion that Mr. Thompson presents a 58% likelihood of violence is of questionable accuracy, it is equally questionable that he presents only a 42% likelihood of no violence. Therefore, lack of knowledge regarding the accuracy or error surrounding a numerical estimate results in a false sense of statistical certainty and potential bias on the part of the decision maker.

A management-oriented model is employed when there is ongoing support, scrutiny, services, and supervision (J. A. Dvoskin, personal communication, May 20, 2008). In addition to identifying risk factors that are amenable to change (i.e., dynamic risk factors), intervention strategies are offered to target each of the identified dynamic risk factors in an effort to reduce the observed risk. Andrews and Bonta (2006) described dynamic correlates of criminal behavior that, when changed, affect the chances of criminal activity as criminogenic needs. Factors linked to criminal behavior include antisocial personality/negative emotionality, antisocial attitudes and cognitions, social supports for crime, substance abuse, inappropriate parental monitoring and disciplining, problems in the school/work context, poor self-control, and lack of prosocial activities.

Noncriminogenic needs are dynamic factors weakly associated with criminal behavior. These factors include vague feelings of personal distress, poor self-esteem, feelings of alienation and exclusion, lack of physical activity, history of victimization, hallucinations, anxiety, stress, disorganized communities, and lack of ambition. Andrews and Bonta (2006) also articulated the need for treatment to be delivered in light of the recipient's ability and learning style, referring to this match as the *responsivity principle.* Characteristics to be considered may include cognitive abilities, personality style, verbal intelligence, cultural background, and social attitudes (Andrews & Bonta, 2006; Conroy & Murrie, 2007).

One instrument that facilitates the identification of risk and treatment needs is the Level of Service Inventory–Revised (LSI-R; Andrews & Bonta, 2006; Melton et al., 2007). This theoretically derived instrument combines the assessment of risk, which is performed via an actuarial algorithm, with the assessment of criminogenic needs. It also informs decision makers about levels of supervision (Andrews & Bonta, 2006). The LSI-R is comprised of 54 items distributed across 10 scales (i.e., criminal history, education/employment histories, financial stability, family/marital status and histories, accommodations/housing, leisure/recreation activities, companions/associates, current and history of alcohol/drug problems, emotional functioning/adjustment, and criminal attitudes/orientation). Research has shown the LSI-R to demonstrate moderate predictive validity with outcome measures such as general/violent recidivism, probation/parole violations, and institutional misconduct (Andrews & Bonta, 2006; Melton et al., 2007). The instrument is intended for use with individuals 16 and older.

Communication associated with the management-oriented model may appear as follows: "It is my clinical opinion that Mr. Jones presents with the following risk factors: (identify salient dynamic/situational/environmental risk factors). It is also my opinion that his risk may be (slightly/moderately/substantially) reduced by (identify intervention strategies to address each risk factor)" (Borum & Verhaagen, 2006; Conroy & Murrie, 2007).

Heilbrun et al. (2000) found that experts in risk assessment highly valued the identification of risk factors and their corresponding risk reduction interventions, especially in high-risk cases. Experts rated as least valuable the approach that described the examinee in terms of "percentage of likelihood" to commit a violent act toward others. Similarly, a study by Heilbrun et al. (2004), which utilized a similar methodology to Heilbrun et al. (2000), found that practitioners highly valued the management style of communication, particularly in high-risk situations and when the observed risk factors were dynamic.

Finally, it is important that examiners be cognizant not to view any risk above none as equivalent. The high-stakes nature of violence risk assessment evaluations must be met with the same objectivity and thorough systematic approach regardless of the setting or retaining party. Maintaining regular consultation with experienced colleagues, conducting empirically based assessments, attending to potential sources of error, and monitoring one's pattern of opinions across cases reduces the opportunity for such bias to occur (Conroy & Murrie, 2007).

CONCLUSION

Violence risk assessment has become a part of the landscape for all mental health practitioners. In the forensic arena, expert witnesses are no longer guaranteed absolute immunity from civil liability. Often, the most salient issue is whether the methods employed were professionally adequate.

The legal–empirical–forensic model of forensic practice should serve as the foundation on which an evaluator's competence is considered. The present chapter addressed critical aspects of current good practice standards that should be employed in any violence risk assessment evaluation, report, or communication.

While the violence risk assessment literature has grown exponentially over the last 30 years, there remains much to learn. Advances must continue in research methodology, the development of actuarial measures and structured professional judgment models of decision making, the identification of static and dynamic risk factors and protective factors, and standards and guidelines for risk assessment. As the field of violence risk assessment continues to evolve, it is hoped that best practice standards and greater cost-effective measures are routinely employed in the assessment and reduction of an individual's risk.

REFERENCES

American Psychiatric Association. (1994). *Diagnostic and statistical manual of mental disorders* (4th ed.). Washington, DC: Author.

American Psychological Association. (2003). Guidelines on multicultural education, training, research, practice, and organizational change for psychologists. *American Psychologist, 58,* 377–402.

Andrews, D. A., & Bonta, J. (2006). *The psychology of criminal conduct* (4th ed.). Cincinnati, OH: Anderson Publishing.

Baxter, P., & Beck, J. (1998). The violent patient. In L. E. Lifson & R. I. Simon (Eds.), *The mental health practitioner and the law: A comprehensive handbook* (pp. 153–165). Cambridge, MA: Harvard University Press.

Bonta, J., Law, M., & Hanson, K. (1998). The prediction of criminal and violent recidivism among mentally disordered offenders: A meta-analysis. *Psychological Bulletin, 123*(2), 123–142.

Borum, R. (1996). Improving the clinical practice of violence risk assessment: Technology, guidelines, and training. *American Psychologist, 51*(9), 945–956.

Borum, R., Otto, R., & Golding, S. (1993, Spring). Improving clinical judgment and decision making in forensic evaluation. *Journal of Psychiatry and Law,* 35–76.

Borum, R., Swartz, M., & Swanson, J. (1996). Assessing and managing violence risk in clinical practice. *Journal of Practical Psychiatry and Behavioral Health, 2*(4), 205–215.

Borum, R., & Verhaagen, D. (2006). *Assessing and managing violence risk in juveniles.* New York: Guilford Press.

Burkell, J. (2004). What are the chances? Evaluating risk and benefit information in consumer health materials. *Journal of the Medical Library Association, 92*(2), 200–208.

Cohen, M. L., Groth, A. N., & Siegel, R. (1978, January). The clinical prediction of dangerousness. *Crime and Delinquency,* 28–39.

Committee on Ethical Guidelines for Forensic Psychologists. (1991). Specialty guidelines for forensic psychologists. *Law and Human Behavior, 15,* 655–665.

Conroy, M. A., & Murrie, D. C. (2007). *Forensic assessment of violence risk: A guide for risk assessment and risk management.* Hoboken, NJ: Wiley.

Craig, R. J. (2003). Assessing personality and psychopathology with interviews. In J. R. Graham & J. A. Naglieri (Eds.), *Assessment psychology* (pp. 487–508). Vol. 10 in I. B. Weiner (Editor-in-Chief), *Handbook of psychology.* Hoboken, NJ: Wiley.

Daubert v. Merrell Dow Pharmaceuticals, 509 U.S. 579 (1993).

Douglas, K. S., & Skeem, J. L. (2005). Violence risk assessment: Getting specific about being dynamic. *Psychology, Public Policy, and Law, 11*(3), 347–383.

Dvoskin, J. A., & Heilbrun, K. (2001). Risk assessment and release decision-making: Toward resolving the great debate. *Journal of the American Academy of Psychiatry and the Law, 29*(1), 6–10.

Ewing, C. P. (2003). Expert testimony: Law and practice. In A. Goldstein (Ed.), *Forensic psychology* (pp. 55–66). Vol. 11 in I. B. Weiner (Editor-in-Chief), *Handbook of psychology.* Hoboken, NJ: Wiley.

Federal Rules of Evidence, Rule 703 (2007).

Frye v. United States, 293 F. 1013 (D.C. Cir. 1923).

Garb, H. N. (1998). *Studying the clinician: Judgment research and psychological assessment.* Washington, DC: American Psychological Association.

Garb, H. N. (2003). Incremental validity and the assessment of psychopathology in adults. *Psychological Assessment, 15*(4), 508–520.

Garb, H. N. (2005). Clinical judgment and decision making. *Annual Review of Clinical Psychology, 1,* 67–89.

Goldstein, A. M. (2003). Overview of forensic psychology. In A. Goldstein (Ed.), *Forensic psychology* (pp. 3–20). Vol. 11 in I. B. Weiner (Editor-in-Chief), *Handbook of psychology.* Hoboken, NJ: Wiley.

Grisso, T., & Appelbaum, P. S. (1992). Is it unethical to offer predictions of future violence? *Law and Human Behavior, 16*(6), 621–633.

Grisso, T., & Appelbaum, P. (1998). *Assessing competence to consent to treatment: A guide for physicians and other health professionals.* New York: Oxford University Press.

Grove, W. M., & Meehl, P. E. (1996). Comparative efficiency of information (subjective, impressionistic) and formal (mechanical, algorithmic) prediction procedures: The clinical-statistical controversy. *Psychology, Public Policy, and Law, 2*(2), 293–323.

Haney, C. (1980). Psychology and legal change: On the limits of a factual jurisprudence. *Law and Human Behavior, 4*(3), 147–199.

Hanson, R. K. (1998). What do we know about sex offender risk assessment? *Psychology, Public Policy, and Law, 4*(1/2), 50–72.

Hanson, R. K, & Bussière, M. T. (1998). Predicting relapse: A meta-analysis of sexual recidivism studies. *Journal of Consulting and Clinical Psychology, 66,* 348–362.

Hanson, R. K., & Morton-Bourgon, K. E. (2005). The characteristics of persistent sexual offenders: A meta-analysis of recidivism studies. *Journal of Consulting and Clinical Psychology, 73,* 1154–1163.

Hart, S. D. (1998). The role of psychopathy in assessing risk for violence: Conceptual and methodological issues. *Legal and Criminological Psychology, 3,* 121–137.

Hart, S. D. (2003). Violence risk assessment: An anchored narrative approach. In M. Vanderhallen, G. Vervaeke, P. J. Van Koppen, & J. Goethals (Eds.), *Much ado about crime: Chapters on psychology and law* (pp. 209–230). Brussels, Belgium: Uitgeverij Politeia NV.

Hart, S. D., Krqpp, P. R., & Laws, D. R. (with Klaver, J., Logan, C., & Watt, K. A.). (2003). *The risk for sexual violence protocol (RSVP): Structured professional guidelines for assessing risk of sexual violence.* Victoria, Vancouver, and Burnaby, Canada: Mental Health, Law, and Policy Institute; Simon Fraser University; Pacific Psychological Assessment Corporation; and Institute Against Family Violence.

Heilbrun, K. (1997). Prediction versus management models relevant to risk assessment: The importance of legal decision-making context. *Law and Human Behavior, 21*(4), 347–359.

Heilbrun, K., Dvoskin, J., Hart, S., & McNiel, D. (1999). Violence risk communication: Implications for research, policy, and practice. *Health, Risk & Society, 1*(1), 91–106.

Heilbrun, K., Marczyk, G. R., & DeMatteo, D. (2002). *Forensic mental health assessment: A casebook.* New York: Oxford University Press.

Heilbrun, K., O'Neill, M. L., Stevens, T. N., Strohman, L. K., Bowman, Q., & Lo, Y. (2004). Assessing normative approaches to communicating violence risk: A national survey of psychologists. *Behavioral Sciences and the Law, 22,* 187–196.

Heilbrun, K., O'Neill, M. L., Strohman, L. K., Bowman, Q., & Philipson, J. (2000). Expert approaches to communicating violence risk. *Law and Human Behavior, 24*(1), 137–148.

Heilbrun, K., Philipson, J., Berman, L., & Warren, J. (1999). Risk communication: Clinicians' reported approaches and perceived values. *Journal of the American Academy of Psychiatry and the Law, 27*(3), 397–406.

Heilbrun, K., Warren, J., & Picarello, K. (2003). Third party information in forensic assessment. In A. Goldstein (Ed.), *Forensic psychology* (pp. 69–86). Vol. 11 in I. B. Weiner (Editor-in-Chief), *Handbook of psychology.* Hoboken, NJ: Wiley.

Hemphill, J. F., & Hart, S. D. (2003). Forensic and clinical issues in the assessment of psychopathy. In A. Goldstein (Ed.), *Forensic psychology* (pp. 87–107). Vol. 11 in I. B. Weiner (Editor-in-Chief), *Handbook of psychology.* Hoboken, NJ: Wiley.

Hersh, K., & Borum, R. (1998). Command hallucinations, compliance, and risk assessment. *Journal of the American Academy of Psychiatry and Law, 26*(3), 353–359.

Hoge, R. D. (2002). Standardized instruments for assessing risk and need in youthful offenders. *Criminal Justice and Behavior, 29*(4), 380–396.

Kozol, H. L., Boucher, R. J., & Garofalo, R. F. (1972, October). The diagnosis and treatment of dangerousness. *Crime and Delinquency,* 371–392.

Kraemer, H. C., Kazdin, A. E., Offord, D. R., Kessler, R. C., Jensen, P. S., & Kupfer, D. J. (1997). Coming to terms with the terms of risk. *Archives of General Psychiatry, 54,* 337–343.

Kwartner, P. P., Lyons, P. M., & Boccaccini, M. T. (2006). Judges' risk communication preferences in risk for future violence cases. *International Journal of Forensic Mental Health, 5*(2), 185–194.

Levine v. Wiss & Co., 97 N.J. 242 (1984).

Link, B. G., & Stueve, A. (1994). Psychotic symptoms and the violent/illegal behavior of mental patients compared to community controls. In J. Monahan & H. J. Steadman (Eds.), *Violence and mental disorder: Developments in risk assessment* (pp. 137–159). Chicago: University of Chicago Press.

Litwack, T. R. (2001). Actuarial versus clinical assessments of dangerousness. *Psychology, Public Policy, and Law, 7*(2), 409–443.

Litwack, T. R., Zapf, P. A., Groscup, J. L., & Hart, S. D. (2005). Violence risk assessment: Research, legal, and clinical considerations. In I. B. Weiner & K. Hess (Eds.), *The handbook of forensic psychology* (3rd ed., pp. 487–533). Hoboken, NJ: Wiley.

Meloy, J. R. (2000). *Violence risk and threat assessment.* San Diego, CA: Specialized Training Services.

Melton, G. B., Petrila, J., Poythress, N. G., & Slobogin, C. (with Lyons, P. M., Jr., & Otto, R. K.). (2007). *Psychological evaluations for the courts: A handbook for mental health professionals and lawyers* (3rd ed.). New York: Guilford Press.

Monahan, J. (1981). *Predicting violent behavior: An assessment of clinical techniques.* Beverly Hills, CA: Sage.

Monahan, J. (1993). Limiting therapist exposure to *Tarasoff* liability: Guidelines for risk containment. *American Psychologist, 48*(3), 242–250.

Monahan, J. (2002). The scientific status of research on clinical and actuarial predictions of violence. In D. Faigman, D. Kaye, M. J. Saks, & J. Sanders (Eds.), *Modern science evidence: The law and science of expert testimony.* St. Paul, MN: West.

Monahan, J. (2003). Violence risk assessment. In A. Goldstein (Ed.), *Forensic psychology* (pp. 527–540). Vol. 11 in I. B. Weiner (Editor-in-Chief), *Handbook of psychology.* Hoboken, NJ: Wiley.

Monahan, J. (2006). A jurisprudence of risk assessment: Forecasting harm among prisoners, predators, and patients. *Virginia Law Review, 92,* 391–435.

Monahan, J., Steadman, H. J., Appelbaum, P. S., Grisso, T., Mulvey, E. P., Roth, L. H., Robbins, P. C., Banks, S., & Silver, E. (2006). The classification of violence risk. *Behavioral Sciences and the Law, 24,* 721–730.

Monahan, J., Steadman, H., Robbins, P., Appelbaum, P., Banks, S., Grisso, T., Heilbrun, K., Mulvey, E., Roth, L., & Silver, E. (2005). An actuarial model of violence risk assessment for persons with mental disorders. *Psychiatric Services, 56,* 810–815.

Monahan, J., Steadman, H. J., Silver, E., Appelbaum, P. S., Robbins, P. C., Mulvey, E. P., Roth, L. H., Grisso, T., & Banks, S. (2001). *Rethinking risk assessment: The MacArthur study of mental disorder and violence.* New York: Oxford University Press.

Monahan, J., & Wexler, D. B. (1978). A definite maybe: Proof and probability in civil commitment. *Law and Human Behavior, 2*(1), 37–42.

Mulvey, E. P., & Lidz, C. W. (1995). Conditional prediction: A model for research on dangerousness to others in a new era. *International Journal of Law and Psychiatry 18*(2), 129–143.

Murphy v. A. A. Mathews, 841 S.W.2d 671 (Mo. 1992).

Otto, R. K. (2000). Assessing and managing violence risk in outpatient settings. *Journal of Clinical Psychology, 56*(10), 1239–1262.

People v. Goldstein, 6 N.Y.3d 119, 843 N.E.2d 727, 810 N.Y.S.2d 100 (2005).

Prentky, R. A., & Burgess, A. W. (2000). *Forensic management of sexual offenders.* New York: Kluwer Academic/Plenum.

Quinsey, V. L., Harris, G. T., Rice, M. E., & Cormier, C. (2006). *Violent offenders: Appraising and managing risk* (2nd ed.). Washington, DC: American Psychological Association.

Rogers, R. (2000). The uncritical acceptance of risk assessment in forensic practice. *Law and Human Behavior, 24*(5), 595–605.

Rogers, R. (2001). *Handbook of diagnostic and structured interviewing.* New York: Guilford Press.

Rogers, R., & Shuman, D. W. (2005). *Fundamentals of forensic practice: Mental health and criminal law.* New York: Springer Publishing.

Slovic, P., Monahan, J., & MacGregor, D. G. (2000). Violence risk assessment and risk communication: The effects of using actual cases, providing instruction, and employing probability versus frequency formats. *Law and Human Behavior, 24*(3), 271–296.

Swanson, J. W., Borum, R., Swartz, M., & Monahan, J. (1996). Psychotic symptoms and disorders and the risk of violent behavior in the community. *Criminal Behavior and Mental Health, 6,* 317–338.

Swanson, J. W., Holzer, C. E., Ganzu, V. K., & Jono, R. T. (1990). Violence and psychiatric disorder in the community: Evidence from the epidemiological catchment area surveys. *Hospital and Community Psychiatry, 41*(7), 761–770.

Tarasoff v. Regents of the University of California, 17 Cal 3d 425, 551 P.2d 334 (1976).

Tseng, W. S., Matthews, D., & Elwyn, T. S. (2004). *Cultural competence in forensic mental health: A guide for psychiatrists, psychologists, and attorneys.* New York: Brunner-Routledge.

Webster, C. D., Douglas, K. S., Eaves, D., & Hart, S. D. (1997). *HCR-20: Assessing risk for violence* (version 2). Burnaby, Canada: Mental Health, Law, and Policy Institute, Simon Fraser University.

Webster, C. D., Hucker, S. J., & Bloom, H. (2002). Transcending the actuarial versus clinical polemic in assessing risk for violence. *Criminal Justice and Behavior, 29*(5), 659–665.

Weissman, H. N., & DeBow, D. M. (2003). Ethical principles and professional competencies. In A. Goldstein (Ed.), *Forensic psychology* (pp. 33–53). Vol. 11 in I. B. Weiner (Editor-in-Chief), *Handbook of psychology.* Hoboken, NJ: Wiley.

Werner, P. D., Rose, T. L., & Yesavage, J. A. (1983). Reliability, accuracy, and decision-making strategy in clinical predictions of imminent dangerousness. *Journal of Consulting and Clinical Psychology, 51*(6), 815–825.

Wong, S.C.P., Gordon, A., & Gu, D. (2007). Assessment and treatment of violence-prone forensic clients: An integrated approach. *British Journal of Psychiatry, 190*(49), 66–74.

World Health Organization. (1992). *International statistical classification of diseases and related health problems* (10th rev.). Geneva, Switzerland: Author.

3

The Utility of Dynamic and Static Factors in Risk Assessment, Prediction, and Treatment

STEPHEN C. P. WONG, MARK E. OLVER, AND KEIRA C. STOCKDALE

The assessment, prediction, and treatment of criminal and violent behaviors are the three major links essential in the rehabilitation of violence-prone forensic clients, the goal of which is to reduce societal violence. The underlying assumptions of this trilogy are that appropriate assessment could predict the risk of violence, which is changeable, and, with appropriate treatment, could be reduced. It follows that risk assessment and prediction should be considered as no more than the prelude for violence reduction treatment: they are necessary but not sufficient requirements for a general violence reduction strategy.

Much attention has been focused on the research and development of the assessment and prediction of violence—in particular, on the development of risk assessment and prediction tools. Paradoxically, much less attention has been paid to the last, but perhaps the key link: the development of violence reduction treatment programs—in particular, treatment for those with co-occurring personality disorders. Violence reduction, rather than violence assessment and prediction per se, should be the overall objective of violence assessment and research (Hart, 1998;

The authors thank Dr. D. Gu for his expert assistance in statistical analyses and data compilation and Correctional Service of Canada for support. The views expressed in this chapter are those of the authors and not necessarily Correctional Service of Canada.

Wong & Gordon, 2006; Wong, Gordon, & Gu, 2007). In a similar vein, Douglas and Skeem (2005) suggested that the next greatest challenge in forensic practice is to develop sound methods for assessing changeable aspects of violence risk or dynamic risk factors or variables and systematic methods for violence risk reduction treatment (see also Dvoskin & Heilbrun, 2001).

This chapter discusses the pros and cons and the utility of dynamic and static factors in risk assessment, prediction, and treatment, including the utility of a number of clinical tools that incorporate static and dynamic factors to assess violent risk. A clinical case illustrates how one of the tools can be used to assess the risk of sexual violence, identify treatment targets in a pedophilic sex offender, and assist in case conceptualization.

STATIC VERSUS DYNAMIC RISK FACTORS

The research focus on violence assessment and prediction sometimes at the exclusion of treatment led to the development of violence risk assessment tools that are useful for predicting violence but far less useful for reducing violence through treatment. These tools focus on assessing what *was*—that is, assessing the person's history using static, historical, or unchangeable factors rather than assessing what *is*, using dynamic or changeable factors. The person's current attitudes and beliefs toward violence, interactions with peer groups, availability of environmental support or lack thereof, use of substances, and so forth can predict risk and are very informative to treatment providers. Static or historical factors, no doubt, are predictive of future violence, because past behaviors are good predictors of future behaviors. However, static factors do not tell us about the person's current functioning and situations that could be precursors of violence, nor can they be used to assess changes in the person. Using static factors to assess violence risk locks the person to the past, tells us little about the person's current functioning, and is not informative to providers of treatment and management services. Although static tools may be prediction friendly, they are not treatment friendly.

On the other hand, dynamic factors such as criminal attitudes, beliefs, and associates as well as availability of community support and services can do just as good a job as static factors in the prediction of violence and recidivism risk (Campbell, French, & Gendreau, 2007; Gendreau, Little, & Goggin, 1996). Results of a recent meta-analysis found no clear difference in the efficacies of risk assessment tools with primarily dynamic factors compared to those with primarily static factors or those with a combination of both in the prediction of violence recidivism among adult offenders (95% confidence intervals or CI_{z+} = 0.16–0.18, 0.14–0.18, and 0.13–0.23, respectively; Campbell et al., 2007). Using dynamic factors to predict violence risk has the additional advantage of identifying precursors of violence, telling us about the individual's current functioning, and identifying for therapists and service providers criminogenic needs that require intervention—that is, a treatment targets. Static and dynamic risk factors could be considered as two sides of the same coin, which is the presence of a pattern of dysfunctional and criminal lifestyle. While dynamic factors assess whether the person's ongoing behaviors and lifestyle are dysfunctional, static factors assess the presence of historical proxies (such as criminal convictions) of the individual's dysfunctional and criminal lifestyle.

Some have argued that dynamic factors are only useful if they can outpredict static variables. Unless a tool is designed solely for the purpose of making risk prediction, little is served by entering tools into a prediction Olympics to determine the gold medal winner. For a dynamic tool, prediction is only one of a number of tasks that that the tool is required to perform. Surely a dynamic tool should have an acceptable level of predictive validity, but prediction is not the be all and end all, and the judgment of the efficacy of the tools should not rest solely on the predictive efficacy of the tool. Dynamic factors do not have to trump the predictive power of static factors or other risk assessment tools to be acceptable. A recent meta-analysis using multilevel regression methodology to compare the predictive efficacy of a number of common risk assessment tools found that much of the difference in predictive efficacy found in other meta-analyses could be attributed to differences in study characteristics rather than in the tools themselves (Yang, Wong, & Coid, 2008). The similarities in predictive efficacies of the tools trump their differences. In essence, there is little, if any, disadvantage to using dynamic variables instead of or in addition to using static variables in doing our work in the assessment, prediction, and reduction of violence and recidivism.

Dynamic variables must fulfill a number of requirements before they can be considered truly dynamic or changeable. According to Kraemer and colleagues (1997), a causal risk factor is one that is manipulable and, when manipulated, can be shown to result in changes in risk in the outcome measures. For example, criminal attitude could be deemed a casual risk factor if reduction in criminal attitude through deliberate manipulations in a treatment program could be linked to reduction in recidivism. However, if there is insufficient evidence to establish clear causal links between risk factors and recidivism changes, a manipulable risk factor should be termed a variable risk factor rather than a causal risk factor. In the present discussion, dynamic risk factors or variables refer to both causal and variable risk factors.

EVOLUTION OF RISK ASSESSMENT TOOLS

Static and dynamic factors have been combined to produce the so-called third-generation risk assessment tools such as the Level of Services Inventory-Revised (Andrews & Bonta, 1995). In comparison, first-generation risk assessment approaches relied on nothing more than unstructured professional opinions or one's gut-feelings, if you will. The predictive validity of first-generation risk assessment for general and violent recidivism is marginal at best (Andrews, Bonta, & Wormith, 2006). Second-generation risk assessments use tools with essentially static predictors or fixed risk markers (Kraemer et al., 1997), such as criminal and family history. Second-generation tools such as the Violence Risk Appraisal Guide (Quinsey, Harris, Rice, & Cormier, 1998), the General Statistical Information for Recidivism (Bonta, Harman, Han, & Cormier, 1996), and the Static 99 (Hanson & Thornton, 1999) have good predictive validity and outperform first-generation methods (Andrews et al., 2006; Grove, Zald, Lebow, Snitz, & Nelson, 2000; Meehl, 1954; Mossman, 1994); however, as indicated above, they have major shortcomings in not being able to inform service providers of the clients' changeable risk factors essential for treatment. Recently, it was proposed that tools with all the third-generation characteristics but that are designed for specific purposes or populations may be deemed fourth-generation tools. Examples are the Level of Service/Case Management Inventory (Andrews, Bonta, & Wormith, 2004) and the Violence Risk Scale (Wong & Gordon, 1999–2003, 2006); the latter was designed to assess violence recidivism, identify treatment targets linked to violence, and the client's treatment readiness of the identified treatment targets.

Structured Professional Judgment

Structured professional judgment (SPJ) refers to an approach that involves systematically assessing a list of risk-related or clinical variables, the ratings of which indicate how closely the individual being assessed approximates the description of the variable. Professional judgment is then used subjectively to weight and combine all the information into an overall judgment of the level of risk. Items are not intended to be summed to arrive at a total score, although many researchers and clinicians have chosen to do so.

One of the best known and researched SPJ tool is the HCR-20, which consists of 10 historical (static) variables, 5 clinical (clinical status and personality) variables, and 5 risk (community support) variables (Webster, Douglas, Eves, & Hart, 1997). Each variable describes a condition (e.g., substance abuse) that can be rated 0, 1, or 2; the higher the rating, the more likely the person has the condition being measured. Some predictors that could be considered as dynamic in nature—for example, relationship stability, employment, mental disorder, and alcohol or drug abuse—are regarded as historical or static predictors in the HCR-20. As such, these predictors are not regarded as open to change. The HCR-20 is biased in favor of historical variables with 10 historical compared to 5 clinical and 5 risk variables. Although the HCR-20 could theoretically reflect change in risk with the use of clinical and risk variables, the manual provides no direction as to how change should be measured or what it is based on. Rescoring the variables is probably the approach one should take to assess change, but there is no direction regarding which variable could be rescored. Despite the above caveats, the HCR-20 has been shown to predict general and violence recidivism in a wide range of forensic clients (Douglas, Yeomans, & Boer, 2005). Although research has demonstrated the ability of the clinical and risk components of the HCR-20 to measure change (Belfrage & Douglas, 2002), research has yet to demonstrate whether changes in HCR-20 scores are related to changes in violence (Douglas & Skeem, 2005). The application of SPJ in sex offender risk assessment is discussed further in a later section.

The Integration of Assessment, Prediction, and Treatment of Violence

If violence reduction treatment is the goal of the assessment–prediction–treatment trilogy, then assessment and prediction of violence should be guided by the theoretical underpinning of violence reduction treatment. In other words, assessment, prediction, and treatment approaches should be closely integrated activities. The "what works" literature—a large body of literature that addresses the issues of effective correctional treatment—has identified the risk–need–responsivity principles as useful guidelines for treatment interventions designed to reduce the risk of recidivism. Treatment approaches, often referred to as correctional treatment, that follow the risk–need–responsivity principles are generally more effective in reducing the risk of recidivism in adult and young offenders than those that do not follow such principles (see Andrews & Bonta, 2003; Andrews et al., 1990).

The *risk* principle states that the intensity of treatment should match the client's risk level: clients with high, medium, and low levels of risk should receive the corresponding intensities of treatment. The *need* principle states that the individual's criminogenic needs—that is, needs linked to violence or criminality, such as criminal attitudes, criminal associates, etc.—must be identified for treatment. Improvements in criminogenic needs should result in violence risk reduction. Treatment of noncriminogenic needs will not reduce violence risk.

The *responsivity* principle states that, to maximize treatment effectiveness, treatment delivery must accommodate clients' idiosyncratic characteristics, such as their cognitive and intellectual abilities, level of motivation and readiness for treatment, cultural background, and so forth. One of the most daunting responsivity factors in correctional treatment is to treat a seemingly unmotivated, noncompliant, and treatment-resistant client—that is, dealing with the general issue of treatment readiness.

Risk assessment, prediction, and treatment must be closely integrated: assessments of the client's risk, need, and responsivity should inform treatment providers of *who* to treat (risk principle), *what* to treat (need principle), and *how* to deliver treatment—in particular, to treatment-resistant clients (responsivity principle). Clinicians who provide correctional treatment require the appropriate tools to assess risk, needs, responsivity, and treatment readiness and to measure treatment change. We use the Violence Risk Scale (VRS) and the Violence Risk Scale–Sex Offender version (VRS-SO) to illustrate the practical utilities of risk assessment tools for forensic clients developed based on the principles discussed above.

THE VIOLENCE RISK SCALE (VRS)

The VRS was developed to assist treatment providers who work with high-risk/-need nonsexual violent offenders to integrate risk assessment/

prediction and treatment (see Wong & Gordon, 2006; Wong, Gordon, & Gu, 2007). Results of VRS assessments can inform service providers of who to treat by identifying high-risk/-need treatment candidates; what to treat by identifying treatment targets—that is, dynamic factors linked to violence; and how to treat by identifying appropriate therapeutic approaches using a modified Stages of Change model (Prochaska, Diclemente, & Norcross, 1992). The VRS is also designed, using the Stages of Change model, to measure how much changes in risks have occurred as a result of treatment. The theoretical basis of the VRS is predicated on the Psychology of Criminal Conduct (PCC; see Andrews & Bonta, 1994, 1998, 2003), the principles of effective correctional treatment, and the Transtheoretical Model of Change (TM).

The VRS Static and Dynamic Variables

The VRS uses 6 static and 20 dynamic variables (see Table 3.1 for a list of the variables) derived primarily from the PCC and is based on the risk–need–responsivity principles (Wong & Gordon, 2006). The VRS dynamic variables are changeable and can be influenced or changed by psychological–social means and/or through treatment interventions. Changes in the dynamic factors are linked to changes in recidivism (Lewis, Olver, & Wong, 2008); the VRS dynamic factors can be deemed causal dynamic factors. A more detailed discussion of how to determine whether a putative dynamic variable is in fact dynamic is given in a latter section.

The VRS static variables can predict recidivism but remain unchanged regardless of treatment interventions.[1] The VRS dynamic and static variables are rated on 4-point Likert scales (0, 1, 2, or 3) based on a careful file review and a semistructured interview. For most variables, higher ratings indicate a closer link to violence in lifetime functioning. Higher ratings on the static variables indicate worse track records of criminality and early experiences. Dynamic variables closely linked to violence (rated 2 or 3) are appropriate targets for violence reduction treatment (the need principle). The total VRS score (the sum of static and dynamic variable ratings) indicates the level of violence risk; the higher the score, the higher the risk. Clients with higher VRS scores should be appropriate candidates for high-intensity intervention (the risk principle). High VRS scores also mean that there are many problem areas linked to violence and criminality. Details about rating and scoring the VRS are set forth in the *VRS Manual* (Wong & Gordon, 1999–2003; also see Wong & Gordon, 2006).

Table 3.1

VIOLENCE RISK SCALE STATIC AND DYNAMIC ITEMS

STATIC ITEMS

- S1 Current age
- S2 Age of first violent conviction
- S3 Number of juvenile convictions
- S4 Violence throughout life span
- S5 Prior release failures/escapes
- S6 Stability of family upbringing

DYNAMIC ITEMS

- D1 Violent lifestyle
- D2 Criminal personality
- D3 Criminal attitudes
- D4 Work ethic
- D5 Criminal peers
- D6 Interpersonal aggression
- D7 Emotional control
- D8 Violence during institutionalization
- D9 Weapon use
- D10 Insight into violence
- D11 Mental illness
- D12 Substance abuse
- D13 Stability of relationships
- D14 Community support
- D15 Released to high-risk situations
- D16 Violence cycle
- D17 Impulsivity
- D18 Cognitive distortion
- D19 Compliance with supervision
- D20 Security of release institution

The VRS uses a scheme based on a modified TM to assess the individual's readiness for treatment and treatment change.[2] Dynamic variables identified as treatment targets (rated 2 or 3) are also rated to determine the stage of change (readiness for treatment) evidenced by the client. The five stages of change are precontemplation, contemplation, preparation, action, and maintenance. Those in the *precontemplation* stage have neither insight nor intention to change in the foreseeable future. They are often in denial and externalize blame. Those in the *contemplation* stage are fence-sitters; they acknowledge their problems but have shown no relevant behavioral change. Those in the *preparation* stage combine intentions to change with relevant behavioral changes to address problems. However, changes tend to be recent and/or quite unstable. Those in the *action* stage actively and consistently modify their behaviors, attitudes, and environment to address their problems; overt behavioral changes are made, commitments followed through, and energies expended to change. In the *maintenance* stage, relapse prevention techniques are used to consolidate, strengthen, and generalize the gains made in the action stage. The operationalizations of the Stages of Change are designed to measure the extent to which the positive coping skills and strategies that the client has learned are stable, sustainable, and generalizable. Progression in treatment from a less advanced to a more advanced stage of change for each treatment target is an indication of improvement, which should lead to risk reduction in that treatment target. Progression through the stages is translated into a quantitative measure of risk reduction for each treatment target (see Wong & Gordon, 2006).

Reliability and Validity of the VRS

The VRS can be rated reliably with interclass correlation coefficients of over 0.90. Dynamic items total scores have a slightly higher correlation with violent reconviction[3] ($r = 0.34$) than static item scores ($r = 0.27$; both with $p < .001$). With receiver operator characteristic (ROC) analyses of VRS scores and recidivism, the area under the curve (AUC), a measure of predictive efficacy independent of base rate differences, for dynamic items at 4.4-year follow-up is around 0.75 ($p < .001$), representing a moderate to high level of predictive validity. Similar results were found with survival analyses. There is a linear relationship between VRS dynamic scores[4] and violence recidivism ($R^2 = 0.97$), indicating a near proportional increase in violence risk with increase in VRS scores. In other words, the more problems the client presents as indicated by an increase in VRS scores, the higher the risk of violence recidivism; this also makes good clinical sense. The results suggest that dynamic factors are effective in predicting violence recidivism—dynamic factors that are also useful for treatment purposes.

Dynamic Risk Profile

The targets for violence reduction treatment are problem areas closely linked to violence. VRS dynamic variables rated as 2 or 3 are appropriate treatment targets. The Dynamic Risk Profile (see Figure 3.1 and Wong & Burt, 2007) is a graphic means of displaying a profile of treatment targets by plotting the percentage of the sample rated 2 or 3 for each VRS dynamic variable against the variables themselves. The dynamic risk profile clearly showed that the sample had multiple problem areas linked to violence, but the incidence rates vary with the problem area. Accordingly, decisions on treatment delivery based on the profile will be more prescriptive and less indiscriminate. The dynamic risk profile is useful for comparisons between groups and for treatment program planning purposes. Managers and lead clinicians can use the information to decide what types of programs need to be designed and delivered to

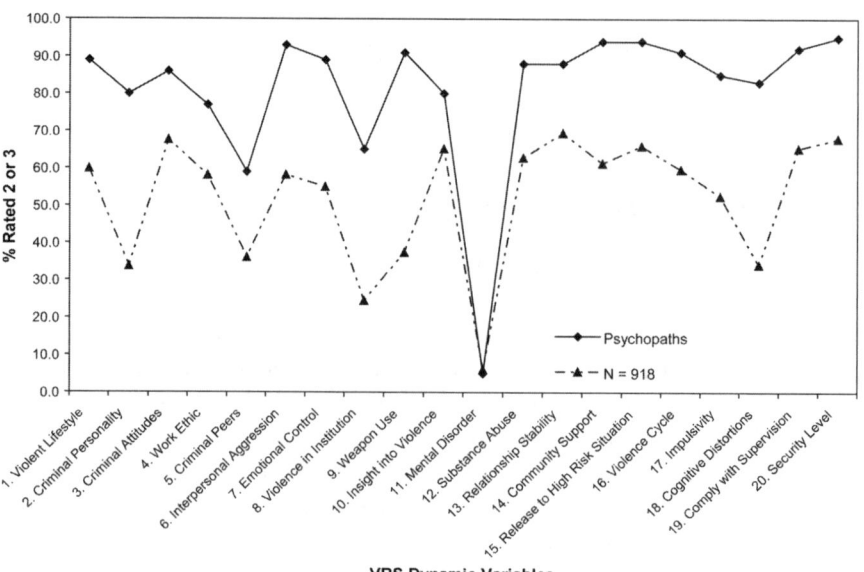

Figure 3.1 Dynamic risk profile of the sample and psychopaths.

address the existing criminogenic needs of a certain population. Overall treatment planning can then be undertaken and resources allocated based on the prevalence of problem areas in the samples of interest (Wong & Gordon, 2006).

A similar profile can be constructed for an individual as part of a comprehensive clinical risk assessment. The ratings (0, 1, 2, or 3) of the 20 dynamic variables, rather than percentages, can be displayed as the individual's dynamic risk or problem–strength profile. Ratings of 0 and, to some extent, 1 are the individual's strengths, and ratings of 2 and 3 are problems/treatment targets. The profile can inform staff of the presence and seriousness of problems for individual treatment planning purposes. Further in-depth investigation may be warranted depending on the presenting problems. Risk reduction interventions can then be formulated based on the individual's risk profile and stage of change. The individual's profile can be reassessed and similarly presented. Violence-prone offenders and psychopaths share many similar problem areas; risk reduction treatment for both groups should be quite similar, although there will be differences in the management of the two groups (Wong & Burt, 2007; Wong & Gordon, 2006; Wong & Hare, 2005).

The foregoing evidence suggests that a risk assessment tool such as the VRS, which consists of primarily dynamic variables, can be designed to be psychometrically sound and treatment friendly. In addition to assessing and predicting violence, it can provide clinicians with useful information to design and deliver risk reduction treatment.

DYNAMIC AND STATIC FACTORS FOR SEX OFFENDERS

Sex offenders have unique characteristics, such as deviance sexual arousal, that must be taken into account in risk assessment, prediction, and treatment as well as in the design of risk assessment tools for sex offenders. The Violence Risk Scale–Sexual Offender version (VRS-SO) was designed to assess the risk, need, and treatment readiness for sex offenders. The VRS-SO uses the same general assessment platform as the VRS—that is, using static and dynamic factors to assess risk and need, 4-point rating scales, Stage of Change ratings, etc. The main difference between the VRS and the VRS-SO is the use of static and dynamic risk factors relevant for sex offenders in the VRS-SO. Similarly, the Violence Risk Scale–Youth Version (VRS-YV) is designed specifically for risk assessment for youths. Both the VRS-SO and VRS-YV are discussed below to illustrate how dynamic and static risk factors can be used for assessment of sex offenders and youths.

Static Variables and Sexual Recidivism

A number of variables can be identified from the sex offender literature that predicts sexual recidivism. Hanson and Bussière's (1998) seminal meta-analysis, for instance, identified predictors of sexual recidivism such as history of prior sexual and nonsexual offenses, unrelated victim, male victim, and the like. Such variables have been combined to form static risk prediction tools, or what Hanson and Morton-Bourgon term *empirical actuarial* approaches, including the Rapid Risk Assessment for Sexual Offense Recidivism (Hanson, 1997), Static 99 (Hanson & Thornton, 1999), Static 2002 (Hanson & Thornton, 2003), Sex Offender Risk Appraisal Guide (Quinsey, Rice, & Harris, 1995), Minnesota Sex Offender Screening Tool–Revised (Epperson et al., 2005), and the Risk Matrix 2000 (Thornton, 2007). Although these measures have demonstrated acceptable to good predictive efficacy for sexual, and, to a lesser degree, general violence, recidivism (e.g., see Langton et al., 2007), they are static tools based on historical information, they do not inform treatment, and they cannot measure changes in risk as we discussed earlier. Sexual recidivism risk is arguably dynamic and can change through intervention. Recent meta-analytic results from the sex offender treatment literature have indicated that appropriate sex offender treatment can reduce sexual recidivism risk, especially interventions using cognitive-behavioral, relapse prevention approaches (Hanson et al., 2002).

Dynamic Variables and Sexual Recidivism

Research has identified dynamic variables that predict sexual recidivism (Beech, Friendship, Erikson, & Hanson, 2002; Dempster & Hart, 2002; Hanson & Harris, 2000; Hudson, Wales, Bakker, & Ward, 2002; Kenny, Keogh, & Seidler, 2001; Thornton, 2002). Hanson and Morton-Bourgon's (2004) meta-analysis identified two domains with strong links to sexual recidivism: sexually deviant interests (e.g., sexual preoccupations, deviant sexual preferences) and an antisocial orientation/criminality (e.g., antisocial personality, substance abuse, release failure). Additional dynamic variables linked to sexual recidivism include attitudes and cognitions supportive of sexual assault and intimacy deficits (Hanson & Morton-Bourgon, 2004).

Static and dynamic variables have also been combined to develop sex offender risk measures such as the Sex Offender Need Assessment Rating (SONAR, Hanson & Harris, 2001), Sexual Violence Risk-20 (Boer, Hart, Kropp, & Webster, 1998), Risk for Sexual Violence Protocol (RSVP; Hart, Kropp, & Laws, 2003), Vermont Assessment of Sex Offender Risk (VASOR; McGrath & Hoke, 2002), and the Violence Risk Scale–Sexual Offender version (VRS-SO; Wong, Olver, Nicholaichuk, & Gordon, 2004–2006). Instruments incorporating static and dynamic variables have important advantages over empirical actuarial measures, including what would deem to be increased content validity—that is, by assessing a greater number of domains of sex offender risk—and having the ability to identify criminogenic needs for sex offender treatment. These instruments with both static and dynamic variables have also demonstrated strong predictive efficacy for sexual reoffending and have similar advantages over static-only tools. Similar to the VRS and unlike other risk assessment tools for sexual offenders, the VRS-SO was designed as a treatment- and change-oriented violence risk assessment tool.

Examples of SPJ for sex offenders include the SVR-20 and RSVP. The SVR-20 consists of 20 static and dynamic items that assess sex offender risk across the broad areas of psychosocial adjustment, sexual offenses, and future plans. The RSVP consists of 22 risk factors that can be grouped across the broad areas of sexual violence history, psychological adjustment, mental disorder, social adjustment, and manageability. In contrast, Hanson and Morton-Bourgon (2007) have used the term *conceptual actuarial* to refer to actuarial tools in which the items are selected based on theory and research. With the conceptual actuarial approach, item ratings are also summed to arrive at a total score, and cutoff scores are provided to inform the overall risk rating. Instruments such as the SONAR, VRS-SO, and VASOR exemplify the conceptual actuarial approach, and adding the items of the SVR-20 to arrive at a risk rating would also be an example of such an approach (Hanson & Morton-Bourgon, 2007).

The VRS-SO Static and Dynamic Variables

The VRS-SO (Wong et al., 2004–2006) was developed to assess sex offender risk using dynamic and static variables linked to sexual recidivism. It was derived from and has the same platform as the VRS, in part to facilitate the transfer of knowledge and skills from one tool to another. The VRS-SO has 7 static and 17 dynamic variables (see Table 3.2 for a

Table 3.2

VIOLENCE RISK SCALE–SEX OFFENDER VERSION STATIC AND DYNAMIC ITEMS

STATIC ITEMS

- S1 Age at release
- S2 Age at first sex offense
- S3 Sex offender type
- S4 Prior sex offenses
- S5 Unrelated victims
- S6 Victim gender
- S7 Prior sentencing dates

DYNAMIC ITEMS

- D1 Sexually deviant lifestyle
- D2 Sexual compulsivity
- D3 Offense planning
- D4 Criminal personality
- D5 Cognitive distortions
- D6 Interpersonal aggression
- D7 Emotional control
- D8 Insight
- D9 Substance abuse
- D10 Community support
- D11 Released to high-risk situation
- D12 Sexual offending cycle
- D13 Impulsivity
- D14 Compliance with community supervision
- D15 Treatment compliance
- D16 Deviant sexual preference
- D17 Intimacy deficits

list of items), and, as in the VRS, each variable is rated on a 4-point scale (0, 1, 2, 3). In general, higher ratings indicate the variable is more closely linked to inappropriate sexual or nonsexual behaviors.

The static items were identified through purely statistical procedures; a set of representative static variables were each correlated with outcome, and the strongest predictors were retained and rescaled on a 4-point scale. The dynamic items were first identified after a detailed review of the risk literature (e.g., Hanson & Harris, 2000; Proulx et al., 1997), including contributions from relapse prevention theory (Pithers, 1993; Ward & Hudson, 1998) and the theory of the psychology of criminal conduct (Andrews & Bonta, 2003). Scale variables were then chosen statistically to maximize the content validity of the scale. As with the VRS, a 2- or 3-point rating on the dynamic variables means the item is linked to increased risk for sexual recidivism—that is, criminogenic—and hence should be targeted for treatment. Stages of Change ratings pre- and posttreatment are identical to the VRS.

A factor analysis of the dynamic items suggested the presence of three broad factors labeled *sexual deviance* (sexually deviant lifestyle, sexual compulsivity, offense planning, sexual offending cycle, deviant sexual preference), *criminality* (criminal personality, interpersonal aggression, substance abuse, community support, impulsivity, compliance with community supervision), and *treatment responsivity* (cognitive distortions, insight, released to high-risk situations, treatment compliance); two of the items (emotional control and intimacy deficits) did not load (see Olver, Wong, Nicholaichuk, & Gordon, 2007). The factor structure of the instrument is consistent with the major risk factor domains identified in the literature (i.e., sexual deviance and antisociality). There is evidence that different types of sex offenders have differential scores on the three factors. For instance, research on the VRS-SO found that child molesters tended to score higher on sexual deviance and lower on criminality compared to rapists, who had the reverse pattern (higher on criminality and lower on sexual deviance), and mixed offenders with quite high scores on both (Olver et al., 2007).

Scores on each of the three factors provide general indications of where the risk of sexual recidivism primarily resides. Further inspection of the items comprising the factors can be used to highlight more specific problem areas for treatment. For instance, some rapists show patterns of deviant arousal (e.g., preference for sex with violence) and thus may require arousal modification interventions. However, for those with no such preference, the focus of intervention may be elsewhere, such as aggressiveness, impulsivity, and lack of community support. Assessment and treatment must be integrated; assessment should inform treatment such that it is focused and prescriptive.

Reliability and Validity of the VRS-SO

A growing body of research supports the validity and reliability of the VRS-SO (Beggs & Grace, 2007; Beyko & Wong, 2005; Olver & Wong, 2006; Olver et al., 2007). Olver et al. (2007) examined the psychometric properties of the VRS-SO in a sample of 321 treated sex offenders. On the basis of detailed file information, the offenders were rated on the VRS-SO items. Followed up for an average of 10 years, approximately 25% of the sample was convicted for a new sex offense during the follow-up. VRS-SO total scores significantly predicted sexual recidivism ($r = 0.34$, area under the curve = 0.72) and demonstrated acceptable interrater reliability (intraclass correlation coefficient = 0.79) and internal consistency ($\alpha = 0.84$).

ARE DYNAMIC VARIABLES ACTUALLY DYNAMIC?

Although much theoretical and empirical work has been done to identify putative dynamic variables linked to nonsexual and sexual offending, little research has specifically addressed the question of whether dynamic variables are actually dynamic—that is, establishing links between changes in the dynamic variables with changes in recidivism in general or sexual recidivism in particular (Douglas & Skeem, 2005; Kraemer et al., 1997).

One way to establish such a link is to assess the putative dynamic variables at two time points to measure change—for example, before and after treatment. The offenders are then followed up after community release to determine the links between observed changes and recidivism. It is key that the assessors of changes must be blind to recidivism outcome to avoid potential confounds and biases. A small collection of studies in the sex offender literature have explicitly done this. Hanson and Harris (2000) compared 208 sex offense recidivists to a sample of 201 nonrecidivists on a large number of dynamic variables. This was a retrospective study in which assessment of the offenders' behaviors were obtained on the variables at two time points (6 months and 1 month) prior to sexually reoffending for the recidivists, or at the two time points prior to data collection for the nonrecidivists. Assessments of the offenders' preoffense behaviors were based on file information and recollections of the offenders' parole officers, many of whom would have knowledge of the recidivism outcomes of offenders they supervised and, therefore, may not be entirely impartial. Hanson and Harris (2000) found that increases in anger between the two time points was associated with increased sexual recidivism; interestingly, recidivists were also more likely than the nonrecidivists to have begun taking antiandrogen medications in the month prior to sexually reoffending. The results from this research informed the development of the SONAR, which consists of five stable factors—sexual self-regulation, general self-regulation, sex offender attitudes, intimacy deficits, and negative social influences—and four acute factors—substance abuse, negative mood, anger, and victim access. Although the stable and the acute factors meaningfully contributed to risk prediction, there was little evidence that changes in these factors were related to sexual recidivism (Hanson, Harris, Scott, & Helmus, 2007, p. 25).

Hudson et al. (2002) correlated the pre–post change scores of several sex offender self-report measures of 242 treated sex offenders and found modest but statistically significant inverse correlations of some of these measures (trait anger, empathy deficits, social discomfort) with sexual recidivism—that is, larger changes were linked to lower sexual recidivism. While the literature examining dynamic sexual violence risk is limited to a few studies, the available findings provide growing support for the changeable nature of dynamic variables and suggest that the improvement or deterioration in sex offender criminogenic need areas is associated with increased or decreased recidivism.

The dynamic nature of the VRS-SO was tested by rating dynamic items of the VRS-SO at the beginning and on completion of treatment (approximately 6 to 8 months apart, on average). Perhaps most significantly, change scores as computed from the dynamic items pre- and posttreatment were found to be significantly inversely related to sexual recidivism after controlling for actuarial risk (i.e., VRS-SO static score) and differences in follow-up time through Cox regression survival analysis, VRS-SO static Wald (1) = 41.33, $p < .001$, $\exp(B) = 1.23$; dynamic change Wald (1) = 3.94, $p < .05$, $\exp(B) = 0.90$. In practical terms, an $\exp(B)$ of 0.90 would be interpreted to mean that every 1-point in change score would predict a 10% decrease in sexual recidivism, after accounting for risk. Furthermore, treatment change was found to predict recidivism better in higher-risk offenders ($r = -0.15$, $p < .05$), who have more to change, than in lower-risk offenders ($r = -0.01$, ns) with less to change—that is, as a result of the floor effect. When change scores were examined on the three factors after controlling for static risk, only sexual deviance change scores were significantly associated with reductions in sexual recidivism, Wald (1) = 3.73, $p = .053$, while static scores continued to be associated with increased recidivism, Wald (1) = 42.14, $p < .001$.

In sum, the change analyses provide support that the VRS-SO dynamic items *are* dynamic—that is, positive changes are linked to reductions in recidivism. The results also are consistent with the risk principle (Andrews & Bonta, 2003), that is, treatment has more impact on higher-risk than lower-risk offenders.

Results of analyses of the VRS change score produce similar results (Lewis et al., 2008). VRS change scores were inversely correlated with violence criminal reconvictions ($r = -0.26$, $p < .001$) after over 6 years of follow-up posttreatment—that is, larger treatment change was linked to lower rates of violence recidivism. The relationship between treatment change and violence recidivism relationship was maintained after controlling for length of follow-up and pretreatment risk level using Cox regression survival analyses.

CASE ILLUSTRATION USING THE VRS-SO

The following clinical case was developed to illustrate the use of the VRS-SO for risk assessment, treatment planning, and evaluating change. Although this case has been informed by previous cases, the details, including the client's name, history, and treatment responses, are fictitious and are intended for illustration purposes only.

Bill, a 36-year-old White man, was serving his first 4-year federal sentence[5] for sexual assault against two teenage boys, aged 13 and 14 years. Bill came from a fairly affluent middle-class background with no reported abuse or neglect growing up. He first learned about sex through erotic magazines he hid around his home. Bill reported being sexually attracted to and had crushes on school-age boys. His first sexual experience occurred when he was about 13 with a neighborhood boy who was about 11. He was also involved in mutual fondling and oral sex with other neighborhood boys. Bill occasionally dated girls in high school, but these relationships were generally short-lived. In his 20s and early 30s, Bill reported living a marginalized existence, drinking heavily, frequently unemployed, and remaining sexually attracted to boys.

Bill received his first conviction for sexual interference at age 22, when he enticed an 11-year-old who was riding his bike home and performed fellatio on him. He complimented the victim, saying he had nice eyes, and, when the boy asked if he had a smoke, Bill invited him back to his home, noticing the boy was unsupervised. Bill used a similar modus operandi with other boys. Bill remained socially isolated, with the exception of the company of the estranged boys he would invite into his home. Here he would entice them with alcohol and soft drugs, and, should they appear willing, he would sexually assault them. Bill rationalized that he was pleasuring the victims because they occasionally ejaculated and they "freely" consented. Even following his fourth sexual conviction, Bill maintained that he had not harmed the victims because they "wanted it," and, if anybody was to blame, it was the irresponsible parents who failed to provide proper supervision. When Bill was arrested, police found a cache of photos of naked boys on Bill's computer hard drive. After a short remand and trial, Bill was found guilty and sentenced to his current term of incarceration. He was recommended to complete sex offender treatment as part of his correctional plan.

Following his admission to treatment, Bill maintained a cautious and skeptical stance toward the prospect of treatment, stating that he simply wished to get it over with so that he could be granted parole and avoid being detained on long-term supervision after completing his sentence. In the pretreatment assessment, Bill reported that most of his sexual fantasies involved boys generally between the ages of 10 and 15, although he reported also having some attraction to young men. He reported masturbating almost daily to these fantasies and admitted to having more victims over the years than he had been convicted for. Despite his drug and alcohol use, Bill reported that he was seldom intoxicated during his sexual offenses; he generally used intoxicants to establish relationships with the victims before sexually assaulting them.

Bill's criminal record indicated three prior convictions for sexual offenses and two unadjudicated charges plus a probation infraction when he was found in the company of minors at a fast food restaurant, thus violating his probation order requiring him not to have unsupervised contact with this group. Bill had four prior sentencing occasions with no convictions for any nonsexual offenses.

Bill denied that he has problems with aggression and anger; however, he reported a history of other emotional problems, including depression and anxiety. He also abused nonprescription medications. Although he reported having had some short-lived gay relationships, Bill never cohabitated with a lover for any meaningful period of time and was frequently lonely and socially withdrawn. Feeling inadequate and self-conscious, Bill reported that the victims filled an emptiness within him through their social contacts during which they would chat, play cards, and drink and "make me feel human again." Although Bill had some family members in the city, he reported that contacts were sporadic and that they drifted further apart as his legal problems grew.

Figure 3.2 presents the first page of a VRS-SO score sheet illustrating Bill's ratings on the static items pretreatment. Bill's item scores reflect the fact that he is a 36-year-old man serving a 4-year sentence, meaning that he will at most be 40 years old when he is released. He was charged for his first sex offense at age 22, is a child molester by virtue of the age of his victims, and has two stayed sexual charges and four prior sexually related convictions. Given that his probation violation seemed sexually motivated, it would be scored as a sex offense in the VRS-SO scoring manual, and in total he would have six prior sexual offenses. Finally, Bill had more than four prior victims, all of whom were unrelated males, and he has four prior sentencing dates. All told, Bill's VRS-SO static score was 15.

Figure 3.3 presents the second page of Bill's VRS-SO score sheet with his ratings on the dynamic items pre- and posttreatment. Bill's VRS-SO dynamic items profile at pretreatment (see left-hand side of the form) indicated that many dynamic items were criminogenic. For the sake of brevity, the scoring rationale for a few representative items on each factor is discussed in detail. First, all of the items on the sexual deviance factor were criminogenic for Bill (i.e., receiving a 2- or 3-point rating). For instance, given that Bill reported being sexually preoccupied with preteen boys, fantasized about this group predominantly, and had an underage pornography collection, he received a score of 3 on the deviant sexual preference item. As well, because he masturbated and fantasized quite frequently, he received a score of 2 on sexual compulsivity; a higher reported frequency of sexual thoughts and behaviors would have generated a score of 3.

Bill had a mixture of high and low scores on items comprising the criminality and treatment responsivity factors. Bill received low scores on several criminality factor items: given that he had basically no concerns with physically or verbally aggressive interpersonal behavior and impulsivity, he received a score of 0 on interpersonal aggression and 0 on impulsivity. However, concerns remained regarding Bill's potential problems with community supervision, receiving a score of 2 on compliance with community supervision, given his past probation violation in which he made contact with children. Although he had some contact with his family, by and large they were estranged, and, having few meaningful supports in the community, Bill received a score of 2 on community support. Although he also abused substances, the use of substances did not

VRS:SO Score Sheet ©

Name: **Bill**
Pre-Treatment Rater: **Dr. M. Olver**
Post-Treatment Rater: **Dr. M. Olver**

Client #: _____
Pre-Treatment Rating Date: **2007 /01/15**
Post-Treatment Rating Date: **2007 /09/14**

Static Factors

Risk Factor[1]		Codes	Score	I or N
S1	Age at Time of Release	Under 25 years	3	
		25 to 34 years	2	
		35 to 44 years	①	
		45 years or older	0	
S2	Age at First Sexual Offense	Under 20 years	3	
		20 to 24 years	②	
		25 to 34 years	1	
		35 years or older	0	
S3	Sex Offender Type	Mixed (both adult and child victims)	3	
		Child molester (child victims only)	②	
		Rapist (adult victims only)	1	
		Incest (related victims predominantly)	0	
S4	Prior Sexual Offenses	4-4+ prior arrests/charges/convictions for a sexual offense	③	
		2-3 prior arrests/charges/convictions for a sexual offense	2	
		1 prior arrests/charge/conviction for a sexual offense	1	
		No prior arrests/charges/convictions for a sexual offense	0	
S5	Unrelated Victims	4 or more unrelated victims	③	
		2-3 unrelated victims	2	
		1 unrelated victim	1	
		No unrelated victims (related victims only)	0	
S6	Number and Gender of Victims	2 or more male victims & any number of female victims	③	
		2 or more female victims *or* 1 female and 1 male victim	2	
		1 male victim only	1	
		1 female victim only	0	
S7	Prior Sentencing Dates	11 or more prior sentencing occasions	3	
		5-10 prior sentencing occasions	2	
		2-4 prior sentencing occasions	①	
		0-1 prior sentencing occasions	0	
Total Static Factor Score		Before Treatment	15	
		After Treatment	15	

1 If it is necessary to omit a Static or Dynamic Factor, the rater should indicate whether the omission is because there is insufficient information (I) or because the item is not applicable (N).

© 2000 Stephen Wong, Mark Olver, Terry Nicholaichuk, & Audrey Gordon

Figure 3.2 Violence Risk Scale–Sex Offender version.

seem to have a strong link to sexual offending. Rather, Bill's substance use seemed to be part of the grooming process, and, as such, he received a score of 1 on substance abuse and a 3 on offence planning.

Finally, Bill's loneliness and lack of fulfilling intimate relationships coupled with an inability to regulate negative emotions (e.g., feelings of depression and inadequacy) suggested that intimacy deficits and, to a

104 Part I Adult Violence

For Stage Of Change:
P/C = Precontemplation/Contemplation
P = Preparation
A = Action
M = Maintenance

Use these symbols to indicate the Stage of Change:
O = Pre-treatment
X = Post-treatment

# of Stages changed:
no change = 0
1 stage = .5
2 stages = 1.0
3 stages = 1.5

DYNAMIC FACTORS AND TOTAL SCORES

		Pre-Tx (a)	F 1†	F 2	F 3	Stage of Change††	# of Stages changed × .5 (b)	Post-Tx (a-b)†††	F 1	F 2	F 3	1 or N
D1	Sexually Deviant Lifestyle	0 1 2 ③	3			(P)C ⋈ A M	1.5 1 ⑤ 0	2.5	2.5			
D2	Sexual Compulsivity	0 1 ② 3	2			(P)C ⋈ A M	1.5 1 ⑤ 0	1.5	1.5			
D3	Offence Planning	0 1 2 ③	3			P(O)⋈ A M	1.5 1 ⑤ 0	2.5	2.5			
D4	Criminal Personality	0 ① 2 3	1			P/C P A M	1.5 1 .5 0	1			1	
D5	Cognitive Distortions	0 1 2 ③			3	(P)⋈ P A M	1.5 1 .5 ⓪	3			3	
D6	Interpersonal Aggression	⓪ 1 2 3			0	P/C P A M	1.5 1 .5 0	0			0	
D7	Emotional Control	0 1 ② 3				P(O)⋈ A M	1.5 1 ⑤ 0	2.5				
D8	Insight	0 1 ② 3		2		(P)⋈ P A M	1.5 1 .5 ⓪	2		2		
D9	Substance Abuse	0 ① 2 3	1			P/C P A M	1.5 1 .5 0	1	1			
D10	Community Support	0 1 ② 3	2			P(O)⋈ A M	1.5 1 ⑤ 0	1.5	1.5			
D11	Release to High Risk Situations	0 1 ② 3		2		(P)C ⋈ A M	1.5 1 ⑤ 0	1.5		1.5		
D12	Sexual Offending Cycle	0 1 2 ③	3			(P)C ⋈ A M	1.5 1 ⑤ 0	2.5	2.5			
D13	Impulsivity	⓪ 1 2 3		0		P/C P A M	1.5 1 .5 0	0		0		
D14	Compliance with Community Superv.	0 1 ② 3		2		(P)⋈ P A M	1.5 1 .5 ⓪	2		2		
D15	Treatment Compliance	0 ① 2 3			1	P/C P A M	1.5 1 .5 0	1			1	
D16	Deviant Sexual Preference	0 1 2 ③	3			(P)C ⋈ A M	1.5 1 ⑤ 0	2.5	2.5			
D17	Intimacy Deficits	0 1 2 ③				(P)⋈ P A M	1.5 1 .5 ⓪	3				

	Pre-Tx:	Factors: 1 2 3		Post-Tx:	Factors: 1 2 3
Total Dynamic Factor Score →	33		Total Dynamic Factor Score →	29	
Total Static Factor Score From Previous Page →	15	14 6 8	Total Static Factor Score From Previous Page →	15	11.5 5.5 7.5
Total Static + Total Dynamic Factor Score →	48		Total Static + Total Dynamic Factor Score →	44	

Indicate if <u>Clinical Override</u> was used: Yes O   No ☒

† To calculate scores for Factors 1 (Sexual Deviancy), 2 (Criminality), & 3 (Treatment Responsivity): Place Pre-Tx score in the corresponding shaded box to the right (Note: D7 is excluded). Tally each column (F1, F2, F3) and enter total score in appropriate box.
†† For treatment purposes, specify whether the client is in Precontemplation or Contemplation stage by circling (O) or marking (X) the 'P' or 'C' stage for pre- and post-treatment, respectively.

Figure 3.3 Violence Risk Scale–Sex Offender version dynamic items score sheet and stages of change ratings for the case of Bill.

certain degree, emotional control were linked to his offending and were thus criminogenic (receiving ratings of 3 and 2 on these items, respectively). In terms of items on the treatment responsivity factor, Bill had clear attitudes and cognitions supportive of sexual offending (e.g., given that he viewed his victims as willing and justified his offending), thus receiving a score of 3 on cognitive distortions. Given that he was cooperative (although reluctant) with treatment and seemed to have some limited understanding of the issues and events contributing to his sexual offending (justifying his behavior), he received a score of 1 on treatment compliance and a 2 on insight.

After rating Bill's static and dynamic items pretreatment, he received a total score of 48, placing him in the high-risk range for sexual offense recidivism. On each of the items deemed criminogenic (i.e., 2- or 3-point rating), Bill was rated as being in the precontemplative or contemplative stage of change given that he had yet to acknowledge his problems or was aware of his problems but reluctant to make changes. Stages of change ratings are only rated on criminogenic items—that is, those rated 2 or 3. For instance, given that Bill was very reluctant to change his deviant fantasies despite their maladaptive nature, he was rated as being in the precontemplative stage of change on deviant sexual preference. Moreover, although Bill knew he was depressed, anxious, and lonely and that such emotional states were linked to his sexual offending, he had yet to make any positive change in his emotional functioning at the outset of treatment, and, as such, he was rated as being in the contemplative stage on emotional control.

Case Conceptualization

The VRS-SO can be used to assist case conceptualization and treatment planning. The static items provide an empirical–actuarial estimate of the offender's risk, reflect the extensiveness of past sexual and nonsexual misconduct, and should show no change with treatment. For Bill, the static variables indicated he is a sexual recidivist, boy-victim child molester who began his offense history rather young and who will be under 40 years of age at the time of his release—all of which are static variables that, in combination, seem to put him at significant risk to reoffend sexually. As well, most of the static variables cannot change, with the exception of more convictions and passage of time (aging). The dynamic items, on the other hand, can be used to elucidate the various elements involved in the persistence and maintenance of sexual offending behavior (i.e., what makes him a multirecidivist, boy-victim child molester?). Specifically, dynamic items dubbed criminogenic can be used to create a dynamic risk profile of individual needs and, hence, areas that should be targeted for intervention. For instance, in Bill's case, he scored particularly high on items comprising the sexual deviance factor, indicating that deviant sexual interests, sexual preoccupations, extensive fantasy, grooming, a strong sex drive, and sexualized lifestyle appeared to play a significant role in his offending. In addition, linked to Bill's offending appeared to be certain items falling under the criminality factor, such as lack of community support, as well as the treatment responsivity factor, including cognitive distortions conducive to sexual offending, exposure to high-risk situations (and, hence, repeated victim access), and little insight about his offending behavior. Perpetuating Bill's offense cycle appeared to be his intimacy deficits, which could have served to exacerbate his pervasive feelings of loneliness, depression, and anxiety, during which he would seek sexual and emotional solace in the company of his victims.

Treatment Program

Treatment consisted of a 12-month, high-intensity inpatient sex offender program and a combination of group and individual therapy. Bill had the opportunity to disclose his offenses in group and benefit from the group's feedback by other treatment participants who also had sexual offences. He completed a detailed crime cycle and learned about the cognitive, behavioral, and emotional dynamics of his sexual offending. Although at first rationalizing and minimizing his molestation of boys, the feedback and challenges he received from other group members, coupled with the constructive and accepting group environment and individual psychotherapy, gradually increased his acceptance of responsibility and accountability for his offending. Bill also completed a detailed relapse prevention plan that articulated his reoffense pathways, high-risk situations, and escape and avoidance strategies to circumvent relapse. In addition to these therapeutic interventions, Bill completed treatment modules that specifically addressed cognitive distortions and attitudes related to sexual offending, healthy relationships and attachments, assertiveness and social skills, victim empathy, and fantasies/healthy sexuality.

Bill underwent phallometric testing as part of his treatment, which confirmed his strong deviant arousal to preteen boys. Importantly, Bill also demonstrated arousal to young men. Bill underwent arousal control sessions, in which he was asked to allow himself to become aroused and then resort to mental strategies in an attempt to decrease his arousal. Although he was eventually able to do this, Bill, not unexpectedly, continued to show deviant arousal when he did not attempt to suppress it. During individual therapy, Bill was encouraged to monitor his fantasies and was counseled on the importance of masturbating to healthy sexual fantasies as a means of heightening healthy sexual interest and controlling deviant arousal. Bill also underwent covert sensitization in an attempt to reduce deviant arousal.

Bill made modest gains in a number of areas. Bill's fantasy monitoring records demonstrated a decrease in the frequency of deviant fantasies and an increase in appropriate adult male homosexual fantasies, and his frequency of masturbation decreased as well. In his work, Bill noticed that whenever he experienced negative affect (loneliness, stress, or feeling overwhelmed), he would sometimes retreat into his fantasy world. Over the course of treatment, he became better at disclosing and discussing his feelings one on one and using other, more appropriate coping strategies. Bill was able to identify cognitive distortions he used to justify his sexual offending behavior and used some effective strategies to challenge them; however, he frequently struggled with relinquishing his justifications and at times dwelled on the physiological displays of sexual excitement shown by his victims during the abuse to excuse and minimize his offending behavior.

As such, the sincerity of Bill's buy-in to treatment was sometimes uncertain. At times, he needed to be reminded to complete homework assignments, and, primarily during the early stages of the program, it was uncertain whether Bill was merely spouting program rhetoric or had actually internalized the material. For the most part, Bill did not seem to have substantial empathy for people or his victims, and he continued to struggle with accepting that his behavior was truly damaging to them. However, he did recognize that child sex offense legislation served a purpose and that he manipulated and exploited his young victims, albeit while making palliative comparisons (e.g., that he would never engage in intercourse with his victims, and all his victims had to do was decline his overtures, which they sometimes did). The covert sensitization work also prompted Bill to contemplate the potentially serious and costly outcomes of his behavior that he could face, some of which he had never considered (e.g., being adjudicated a dangerous offender upon recidivating).

Bill agreed to attend a maintenance outpatient sex offender program in the community following his release (imposed as a special condition by his case management team), although he expressed mild reluctance to follow through on this, given that he had already successfully completed a high-intensity treatment program and was not sure whether more treatment was necessary. Bill's case management team also worked hard to establish supports for him in the community, and he reestablished some contact with an older sister (providing her with a copy of his relapse prevention plan), who provided her commitment to support him. In the course of his work on intimate relationships and attachments, the supportive treatment environment, and individual work, Bill began to develop an increasing level of trust. As such, an additional component of his release planning involved establishing links to the gay community so that Bill may have an opportunity to develop further healthy supports.

In summary, following the completion of treatment, Bill was judged to have made varying gains in all of his criminogenic need areas. However, Bill was judged to have advanced to the preparation stage on several of his dynamic risk factors, given that his changes were relatively recent (i.e., made over the course of a 12-month treatment program) and he had not yet had any opportunity to practice his skills in real-world contexts. During times of emotional distress, Bill would occasionally lapse, although with continued support he would regain control. For instance, Bill reported reductions in the frequency of deviant fantasy and increases in the frequency of appropriate sexual fantasies (i.e., consenting adult homosexual fantasies); however, given that he would lapse into deviant fantasy on occasion and had not demonstrated greater consistency in his arousal control and appropriate fantasies, he was considered to have only progressed to the preparation stage. Similarly, although he could discuss painful feelings and emotions with treatment staff to "drain off negative affect," on occasion he had coped with negative feelings in treatment through social isolation and was again appraised to be in the preparation stage on emotional control.

As illustrated in Figure 3.3, at posttreatment, Bill's VRS-SO score changed by four points (roughly one-half of a standard deviation) as he moved to the preparation stage on eight of the criminogenic items. Although Bill continued to fall within the high-risk range (with a score of 44) at the end of treatment, he fell within the lower end of this risk category and had demonstrated some important changes. It is important to emphasize that, in many ways, this reflects the reality of a repeat sex offender, who can hardly be expected to be radically transformed after a 12-month program. This being said, a continued reduction in Bill's risk would be anticipated should he complete a maintenance sex offender group and continue to demonstrate sustained behavior change in his dynamic risk factors into the community. For Bill to move into action stages for most of the criminogenic factors, he must demonstrate sustained changes over a significant period of time. Moving into the maintenance stage would require the generalization of the changes to real-life situations and for Bill to have withstood significant challenges with little or no relapse.

STATIC AND DYNAMIC PREDICTORS OF YOUTH VIOLENCE

Violence among young people left an estimated 199,000 youths dead in 2000 (Krug, Dahlberg, Mercy, Zwi, & Lorazano, 2002). For every young person killed as a result of violence perpetuated by youth, an estimated 20 to 40 receive injuries requiring hospital treatment, and many more suffer from a range of physical, sexual, reproductive, and mental health problems (Krug et al., 2002). Needless to say, violence among youth exacts substantial social and financial costs.

Current intervention efforts for youths include a wide range of legislative and judicial remedies, community-based activities, and individual approaches. In North America, most programs for violent youths are aimed at those at risk for future violence. As such, service providers have to assess the youth's risk for violence for case management and treatment planning purposes. This section briefly reviews static and dynamic predictors of violence and general recidivism among youths and common youth risk assessment measures, including discussions on the integration of assessment and risk reduction treatment in youth. An experimental tool specifically designed for this purpose, the Violence Risk Scale–Youth Version (VRS-YV; Wong, Lewis, & Gordon, 2004), is used to illustrate the use of static and dynamic risk factors in the assessment of youth violence.

Findings from several longitudinal studies, meta-analytic reviews, and large scale recidivism projects have identified several correlates of violence and general recidivism among youths. Although a detailed review of this literature is beyond the scope of this chapter, common static predictors include criminal history, young age at first conviction, past weapon use, ethnicity, community disorganization, and instability in family upbringing such as abuse, neglect, exposure to domestic violence, and residential mobility (Cottle, Lee, & Heilbrun, 2001; Derzon, 2001; Herrenkohl et al., 2000; Latimer, Kleinknecht, Hung, & Gabor, 2003). Several putatively dynamic variables have also been identified from this literature including delinquent peers (including gang membership), family criminal activity, antisocial attitudes, school problems, externalizing pathology (e.g., impulsivity), and substance abuse/dependence among others (Cottle et al., 2001; Derzon, 2001; Farrington, Jolliffe, Loeber, Stouthamer-Loeber, & Kalb, 2001; Heilbrun et al., 2000; Herrenkohl et al., 2000; Hoge, Andrews, & Leschied, 1994; Latimer et al., 2003). Still, the majority of this large literature has focused on generalized delinquency rather than on youth violence per se, and males have been the primary target of investigation.

It is evident that a substantial amount of overlap and continuity exist in the static and dynamic recidivism predictors between youths and adults. However, there are potential differences over the course of development along age and gender lines; research has demonstrated some risk variables to be more prominent than others at certain developmental periods for males and females. For instance, given the increasingly influential role played by one's peer group during adolescence, having criminal peers, who serve to role model and reinforce criminal attitudes and behaviors, is a particularly salient predictor among youths. Data gathered from a New Zealand birth cohort ($N = 1,265$) found clear and consistent trends for increasing affiliations with deviant peers to be associated with increasing rates of violent crime at four age intervals for both genders (Fergusson, Swain-Campbell, & Horwood, 2002); interestingly, however, the strength of the association decreased with age, suggesting that criminal peers may have a greater impact on risk for violent behavior among younger youth. Gang membership has also been found to make a unique contribution above and beyond the influence of antisocial peers and has been found to be one of the strongest predictors of violent behavior, particularly among male youths (e.g., Thornberry, 1998).

Moreover, a constellation of predictors external to the individual, although predictive for adults, appear to be particularly salient for youth. These include social/contextual or systemic factors (i.e., family, school, and community variables). The importance of such variables is well supported in the fields of child development and developmental psychopathology (e.g., Bronfenbrenner, 1979), and empirical research has shown that juvenile antisocial behavior is influenced by a reciprocal interplay between characteristics of the individual youth and the social systems in which he or she is embedded (Henggeler, Schoewnwald, Borduin, Rowland, & Cunningham, 1998). For instance, using data obtained from the National Longitudinal Survey of Children and Youth ($N = 1,368$), Latimer et al. (2003) identified several core correlates of self-reported delinquency among Canadian boys and girls aged 12 to 15 years, including inconsistent/inadequate parenting, history of victimization, and negative school attachment. Violent offending was positively correlated with witnessing violence in the home and parental abuse and was negatively correlated with parental monitoring and parental nurturance.

These static and dynamic predictors have been combined to form risk assessment measures for young offenders. These are generally youth-adapted versions of adult measures, with modifications based on developmental considerations unique to the young offender population, such as those mentioned above. For instance, multiple variations of the Level of Services Inventory (LSI) and its revised version (LSI-R; Andrews & Bonta, 1995) have been developed for young offenders, including the Youth Level of Services/Case Management Inventory (YLS/CMI; Hoge & Andrews, 2003). The YLS/CMI is a 42-item clinician-rated measure designed to assess risk/need characteristics of young offenders across eight criminogenic domains: prior and current offenses/dispositions, education/employment, family circumstances/parenting, leisure/recreation, peer relations, attitudes/orientation, substance abuse, and personality/behavior. Psychometric research on the YLS/CMI and other youth-adapted variations have found these measures to be strong predictors of general recidivism (Catchpole & Gretton, 2003; Ilacqua, Coulson, Lombardo, & Nutbrown, 1999; Jung & Rawana, 1999) and violent recidivism (Catchpole & Gretton, 2003).

Another standardized forensic instrument often used with young offenders is the Psychopathy Checklist: Youth Version (PCL:YV; Forth, Kosson, & Hare, 2003). In contrast to the family of youth adapted variants of the LSI, which tap a broad range of criminogenic needs to be targeted for services, the PCL:YV assesses a more specialized set of constructs associated with violence and general criminality that are arguably more static than dynamic—that is, they capture the behavioral and personality features of psychopathy. Although the assessment of features of psychopathy among youth have been controversial (Edens, Skeem, Cruise, & Cauffman, 2001), ongoing research supports the criterion-related validity of the PCL:YV, and other youth adaptations of the PCL-R, for various criminal behavioral phenomena such as increased institutional misconducts (Brandt, Kennedy, Patrick, & Curtin, 1997), violent and general recidivism (Catchpole & Gretton, 2003; Edens, Campbell, & Weir, 2007; Gretton, McBride, Hare, O'Shaughnessy, & Kumka, 2001), and adult criminality (Gretton, Hare, & Catchpole, 2004).

Although instruments such as the YLS/CMI and the PCL:YV have been shown to be strong predictors of recidivism with youth, an instrument designed specifically to assess violence risk with young offenders is the Structured Assessment of Violence Risk in Youth (SAVRY; Borum, Bartel, & Forth, 2002), a multi-item clinician-rated measure composed of 10 historical risk items, 6 social-contextual risk items, 8 individual-clinical risk items, and 6 protective factors. A summary risk rating of low, medium, or high risk can be assigned based either on a summation of the items or through using SPJ. Although little data are available concerning the psychometric properties of the SAVRY, some preliminary research supports its predictive validity for violence and general recidivism (e.g., Catchpole & Gretton, 2003).

Violence Risk in Youths: Linking Assessment and Treatment

Although appraising a youth's risk for violence is important information for decision makers and service providers, this in itself is insufficient. Not only is it important to identify youths who are at high risk for future violence, it is also important to identify the risk factors or criminogenic needs that contribute to their violence risk, as well as the responsivity factors that may impact the successful delivery of treatment services. These factors, in turn, can be targeted for intervention (e.g., addictions counseling, targeted interventions such as relapse prevention, anger management, etc.) to lower the youth's risk and hence reduce further violence victimization. As such, violence risk assessments should inform community supervision, access to services, and treatment planning to prevent and reduce violence recidivism.

The literature has demonstrated that certain forms of treatment can be effective in reducing violence and general recidivism in youths. For instance, Lipsey's (1992) meta-analysis of nearly 400 juvenile offender treatment studies demonstrated modest reductions in juvenile recidivism (about 10%) across all treatments and larger reductions (about 20%) for behaviorally specific and structured approaches. Moreover, Dowden and Andrews (2000) conducted a meta-analysis of 35 studies examining the effectiveness of treatment specifically for reducing violence. Although separate findings were not presented for young offender programs, over a quarter of the effect sizes were generated from young offender samples. Treatment programs that generally adhered to the principles of risk, need, and responsivity yielded the largest reductions in violence recidivism (15% and 20%, respectively). Examples of young offender treatment programs that seem to subscribe to risk, need, and responsivity include multisystemic therapy (Henggeler et al., 1998), wraparound approaches (VanDenBerg & Grealish, 1996), and functional family therapy (Barton & Alexander, 1980), among others.

The emergence of youth risk measures with good predictive accuracy for violence and general recidivism is encouraging; however, some of the current measures reviewed do not specifically assess violence risk and rather tend to focus on general risk-need. Other measures, such as the PCL:YV (which, as with its adult predecessor, was not developed specifically to assess risk), are limited in their ability to inform risk reduction treatment. Although violence-specific risk measures for youths have been developed that include both static and dynamic risk factors (e.g., SAVRY), there has remained an ongoing need for a violence-specific measure for youths that can assess risk for violence, identify targets for treatment, and evaluate changes in risk as a function of treatment or experience.

The Violence Risk Scale-Youth Version

The Violence Risk Scale–Youth Version (Wong et al., 2004), modeled after the VRS and VRS-SO, is a psychometric tool designed to integrate the assessment of risk, need, responsivity, and treatment change into a single tool for youth at risk for violence. Similar to the adult and sex offender versions, the VRS-YV is a 23-item clinician-rated measure comprised of both static and dynamic items (see Table 3.3 for a list of items) for which change is assessed using an adaptation of Prochaska et al.'s (1992) transtheoretical model of change. All items are empirically, conceptually, or theoretically related to violence risk in youths and are rated according to the youth's developmental level. Ratings are also made on a 4-point (0, 1, 2, 3) scale with higher values indicating increased risk for violence.

The VRS-YV was developed to assist forensic service providers in (1) determining a youth's initial risk for engaging in violence; (2) identifying factors linked to violence to be addressed in treatment; (3) assessing responsivity factors such as the youth's readiness to change; and (4) evaluating changes in risk (or lack thereof) as a result of treatment or experience. It is important to note that, while other instruments exist to assess dynamic factors relevant to offending in youth, they lack a coherent theoretical mechanism for conceptualizing and assessing changes in risk. Moreover, the VRS-YV has the additional advantage of assessing dynamic factors that are specific to violence in a treatment-friendly and developmentally sensitive manner. In comparison to the adult version, greater emphasis is placed on social/contextual or systemic factors (i.e.,

Table 3.3

VIOLENCE RISK SCALE–YOUTH VERSION STATIC AND DYNAMIC ITEMS

STATIC ITEMS

S1 Early onset of serious antisocial behaviors
S2 Criminality
S3 Instability of family upbringing
S4 Exposure to antisocial behavior in the family

DYNAMIC ITEMS

D1 Violent lifestyle
D2 Callous and unemotional
D3 Criminal attitudes
D4 Negative attitude toward education
D5 Antisocial peers
D6 Interpersonal aggression
D7 Poor emotional control
D8 Violence during institutionalization
D9 Weapon use
D10 Lack of insight into cause of violence
D11 Mental disorder
D12 Substance abuse
D13 Impulsivity/attention deficits
D14 Cognitive distortions
D15 Poor parent–child interaction
D16 Family stress
D17 Social isolation
D18 Community disorganization
D19 Poor compliance

family, school, and community variables). Thus, all VRS-YV items are empirically, conceptually, and/or theoretically related to violence risk in youths.

Research to assess the reliability and validity of this clinical tool has produced promising results. Preliminary research on the VRS-YV was carried out using a sample of 133 adjudicated male and female youths who were charged or convicted for violent offenses in the province of Saskatchewan (Stockdale, 2008; Stockdale, Olver, & Wong, 2007). VRS-YV total scores demonstrated high interrater reliability (intraclass correlation coefficient = 0.90) on 23 randomly selected cases, as well as good internal consistency (α = 0.91) overall. Outcome data were available for a subsample of 62 youths (average follow-up = 25.8 months), and VRS-YV total scores significantly predicted violent recidivism (r = 0.45, area under the curve = 0.78) and general recidivism (r = 0.52, area under the curve = 0.81). There was also initial evidence to show that the VRS-YV dynamic items can change in a subsample of youths (n = 39) who had participated in treatment services, although less than half of these youths had outcome data available, which precluded drawing firm conclusions about the relationship of change to reductions in violence. While research is ongoing, these efforts provide initial support for the validity and reliability of the VRS-YV as a tool to assess violence risk in young offenders.

NOTES

1. Values for current age and prior release failures or escapes could change and are, therefore, exceptions.
2. The Stages of Change model was modified to ensure that ratings indicating risk reduction are given only when relevant and sustainable behavioral changes are clearly observed.
3. A complete list of all violent and nonviolent convictions is available from the authors.
4. VRS divided into 5-point bins and plotted against percent violence recidivism.
5. Sentences of 2 years or more are under federal jurisdiction (federal sentences) in contrast with provincial sentences of less than 2 years.

REFERENCES

Andrews, D. A., & Bonta, J. (1994). *The psychology of criminal conduct*. Cincinnati, OH: Anderson.

Andrews, D. A., & Bonta, J. (1995). *The LSI-R: The Level of Service Inventory-Revised*. Toronto, Canada: Multi-Health Systems.

Andrews, D. A., & Bonta, J. (1998). *The psychology of criminal conduct* (2nd ed.). Cincinnati, OH: Anderson.

Andrews, D. A., & Bonta, J. (2003). *The psychology of criminal conduct* (3rd ed.). Cincinnati, OH: Anderson.

Andrews, D. A., Bonta, J., & Wormith, J. S. (2004). *The Level of Service/Case Management Inventory (LS/CMI)*. Toronto, Canada: Multi-Health Systems.

Andrews, D. A., Bonta, J., & Wormith, J. S. (2006). The recent past and near future of risk and/or need assessment. *Crime and Delinquency, 52,* 7–22.

Andrews, D. A., Zinger, I., Hoge, R. D., Bonta, J., Gendreau, P., & Cullen, F. T. (1990). Does correctional treatment work? A clinically relevant and psychologically informed meta-analysis. *Criminology, 28,* 369–404.

Barton, C., & Alexander, J. F. (1980). Functional family therapy. In A. S. Gurman & D. P. Kniskern (Eds.), *Handbook of family therapy* (pp. 403–443). New York: Brunner/Mazel.

Beech, A., Friendship, C., Erikson, M., & Hanson, R. K. (2002). The relationship between static and dynamic factors and reconviction in a sample of U.K. child abusers. *Sexual Abuse: A Journal of Research and Treatment, 14,* 155–167.

Beggs, S. M., & Grace, R. C. (2007). *Measuring dynamic risk with the Violence Risk Scale–Sexual Offender Version: An independent validation study.* Manuscript in preparation.

Belfrage, H., & Douglas, K. S. (2002). Treatment effects on forensic psychiatric patients measured with the HCR-20 violence risk assessment scheme. *International Journal of Forensic Mental Health, 1,* 25–36.

Beyko, M., & Wong, S.C.P. (2005). Predictors of treatment attrition as indicators for program improvement not offender shortcomings: A study of sex offender treatment attrition. *Sexual Abuse: A Journal of Research and Treatment, 17,* 375–389.

Boer, D. P., Hart, S. D., Kropp, P. R., & Webster, C. D. (1997). *Manual for the Sexual Violence Risk-20: Professional guidelines for assessing risk of sexual violence.* Vancouver, Canada: Institute Against Family Violence and the Mental Health, Law, and Policy Institute, Simon Fraser University.

Bonta, J., Harman, W. G., Han, R. G., & Cormier, R. B. (1996). The prediction of recidivism among federally sentenced offenders: A re-validation of the SIR scale. *Canadian Journal of Criminology, 38,* 61–79.

Borum, R., Bartel, P., & Forth, A. (2002). *Manual for the Structured Assessment of Violence Risk in Youth (SAVRY). Consultation version.* Tampa: Florida Mental Health Institute, University of South Florida.

Brandt, J. R., Kennedy, W. A., Patrick, C. J., & Curtin, J. J. (1997). Assessment of psychopathy in a population of incarcerated adolescent offenders. *Psychological Assessment, 9,* 429–435.

Bronfenbrenner, U. (1979). *The ecology of human development.* Cambridge, MA: Harvard University Press.

Campbell, M. A., French, S., & Gendreau, P. (2007). *Assessing the utility of risk assessment tools and personality measures in the prediction of violent recidivism in adult offenders.* Report Prepared for the Department of Public Safety and Emergency Preparedness Canada. Saint John, New Brunswick, Canada: Centre of Criminal Justice Studies, University of New Brunswick.

Catchpole, R., & Gretton, H. (2003). The predictive validity of risk assessment with violent young offenders: A 1-year examination of criminal outcome. *Criminal Justice and Behavior, 30,* 688–708.

Cottle, C., Lee, R., & Heilbrun, K. (2001). The prediction of criminal recidivism in juveniles: A meta-analysis. *Criminal Justice and Behavior, 28,* 367–394.

Dempster, R. J., & Hart, S. D. (2002). The relative utility of fixed and variable risk factors in discriminating sexual recidivists and nonrecidivists. *Sexual Abuse: A Journal of Research and Treatment, 14,* 121–138.

Derzon, J. (2001). Antisocial behavior and the prediction of violence: A meta-analysis. *Psychology in the Schools, 38*, 93–106.

Douglas, K., & Skeem, J. (2005). Violence risk assessment: Getting specific about being dynamic. *Psychology, Public Policy, and Law, 11*, 347–383.

Douglas, K. S., Yeomans, M., & Boer, D. P. (2005). Comparative validity analysis of multiple measures of violence risk in a sample of criminal offenders. *Criminal Justice and Behavior, 32*, 479–510.

Dowden, C., & Andrews, D. A. (2000). Effective correctional treatment and violent reoffending: A meta-analysis. *Canadian Journal of Criminology, 42*, 449–476.

Dvoskin, J. A., & Heilbrun, K. (2001). Risk assessment and release decision-making: Towards resolving the great debate. *Journal of the American Academy of Psychiatry and the Law, 29*, 6–10.

Edens, J. F., Campbell, J. S., & Weir, J. M. (2007). Youth psychopathy and criminal recidivism: A meta-analysis of the psychopathy checklist measures. *Law and Human Behavior, 31*, 53–75.

Edens, J. F., Skeem, K. L., Cruise, K. R., & Caufmann, E. (2001). Assessment of "juvenile psychopathy" and its association with violence: A critical review. *Behavioral Sciences and the Law, 19*, 53–80.

Epperson, D. L., Kaul, J. D., Goldman, R., Huot, S. J., Hesselton, D., & Alexander, W. (2005). *Minnesota Sex Offender Screening Tool Revised (MnSOST-R)*. St Paul: Minnesota Department of Corrections.

Farrington, D. P., Jolliffe, D., Loeber, R., Stouthamer-Loeber, M., & Kalb, L. M. (2001). The concentration of offenders in families, and family criminality in the prediction of boys' delinquency. *Journal of Adolescence, 24*, 579–596.

Fergusson, D. M., Swain-Campbell, N. R., & Horwood, L. J. (2002). Deviant peer affiliations, crime and substance use: A fixed effects regression analysis. *Journal of Abnormal Child Psychology, 30*, 419–430.

Forth, A. E., Kosson, D., & Hare, R. D. (2003). *The Psychopathy Checklist: Youth Version (PCL:YV)*. Toronto, Canada: Multi-Health Systems.

Gendreau, P., Little, T., & Goggin, C. (1996). A meta-analysis of the predictors of adult offender recidivism: What works! *Criminology, 34*, 575–607.

Gretton, H. M., Hare, R. D., & Catchpole, R.E.H. (2004). Psychopathy and offending from adolescence to adulthood: A 10-year follow-up. *Journal of Consulting and Clinical Psychology, 72*, 636–645.

Gretton, H. M., McBride, M., Hare, R. D., O'Shaughnessy, R., & Kumka, G. (2001). Psychopathy and recidivism in adolescent sex offenders. *Criminal Justice and Behavior, 28*, 427–449.

Grove, W. M., Zald, D. H., Lebow, B. S., Snitz, B. E., & Nelson, C. (2000). Clinical versus mechanical prediction: A meta-analysis. *Psychological Assessment, 12*, 19–30.

Hanson, R. K. (1997). *The development of a brief actuarial scale for sexual offense recidivism*. (User Report 97–04). Ottawa: Department of the Solicitor General of Canada.

Hanson, R. K., & Bussière, M. T. (1998). Predicting relapse: A meta-analysis of sexual offender recidivism studies. *Journal of Consulting and Clinical Psychology, 66*, 348–362.

Hanson, R. K., Gordon, A., Harris, A.J.R., Marques, J. K., Murphy, W., Quinsey, V. L., & Seto, M. C. (2002). First report of the Collaborative Data Outcome Project on the effectiveness of psychological treatment for sexual offenders. *Sexual Abuse: A Journal of Research and Treatment, 14*, 169–194.

Hanson, R. K., & Harris, A.J.R. (2000). Where should we intervene? Dynamic predictors of sexual offense recidivism. *Criminal Justice and Behavior, 27,* 6–35.

Hanson, R. K., & Harris, A.J.R. (2001). A structured approach to evaluating change among sexual offenders. *Sexual Abuse: A Journal of Research and Treatment, 13,* 105–122.

Hanson, R. K., Harris, A.J.R., Scott, T-L., & Helmus, L. (2007). *Assessing the risk of sexual offenders on community supervision: The dynamic supervision project.* (User-Report 2007–05.) Ottawa: Public Safety and Emergency Preparedness Canada.

Hanson, R. K., & Morton-Bourgon, K. (2004). *Predictors of sexual recidivism: An updated meta-analysis.* (User Report 2004–02). Ottawa: Public Safety and Emergency Preparedness Canada.

Hanson, R. K., & Morton-Bourgon, K. (2007). *The accuracy of recidivism risk assessments for sexual offenders: A meta-analysis* (User Report 2007–01). Ottawa: Public Safety and Emergency Preparedness Canada.

Hanson, R. K., & Thornton, D. (1999). *Static 99: Improving actuarial risk assessments for sex offenders.* (User Report 99–02). Ottawa: Department of the Solicitor General of Canada.

Hanson, R. K., & Thornton, D. (2003). *Notes on the development of Static-2002.* (User Report 2003–01). Ottawa: Department of the Solicitor General of Canada.

Hart, S. D. (1998). The role of psychopathy in assessing risk for violence: Conceptual and methodological issues. *Legal and Criminological Psychology, 3,* 121–137.

Hart, S. D., Kropp, P. R., & Laws, D. R. (2003). *The Risk for Sexual Violence Protocol (RSVP)—Structured professional guidelines for assessing risk of sexual violence.* Burnaby, Canada: Simon Fraser University, Mental Health, Law and Policy Institute.

Heilbrun, K., Brock, W., Waite, D., Lanier, A., Schmid, M., Witte, G., et al. (2000). Risk factors for juvenile criminal recidivism: The post-release community adjustment of juvenile offenders. *Criminal Justice and Behavior, 27,* 275–291.

Henggeler, S., Schoenwald, S., Borduin, C., Rowland, M., & Cunningham, P. (1998). *Multisystemic treatment of antisocial behavior in children and adolescents.* New York: Guilford Press.

Herrenkohl, T. I., Maguin, E., Hill, K. G., Hawkins, J. D., Abbott, R. D., & Catalano, R. F. (2000). Developmental risk factors for youth violence. *Journal of Adolescent Health, 26,* 176–186.

Hoge, R. D., & Andrews, D. A. (2003). *The Youth Level of Service/Case Management Inventory.* Toronto, Canada: Multi-Health Systems.

Hoge, R.D., Andrews, D. A., & Leschied, A. W. (1994). Tests of three hypotheses regarding the predictors of delinquency. *Journal of Abnormal Child Psychology, 22,* 547–559.

Hudson, S. M., Wales, D. S., Bakker, L., & Ward, T. (2002). Dynamic risk factors: The Kia Marama evaluation. *Sexual Abuse: A Journal of Research and Treatment, 14,* 103–119.

Ilacqua, G. E., Coulson, G. E., Lombardo, D., & Nutbrown, V. (1999). Predictive validity of the Young Offender Level of Service Inventory for criminal recidivism of male and female young offenders. *Psychological Reports, 84,* 1214–1218.

Jung, S., & Rawana, E. (1999). Risk and need assessment of juvenile offenders. *Criminal Justice and Behavior, 26,* 69–89.

Kenny, D. T., Keogh, T., & Seidler, K. (2001). Predictors of recidivism in Australian juvenile sex offenders: Implications for treatment. *Sexual Abuse: A Journal of Research and Treatment, 13*, 131–148.

Kraemer, H. C., Kazdin, A. E., Offord, D. R., Kessler, R. C., Jensen, P. S., & Kupfer, D. J. (1997). Coming to terms with the terms of risk. *Archives of General Psychiatry, 54*, 337–343.

Krug, E., Dahlberg, L. L., Mercy, J. A., Zwi, A. B., & Lorazano, R. (2002). *World report on violence and health*. Geneva, Switzerland: World Health Organization.

Langton, C. M., Barbaree, H. E., Seto, M. C, Peacock, E. J., Harkins, L., & Hansen, K. T. (2007). Actuarial assessment of risk for reoffense among adult sex offenders. Evaluating the predictive accuracy of the Static 2002 and five other instruments. *Criminal Justice and Behavior, 34*, 37–59.

Latimer, J., Kleinknecht, S., Hung, K., & Gabor, T. (2003). *The correlates of self-reported delinquency: Analysis of the National Longitudinal Survey of Children and Youth*. Ottawa: Research and Statistics Division, Department of Justice Canada.

Lewis, K., Olver, M. E., & Wong, S.C.P. (2008). *The Violence Risk Scale: Validity, measurement of treatment changes, and violent recidivism in a high risk and personality disordered sample of male offenders*. Manuscript in preparation.

Lipsey, M. (1992). The effect of treatment on juvenile delinquents: Results from meta-analysis. In F. Losel, D. Bender, & T. Bliesener (Eds.), *Psychology and law: International perspectives* (pp. 131–143). Berlin: European Association of Psychology and Law.

McGrath, R. J., & Hoke, S. E. (2002). *Vermont Assessment of Sex Offender Risk manual. Research edition 2001*. Waterbury, VT: Author.

Meehl, P. E. (1954). *Clinical vs. statistical prediction*. Minneapolis: University of Minnesota Press.

Mossman, D. (1994). Assessing predictions of violence: Being accurate about accuracy. *Journal of Consulting and Clinical Psychology, 62*, 783–792.

Olver, M. E., & Wong, S.C.P. (2006). Psychopathy, sexual deviance, and recidivism. *Sexual Abuse: A Journal of Research and Treatment, 18*, 65–82.

Olver, M. E., Wong, S.C.P., Nicholaichuk, T., & Gordon, A. (2007). The validity and reliability of the Violence Risk Scale–Sexual Offender version: Assessing sex offender risk and evaluating therapeutic change. *Psychological Assessment, 19*, 318–329.

Pithers, W. D. (1993). Treatment of rapists: Reinterpretation of early outcome data and exploratory constructs to enhance therapeutic efficacy. In G.C.N. Hall, R. Hirschman, J. R. Graham, & M. S. Zaragoza (Eds.), *Sexual aggression: Issues in etiology, assessment, and treatment* (pp. 167–196). Philadelphia: Taylor & Francis.

Prochaska, J., DiClimente, C., & Norcross, J. (1992). In search of how people change: Applications to addictive behaviors. *American Psychologist, 47*, 1102–1114.

Proulx, J., Pellerin, B., Paradis, Y., McKibben, A., Aubut, J., & Ouimet, M. (1997). Static and dynamic predictors of recidivism. *Journal of Interpersonal Violence, 10*, 85–105.

Quinsey, V. L., Harris, G. T., Rice, M. E., & Cormier, C. A. (1998). *Violent offenders: Appraising and managing risk*. Washington, DC: American Psychological Association.

Quinsey, V. L., Rice, M. E., & Harris, G. T. (1995). Actuarial prediction of sexual recidivism. *Journal of Interpersonal Violence, 10*, 85–105.

Stockdale, K. C. (2008). *The validity and reliability of the Violence Risk Scale–Youth Version (VRS-YV)*. Unpublished doctoral dissertation, University of Saskatchewan, Saskatoon.

Stockdale, K. C., Olver, M. E., & Wong, S.C.P. (2007). Assessment and treatment of violent youth: Evaluating changes in risk with service provision. In M. E. Olver (Chair), *Evaluating specialized clinical services with high risk, high needs offenders*. Symposium conducted at the 68th annual meeting of the Canadian Psychological Association, Ottawa.

Thornberry, T. P. (1998). Membership in youth gangs and involvement in serious and violent offending. In R. Loeber & D. P. Farrington (Eds.), *Serious and violent juvenile offenders: Risk factors and successful interventions* (pp. 147–166). Thousand Oaks, CA: Sage Publications.

Thornton, D. (2002). Constructing and testing a framework for dynamic risk assessment. *Sexual Abuse: A Journal of Research and Treatment, 14,* 139–153.

Thornton, D. (2007). *Scoring guide for risk matrix 2000.9/SVC.* Unpublished manuscript.

VanDenBerg, J., & Grealish, M. (1996). Individualized services and supports though the wraparound process: Philosophy and procedures. *Journal of Child and Family Studies, 5,* 7–21.

Ward, T., & Hudson, S. M. (1998). A model of the relapse process in sex offenders. *Journal of Interpersonal Violence, 13,* 700–725.

Webster, C. D., Douglas, K. S., Eves, D., & Hart, S. D. (1997). *HCR-20: Assessing risk for violence* (version 2). Burnaby, Canada: Mental Health, Law, and Policy Institute, Simon Fraser University.

Wong, S.C.P., & Burt, G. (2007). The heterogeneity of incarcerated psychopaths: Differences in risk, need, recidivism and management approaches. In J. Yuille & H. Herve (Eds.), *The psychopath: Theory research and practice* (pp. 461–484). Mahwah, NJ: Erlbaum.

Wong, S.C.P., & Gordon, A. (2006). The validity and reliability of the Violence Risk Scale: A treatment-friendly violence risk assessment tool. *Psychology, Public Policy, and Law, 12,* 279–309.

Wong, S.C.P., & Gordon, A. (1999–2003). *Violence Risk Scale* (Available from the authors, Department of Psychology, University of Saskatchewan, Saskatoon, Saskatchewan, S7N 5A5).

Wong, S.C.P., Gordon, A., & Gu, D. (2007). Assessment and treatment of violence prone forensic clients: An integrated approach. *British Journal of Psychiatry, 190*(Suppl. 49), s66–s74.

Wong, S.C.P., & Hare, R. D. (2005). *Guidelines for a treatment program for psychopaths.* Toronto, Canada: Multi-Health Systems.

Wong, S.C.P., Lewis, K., & Gordon, A. (2004). *The Violence Risk Scale: Youth Version (VRS:YV)* (Available from the authors, Department of Psychology, University of Saskatchewan, Saskatoon, Saskatchewan, S7N 5A5).

Wong, S.C.P., Olver, M., Nicholaichuk, T., & Gordon, A. (2004–2006). *Violence Risk Scale–Sexual Offender version* (Available from the authors, Department of Psychology, University of Saskatchewan, Saskatoon, Saskatchewan, S7N 5A5).

Yang, M., Wong, S.C.P., & Coid, J. (2008). *The efficacy of violence prediction: A meta-analytic comparison of commonly-used risk assessment instruments using multilevel regression analysis.* Manuscript submitted for publication.

4

Contextualizing Women's Violence: Gender-Responsive Assessment and Treatment

JUDITH S. WILLISON AND YVONNE L. LUTTER

Charlene is convicted for assaulting another young woman in her impoverished, urban neighborhood with whom she had an ongoing conflict. She is a 20-year-old Black woman who minimizes her history of childhood neglect and abuse. With a string of assaults behind her and time spent in a juvenile justice facility, she believes violence is just a part of life in her world.

Ella is a biracial woman in her early 20s, serving time in prison for aggravated assault after stabbing her stepdaughter's rapist, who was a friend of the family. Ella asserts that she would attack him again to protect the child. She recalls her own brutal childhood history of sexual and physical abuse in a home characterized by violence, drugs, and criminality.

Rita, a 53-year-old Hispanic woman, is in the ninth year of a 10-year sentence for manslaughter, having fatally stabbed her husband after enduring many years of domestic violence. Her experiences of childhood abuse and resulting drug addiction led her to prostitution to support her habit. Rita's docile, grandmotherly presentation belies her underlying rage.

Women's violent crime differs significantly from men's. The stories of the three women above, whose identities have been altered to protect their confidentiality, illustrate some of these differences. Charlene typifies the approximately 74% of women arrested for violent crime who are charged with assault (Uniform Crime Reports, 2002). A striking three-quarters of these assaults are perpetrated against female acquaintances (Catalano, 2006; Greenfeld & Snell, 1999). Ella's crime illustrates the high frequency with which female violent offenders have a prior relationship with their victim: 62% of female violent offenders had such a relationship, whereas about 36% of male violent offenders did (Greenfeld & Snell, 1999). Ella is one of the 23% of female violent offenders arrested for aggravated assault (Uniform Crime Reports, 2002). Rita's crime reflects the fact that most female homicide victims are family members, and women are twice as likely to kill an intimate partner as opposed to a relative (Greenfeld & Snell, 1999). These women's realities are only three of the many that represent women's violent crime. Their stories will be followed throughout this chapter to illustrate the importance of risk assessment and treatment interventions specific to women.

This chapter discusses risk assessment and treatment of female violence and provides a model that incorporates recent advances in evidence-based practices. Gender responsiveness in assessment, treatment, and program design for female offenders involves recognizing the complex roots of violence in women's lives and the unique ways in which women learn and change (Covington & Bloom, 2006). Reflecting the authors' practice experience, this chapter primarily considers women who are incarcerated. Before offering data regarding the scope, prevalence, and etiologic risk factors for women's violence, we consider several of the more pertinent contextual issues.

CONTEXTUAL ISSUES IN THE APPROACH TO WOMEN'S VIOLENCE

There are a number of differences between women and men's violence. Women's violence is more often perpetrated against acquaintances or family and more often occurs in the home (Greenfeld & Snell, 1999; Robbins, Monahan, & Silver, 2003); results in less serious injuries; is far less frequently sexual in nature (Uniform Crime Reports, 2004); and is characterized as reactive or defensive in the context of dangerous domestic violence more often than men's violence (Pollock & Davis, 2005). Further, incarcerated women consistently report a higher incidence of violent victimization and suffer from higher rates of posttraumatic stress disorder (PTSD) than do male offenders or women in the general population (Chesney-Lind & Pasko, 2004; Zlotnick, 1997).

These differences have been poorly understood. Until recently, women who entered the criminal justice system for violent offenses have been missing from the assessment and intervention literature. When they have been included, the complexity of the relationship between the female offender's status as both perpetrator and victim has generally been oversimplified. Yet the prevalence of this dual status is undeniable and profoundly impacts the expression of violence in women and their course of treatment.

One-third of female sentenced state prisoners are incarcerated for violent offenses compared to over half (53%) of male offenders (Harrison & Beck, 2006). Because the majority of women in prison are survivors of violent victimization, the focus of this chapter is to explore what sets apart women who themselves turned to violence. This is a complicated task, partly because criminological theory has focused almost exclusively on men (Belknap, 2007). This is, to some extent, due to the low incidence of women's violence. While women comprise more than half (51.6%) of the U.S. population age 10 or older, the Bureau of Justice Statistics reports that only 14% of all violent crime in the United States can be attributed to women. One out of every 9 male offenders has perpetrated a violent crime, while one out of every 56 female offenders has, a per-capita rate six times less than that for males (Greenfeld & Snell, 1999). These factors, coupled with a criminal justice system designed for and largely administered by men, contribute to woefully inadequate responses to women's criminality (Covington & Bloom, 2006; Gilfus, 2006; Sokoloff, 2005). Forensic mental health professionals are at a serious disadvantage when charged with conducting violence risk assessments and designing treatment programs for women who have been violent.

Female Offenders and the Violent Crimes They Commit

Nationally, the rates of incarceration for women of color are disproportionate. Black and Hispanic women comprise 25% of the total national female population but make up almost half of the women incarcerated in the United States (Harrison & Beck, 2006; Sokoloff, 2005). As with other groups overrepresented among incarcerated populations, socioeconomic status is a robust mediating variable. Half of female offenders are unemployed at the time of arrest, and the largest percentage of those are women of color between the ages of 25 and 34 (Meichenbaum, 2001). The relationship is clarified by research showing that, when socioeconomic status is controlled, race is not significantly correlated with violence (Free, 2003; Herivel & Wright, 2003; Monahan, 2002). These findings underscore the juncture of race and class that is reflected in the typical characteristics of women who are incarcerated (van Wormer & Kaplan, 2006). Female offenders are generally poor; are heads of households and mothers of younger children; lack adequate education and vocational training; are often in poor health; suffer from serious substance abuse disorders; demonstrate mental health problems; and are victims of interpersonal and community violence (Covington & Bloom, 2006; Greenfeld & Snell, 1999; Sokoloff, 2005).

Of women arrested for violent crime, the vast majority are charged with assault—three-quarters with simple assault and nearly one-quarter with aggravated assault (Sokoloff, 2005; Uniform Crime Reports, 2002). Most of these assaults are against female acquaintances (Greenfeld & Snell, 1999), are intraracial, and preceded by an argument around personal respect, protecting others, or jealousy and conflict concerning a male partner. Violence was mutual in 40% of the cases, and the assailant was using alcohol in 35% of the assaults (Hirschinger et al., 2003). Rates of homicide and robbery for women are low and have continued to diminish, while rates of assault have increased (Greenfeld & Snell, 1999; Pollock & Davis, 2005). This may, in part, reflect the trend in law enforcement and the judiciary of arresting and prosecuting women in domestic violence situations (Henning, Jones, & Holdford, 2003; Stuart, Moore, Coop, Ramsey, & Kahler, 2006).

Women's violence often occurs in the home. Mothers acting alone are responsible for approximately 40% of reported child abuse and neglect cases (U.S. Department of Health and Human Services, 2007), an unremarkable figure given how often women figure as primary caretakers for children. Women are at least five times more likely to be the victims of intimate partner violence (IPV) than men (Rennison, 2001). Although a small percentage of women are considered the primary aggressors in IPV, men's violence tends to be more frequent and serious, while women's violence more often occurs in the context of self-defense (Dobash & Dobash, 2004). IPV among lesbian couples appears to occur at roughly the same frequency as among heterosexual couples (Miller, Greene, Causby, White, & Lockhart, 2001; Ristock, 2003) with a pattern of coercion, control, and initiation of abuse by the primary abuser (McClennen, 2005; Peterman & Dixon, 2003). Abusive tactics unique to same-sex couples include threats to expose the victim's sexual orientation and factitious charges of mutual battering to increase the primary victim's isolation (West, 2004).

Homicide accounts for about 0.4% of arrests for all female violent crime (Uniform Crime Reports, 2002) and 12% of women in state prisons (Harrison & Beck, 2006). Rates of homicides committed by women have been steadily decreasing since 1980, and the per-capita murder rate for female offenders in 1998 was the lowest it had been in a generation, since 1976. The only group of women perpetrators among whom the homicide rate has been increasing is women ages 18 to 24 (Greenfeld & Snell, 1999). Approximately 33% of female murder victims are killed by a male intimate, whereas 4% of male murder victims are killed by a female intimate (Rennison, 2003). Brownstein, Spunt, Crimmins, and Langley (2006) found that 8.8% of homicides committed by females were related to the drug market, the majority of which occurred within the context of the offender's relationship to a man despite the fact that economic motivations were present.

An estimated 1,530 children died in 2006 as a result of abuse or neglect, with most of these fatalities involving children under the age of 4. When mothers are responsible for fatal child maltreatment, it is more often through acute or chronic neglect rather than abuse (Child Welfare Information Gateway, 2008). About one-quarter (28.5%) of these deaths were caused by mothers acting alone (U.S. Department of Health and Human Services, 2007). Mothers and stepmothers are responsible for committing about half of all murders of children by parents/stepparents, and women are more likely to murder children during infancy, while men are more likely to murder school-aged children (Greenfeld & Snell, 2000).

Finally, women are far less likely to be sexually invested in violence than men. Between 1993 and 1997, women made up 2% of all sexual offenders (Greenfeld & Snell, 1999). Women sex offenders are most likely to be White and often have codefendants who are male. They are more likely to choose child and adolescent victims who are related to them or whom they know (Oliver, 2007). To better understand women's violent behavior, we will outline the risk factors that are associated with women's violence.

ETIOLOGY OF WOMEN'S VIOLENCE

A constellation of traumatic experiences and environmental risk factors most often land women in the criminal justice system (Chesney-Lind & Pasko, 2004; Covington & Bloom, 2006), and a specific set of risk factors has been demonstrated for the small subgroup of female offenders who have been violent. Rita's pathway to prison, which reflects many of these risk factors, is all too common.

Rita grew up a victim of frequent physical abuse at the hands of an alcoholic father who also regularly beat her mother. Her parents were uneducated, and the family was poor. Pregnant at age 16, Rita dropped out of school to marry the baby's father and at 18 had a second daughter. Her husband, who had begun to beat Rita, introduced her to drugs, which gave Rita emotional respite from the effects of the domestic violence and the emerging flashbacks of being abused as a child. Within a year of her release from a psychiatric hospital following a suicide attempt, Rita was addicted to crack cocaine and entered the sex industry to support her habit. Arrested for prostitution and drug possession, she was placed on probation, only to relapse and return to the streets. Eventually, Rita served a 2-year prison term. Ten years later, her life was a nightmare of social isolation, increasing domestic violence, and sexual humiliation with her second husband. One night, when the couple had been drinking and using crack cocaine, her husband's sexual demands escalated together with his physical abuse, Rita grabbed a kitchen knife and stabbed him and he died from his wounds. Jailed on a murder charge, she again attempted suicide and nearly succeeded. Prison mental health staff diagnosed Rita with PTSD, cocaine dependence, and major depression. Now a grandmother, Rita laments the fact that her daughter, like her and her mother before her, is in an abusive relationship.

Risk Factors for Women's Violence

Rita's story reflects the gendered phenomena of women's violence. Although many of the risk factors for violent male offending hold true for women, the route to violent acts diverges sharply given women's more frequent experiences of childhood abuse, adult victimization, and resulting trauma-related psychological and behavioral difficulties (Crimmins, Langley, Brownstein, & Spunt, 1997; Eronen, 1995; Leenaars, 2005; Oliver, 2007). In addition, women have significantly fewer economic resources than men prior to incarceration (Greenfeld & Snell, 1999). Unsafe family situations lead girls to run away from home, where they then find themselves with no financial or social supports. Recruitment into the sex industry and the drug trade, as a result of economic necessity and lack of skills, are often the next steps on young women's pathways to violence. Relationships with, and economic dependence on, abusive men involved with crime often complete the picture (Gilfus, 2002; Steffensmeier & Schwartz, 2004; van Wormer & Kaplan, 2006).

Childhood Experiences Including Abuse and Trauma

Childhood physical abuse is strongly associated with violent behavior later in women's lives (Monahan et al., 2001; Pollock, Mullings, & Crouch, 2006). The majority of women convicted of assaulting their male partner were physically abused as children (Henning et al., 2003), and women who were physically abused by their mothers are more likely to abuse their own children, suggesting a gender-specific model of intergenerational transmission of abusive behavior (Coohey, 2004). Childhood maltreatment, witnessing family violence, parental substance abuse, and/or criminality also correlate with violence in adulthood for women.

These childhood risk factors are influenced by various intervening variables, such as socioeconomic status, experiencing community violence, being the victim of adult IPV, and psychological difficulties, particularly maternal depression (Banyard, Williams, & Siegel, 2003; Feerick, Haugaard, & Hien, 2002; Siegel, 2000; Weizmann-Henelius, Viemero, & Eronen, 2004). Research supports the hypothesis that cumulative maternal trauma is associated with parenting difficulties, including child abuse potential, punitiveness, psychological aggression, and physical discipline (Banyard et al., 2003; Cohen, Hien, & Batchelder, 2008).

Substance Abuse and Dependence

Women who abuse substances report a higher exposure to interpersonal trauma (Cohen et al., 2008), and many of these women report using drugs and alcohol to dull trauma-related symptoms (Gilfus, 2002; Mullings, Pollock, & Crouch, 2002). This can often lead to full-blown addictive disorders and the criminal behaviors necessary to support addiction. Almost half of female offenders are under the influence of drugs or alcohol at the time of their violent offense (Greenfeld & Snell, 2000). Research indicates a strong connection between women's use of alcohol and drugs and their aggressive behavior, particularly in intimate relationships (Chase, O'Farrell, Murphy, Fals-Stewart, & Murphy, 2003; Feerick et al., 2002; Weizmann-Henelius et al., 2004). Substance abuse has also been linked to poorer parenting skills and the use of aggressive discipline, and research has shown that children are at twice the risk of abuse if their parents abuse drugs or alcohol (Cohen et al., 2008).

Mental Disorder

Women's expression of violence risk in relation to mental illness differs in some regards from that of men's. Women are less likely than men to respond to threatening delusions with violence (Teasdale, Silver, & Monahan, 2006). Female psychiatric patients discharged to the community are more likely to be violent in the home and toward a family member but generally commit less serious violence than male psychiatric patients (Robbins et al., 2003).

Diagnosis may represent a significant factor correlated with rates of violence for female psychiatric patients. Those patients carrying an Axis I diagnosis are less likely to be violent postdischarge than those patients carrying an Axis II personality or adjustment disorder. A diagnosis of schizophrenia is associated with lower rates of violence than depression or bipolar disorder. Patients diagnosed with a co-occurring substance abuse disorder were two to three times more likely to engage in violence (Monahan et al., 2001). Higher levels of Axis I psychopathology are found in women who are court referred to batterer's programs than women in the general population, which may be related to the experience of also being a victim of IPV (Stuart et al., 2006).

Critical risk factors for women's violence include personality disorder, impulsivity, and relationship instability (de Vogel & de Ruiter, 2005), and higher rates of personality disorders have been found in violent female offenders than in nonviolent female offenders (Strand & Belfrage, 2001; Weizmann-Henelius et al., 2004). It makes clinical sense that women with disorders of affective dysregulation such as borderline personality disorder, often implicated in complex PTSD and associated with struggles to maintain a sense of self-integrity in intimate relationships, are at higher risk for acting-out behaviors when something goes awry in those relationships. Emotional regulation deficits are associated with female aggression toward children (Cohen et al., 2008). This may well be the link between cumulative exposure to interpersonal trauma and child abuse potential.

Intimate Partner Violence and Adult Trauma

Being in an abusive relationship increases a woman's risk for behaving violently herself (Siegel, 2000), including an increased risk for perpetrating child abuse (Cohen et al., 2008). This can be explained by women's use of violence as self-defense (Das Dasgupta, 2001; Meichenbaum,

2001) and the association between violent behavior and high levels of prior violent victimization (Leisring, Dowd, & Rosenbaum, 2003). Men are more likely to be the primary aggressors in heterosexual IPV (Dobash & Dobash, 2004; Hamberger & Potente, 1994), while intervention programs in the community have found that most female primary aggressors of IPV were in lesbian relationships (Hamlett, 1998).

As with male batterers, the need for control has been found to be the strongest predictor of physical violence in lesbian IPV (Miller et al., 2001). Perpetrators of IPV in lesbian relationships appear to be motivated by issues of dependency, jealousy, and fear of abandonment, and substance abuse and social isolation are also contributing factors (Margolis & Leeder, 1995; Renzetti, 1992).

Battered women who kill abusive partners appear to differ from battered women who do not only in the amount of violence they have endured and the severity of resulting trauma (Hattendorf, Ottens, & Lomax, 1999). Women in relationships with men who more often abuse them and/or their children and women who perceive more imminent danger, including intense, specific death threats, are more likely to kill their abusive partners (Belknap, 2007; O'Keefe, 1997).

GENDER-RESPONSIVE VIOLENCE RISK ASSESSMENT

Research has established the relationship between the individual and environmental, as well as childhood and adult, risk factors for female violence identified in the previous section. Therefore, there is a need for a violence risk assessment approach that addresses the interrelated nature of these factors (Monahan et al., 2001). Violence risk assessment aids in forensic evaluations, behavioral management, and treatment planning.

A recent study found that mental health practitioners, regardless of professional affiliation or gender, tend to underestimate women's potential for violence (Skeem et al., 2005). It is unclear why we misjudge this. Perhaps the cultural prohibitions against aggression in women contribute to minimization of the reality of their capacity for violence. The implications for potential harm, as well as for treatment, underscore the need for forensic mental health professionals to learn skills specific to assessment of women's risk for violence.

Because actuarial risk assessment instruments have principally been normed on men, forensic mental health professionals need to be aware that the level of ambiguity when using a standardized risk assessment tool may be greater with women. A complete clinical interview is imperative with the use of any actuarial risk assessment tool, because data gleaned in interviews contextualizes test results and must inform the clinician's use of the tool (Maden, 2004). Risk assessment of women's potential for violence needs to be tailored to gender-specific experiences, including violent victimization, investment in and influence of interpersonal relationships, and reaction to loss of these relationships (Chesney-Lind & Pasko, 2004; de Vogel & de Ruiter, 2005). In addition, the contextual nature of women's risk for violence requires not only an assessment of individual pathology but also of oppressive environmental influences, interpersonal relationships, strengths, and supports.

Types of Gender-Responsive Violence Risk Assessment

Structured Interviews

Gender-specific issues relevant to violence risk assessment include the fact that women are typically primary caretakers for children. The majority of incarcerated women have children, and up to 75% have children living at home at the time of their arrest (Pollock, 1998). Their children's welfare is a paramount concern for women offenders, and plans for their children's care and safety are crucial in initial and ongoing assessment. The client's capacity to communicate with her children and their caretakers can impact her mental status and level of behavioral control, as well as motivation for treatment. While 60% of incarcerated mothers maintain weekly contact with their children, half never see their children due to long distances, security procedures, and confounded relationships with the child's primary caregiver. Most children of incarcerated mothers end up in the care of family members and 10% go into foster care. The Adoption and Safe Families Act (1997) stipulates that if a child is in foster care for 15 of 22 months, then parental rights can be terminated. For female offenders, whose average sentence is between 18 months and 4 years, this represents a real concern (Travis & Waul, 2003). Medical problems specific to women, including pregnancy, sexually transmitted diseases, and trauma-related somatic problems, can also impact mental status and behavioral stability and should be included in risk assessment.

Meichenbaum (2001) describes a comprehensive Case Conceptualization Model for violence risk assessment, grounded in research on IPV. He emphasizes the importance of exploring motivations underlying the use of violence, as well as types and patterns of aggression across relational situations. He describes three types of interpersonal violence: self-defense, proactive or premeditated aggression, and reactive or affectively dysregulated aggression. This paradigm seems particularly relevant to the assessment of women who are arrested or convicted of IPV or child abuse due to the role of significant relationship issues and emotion regulation deficits.

In assessments of IPV, identification of the primary aggressor and a categorization of the woman's role are essential. These roles may include battered women who use violence mainly in self-defense; women who use violence to have power over their partners and are the primary aggressors; and women who use violence when they feel threatened, in an attempt to reduce their chances of being victimized again (Hamlett, 1998). Determination of the primary aggressor includes assessment of relationship dynamics, individual risk factors, and environmental variables (Henning et al., 2003; Swan & Snow, 2002). The clinician's understanding of the woman's reason for using force in intimate relationships identifies salient problem areas to target during the treatment process (Hamlett, 1998).

In all assessments of women's risk for violence, it is critical to gather details about the context of women's past aggressive behavior. Questions may include: Were fights in school provoked by conflict with other girls? Was she acting primarily in self-defense, as part of a gang, or in the context of an ongoing dispute with a classmate? Did the restraining order against her occur after she filed domestic violence charges against a partner? Was her violence related to economic or other stressors?

The context of the index crime should be explored in detail. What was the woman's relationship to her victim and to the codefendant, if applicable? Who was involved and present at the time of the violence? Did her violence occur in the context of IPV? Did she feel her children were in danger? What sort of history did she and the victim and codefendant have together? What was the precipitant to the incident?

A unique component of the Case Conceptualization Model that makes it particularly useful in working with women is its emphasis on strengths, assessment of personal resources, and social and cultural supports (Meichenbaum, 2001). Protective factors that mediate risk for violence—supportive networks with others, strong relationships with children and family, economic resources, educational achievements, vocational skills, and intrapersonal assets such as intelligence, verbal expressiveness, and emotional resourcefulness—should all be configured into a thorough assessment.

Questions that seek to identify strengths may include: Who are the woman's family and other supports? What role does religion/spirituality play in her life, and what guidelines does her practice provide for behavior toward self and others related to harm? What stops her from acting out when angry? Who supports her in remaining nonviolent? Because dedication to children is often a major incentive for maintaining a commitment to recovery and nonviolence, it is essential to ask questions regarding the welfare of the offender's children, frequency of contact, and opportunities for ongoing visits.

Finally, Meichenbaum's (2001) model links the assessment process to treatment through its emphasis on therapeutic engagement with the client during assessment. Through this collaboration, the clinician and client identify barriers in the pursuit of the individual's short- and long-term goals. What goals related to family, friends, employment, education, and other life goals does she have? How has violence gotten in the way of her achieving those goals? How has she overcome those obstacles previously?

Actuarial Violence Risk Assessment Tools

The Psychopathy Checklist–Revised (PCL-R; Hare, 1991) is the most widely used assessment measure to assess the construct of psychopathy, which has been linked to recidivism. Most of the studies on the PCL-R have been based on White males, however, raising the obvious question of how data from this assessment tool may be legitimately used in regard to women. The lower overall prevalence of psychopathy and lower scores on specific checklist items among women has caused speculation that both the etiology of psychopathy and its expression may vary by gender (Salekin, Rogers, & Sewell, 1997; Vitale & Newman, 2001; Warren et al., 2005). Results of one study of over 500 incarcerated females found that the instrument's reliability and validity were consistent across gender and between Black and White females (Vitale, Smith, Brinkely, & Newman, 2002).

The limited evidence to date suggests that the construct of psychopathy may apply to women, but at significantly lower rates than among men. Further, the expression of psychopathy among women appears to differ from its presentation among men. Women who score high on psychopathy are more likely to have personality disorders, and women who live an unstable and antisocial lifestyle are more likely to present with anxiety and depression than men (Weizmann-Henelius et al.,

2004). Although it is clear that much remains to be studied in terms of how the construct of psychopathy relates to violent behavior in women, limited existing research supports assessment for both mood and personality disorders as potential indicators of a risk for violent behavior.

The Historical, Clinical, Risk Management-20 (HCR-20) (Webster, Douglas, Eaves, & Hart, 1997) is another commonly used assessment checklist that structures and informs clinical judgment regarding potential violence risk. Research on the HCR-20 as a risk assessment and management tool indicates that the instrument has good validity for predicting inpatient violence across gender, but only moderate predictive validity for women in the community (de Vogel & de Ruiter, 2005). The HCR-20 consists of 20 items in three categories: fixed, *historical* factors such as previous violence, employment problems, and substance abuse; current *clinical* concerns such as lack of insight, impulsivity, and unresponsiveness to treatment; and future *risk management* issues such as feasibility of goals, lack of personal support, and exposure to destabilizing factors. Additionally, the *HCR-20 Violence Risk Management Companion Guide* (Douglas, Webster, Hart, Eaves, & Ogloff, 2001) offers intervention strategies that target identified clinical variables and risk factors. These interventions are designed to enhance stabilization, thereby reducing the individual's overall risk of violence.

Low scores on the HCR-20 may suggest lower risk for recidivism and violence and simultaneously describe protective factors. For example, a woman with no mental illness, no problems with employment, and a low probability of exposure to destabilizing forces can be described as someone with a solid work history and stable mental health whose life situation is generally secure. Because the HCR-20 can be used to identify protective factors, highlight contextual issues, and shape the focus of treatment, it is an especially valuable tool in working with women at risk for violent behavior.

LINKING VIOLENCE RISK ASSESSMENT TO TREATMENT

Both structured interviews and formal risk assessment tools assist in formulating an initial and ongoing treatment plan. The use of a matrix that can be conceptualized along two dimensions—level of risk (high, low) and level of motivation/amenability to treatment (high, low)—can help to identify appropriate interventions (H. Conyngham, personal communication, 2004). Charlene's case illustrates a client in a prison mental health program who, upon entering treatment, fell in the category of high risk, low motivation, as evidenced by her high scores on the HCR-20 clinical factors—limited insight, impulsiveness, antisocial attitudes, and a lack of commitment to treatment. Personality testing was consistent with her high PCL-R scores on need for stimulation, poor behavioral controls, irresponsibility, juvenile delinquency, and failure to accept responsibility.

Initially, Charlene approached her 3-year sentence for assault and battery as something to be tolerated rather than an opportunity for positive growth. Charlene met diagnostic criteria for PTSD, polysubstance abuse, and a personality disorder reflected in her inability to manage powerful emotions, her cognitive distortions, and faulty decision making. These issues led to self-injurious behavior and numerous fights during her adjustment to the facility. A young woman, Charlene had not successfully mastered crucial developmental tasks: without a high school education, she remained unemployed, living with friends who were involved in the drug trade. Charlene was also faced with the consequences of unaddressed trauma symptoms that she masked with substances. She lacked social skills, and her antisocial behaviors were reinforced by her peers. Charlene's relationship with an aunt was the only one supporting her latent desire to pursue education, employment, and treatment.

Charlene's problem behaviors were curtailed through interdepartmental management and supervision following the HCR-20 initial risk management strategies of environmental controls and safety planning. This included random drug testing and medical checks for signs of self-mutilation, weekly supervised phone contact with her aunt (to bolster this prosocial influence), closely supervised programming, and frequent mental health contact to determine her need for placement in a mental health unit. Charlene began to experience positive consequences for her efforts to change her behavior, which reinforced her willingness to participate in treatment. Individual interventions were then geared toward providing psychoeducation about her diagnoses, enhancing her capacity for self-care, and supporting her personal responsibility for emotion regulation. Her motivation was enhanced through interactions with prosocial peers. Following Charlene's progress demonstrates the relationship between risk assessment, risk management, and treatment planning. Interventions are tailored to reduce risk factors and promote protective factors in order to reduce overall risk of violent behavior.

Gender-Responsive Intervention

The main principle of gender-responsive intervention requires that women's unique experiences as women be considered in the design and implementation of treatment. It is only recently that the need for gender-specific programming for female offenders, founded in relational and trauma-sensitive theories, has been recognized (Bloom, Owen, & Covington, 2003). What follows are the main elements of a gender-responsive approach as applied to the treatment of women who have been violent.

A Relational and Strengths-Based Model of Treatment

Gender-responsive programming addresses not only the lived experiences of women, but the unique ways in which women learn and heal. Relational theory posits that the goal of female adult development is not independence, as men's psychological development has been commonly understood, but rather relatedness and a sense of connection with others (Miller, 1986). Research has shown that women's growth occurs through healthy relationships characterized by mutuality and empowerment (Jordan & Hartling, 2002). For the woman who has acted violently, effective treatment addresses the breaches and violations that have occurred in her relationships and provides opportunities for her to repair connections and build healthy and safe relationships. This can only transpire within an interactional environment that supports responsibility for prosocial behavior (DeCou, 2001) and offers opportunities for genuine relational experiences (DeCou & Van Wright, 2002).

It is especially important in secure settings to understand women's relational capacities, such as emotional expression, as assets (Covington & Bloom, 2006) and to make use of intervention models that recognize women's mental health issues and behavioral dyscontrol as rooted in their social and relational world (Jeffcote & Travers, 2004). Both women's internalization and externalization of aggression are often in direct response to a disconnection with others. The inmate who cuts herself rather than hit her girlfriend during a conflict is demonstrating a more prosocial, albeit maladaptive, way of coping with her feelings of frustration and anger. Rather than using physical restraint and/or isolation as a response to violence, women generally respond more positively to controlled social encounters where they can practice skills and gain support. A gender-sensitive response to this woman would involve validating her feelings, supporting her choice to be nonviolent toward others, and exploring more adaptive strategies for coping with intense emotions such as journaling or talking with others. Women's motivation for self-restraint is enhanced when their relational experiences are characterized by respect and validation (DeCou, 2001).

When the therapy process privileges and emphasizes women's relational ties and responsibilities, clients are better able to embrace genuine accountability for their violence and a commitment to nonviolence. For this reason, and to foster supportive social networks, treatment must include structures for acknowledging and enhancing women's relationships with children, family, and prosocial peers (Covington & Bloom, 2006). Consider Ella, who takes full responsibility for stabbing her stepdaughter's rapist. Upon entering treatment, she is unable to identify a nonviolent alternative solution she could have chosen. She struggles to keep her rage in check and her despair at bay—longing for contact with her three young children, now kept from her by her estranged husband. Ella says her children are "the reason I keep going," and her engagement in treatment is motivated by her wish to see them again and to be a positive role model. Children are often the most powerful motivator for change in working with women who have been violent, and treatment must attend to building parenting skills, development of a realistic approach to parenting, and managing depression related to harm done to children by the mother and a severing of the mothering role (Pollock, 1998).

Trauma-Informed Interventions in a Safe Environment

Because of the prevalence of trauma in the histories of most female offenders, treatment must be provided in a safe environment, with minimal risk of retraumatization and with maximum support for healthy coping skills (Covington & Bloom, 2006; Harris & Fallot, 2001). This is a challenge in all secure forensic settings and especially within correctional settings that are not designed for treatment. In women's facilities, staff sexual misconduct can be a serious concern, contributing to retraumatization (van Wormer & Kaplan, 2006). But even under the most professional circumstances, some security procedures can have an adverse effect on women with a history of trauma and violent behavior. The effectiveness of treatment depends on the development of an environment of containment and safety with a judicious use of external controls.

Monique, a correctional officer with years of experience, approaches Charlene slowly, her voice firm but calm, directing the young inmate to take off her clothes for the strip search that follows visitation. Charlene's abuse history is well known to security staff from their experiences supervising her after episodes of self-harm. In the past, Charlene has fought staff to avoid the humiliation of being strip searched. Today, however, is different. With mental health staff close by, Monique assures Charlene in a matter-of-fact manner that the strip search is simply a routine procedure and walks her through it step by step. Charlene removes one piece of clothing at a time, hands it to Monique who shakes it out and returns it to her in exchange for another item. Monique maintains a safe interaction for all involved, tacitly acknowledging Charlene's history of shame and humiliation, her need for dignity, and her fear of being out of control.

A history of childhood victimization is associated with an array of adjustment problems for women in forensic settings, including self-harm, suicidal ideation, hostility, anger, aggression, and paranoia (Kubiak, 2004). Some women who struggle with behavioral dyscontrol experience secure settings as an external holding environment able to contain their rage. "I know what I'm capable of" is a common refrain among women whose violence has brought them to prison, where they seek out mental health to find alternative ways to cope with interpersonal conflict. However, some women experience these same settings as threatening, where routine procedures and a lack of control can trigger symptoms related to past victimization (Covington & Bloom, 2006; DeCou, 2001), including violent outbursts. For example, Rita was found with drugs and subsequently placed in segregation. As a survivor of chronic, severe domestic violence with a diagnosis of PTSD, the extreme isolation of segregation led to increased symptoms of intrusive memories and nightmares, eventually resulting in an incident of self-harm and lashing out at correctional officers.

The treatment environment must be designed to contain self-harming and violent behaviors while maintaining a sense of personal safety and dignity. Seclusion, restraints, and other interventions should be implemented in a way that takes into account the woman's trauma history and preserves her personal boundaries as much as possible (DeCou, 2001).

Integrated Treatment Approach

Effective intervention programs for violent female offenders must address the coexisting issues of trauma recovery, substance abuse, and mental health needs (Covington & Bloom, 2006; Marcus-Mendoza & Wright, 2004) because most female offenders present with these concerns (DeCou & Van Wright, 2002). Women's violence is often associated with this tripartite constellation, and effective intervention targets each set of problems with an understanding of their interrelatedness. Trauma-related conditions and addiction are often manifested through somatic discomfort and affective and behavioral dyscontrol, and dually diagnosed women in prison generally present as more functionally impaired, presenting with more psychiatric symptoms, medical concerns, and interpersonal problems (Battle, Zlotnick, Najavits, Gutierrez, & Winsor, 2002). An integrated treatment model takes into account co-occurring disorders and the subsequent behavioral problems that often arise.

Initially, Rita moved into the residential substance abuse treatment program in the prison in an effort to avoid the stress of living in the general population with so many other inmates. However, after she was oriented to the program, she became genuinely interested in learning new skills to address her chronic substance use. Unfortunately, the program used a traditional model of confrontation. Problems other than addiction were not addressed, and psychotropic medication was frowned upon. While it was generally acknowledged that clients had a history of trauma, the addictions staff lacked an understanding of its implications for treatment and sobriety. Rita stopped taking her antidepressant medication, her mood deteriorated, she cried daily, and she became increasingly irritable. Her symptoms of PTSD also increased as she struggled to separate her past abuse from current triggers. Eventually, she left the program, saying, "I got tired of being yelled at—I took enough of that from my husband."

In contrast, an integrated approach allows for stabilization of symptoms; psychoeducational interventions to help women understand the relationship between trauma, addiction, and mental health problems; and opportunities to learn new skills to better regulate affect and behavior. Two years after Rita left the residential substance abuse program, staff embarked on an evaluation of the program's gender responsiveness. As a result of this review, addictions staff initiated weekly consultations with the mental health program to address residents' mental health issues. Addictions staff also completed training on trauma to better understand the interplay between addiction, trauma history, and PTSD. And, finally, this residential program incorporated a dual-diagnosis group for women with mental illness who were prescribed psychotropic medication. In these ways the program validated the importance of mental health self-care as a critical component of sobriety and relapse prevention.

In summary, clinical interventions that are based on a relational and strengths-based model, are trauma sensitive and provided in a safe environment, and integrate substance abuse, trauma, and mental health treatment are the most effective with women who have been violent.

Forensic Treatment Issues With Women Who Have Used Violence

The following section addresses specific forensic issues such as the complicated nature of the therapeutic relationship in forensic settings with women who have been violent and techniques to promote personal responsibility through a solution-focused, cognitive-behavioral approach that utilizes contingencies and consequences.

The Therapeutic Relationship

Establishing emotional and behavioral stability is the first step in building a therapeutic relationship with women who have been violent. Maintaining the safety of the client and those around her is the primary treatment goal. Therefore, it is critical to lay out the parameters of treatment and review the limits of confidentiality. Regardless of the setting, the forensic mental health provider has a mandate to report issues of safety. While the client must gauge what the legal or other consequences may be of disclosures in treatment, the therapist has to continually assess issues of malingering, secondary gain, duty to protect concerns, and personal safety. For example, a woman brings a makeshift weapon into a therapy session, ostensibly to give it to the clinician as an external control on her behavior so that others don't get harmed. The clinician wants to reinforce the client's use of therapy to reduce her violence risk; however, there is an obligation to report these safety concerns. The clinician may be concerned that, by reporting her client's good-faith gesture to turn in a weapon, she will jeopardize a fragile therapeutic alliance that took months to establish. This balance of obligations to public safety and therapeutic alliance can take its toll on forensic clinicians. Consistent supervision and team support are essential to sustain sound clinical judgment and effective interventions in the service of safety.

Although the primary goals of treatment with women who have used violence include symptom management, skills acquisition, and behavioral change, none of these goals can be achieved without first establishing a therapeutic relationship. Trust is difficult enough for survivors of violent victimization, but for women who inhabit the dual status of also having used violence, the issue may be further compounded by their feelings of being unacceptable social outcasts because of their violent behavior and their difficulty managing relationships safely and respectfully.

A victim of severe child abuse, Ella was fiercely protective of her own children and had vowed not to be like her parents. As a child, she chose a self-reliant isolation. As an inmate, she presented herself as untouchable, yet her self-loathing was palpable. Ella had a pattern of driving peers away with her aggression and then feeling rejected; thus, her only lasting relationships were with her children. Leading up to the first anniversary of the day she stabbed her stepdaughter's rapist, Ella spent two weeks on a mental health watch where she raged and cried, throwing food and drink, hitting the wall, rejecting all efforts to reach her. This marked the start of her recovery as she began to face her history, her violence, and its consequences. Furious at the man she assaulted for raping her stepdaughter, she initially sought to justify her attack. But as she considered the impact of her violence on her children as well as the offender and his family, she began to doubt her judgment.

Her therapist accepted Ella's distress as understandable given the circumstances of her survival, while persistently challenging her assumptions about herself and her behavioral choices. With guidance, Ella began to examine her isolation and distorted thinking and her responsibility for hurting another person. The therapeutic relationship evolved slowly, developing a common language that allowed for the development of mutually created goals. With some trepidation, Ella began to engage with other inmates in anger management and trauma survivors' psychoeducation groups, slowly letting down her guard as others shared their own painful histories and acts of rage.

Developing a therapeutic relationship with women who have used violence requires a level of clinical and emotional sophistication often not learned in graduate school. As supervisors, we see forensic clinicians struggle not to overidentify with the helpless victim who minimizes her responsibility and is paralyzed by her own powerlessness. The other end of this dangerous polarization is taking on a punitive, overcontrolling and judgmental stance that does not promote reflection and positive personal change. The essential therapeutic challenge, then, is to hold the offender personally accountable for her violence, expect her to change her unacceptable behavior, and simultaneously validate the untenable choices she faced in her life.

The Therapeutic Environment

It is recognized in correctional and mental health circles that working with female clients in residential settings is particularly challenging. This difficulty stems, in part, from the challenge of managing the often emotionally charged relationships created by groups of troubled women living together (DeCou, 2001). It also reflects the inadequacy of programs designed specifically for men and used with women. Forensic mental health professionals must address the unique ways in which women express emotions and aggression toward each other.

The term *relational aggression* (Crick & Grotpeter, 1995), perhaps better called hostility, is used here to describe verbal but not physical aggression. These behaviors include using a social context to bully, exclude, spread rumors, and expose secrets, which compounds the emotional intensity of secure environments. The problem of holding aggressors of this type of covert hostility accountable is that it can provoke incidents of emotional outbursts, self-harm, and physical altercations. For example, Ella was told that an inmate she considered a close friend had informed a correctional officer that Ella had a weapon in her cell. Furious, she denied this and insisted that her cell be searched to prove she was telling the truth. Ella sought out mental health, presenting in tears of frustration at the lies being told about her, stating she wanted to retaliate and teach the woman a lesson to "keep my name out of her mouth." The experience of a friend spreading rumors about Ella was intolerable to her and impacted her sense of trust, identity, and control. Forensic mental health professionals will benefit from studying these forms of relational hostility. Interventions that assist women in managing conflict without resorting to covertly hostile tactics by using effective social skills will reduce the tension level in the program as a whole as well as for the mental health practitioner.

Women seek mental health contact more often and engage in more intense therapeutic relationships than men. The forensic mental health clinician is best served by adopting a relational approach to understanding and managing the intensity of the treatment environment and the therapeutic relationship (Jeffcote & Travers, 2004). Understanding that women may lack the interpersonal skills necessary to maintain the relationships that are so primary for them can guide the clinician in targeting social skills related to healthy relationships. This relational stance is a much-needed contextual framework for maintaining the therapeutic relationship and the therapeutic environment during times of emotional upheaval for clients. Frequent training and opportunities for case conferencing difficult treatment dilemmas is essential for team building and clinical skill development in these settings.

Personal Agency and the Change Process

Forensic mental health professionals are accustomed to receiving criticism that, by seeking to *understand the reasons* a client is violent, they are *excusing* the violent behavior. We believe, however, that understanding the causes of violence is essential in the process of identifying risk factors and working to combat them in the service of future violence prevention. When clinicians acknowledge a woman's history of victimization, this does not imply that she evades all responsibility for her own behavioral choices or is unable to regain personal power and agency (Denneby & Severs, 2003). Rather, when we acknowledge the profound influence of multiple oppressions, her "level of burden" (Covington, 2003) or identified problem areas, we can ally with the client in order to overcome the obstacles to nonviolence that have been put in her way. Women often express guilt about their violent behavior but lack the sense of personal agency to make different choices.

The therapeutic process involves helping the client examine the obstacles to nonviolence in her life and the impact of her actions on others as well as enhancing motivation for changing behaviors. We have found a number of therapeutic approaches helpful in addressing the process of change with women who have been violent. One of these models includes perspectives from narrative therapy that provide opportunities for women to recognize the impact of multiple influences on individual behavior. A theory of restraint (Jenkins, 2001) can be applied to working with women in identifying obstacles to nonviolence including sociocultural barriers, those related to women's gendered experiences, and developmental, family, and individual issues. Through this process of contextualizing women's violence, therapist and client work together to overcome these restraints, and the client's sense of personal agency in relation to recovering from trauma is enhanced (Sach, 2006). This approach allows the therapist to join with the client in recognizing and overcoming obstacles to changing violent behavior.

The second approach is the Transtheoretical Model (TTM), which conceptualizes readiness for change as a target of intervention (Prochaska, DiClemente, & Norcross, 1992). An individual is understood as moving between the precontemplative, contemplative, preparation, action, and maintenance stages of change. A study by Babcock, Canady, Senior, and Eckhardt (2003) found that the TTM applied to women court-ordered into batterer intervention programs. Although women were more likely than men to acknowledge their abusive behaviors, both men and women were in the precontemplative or contemplative stages of change upon entering treatment. (In the precontemplative stage of change, the individual does not yet identify a behavior problem; in the contemplative stage, the individual is aware of the problem and interested in change but lacks the skills and dedication to change.) These findings point to the need for interventions such as motivational interviewing (Miller & Rollnick, 2002) to target specific stages of change and assist clients in gaining the skills necessary to make durable behavior change.

The third approach that informs our work is dialectical behavior therapy (DBT) (Linehan, 1993). DBT has been adapted for a variety of inpatient, outpatient, and forensic settings and shown to reduce self-injury, suicidal, aggressive, or other impulsive behaviors of patients who present with complex diagnostic pictures. Designed for women who suffer from borderline personality disorder, DBT has also been found to be effective with women diagnosed with co-occurring disorders including PTSD and substance abuse (Kröger, Schweiger, Sipos, & Ruediger, 2006; Verheul et al., 2003). DBT has particular utility for addressing the affective dysregulation, or emotionally reactive volatility, implicated in both interpersonal violence and child abuse.

DBT is unique in that there are three essential components to the treatment model: individual therapy, skills group therapy, and consultation group supervision and training. DBT targets self-injurious, suicidal, or acting out/aggressive behaviors followed by therapy-interfering behavior, and quality-of-life issues. DBT skills include four basic skills modules: core mindfulness, emotional regulation, interpersonal effectiveness, and distress tolerance. Individual and group DBT therapists receive support, guidance, and supervision in the use of the model through group supervision and training.

We will illustrate these approaches through a discussion of clinical work with Charlene. For clients who live in socioeconomically disadvantaged communities where violence is common, there are often obstacles to recognizing and choosing nonaggressive responses to interpersonal conflict. Charlene had not previously considered giving up fighting and using drugs—survival mechanisms in her community. She appeared to be in the precontemplation stage of the change process, and motivational interviewing interventions were therefore tailored to capitalize on any ambivalence she had about using violent behavior. Charlene was encouraged to identify the negative consequences of her actions in the immediate community of the prison (such as isolation, chronic conflict with other women, and loss of privileges) and slowly began to reconsider her use of violence toward herself and others.

Charlene was sensitive to criticism and responded quickly and aggressively to perceived slights. Her behaviors, including substance abuse, self-harm, and violence toward others, could be understood as impulsive efforts to regulate her aroused emotional states. Treating her impulsivity began by targeting her destructive behaviors and developing a goal to reduce incidents of aggression. Charlene and her therapist used a DBT technique called behavioral chain analysis to painstakingly analyze episodes of aggressive behavior. Charlene learned to identify precipitants; environmental stressors; her thoughts and feelings before, during, and after her aggression; consequences; choice points in the sequences of events; and alternative behavioral options (Linehan, 1993). Once she had gained control over her behavioral choices, Charlene blamed others less often, expressing responsibility for her actions and pride in her mastery of a previously chaotic emotional life.

Addressing Charlene's entrenched antisocial beliefs and distorted thinking was a complicated task. As Charlene's sense of her own goals and preferred ways of living emerged, she became more aware of her personal agency and her accountability both to herself and to others. Her therapist asked Charlene to imagine the emotional impact on the officer who removed the noose from her neck after a suicide attempt. This exercise in empathy helped Charlene consider the effects of her behavior on others as an integral element of decision making. Ultimately, she sought out the officer to make amends.

Group Interventions

Group intervention is a forum for problem solving that meets the relational needs of women by providing an opportunity to develop prosocial, supportive relationships; gain a sense of belonging; and provide mutual aid. The facilitated social interactions in group offer women the best opportunity to acquire life skills for managing the everyday stresses of institutional living in order to prevent crisis reactions such as self-injury or impulsive violence. In addition, group treatment offers possibilities for immediate and direct peer feedback, particularly important in the process of understanding the consequences of and taking responsibility for one's actions. Social skill deficits can be addressed through the modeling, development, and practice of healthy peer relationships. Groups present opportunities to learn and practice prosocial skills, effective parenting strategies, techniques for the management of emotions and symptoms of mental illness, self-care, and coping skills (Pollock, 1998). The maladaptive and negative interpersonal patterns presented by many women who have been violent can be identified and addressed in the unique setting of a group.

Readiness for group can be a concern for high-risk/high-need, multiply diagnosed women. Often, women who have used violence struggle in early treatment to tolerate group environments because they have difficulty managing affect and interpersonal conflict. For these women, preparation for group treatment should include stabilization strategies such as medication management and individual therapy with a focus on enhancing commitment to treatment, understanding one's diagnosis, and acquiring distress tolerance and interpersonal effectiveness skills. Providing psychoeducation that addresses the nature of group therapy, including expectations and norms for participation, is also essential. For many women coping with behavioral instability, group therapy should be considered an adjunct to individual treatment.

Specific gender-responsive treatment curricula can be modified in terms of frequency of delivery and applicability to milieu development for varying levels of care. For example, in a residential treatment unit, dedicated unit staff can be trained in the treatment model, and services can be delivered with greater frequency. While evidence-based, gender-specific curricula targeting violent behavior do not exist for women, the following curricula are particularly effective in addressing related issues of trauma, substance abuse, and mental health and, in the authors' experience, are useful as part of a comprehensive treatment program for women who have used violence.

A treatment curriculum found to be effective for incarcerated women is *Seeking Safety* (Najavits, 2002). Used in either individual or group formats, *Seeking Safety* addresses safety from the use of substances, in relationships, and from extreme psychiatric symptoms or self-destructive behaviors. The curriculum includes topics in cognitive, behavioral, and interpersonal spheres, offering integrated treatment of trauma and substance abuse. Designed to enhance functioning, *Seeking Safety* has been found to reduce suicidal risk, social adjustment problems, depression, substance abuse, and trauma-related symptoms (Zlotnick, Najavits, & Rohsenow, 2003).

Another group curriculum is *Beyond Trauma: A Healing Journey for Women,* developed by Stephanie Covington (2003), that addresses the relationship between trauma and substance abuse and is based on the principles of relational therapy. It includes psychoeducation regarding trauma, coping skills, self-care, managing symptoms of trauma, and developing emotional health using cognitive behavioral techniques. *Helping Women Recover,* also developed by Stephanie Covington (1999), is a psychoeducational group curriculum for substance abuse based on clinical research that emphasizes the central role of connection and empowerment in women's recovery. The curriculum seeks to help women recognize cognitive distortions, identify and manage their emotions, and change their addictive behavior.

Issues of women's violence can arise in any of these group formats, and the dual status of survivor and perpetrator often permeates the work. Ella sits in the back of the group therapy room, her awkwardness apparent to all. This is her third session of a group focused on recovering from trauma, no more comfortable for her than the first. The discussion focuses on accepting responsibility for one's healing and self-care in the process of coming to terms with having been victimized. Suddenly, a young woman, Teresa, blurts out her regret for the injuries she inflicted on her 8-month-old baby in a methamphetamine-induced rage. The room goes silent. Some participants look to the therapist for help. Others make an attempt at offering comfort to Teresa. Then, Ella erupts at the therapist. "How could you let her in the group? She's a perpetrator!" Here is the point where the false dichotomy of the abuser–victim dynamic melds into the gray of real human experience. Teresa looks anxious, confused. With the curriculum effectively derailed, the group therapist guides the discussion toward a critical turn, where she encourages each group member to examine her dual status as victim and perpetrator.

Each group member is struggling with her own history and crime. Ella's overidentification with her childhood victimization interferes with her taking responsibility for her own perpetration of violence, which she justifies as protecting children. Teresa, on the other hand, herself a victim of molestation by her grandfather, has apparently disclosed her own abusive behavior in an attempt to make restitution and find absolution. The group argues vehemently. Teresa should be asked to leave, one member asserts. Another member counters that Teresa was acting out her own victimization and should not be held accountable for her violence. Ella refuses to let her off the hook, and the implications of Teresa remaining in the group begin to become clearer for the other group members. How can a woman be the victim of child abuse and commit such a horrific act against her own child? Is it possible to understand this abusive behavior? What would it mean to do so? The group therapist challenges the women to address the complexity of what it means to be both victim and perpetrator of violence and points out that Teresa has provided the group with a rich opportunity to explore the issues of responsibility, personal agency and change, self-acceptance, and restoration. Provided with a context for their struggle, the group members begin to accept each other and the therapeutic process. As this example illustrates, the group therapist must possess the sophistication and skill to facilitate the group's process through complicated territory.

The one treatment curriculum that has been modified to specifically address antisocial and aggressive behaviors of forensic patients is DBT (McCann, Ball, & Ivanoff, 2000). Based on a biosocial theory of antisocial personality disorder, an elevated role of the treatment team and group is promoted, and altered targets for stage one are established, including behaviors that harm others. An advanced forensic DBT group includes a crime review in which each group member presents a sequential behavioral analysis of her crime to the group. The group member is expected to present a description of the crime from her own as well as the victim's perspective, identify precipitating factors, address any possible strategies for repair and make amends, and develop a relapse prevention plan. The group then enacts a role play to enhance empathy for the victim. Although no research currently exists evaluating the effectiveness of the forensic DBT treatment model with women who have been violent, this approach appears to have significant potential given the DBT model's previous success in reducing women's self-injurious behaviors.

Community Reentry

The likelihood of female offenders having a history of repetitive physical and sexual traumas may adversely affect both their adjustment to incarceration and their postincarceration outcomes (Kubiak, 2004). Forensic mental health clinicians must consider discharge planning a relevant issue from the beginning of treatment in order to assist the client in gaining the skills necessary to live successfully in the community. Lack of occupational skills, transportation problems, the pressures of reuniting with families, child care responsibilities, poor social supports, and difficulty accessing needed medical, psychiatric, and mental health care all confound a woman's successful reentry. If she is facing more severe concerns such as custody problems, issues with child protective services, the loss of children through termination of parental rights, or returning to a violent relationship or a drug-involved community without proper supports, then her risk for recidivism will likely increase dramatically. A thorough discharge plan will address each of these factors as a potential risk for violence and recidivism.

Charlene identified goals to accomplish prior to her release to prepare her for reentry into the community. She planned to complete a residential substance abuse program and vocational training while continuing therapy. When she is released from the treatment facility, Charlene will return to the same community where opportunities are limited. She will be faced with the same peers she spent time with before her incarceration who are still involved in drugs and violence. Charlene has actively problem solved about how to use her strength and determination to choose prosocial alternatives and has expressed an interest in getting involved with a youth group to help other young people avoid the troubled path she took. With outpatient substance abuse and mental health treatment in place, and access to supportive social and financial resources, Charlene's chances of succeeding are vastly improved.

CONCLUSION

Women's violence is inextricably embedded in the ecology of women's lives, their social frame of reference, and their relationships (Gilfus, 2006). Women's roles as caregivers, mothers, wives, daughters, sisters, and lovers shape their opportunities and life choices. Women's violence diverges from male violence in the context of these unique gendered experiences and their investment in relationships, requiring gender-responsive assessment and intervention.

As this chapter has demonstrated, the small subset of female offenders who use violence is, of course, not homogeneous. It appears that most, although not all, women who use violence do so, at least in part, as a self-protective survival mechanism against either interpersonal or environmental threats. We have seen that young women are at greater risk, and perhaps those who turn to violence have experienced more serious violent victimization and have fewer social and economic resources than those who do not (Pollock & Davis, 2005). Due to the presence of risk factors and the absence of mediating protective factors, these women appear unable to develop adequate prosocial resilience. Thus, they resort to violence. For example, some women's violence has been understood as "violent resistance" (Muftic, Bouffard, & Bouffard, 2007, p. 766) in the context of intimate partner violence, which is distinguished from women's violence when they are the primary aggressor in IPV.

The relational and social context of women's offending includes the complicated relationship between women's experiences of violent victimization and their own aggressive and antisocial behavior (Chesney-Lind & Pasko, 2004; Gilfus, 2006). Like Ella, some women perceive violence as their only recourse to stop abuse. Charlene's violence was condoned by her peers and occurred in a community lacking conventional routes to educational, occupational, and financial success. And for others, such as Rita, mental health issues including trauma-related symptoms and addiction, coupled with extreme isolation, engender violence against abusive intimate partners.

Although there is no disagreement that women are far more often the victims of violence than the perpetrators, recent reports suggest that rates of violence committed by both girls and women have risen. However, policies throughout the justice system, in law enforcement and sentencing, that reflect the current national emphasis on punishment may be skewing the data (Steffensmeier & Schwartz, 2004). Although alterations in policy have undoubtedly brought more serious attention to incarcerated women in general, it is likely that the frequency and severity of women's violence has not significantly changed. The reality is that, while the incarceration rate for women increased seven-fold between 1980 and 2001 (Sokoloff, 2005), the numbers of women actually imprisoned for violent crimes fell from 49% of all female prisoners in 1979 to 34.8% in 2005 (Harrison & Beck, 2006; Steffensmeier & Schwartz, 2004).

Pollock and Davis (2005) argue that women are portrayed as more violent in research, literature, and the media despite the actual decrease in violent crime. This occurs through a variety of mechanisms, including the description of verbal aggression as violence and the downplaying of policy changes impacting arrest and conviction rates. In addition, the media sensationalizes atypical, extremely violent individual incidents (Belknap, 2007; van Wormer & Kaplan, 2006). These phenomena perpetuate a misunderstanding of women's criminal behavior, contribute to inadequate interventions, and, in effect, beget higher rates of women's violence.

The women who forensic mental health practitioners serve are at the center of these controversies. The response of law enforcement, the judiciary, and the human service community is impacted by how women's violence is understood. Forensic mental health practitioners, including clinicians, researchers, and administrators, will better serve the interests of public safety and the clients and families we treat, if we avail ourselves of a richer and more accurate understanding of the contextual phenomena of women's violence.

REFERENCES

Babcock, J. C., Canady, B. E., Senior, A., & Eckhardt, C. I. (2003). Applying the transtheoretical model to female and male perpetrators of intimate partner violence: Gender differences in stages of processes of change. *Violence and Victims, 20*(2), 235–250.

Banyard, V. L., Williams, L. M., & Siegel, J. A. (2003). The impact of complex trauma and depression on parenting: An exploration of mediating risk and protective factors. *Child Maltreatment, 8,* 334–349.

Battle, C. L., Zlotnick, C., Najavits, L. M., Gutierrez, M., & Winsor, C. (2002). Posttraumatic stress disorder and substance use disorder among incarcerated women. In P. Ouimette & P. J. Brown (Eds.), *Trauma and substance abuse: Causes, consequences, and treatment of comorbid disorders* (pp. 209–226).Washington, DC: American Psychological Association Press.

Belknap, J. (2007). *The invisible woman: Gender, crime, and justice* (3rd ed.). Belmont, CA: Thomson Wadsworth.

Bloom, B., Owen. B., & Covington, S. (2003). *Gender-responsive strategies: Research, practice, and guiding principles for women offenders.* Washington, DC: National Institute of Corrections, U.S. Department of Justice.

Brownstein, H. H., Spunt, B. J., Crimmins, S. M., Langley, S. C. (2006). Women who kill in drug market situations. In L. F. Alarid & P. Cromwell (Eds.), *In her own words: Women offenders' views on crime and victimization* (pp. 225–236). Los Angeles: Roxbury.

Catalano, S. M. (2006). *National Crime Victimization Survey: Criminal victimization, 2005.* Washington, DC: U.S. Department of Justice.

Chase, K. A., O'Farrell, T. J., Murphy, C. M., Fals-Stewart, W., & Murphy, M. (2003). Factors associated with partner violence among female alcoholic patients and their male partners. *Journal of Studies on Alcohol, 64,* 137–149.

Chesney-Lind, M., & Pasko, L. (2004). *The female offender: Girls, women, and crime* (2nd ed.). Thousand Oaks, CA: Sage.

Child Welfare Information Gateway. (2008). *Child abuse and neglect fatalities: Statistics and interventions.* U.S. Department of Health and Human Services, Administration for Children and Families. Retrieved November 30, 2008, from http://www.childwelfare.gov/pubs/factsheets/fatality.cfm

Cohen, L. R., Hien, D. A., & Batchelder, S. (2008). The impact of cumulative maternal trauma and diagnosis on parenting behavior. *Child Maltreatment, 13,* 27–38.

Coohey, C. (2004). Battered mothers who physically abuse their children. *Journal of Interpersonal Violence, 19,* 943–952.

Covington, S. (1999). *Helping women recover: A program for treating addiction.* San Francisco, CA: Jossey Bass.

Covington, S. (2003). *Beyond trauma: A healing journey for women.* Center City, MN: Hazelden.

Covington, S., & Bloom, B. (2006). Gender responsive treatment and services in correctional settings. *Women and Therapy, 29*(3/4), 9–33.

Crick, N. R., & Grotpeter, J. K. (1995). Relational aggression, gender, and social-psychological adjustment. *Child Development, 66,* 710–722.

Crimmins, S., Langley, S., Brownstein, H., & Spunt, B. J. (1997). Convicted women who have killed children: A self psychology perspective. *Journal of Interpersonal Violence, 12*(1), 49–60.

Das Dasgupta, S. (2001, February). Towards an understanding of women's use of non-lethal violence in intimate heterosexual relationships. Harrisburg: Pennsylvania Coalition Against Domestic Violence. VAWnet, *Applied Research Forum,* National Electronic Network on Violence Against Women. Retrieved September 18, 2007, from http://www.vawnet.org

DeCou, K. (2001). Incarcerated women and self-harm—Security or sanity. In G. Landsberg & A. Smiley (Eds.), *Forensic mental health: Working with offenders with mental illness* (pp. 36-1–36-15). Kingston, NJ: Civic Research Press.

DeCou, K., & Van Wright, S. (2002). A gender-specific intervention model for incarcerated women: Women's V.O.I.C.E.S. (Validation Opportunity Inspiration Communication Empowerment Safety). In G. Landsberg, M. Rock, L.K.W. Berg, & A. Smiley (Eds.), *Serving mentally ill offenders: Challenges and opportunities for mental health professionals* (pp. 172–190). New York: Springer Publishing.

Denneby, G., & Severs, M. (2003). Working with women who abuse. In K. McMaster & A. Wells (Eds.), *Innovative approaches to stopping family violence* (pp. 37–56). Wellington, New Zealand: Steele Roberts.

de Vogel, V., & de Ruiter, C. (2005). The HCR-20 in personality disordered female offenders: A comparison with a matched sample of males. *Clinical Psychology and Psychotherapy, 12,* 226–240.

Dobash, R. P., & Dobash, R. E. (2004). Women's violence to men in intimate relationships: Working on a puzzle. *British Journal of Criminology, 44*(3), 324–349.

Douglas, K. S., Webster, C. D., Hart, S. D., Eaves, D., & Ogloff, J.R.P. (2001). *HCR-20 violence risk management companion guide.* Burnaby, Canada: Mental Health, Law, and Policy Institute, Simon Fraser University.

Eronen, M. (1995). Mental disorders and homicidal behavior in female subjects. *American Journal of Psychiatry, 152*(8), 1216–1219.

Feerick, M., Haugaard, J., & Hien, D. (2002) Childhood maltreatment and adulthood violence: The contribution of attachment and drug abuse. *Child Maltreatment, 2,* 226–240.

Free, M. (2003). *Racial issues in criminal justice: The case of African Americans.* Westport, CT: Praeger.

Gilfus, M. (2002, December). Women's experiences of abuse as a risk factor for incarceration. Harrisburg: Pennsylvania Coalition Against Domestic Violence. VAWnet,

Applied Research Forum, National Electronic Network on Violence Against Women. Retrieved August 25, 2007, from http://www.vawnet.org

Gilfus, M. (2006). From victims to survivors to offenders: Women's routes of entry and immersion into street crime. In L. F. Alarid & P. Cromwell (Eds.), *In her own words: Women offenders' views on crime and victimization* (pp. 5–14). Los Angeles: Roxbury.

Greenfeld, L. A., & Snell, T. L. (1999). *Women offenders*. Bureau of Justice Statistics Special Report. Washington DC: U.S. Department of Justice.

Greenfeld, L. A., & Snell, T. L. (2000). About female offenders. *Women Police, 34*(1), 43–44.

Hamberger, K., & Potente, T. (1994). Counseling heterosexual women arrested for domestic violence: Implications for theory and practice. *Violence & Victims, 9*(2), 125–137.

Hamlett, N. (1998). *Women who abuse in intimate relationships (a manual)*. Minneapolis, MN: Domestic Abuse Project.

Hare, R. D. (1991). *The Hare Psychopathy Checklist–Revised (PCL-R)*. Toronto, Canada: Multi-Health Systems.

Harris, M., & Fallot, R. D. (2001). *Using trauma theory to design service systems*. San Francisco, CA: Jossey-Bass.

Harrison, P. M., & Beck, A. J. (2006). *Prisoners in 2005*. Washington, DC: U.S. Department of Justice, Bureau of Justice Statistics.

Hattendorf, J., Ottens, A. J., & Lomax, R. G. (1999). Type and severity of abuse and posttraumatic stress disorder symptoms reported by women who killed abusive partners. *Violence Against Women, 5*(3), 292–312.

Henning, K., Jones, A., & Holdford, R. (2003). Treatment needs of women arrested for domestic violence: A comparison with male offenders. *Journal of Interpersonal Violence, 18*(8), 839–856.

Herivel, T., and Wright, P. (Eds.). (2003). *Prison nation: The warehousing of America's poor*. New York: Routledge.

Hirschinger, N. B., Grisso, J. A., Wallace, D. B., McCollum, K. F., Schwarz, D. F., Sammel, M. D., et al. (2003). A case-control study of female-to-female nonintimate violence in an urban area. *American Journal of Public Health, 93*(7), 1098–1103.

Jeffcote, N., & Travers, R. (2004). Thinking about the needs of women in secure settings. In N. Jeffcote & T. Watson (Eds.), *Working therapeutically with women in secure mental health settings* (pp. 19–30). New York: Jessica Kingsley Publishers.

Jenkins, A. (2001). *Invitations to responsibility: The therapeutic engagement of men who are violent and abusive*. Adelaide, Australia: Dulwich Centre.

Jordan, J., & Hartling, L. (2002). New developments in relational-cultural theory. In M. Ballou & L. Brown (Eds.), *Rethinking mental health and disorder: Feminist perspectives* (pp. 48–70). New York: Guilford Press.

Kröger, C., Schweiger, U., Sipos, V., & Ruediger, A. (2006). Effectiveness of dialectical behavior therapy for borderline personality disorder in an inpatient setting. *Behavior Research and Therapy, 44*(8), 1211–1217.

Kubiak, S. P. (2004). The effects of PTSD on treatment adherence, drug relapse, and criminal recidivism in a sample of incarcerated men and women. *Research on Social Work Practice, 14*(6), 424–433.

Leenaars, P.E.M. (2005). Differences between violent male and violent female forensic psychiatric outpatients: Consequences for treatment. *Psychology, Crime & Law, 11*(4), 445–455.

Leisring, P. A., Dowd, L., & Rosenbaum, A. (2003). Treatment of partner aggressive women. In D. Dutton & D. Sonkin (Eds.), *Intimate violence: Contemporary treatment innovations* (pp. 257–277). New York: Haworth Maltreatment & Trauma Press.

Linehan, M. M. (1993). *Cognitive-behavioral treatment of borderline personality disorder.* New York: Guilford Press.

Maden, T. (2004). Women and risk. In N. Jeffcote & T. Watson (Eds.), *Working therapeutically with women in secure mental health settings* (pp. 66–77). New York: Jessica Kingsley Publishers.

Marcus-Mendoza, S., & Wright, E. (2004). Decontextualizing female criminality: Treating abused women in prison in the United States. *Feminism & Psychology, 14,* 250–255.

Margolis, L., & Leeder, E. (1995). Violence at the door: Treatment of lesbian batterers. *Violence Against Women, 1*(2), 139–157.

McCann, R., Ball, E., & Ivanoff A. (2000). DBT with an inpatient forensic population: The CMHIP forensic model. *Cognitive and Behavioral Practice, 7,* 447–456.

McClennen J. C. (2005). Domestic violence between same-gender-partners: Recent findings and future research. *Journal of Interpersonal Violence, 20*(2), 149–154.

Meichenbaum, D. (2001). *Treatment of individuals with anger control problems and aggressive behaviors: A clinical handbook.* Clearwater, FL: Institute Press.

Miller, J. B. (1986). *Toward a new psychology of women.* Boston: Beacon Press.

Miller, D. H., Greene, K., Causby, V., White, B. W., & Lockhart, L. L. (2001). Domestic violence in lesbian relationships. *Women and Therapy, 23*(3), 107–127.

Miller, W., & Rollnick, S. (2002). *Motivational interviewing: Preparing people to change addictive behavior* (2nd ed.). New York: Guilford Press.

Monahan, J. (2002). The MacArthur studies of violence risk. *Criminal Behaviour and Mental Health, 12,* S67–S72.

Monahan, J., Steadman, H. J., Silver, E., Applebaum, P. S., Robbins, P. C., Mulvey, E. P., et al. (2001). *Rethinking risk assessment: The MacArthur study of mental disorder and violence.* New York: Oxford University Press.

Muftic, L. R., Bouffard, J. A., & Bouffard, L. A. (2007). An exploratory study of women arrested for intimate partner violence: Violent women or violent resistance? *Journal of Interpersonal Violence, 22,* 753–774.

Mullings, J. L., Pollock, J. M., & Crouch, B. M. (2002). Drugs and criminality: Results from the Texas women inmates study. *Women & Criminal Justice, 13*(4), 69–97.

Najavits, L. M. (2002). *Seeking safety: A treatment manual for PTSD and substance abuse.* New York: Guilford Press.

O'Keefe, M. (1997). Incarcerated battered women: A comparison of battered women who killed their abuser and those incarcerated for other offenses. *Journal of Family Violence, 12*(1), 1–19.

Oliver, B. E. (2007). Preventing female-perpetrated sexual abuse. *Trauma, Violence, & Abuse, 8*(1), 19–32.

Peterman, L. M., & Dixon, C. G. (2003). Domestic violence between same-sex partners: Implications for counseling. Journal *of Counseling and Development, 81*(1), 40–47.

Pollock, J. (1998). *Counseling women in prison.* Thousand Oaks, CA: Sage.
Pollock, J. M., & Davis, S. M. (2005). The continuing myth of the violent female offender. *Criminal Justice Review, 30*(1), 5–29.
Pollock, J. M., Mullings, J. L., & Crouch, B. M. (2006). Violent women: Findings from the Texas women inmates study. *Journal of Interpersonal Violence, 21,* 485–502.
Prochaska, J. O., DiClemente, C. C., & Norcross, J. C. (1992). In search of how people change: Applications to addictive behavior. *American Psychologist, 47,* 1102–1114.
Rennison, C. M. (2001). *Criminal victimization 2000: Changes 1999–2000 with trends 1993–2000.* Bureau of Justice Statistics, National Crime Victimization Survey. Washington, DC: U.S. Department of Justice.
Rennison, C. M. (2003). *Intimate partner violence, 1993–2001.* Bureau of Justice Statistics Crime Data Brief. Washington, DC: U.S. Department of Justice.
Renzetti, C. M. (1992). *Violent betrayal: Partner abuse in lesbian relationships.* Newbury Park, CA: Sage.
Ristock, J. L. (2003). Exploring dynamics of abusive lesbian relationships: Preliminary analysis of a multisite, qualitative study 1. *American Journal of Community Psychology, 31*(3/4), 329.
Robbins, P. C., Monahan, J., & Silver, J. (2003). Mental disorder, violence, and gender. *Law and Human Behavior, 27*(6), 561–571.
Sach, J. (2006). Conversations in groups with women about their experiences of using anger, abuse and violence. *International Journal of Narrative Therapy and Community Work, 4,* 32–44.
Salekin, R. T., Rogers, R., & Sewell, K. W. (1997). Construct validity of psychopathy in a female offender sample: A multitrait-multimethod evaluation. *Journal of Abnormal Psychology, 106*(4), 576–585.
Siegel, J. A. (2000). Aggressive behavior among women sexually abused as children. *Violence and Victims, 15*(3), 235–255.
Skeem, J., Schubert, C., Stowman, S., Beeson, S., Mulvey, E., Gardner, W., et al. (2005). Gender and risk assessment accuracy: Underestimating women's violence potential. *Law and Human Behavior, 29*(2), 173–186.
Sokoloff, N. J. (2005). Women prisoners at the dawn of the 21st century. *Women & Criminal Justice, 16*(1/2), 127–137.
Steffensmeier, D., & Schwartz, J. (2004). Trends in female crime: Is crime still a man's world? In B. Raffel Price & N. J. Sokoloff (Eds.), *The criminal justice system and women: Offenders, prisoners, victims and workers* (3rd ed., pp. 95–111). New York: McGraw-Hill.
Strand, S., & Belfrage, H. (2001). Comparison of HCR-20 scores in violent mentally disordered men and women: Gender differences and similarities. *Psychology, Crime & Law, 7,* 71–79.
Stuart, G. L., Moore, T. M., Coop, G. K., Ramsey, S. E., & Kahler, C. W. (2006). Psychopathology in women arrested for domestic violence. *Journal of Interpersonal Violence, 21*(3), 376–389.
Swan, S. C., & Snow, D. L. (2002). A typology of women's use of violence in intimate relationships. *Violence Against Women, 8,* 286–319.
Teasdale, B., Silver, E., & Monahan, J. (2006). Gender, threat/control-override delusions and violence. *Law and Human Behavior, 30,* 649–658.

Travis, J., & Waul, M. (Eds.). (2003). *Prisoners once removed: The impact of incarceration and reentry on children, families, and communities.* Washington, DC: Urban Institute Press.

Uniform Crime Reports. (2002). Retrieved August 23, 2007, from http://www.fbi.gov/ucr.html

Uniform Crime Reports. (2004). Retrieved August 23, 2007, from http://www.fbi.gov/ucr.html

U.S. Department of Health and Human Services. (2007). *Child maltreatment, 2005.* Administration for Children and Families. Retrieved December 16, 2007, from http://www.acf.hhs.gov/programs/cb/pubs/cm05

van Wormer, K., & Kaplan, L. E. (2006). Results of a national survey of wardens in women's prisons: The case for gender specific treatment. *Women & Therapy, 29*(1/2), 133–151.

Verheul, R., Van Den Bosch, L.M.C., Koeter, M.W.J., De Ridder, M.A.J., Stijnen, T., & Van Den Brink, W. (2003). Dialectical behavior therapy for women with borderline personality disorder, 12-month, randomized clinical trial in The Netherlands. *British Journal of Psychiatry, 182,* 135–140.

Vitale, J. E., & Newman, J. P. (2001). Using the Psychopathy Checklist–Revised with female samples: Reliability, validity, and implications for clinical utility. *Clinical Psychology: Science and Practice, 8*(1), 117–132.

Vitale, J. E., Smith, S. S., Brinkley, C. A., & Newman, J. P. (2002). The reliability and validity of the Psychopathy Checklist–Revised in a sample of female offenders. *Criminal Justice and Behavior, 29*(2), 202–231.

Warren, J. I., South, S. C., Burnette, M. L., Rogers, A., Friend, R., Bale, R., et al. (2005). Understanding the risk factors for violence and criminality in women: The concurrent validity of the PCL-R and HCR-20. *International Journal of Law and Psychiatry, 28,* 269–289.

Webster, C. D., Douglas, K. S., Eaves, D., & Hart, S. D. (1997). *HCR-20 assessing risk for violence* (version 2). Burnaby, Canada: Mental Health, Law, and Policy Institute, Simon Fraser University.

Weizmann-Henelius, G., Viemero, V., & Eronen, M. (2004). Psychological risk markers in violent female behavior. *International Journal of Forensic Mental Health, 3*(2), 185–196.

West, C. (2004). Leaving a second closet: Outing partner violence in same-sex couples. In B. Raffel Price & N. J. Sokoloff (Eds.), *The criminal justice system and women: Offenders, prisoners, victims and Workers* (3rd ed., pp. 375–389). New York: McGraw-Hill.

Zlotnick, C. (1997). Posttraumatic stress disorder (PTSD), PTSD comorbidity, and childhood abuse among incarcerated women. *Journal of Nervous and Mental Disease, 185*(12), 761–763.

Zlotnick, C., Najavits, L. M., & Rohsenow, D. J. (2003). A cognitive-behavioral treatment for incarcerated women with substance use disorder and posttraumatic stress disorder: Findings from a pilot study. *Journal of Substance Abuse Treatment, 25,* 99–105.

5 Intimate Partner Violence

GRETCHEN E. ELY AND CHRIS FLAHERTY

Violence between intimate partners in the United States is a problem of epidemic proportions and one of serious public health concern. The consequences of intimate partner violence (IPV) for victims, families, and society are numerous. From an economic standpoint alone, it has been conservatively estimated that nonlethal IPV results in financial losses of approximately $150 million per year (Greenfield et al., cited in Arias, Dankwort, Douglas, Dutton, & Stein, 2002). Of the $150 million spent annually, medical expenses account for approximately 40% of these costs, property loss for another 44%, and lost pay for the remainder (Arias et al., 2002). Estimates from the Centers for Disease Control (2003) indicate even higher costs, at $4.1 billion annually in health and mental health expenditures and $1.8 billion in lost productivity. These increased medical costs are most often incurred by female victims of partner violence; women who are victims of partner violence report 60% more physical and mental health problems compared to women who are not involved in partner violence (Campbell et al., 2002). Furthermore, women require more medical attention, take more time off from work, and spend more days in bed than men as a result of partner violence victimization (Arias et al., 2002). Additionally, women involved in partner violence are more likely than men to be hospitalized, raped, injured, stalked, coerced, and murdered (Westbrook, 2007).

Despite these documented detrimental consequences and the fact that IPV occurs in all societies and varies by culture, IPV is continually ignored, trivialized, and rationalized by professionals, institutions, and society, severely inhibiting prevention efforts (Sharma, 1997).

INCIDENCE RATES

Current estimates of the rates of IPV indicate that 1.5 million women are sexually or physically assaulted by an intimate partner each year in the United States (Tjaden & Thoennes, 1998). The highest rates of intimate partner violence occur among women between ages 16 and 24; almost 1 in every 50 women in this age group will be victimized (the 1998 National Crime Victimization Survey, cited in Waul, 2000). In a study of over 11,000 heterosexual young adults ages 18 to 28, 24% reported violence in their intimate relationships, and half of those who experienced violence were involved in relationships that were identified as mutually or reciprocally violent (Whitaker, Haileyesus, Swahn, & Saltzman, 2007). For some, abuse is primarily psychological, as evidenced by results from a study indicating that major verbal aggression from a partner was reported by 13.5% of female members of a managed care organization in New Mexico (Tollestrup et al., 1999). Almost 7% of respondents in this same study reported also experiencing physical aggression from a partner.

It has been reported that approximately 834,700 men are physically assaulted and/or raped by intimate partners in the United States every year (Tjaden & Thoennes, 1998). However, not only is the victimization rate among men significantly lower than among women, but the differences between women's rates of physical and/or sexual assault victimization becomes greater as the severity of assault increases (Tjaden & Thoennes, 1998).

Due to the facts that no national database for tracking annual rates of partner violence exists and studies of partner violence often contain methodological problems, accurate prevalence rates are difficult to discern. Some studies include both members of a dyad in their study samples, thus potentially doubling the data when respondents are asked about the presence of abuse in their relationships (Burke & Follingstad, 1999). Many studies do not separate out victims from perpetrators, which is necessary to accurately estimate the presence of abuse and to determine the use of force in self-defense (Burke & Follingstad, 1999).

EFFECTS OF IPV

Unfortunately, IPV is a problem that is perpetuated by our society. A lack of policy responses, societal norms that encourage ignoring and/or accepting IPV, and rigid gender role expectations promote a cultural environment that perpetuates IPV (Mears, 2003). The effects of such violence are staggering and may continue on long after the IPV ceases. For example, women who were involved in partner violence during their transition to adulthood were found to be more likely to be unemployed up to 5 years after exiting the public welfare system (Lindhorst, Oxford, & Gillmore, 2007).

Health Effects

Partner violence puts women at risk for the negative health outcomes of physical injury, according to the World Health Organization (Turmen, 1998). Women exposed to IPV have been found to engage in less-healthy behaviors and need more health services compared to women not exposed to IPV (Tomasulo & McNamara, 2007). Women across cultures report illnesses, bruises, lesions, loss of teeth, fatigue, loss of sleep, unwanted pregnancy, shortened life expectancy, and exposure to and contraction of sexually transmitted diseases, especially HIV/AIDS associated with exposure to IPV (Diaz-Olavarrieta, Paz, De la Cadena, & Campbell, 2001; Ellsberg, Caldera, Herrera, Winkvist, & Kullgren, 1999; Fischbach & Herbert, 1997; Glantz, Halperin, & Hunt, 1998; Haniff, 1998).

Some of the most serious health effects of partner violence surround the relationships between partner violence and pregnancy (Ely, Dulmus, & Wodarski, 2004) and other reproductive health problems. Many studies indicate that IPV is occurring in 3% to 13% of pregnant women (Campbell, 2002). Pregnant women are found to be at higher risk for involvement in IPV, especially IPV ending in homicide (Shadigian & Bauer, 2004), as IPV frequently escalates during pregnancy with serious consequences to mother and baby, including death to both parties (Anderson, Marshak, & Hebbeler, 2002). One study found that the risk of a pregnant woman being the victim of murder or attempted murder is tripled in women who are also involved in IPV (McFarlane, Campbell, Sharps, & Watson, 2002). The existence of pregnancy has also been found to increase the risk of assault for Spanish-speaking women in the United States (Wiist & McFarlane, 1998), Hispanic women (Jasinski & Kantor, 2001), and Latina migrant farm workers (Van Hightower, Gorton, & DeMoss, 2000).

A recent comprehensive review of the sexual health literature from 1966 to 2006 revealed that IPV was associated with lack of condom use, sexual risk taking, multiple sexual partners, sexual dysfunction, unplanned pregnancy, painful menses, sexual pain, and sexually transmitted infections in women, demonstrating the serious and long-standing reproductive health effects experienced by female victims of IPV (Coker, 2007). Results from another study of Black, Hispanic, and White women indicate that 68% of physically abused women also reported sexual assault by an intimate partner, 15% attributed a sexually transmitted disease to the sexual assault, and 20% reported a rape-related pregnancy (McFarlane et al., 2005). A review of 35 studies examining the relationship between HIV/AIDS and IPV in women found that IPV puts women at a significant disadvantage related to requesting safer sex practices, and HIV-positive women experience IPV that is more frequent and more severe (Gielen et al., 2007).

Mental Health Effects

The World Health Organization indicates that women are at risk internationally for mental health problems related to IPV (Turmen, 1998). In the United States and across cultures, women exposed to IPV suffer from high rates of emotional abuse leading to problems such as mental harm, posttraumatic stress disorder (PTSD), depression and other mental disorders, emotional distress, sleeping and eating disorders, general fear, increased alcohol use, suicide and suicide attempts, and other psychological effects and trauma (Diaz-Olavarrieta et al., 2001; Ellsberg et al., 1999; Fischbach & Herbert, 1997; Glantz et al., 1998; Haniff, 1998; Johnson, Palmeiri, Jackson, & Hobfall, 2007; Mears, 2003; O'Leary, 2000; Thompson, Kaslow, & Kingree, 2002). Exposure to IPV was significantly associated with the adoption of a negative psychological perspective and problems with mental health in a sample of 148 rural women seeking services in a community health center (Tomasulo & McNamara, 2007).

Women who report sexual abuse in an intimate relationship are also more likely to have higher PTSD scores compared to nonabused women (McFarlane et al., 2005). In a recent study examining the long-term effects of IPV on women who suffer from PTSD, findings indicate that PTSD symptoms in victims are associated with ongoing emotional resource losses that continue after involvement in IPV has ceased (Johnson et al., 2007).

FACTORS ASSOCIATED WITH IPV INVOLVEMENT

Factors such as stressful life events, family conflicts, cultural norms of male dominance, and families being socialized toward violence have been found to contribute to involvement in IPV (Sharma, 1997; Straus & Gelles, 1990; Straus & Smith, 1990). Women in focus groups who had been free of partner violence for at least 6 months indicated that once partner violence began, it escalated over time (Short et al., 2000), supporting the assertion that prior involvement in IPV is a risk factor for future involvement in IPV.

In a recent study comparing male nondrinkers to males who use alcohol at various levels, findings indicate that those engaged in heavy drinking within the past 30 days are six times more likely to report involvement in a mutually violent intimate relationship (Cunradi, 2007). Results from this same study also indicate that male drinkers who are not categorized as heavy drinkers are still two to three times more likely to report involvement in mutually violent relationships. Female subjects in this study who were characterized as heavy drinkers were also six times more likely to report involvement in IPV compared to nondrinkers. Results from other studies support the association between substance use and IPV, as individuals in substance abuse treatment programs have been found to be at high risk for involvement in IPV (Chermack, Fuller, & Blow, 2000). Thus, it is suggested that batterer programs might be more effective if offered in conjunction with substance abuse programs (Stuart, Moore, Ramsey, & Kahler, 2003), as results from another study revealed that unsuccessful participants of a court referred batterer program were more likely to be using alcohol at the time of arrest compared to participants who successfully completed the program (Yarbrough & Blanton, 2000).

Factors outside of one's personal control have been associated with IPV involvement in many study results. For instance, almost two-thirds (62%) of women in one study who reported experiencing child abuse also reported IPV as an adult, compared to 25% of adults who experienced violence and had no history of child abuse (Waul, 2000). It is also documented that rates of partner violence are higher in women who receive public welfare assistance (Tolman & Raphael, 2000). Living conditions have also been found to play a role in involvement in IPV, as findings from a recent study indicate that mutually violent relationships were more likely to occur in neighborhoods associated with high levels of crime and other types of social disorder (Cunradi, 2007).

The factors that lead men to perpetrate partner violence remain unclear. Men in one study reported a tendency to minimize conflict and blame the partner when self-describing their recent involvement in partner violence (Scott & Straus, 2007). Batterers in another study with a higher propensity toward physical assault also reported difficulty identifying with the perspectives of others and difficulty dealing with the negative emotions of others, indicating that lack of empathy is associated with battering behavior in males (Covell, Huss, & Langhinrichsen-Rohling, 2007). Other recent research results indicate that antisocial batterers possess different personality characteristics compared to antisocial males with criminal backgrounds who have not been involved in partner violence (Swogger, Walsh, & Kosson, 2007). Results from another study indicate that problem gambling by the male partner was also associated with involvement in IPV (Mulleman, DenOtter, Wadman, Tran, & Anderson, 2001).

IPV IN UNDERRECOGNIZED POPULATIONS

Although a significant body of literature has begun to develop related to IPV in heterosexual couples, research is lacking on how IPV manifests in the lesbian, gay, bisexual, and transgender (LGBT) community. Furthermore, populations in these communities are marginalized and often underrecognized by those providing domestic violence assistance and those doing research in this area.

Despite this lack of attention, the literature available does indicate that IPV is a significant problem in the LGBT community. Study results indicate that IPV in the LGBT community is prominent, as rates are as high or higher than rates in heterosexual women (Burke & Follingstad, 1999; Greenwood et al., 2002; Tjaden & Thoennes, 2000). In a study of 58 LGBT clients receiving counseling services for IPV, 41% of respondents report being forced by a partner to have sex, and 28% report feeling it was unsafe to request safer sex practices; 19% reported sexual abuse, 21% report physical abuse, and 32% report verbal abuse as a result of requesting safer sex practices (Heintz & Melendez, 2006). Results from another study indicate that abuse tactics of female perpetrators of IPV in same-sex relationships differ very little from abuse tactics of male perpetrators, while victims of such abuse are often discouraged from applying for legal abuse protections, even in model programs (Brasile, 2004). Results such as these clearly indicate a need to acknowledge and address IPV in the LGBT community as well as a need to train social workers to provide culturally competent services to this population.

The relationship between homelessness and IPV is also understudied. Results from one study indicate that IPV in homeless adults is so prevalent that it seems a normative consequence of homelessness (Boris, Heller, Shepard, & Zeanah, 2002). In a study of 60 young adults ages 18 to 21 residing in an urban homeless shelter, 70% reported a history of physical partner violence (Boris et al., 2002). Although it is difficult to access homeless populations for research, results from this study indicate that IPV is prevalent in this population, and more research needs to be developed so that effective interventions may be implemented.

Immigrant women are also an underrecognized population related to IPV. Women who immigrate to the United States may experience IPV in unique ways, and cultural factors that contribute to IPV in their home countries may follow them even after they settle in the United States (Ely, 2004). One particularly important factor for social workers to consider when working with immigrant women involved in IPV is their immigration status. Immigrant women often enter the United States as dependents of a male, and attempts to separate a woman from a husband and his family may result in losing the ability to remain in the United States (Merchant, 2000). Oppressive immigration laws make it difficult, if not impossible, for dependent immigrant women to file charges against abusive partners without risk to themselves of deportation (Dasgupta, 2000; Kurien, 2001). Language barriers in law enforcement and social service provisions further decrease the likelihood that immigrant women will pursue relief from a domestically abusive situation (Dasgupta, 2000). Yoshihama (2000) indicates that women of Japanese decent in the United States report feeling pressured to endure violence because of cultural misunderstandings and lack of available services for non-English-speaking women. South Asian immigrant women report that they are afraid to seek domestic violence services from community agencies or the criminal justice system (Dasgupta, 2000). It is also important to note that IPV may manifest itself in distinctive ways that are unfamiliar to social workers in the United States. Such unique types of violence include honor killings, dowry killings, woman burning, nonconsensual sex-selection abortions, public beatings, public verbal abuse, acid throwing and stoning, lack of access to education and medical care, forced prostitution, genital mutilation, and bonded labor (Faquir, 2001; Singh & Unnithan, 1999; U.S. Government Printing Office, 2000; Vindhya, 2000).

INTERVENTIONS FOR VICTIMS

Assessment and Screening

An intervention approach that might be most effective for preventing injuries and further involvement in IPV is having medical professionals screen for the problem in their patients. In fact, abuse screening may be the most effective intervention available for preventing IPV in pregnant women (McFarlane, Soeken, & Wiist, 2000). Medical professionals have a unique opportunity to intervene and prevent future involvement in IPV in patients presenting in their offices as a result of physical involvement in IPV (Mears, 2003). Doctors and other medical professionals should do all they can to identify IPV and make referrals to social agencies, where patients can get help for IPV (Rhodes & Levinson, 2003). Helping professionals in medical settings should make a point to ask patients about abuse, provide validating messages when the abuse is revealed, acknowledge that IPV is wrong, confirm patients' self-worth, and document the symptoms and disclosures of abuse (Gerbert et al., 2002). Universal screening for IPV is recommended by medical professionals in both urban and rural health care settings (Bauer & Shadigian, 2002; Ulbrich & Stockdale, 2002), and referral information and patient handouts are seen as valuable tools for use by physicians who identify IPV in their patients (Taylor et al., 2007).

Screening for IPV can and should be implemented in a variety of health care settings, including gynecology offices, primary care offices, and emergency settings, as well as in pediatric offices, because it has been documented that women with children are frequently victims of IPV (Phelan, 2007). It is also recommended that screening for partner violence occur throughout all stages of cases involved in the child welfare system (Hazen et al., 2007).

Screening is also recommended for pregnant women, and it is suggested that it should occur throughout the pregnancy, not simply at one point in time (Anderson et al., 2002) in order to avert lethal consequences (McFarlane et al., 2000). It is recommended that assessment for IPV in pregnant women should be conducted at the first prenatal visit, once during each trimester, and at delivery, because patients need to be given time to build trust in their providers as well as given many opportunities to disclose abuse in a supportive setting (Anderson et al., 2002).

IPV screenings also should be a part of routine medical appointments when assessing for other common conditions such as hypertension, diabetes, and drug/alcohol use (Johnson, Haider, Ellis, Hay, & Lindow, 2003). In one study where IPV screening was implemented in a family planning clinic, 11.5% of the participants screened reported involvement in IPV (Shattuck, 2002). This screening gave the clinic staff an opportunity to intervene when such an opportunity had not been present before the implementation of the screening process. Results from another emergency room study of 4,641 women indicate that routine screening for IPV in emergency rooms increases the likelihood that women who are involved in IPV will get needed interventions (Glass, Dearwater, & Campbell, 2001).

The types of instruments used for screening and the environment in which the screening takes place are also important components of effective assessment of IPV. The use of a sensitive, efficient, and easy-to-administer screening tool is a key component to identifying IPV in medical patients, while also demonstrating to the patient the importance of intervening when one is experiencing IPV (Phelan, 2007). Health care professionals recommend that written questionnaires and computer-based questionnaires are preferable methods of screening in health settings, because they are confidential, easy to administer, and can be filled out by patients while they are waiting to see their provider (Phelan, 2007). Rapid assessment instruments, such as the Partner Violence Screen (PVS), are recommended for use during emergency room visits; it has been documented that the PVS can help detect IPV 65% to 71% of the time (Feldhaus et al., 1997). Thus, use of screening instruments such as the PVS can detect a large number of women suffering from IPV and give professionals a chance to prevent many incidences of revictimization (Feldhaus et al., 1997). Others recommend the 29-item Abuse Behavior Inventory developed by Shepard and Campbell (1992) as an effective instrument for assessing for both verbal and physical abuse in medical patients (Zink, Klesges, Levin, & Putnam, 2007).

While choosing the appropriate instrument for screening has been identified as important, social workers also must consider how the person screening for IPV and where the screening takes place may impact the screening process. Screenings should be conducted by a professional who is educated about the dynamics of IPV and who has been taught how to use the screening instrument (Shadigian & Bauer, 2004). Results from a study of 140 female victims of IPV indicate that women prefer to be screened by another woman who is the same race, age 30 to 50 years old, and without anyone else present in the room (Thackerary, Seltzner,

Downs, & Miller,, 2007). Such results point to the impact that screener competence, characteristics, and environment can have on the comfort level of those disclosing IPV (Thackerary et al., 2007). Thus, social workers screening for IPV should be familiar with the characteristics that improve victim comfort and should strive to provide multiple opportunities for disclosure in a safe, respectful, and culturally competent manner (Thackerary et al., 2007).

Shelter, Counseling, and Other Community Services

Results of an analysis of 22 studies on the topic of preventing IPV indicate that women who spend at least one night in a shelter and receive counseling and other advocacy services experience a decrease in rates of IPV (Wathen & MacMillan, 2003). In another study, counseling reportedly reduced the severity of involvement in IPV across time for a group of Hispanic women who were pregnant at the initial time of intervention (McFarlane et al., 2000). In another study of 81 women who received case management and counseling services at a domestic violence shelter, results indicate that, after three contacts with the shelter services, victims reported that incidences of IPV had decreased (McNamara, Ertl, Marsh, & Walker, 1997). In another study of a domestic violence program in an urban Indian health center, intervention approaches that were most successful at preventing further involvement in IPV were identified as home visits combined with a domestic violence support group that incorporated values from the native Indian culture (Norton & Manson, 1997).

Orders of Protection

Some controversy surrounds whether orders of protection are successful at preventing further incidences of IPV. If a defendant will abide by an order of protection, the victim can be provided safety and resources; however, if the defendant ignores the order, the only avenue for the victim is to have the defendant arrested for contempt and put back into the court system. Research suggests, however, that orders of protection do serve to reduce incidents of IPV in some cases (McFarlane, Malecha, et al., 2002).

According to research on protection order petitioners, women who sought court intervention had typically experienced severe abuse over an extended period of time and were seeking protection orders to interrupt the abuse (Waul, 2000). Based on this knowledge, many courts are offering extra assistance to those requesting orders of protection to prevent further incidences of IPV. Waul (2000) conducted a study examining the handling of orders of protection in the Domestic Violence Intake Center in the District of Columbia to see whether the method of obtaining orders of protection had any impact on the likelihood of a woman returning to court to obtain a permanent protection order. The results of the study indicate that a centralized case processing system can help encourage women to continue involvement in the court process by providing direct assistance to petitioners (Waul, 2000). Thus, permanent orders of protection and continued involvement in the court system were considered successful interventions for preventing further involvement in IPV (Waul, 2000). Another study of immigrant women found that contact with the justice system to obtain an order of protection resulted in a significant reduction in levels of IPV, and these results were maintained at 6-month follow-up (McFarlane, Malecha, et al., 2002).

Domestic Violence Courts

A number of states have created domestic violence courts that are separate systems from regular criminal courts. One of the distinguishing features of domestic violence courts is the assignment of cases to specialized judges and the use of specialized personnel, who typically have specialized training in issues related to handling IPV cases (Karan et al., cited in Weber, 2000). Some of these domestic violence courts use a "combined calendar" in which both civil and criminal IPV matters are heard (Weber, 2000). Screening court cases for domestic violence takes place by trained personnel. Some courts have specialized units staffed by personnel with experience in working with victims and perpetrators to assist litigants in filling out forms, provide an orientation to the legal system, and escort parties through the courtroom process (Weber, 2000). Additionally, domestic violence courts strictly monitor defendants' compliance with court orders. In a study of one city's domestic violence court, dismissal rates declined almost 60%, and probation violation rates of defendants were nearly half the typical rates during the first 2 years of operation (Kaye & Knipps, 2000). Another study examined the relationship between women's receipt of counseling services, protective orders, partner's subsequent arrests, and police contacts (Weisz, Tolman, & Bennett, 1998). Results from this study indicate that, when victims received battered women's counseling services or had a protective order, a completed court case was more likely and the number of perpetrator arrests rose, thus reducing continued victim involvement in IPV.

Central to the legal process is the prosecution of domestic violence cases. Without effective prosecution, victims of intimate partner violence will not receive legal assistance and their involvement in IPV will continue. For example, in Quincy, Massachusetts, the domestic violence district court is a full enforcement, proactive approach to partner violence that is considered a national model (Brasile, 2004). This approach is characterized by outreach and advocacy for women victims, mandatory arrest policies, and a no-drop prosecution policy (Brasile, 2004). All of these efforts take place under the watchful eye of advocates who focus their concerns on the protection of women who are victims of IPV (Brasile, 2004).

In light of study results suggesting that many violent relationships are mutually violent, prevention approaches designed to address the escalation of partner violence may also need to take into account the unique needs of partners who are identified to be mutually violent (Whitaker et al., 2007). While male-to-female partner violence is an obvious detriment to public health, female-perpetrated violence should not be ignored, because it puts women at risk of dangerous retaliation by men, and it perpetuates the cultural perception that female-to-male violence is acceptable (Straus, 2005).

INTERVENTIONS FOR PERPETRATORS

Standards that have been developed for batterer intervention programs typically include counseling techniques designed to counter perpetrator denial and minimization of their actions, while also encouraging them to take personal responsibility for their actions, because clinicians have long recognized the role that denial, minimization, and blaming play in the continuation of the cycle of violence (Austin & Dankwort, 1999; Scott & Strauss, 2007). In an attempt to reduce intimate partner violence, many batterers are ordered by the courts to participate in such treatment programs. Debate continues over whether court-referred batterer programs are effective at preventing perpetrators from becoming involved in future incidents of IPV (Rosenbaum, Gearan, & Ondovic, 2002).

One study examined the relationship between referral sources, participant characteristics, treatment length, treatment completion, and recidivism in a sample of 326 men who had completed at least one section of a program designed to treat perpetrators of IPV (Rosenbaum et al., 2002). Study results revealed that court-referred men had significantly higher treatment completion rates than self-referred men. In this study, treatment completion was associated with significantly lower rates of recidivism for court-referred perpetrators compared to self-referred perpetrators.

In contrast, results from a recent study examining program completion rates for immigrant and nonimmigrant men indicate that 46% of immigrant men and 62% of nonimmigrant men do not complete their batterer intervention programs, regardless of the method of referral (Rothman, Gupta, Pavlos, Dang, & Coutinho, 2007). Furthermore, a meta-analysis of randomized controlled evaluations of commonly used cognitive-behavioral treatments for male batterers of female victims found insufficient evidence to draw conclusions about effectiveness. The authors recommend further evaluation of such interventions using large-scale randomized studies (Smedslund, Dalsbø, Steiro, Winsvold, & Clench-Aas, 2007). Thus, it remains a frustrating situation for social work practitioners, because current research does not provide conclusive evidence related to what is the best way to proceed with interventions for perpetrators.

INTERVENTION APPROACHES FOR SOCIAL WORKERS

Although an extensive body of literature related to IPV exists, there is still much that the social work field does not know about the problem of IPV. It is certain, however, that the problem exists in epidemic proportions, and social workers in all areas of practice should be prepared to encounter clients who are affected by IPV. In *The Social Work and Human Services Treatment Planner* (Wodarski, Rapp-Pagliccí, Dulmus, & Jongsma, 2001), the authors recommend some basic best practice approaches that can be utilized by social workers in any setting who discover clients affected by IPV. Their recommendations include brief intervention approaches that are beneficial for social workers in all settings to become familiar with, because no social worker knows when IPV may become an issue in his or her practice. The following intervention steps are recommended as helpful ways for practitioners to address IPV in clients and families:

1. Interview both partners separately to determine history of abuse.
2. Determine whether it is safe for partners to continue to live together (if partners are living in the same home).

3. Refer the victim to shelter services if an imminent threat exists.
4. Recommend and help facilitate separation when it is determined that partners should not live together.
5. Help victim assess her (or his) financial stability and refer to vocational services as needed.
6. Assist victim to develop a decision matrix about whether to remain in the relationship.
7. Establish safety plans for victims who decide not to exit the relationship.
8. Affirm and reinforce the victim's right to safe and confidential social services.
9. Teach partners to recognize the triggers that lead to abuse.

In addition to the above recommendations from Wodarski and colleagues (2001), social workers should become familiar with all the IPV resources and hotlines available in their communities, so that referrals can be made for any problems related to IPV that are reported.

CONCLUSION

Intimate partner violence is a pervasive and costly social phenomenon in the United States, cutting across racial, ethnic, and socioeconomic lines and affecting LBGT as well as heterosexual couples. IPV typically occurs behind closed doors, and society has been loathe to respond assertively to what has historically been viewed as a private matter. Consequently, accurate prevalence and incidence estimates are difficult to obtain. Current best estimates indicate that 1.5 million women are assaulted each year (Tjaden & Thoennes, 1998) and that nearly 1 in 50 will be victimized by age 24 (Waul, 2000).

The human and economic costs of IPV are enormous. Victims are at increased risk for a host of adverse physical and emotional problems, including physical injury, sexually transmitted infection, unwanted pregnancy, fetal loss, depression, posttraumatic stress disorder, and substance use disorders to name a few. Many will ultimately die at the hands of their abusers. Aside from the human toll, IPV costs the nation billions of dollars annually due to lost productivity and increased demand on health and mental health services (Arias et al., 2002; Centers for Disease Control, 2003).

Numerous factors contribute to the intractability of IPV. Cultural norms that encourage male dominance and rigid gender roles create an environment in which IPV may be accepted and kept secret. Men who have been raised in violent homes or violent neighborhoods (Cunradi, 2007; Sharma, 1997; Straus & Gelles, 1990; Straus & Smith, 1990), who abuse substances (Cunradi, 2007), and/or have difficulty empathizing with others (Covell et al., 2007) are at risk for perpetrating IPV. Likewise, women who were abused as children are more likely to find themselves in violent adult relationships (Waul, 2000).

Individuals from historically oppressed populations may be even more vulnerable to IPV. Evidence indicates that IPV is as prevalent, or perhaps more prevalent, in the LGBT community as it is in heterosexual populations (Burke & Follingstad, 1999; Greenwood et al., 2002; Tjaden & Thoennes, 2000). However, LGBT victims may be especially reluctant to seek professional help. Immigrant women may hail from societies that are even more rigid in terms of gender roles and notions of male dominance and family privacy. They may be unaware of their rights to access legal remedies and may rightly fear deportation as a result of disclosing abuse (Dasgupta, 2000; Kurien, 2001). Homeless individuals may be the most vulnerable of all subgroups, with victimization being the norm rather than the exception (Boris et al., 2002).

Intervention into IPV requires a combination of accurate and widely implemented screening procedures; provision of support services and counseling to victims; and legally leveraged, evidence-based treatments for perpetrators. Medical settings provide key points of access to victims of IPV. Doctors and other medical professionals should implement valid, easy-to-use screening tools and should administer these at various points along the continuum of care, not just at initial contact.

Identified victims of IPV may need emergency shelter, emergency orders of protection, counseling, and other advocacy services. Clinicians who provide direct services to victims of IPV need specialized training regarding the dynamics of IPV, risk assessment techniques, and evidence-based therapies.

Perpetrators of IPV require specialized treatment programs, often with mandate and ongoing monitoring by criminal courts or specialized domestic violence courts. Typical treatments seek to counter denial, encourage acceptance of personal responsibility, and confront minimization and victim blaming. Evidence regarding the effectiveness of commonly used cognitive-behavioral interventions for male perpetrators has been equivocal (Smedslund et al., 2007). Researchers have called for further rigorous evaluations of such treatments. Additionally, specialized treatments may be required for partners identified as being mutually violent (Whitaker et al., 2007).

Finally, social workers can strive to redress social conditions through advocacy and research efforts that discourage the perpetration and concealment of intimate partner violence. Social policies that perpetuate power inequities between genders, marginalize groups of people based on their sexual orientations, or create an atmosphere of fear and mistrust among minority and immigrant populations should be challenged.

REFERENCES

Anderson, B. A., Marshak, H. H., & Hebbeler, D. L. (2002). Identifying intimate partner violence at entry to prenatal care: Clustering routine clinical information. *Journal of Midwifery & Women's Health, 47*(5), 353–359.

Arias, I., Dankwort, J., Douglas, U., Dutton, M., & Stein, K. (2002). Preventing injuries & abuse: Violence against women: The state of batterer prevention programs. *Journal of Law, Medicine & Ethics, 30,* 157–164.

Austin, J. B., & Dankwort, J. (1999). Standards for batterer programs: A review and analysis. *Journal of Interpersonal Violence, 14,* 152–168.

Bauer, S. T., & Shadigian, E. M. (2002). Screening for partner violence makes a difference and saves lives. *British Medical Journal, 325,* 1418–1420.

Boris, N. W., Heller, S. S., Shepard, T., & Zeanah, C. H. (2002). Partner violence among homeless young adults: Measurement issues and associations. *Journal of Adolescent Health, 30,* 355–363.

Brasile, S. (2004). Comparison of abuse alleged by same- and opposite-gender litigants as cited in requests for abuse prevention orders. *Journal of Family Violence, 19*(1), 59–68.

Burke, L. K., & Follingstad, D. R. (1999). Violence in lesbian and gay relationships: Theory, prevalence, and correlational factors. *Clinical Psychology Review, 19,* 487–512.

Campbell, J., Jones, A., Dienemann, J., Kub, J., Schollenberger, J., & O'Campo, P. (2002). Intimate partner violence and physical health consequences. *Archives of Internal Medicine, 162,* 1157–1163.

Campbell, J. C. (2002). Health consequences of intimate partner violence. *The Lancet, 359*(9314), 1331–1336.

Centers for Disease Control. (2003). *Costs of intimate partner violence against women in the United States.* Retrieved August 31, 2007, from http://www.cdc.gov/ncipc/pub-res

Chermack, S. T., Fuller, B. E., & Blow, F. C. (2000). Predictors of expressed partner and nonpartner violence among patients in substance abuse treatment. *Drug and Alcohol Dependency, 58,* 43–54.

Coker, A. L. (2007). Does physical intimate partner violence affect sexual health? *Trauma, Violence & Abuse: A Review Journal, 8*(2), 149–177.

Covell, C. N., Huss, M. T., & Langhinrichsen-Rohling, J. (2007). Empathic deficits among male batterers: A multidimensional approach. *Journal of Family Violence, 22,* 165–174.

Cunradi, C. B. (2007). Drinking level, neighborhood social disorder, and mutual intimate partner violence. *Alcoholism: Clinical and Experimental Research, 31*(6), 1012–1019.

Dasgupta, S. D. (2000). Charting the course: An overview of domestic violence in the South Asian community in the United States. *Journal of Social Distress and the Homeless, 9,* 173–185.

Diaz-Olavarrieta, C., Paz, F., De la Cadena, C. G., & Campbell, J. (2001). Prevalence of intimate partner abuse among nurses and nurses' aides in Mexico. *Archives of Medical Research, 32,* 79–87.

Ellsberg, M., Caldera, T., Herrera, A., Winkvist, A., & Kullgren, G. (1999). Domestic violence and emotional distress among Nicaraguan women: Results from a population based study. *American Psychologist, 54,* 30–37.

Ely, G. E. (2004). Domestic violence and immigrant communities in the United States: A review of women's unique needs and recommendations for social work practice and research. *Stress, Trauma & Crisis: An International Journal, 7,* 223–241.

Ely, G. E., Dulmus, C. N., & Wodarski, J. S. (2004). Domestic violence: A literature review reflecting an international crisis. *Stress, Trauma & Crisis: An International Journal, 7,* 77–91.

Faquir, F. (2001). Intrafamily femicide in the defense of honour: The case of Jordan. *Third World Quarterly, 22,* 65–83.

Feldhaus, K. M., Koziol-McLain, J., Amsbury, H. L., Norton, I. M., Lowenstein, S. R., & Abbott, J. T. (1997). Accuracy of 3 brief screening questions for detecting partner violence in the emergency department. *Journal of the American Medical Association, 277,* 1357–1361.

Fischbach, R. L., & Herbert, B. (1997). Domestic violence and mental health: Correlates and conundrums within and across cultures. *Social Science & Medicine, 45,* 1161–1177.

Gerbert, B., Moe, J., Caspers, N., Salber, P., Feldman, M., Herzig, K., et al. (2002). Physicians' response to victims of domestic violence: Toward a model of care. *Women & Health,* February/March, 1–22.

Gielen, A. C., Ghandour, R. M., Burke, J. G., Mahoney, P., McDonnell, K. A., & O'Campo, P. (2007). HIV AIDS and intimate partner violence: Intersecting women's health issues in the United States. *Trauma, Violence & Abuse: A Review Journal, 8*(2), 178–198.

Glantz, N. M., Halperin, D. C., & Hunt, L. M. (1998). Studying domestic violence in Chipas, Mexico. *Qualitative Health Research, 8,* 377–392.

Glass, N., Dearwater, S., & Campbell, J. (2001). Intimate partner violence screening and intervention: Data from eleven Pennsylvania and California community hospital emergency departments. *Journal of Emergency Nursing, 27,* 141–149.

Greenwood, G. L., Relf, M. V., Huang, B., Pollack, L. M., Canchola, J. A., & Catania, J. A. (2002). Battering victimization among a probability-based sample of men who have sex with men. *American Journal of Public Health, 92*(12), 1964–1969.

Haniff, N. Z. (1998). Male violence against men and women in the Carribean: The case of Jamaica. *Journal of Comparative Family Studies, 29,* 361–369.

Hazen, A. L., Connelly, C. D., Edelson, J. L., Kelleher, K. J., Landverk, J. A., Coben, J. H., et al. (2007). Assessment of intimate partner violence by child welfare services. *Children and Youth Services Review, 29*, 490–500.

Heintz, A. J., & Melendez, R. M. (2006). Intimate partner violence and HIV/STD risk among lesbian, gay, bisexual, and transgender individuals. *Journal of Interpersonal Violence, 21*(2), 193–208.

Jasinski, J. L., & Kantor, G. K. (2001). Pregnancy, stress and wife assault: Ethnic differences in prevalence, severity, and onset in a national sample. *Violence and Victims, 16*, 219–233.

Johnson, D. M., Palmeiri, P. A., Jackson, A. P., & Hobfall, S. E. (2007). Emotional numbing weakens abused inner-city women's resiliency resources. *Journal of Traumatic Stress, 20*(2), 197–206.

Johnson, J. K., Haider, F., Ellis, K., Hay, D. M., & Lindow, S. W. (2003). The prevalence of domestic violence in pregnant women. *British Journal of Obstetrics and Gynaecology, 110*, 272–275.

Kaye, J. S., & Knipps, S. K. (2000). Judicial responses to domestic violence: The case for a problem solving approach. *Western State University Law Review, 27*, 1–13.

Kurien, P. (2001). Religion, ethnicity and politics: Hindu and Muslim Indian immigrants in the United States. *Ethnic & Racial Studies, 24*, 263–293.

Lindhorst, T., Oxford, M., & Gillmore, M. R. (2007). Longitudinal effects of domestic violence on employment and welfare outcomes. *Journal of Interpersonal Violence, 22*(7), 812–828.

McFarlane, J., Campbell, J. C., Sharps, P., & Watson, K. (2002). Abuse during pregnancy and femicide: Urgent implications for women's health. *Obstetrics & Gynecology, 100*(1), 27–36.

McFarlane, J., Malecha, A., Gist, J., Watson, K., Batten, E., Hall, I., et al. (2002). Intimate partner violence against immigrant women: Measuring the effectiveness of protection orders. *American Journal of Family Law, 16*, 244–253.

McFarlane, J., Malecha, A., Watson, K., Gist, J., Batten, E., Hall, I., et al. (2005). Intimate partner sexual assault against women: Frequency, health consequences, and treatment outcomes. *Obstetrics & Gynecology, 105*(1), 99–108.

McFarlane, J., Soeken, K., & Wiist, W. (2000). An evaluation of interventions to decrease intimate partner violence to pregnant women. *Public Health Nursing, 17*, 443–451.

McNamara, J. R., Ertl, M. A., Marsh, S., & Walker, S. (1997). Short-term response to counseling and case management intervention in a domestic violence shelter. *Psychological Reports, 81*, 1243–1251.

Mears, D. P. (2003). Research and interventions to reduce domestic violence revictimization. *Trauma, Violence & Abuse: A Review Journal, 4*, 127–147.

Merchant, M. (2000). A comparative study of agencies assisting domestic violence victims: Does the South Asian community have special needs? *Journal of Social Distress and the Homeless, 9*, 249–259.

Mulleman, R. L., DenOtter, T., Wadman, M. C., Tran, T. P., & Anderson, J. (2001). Problem gambling in the partners of the emergency department patient as a risk factor for intimate partner violence. *Journal of Emergency Medicine, 23*, 307–312.

Norton, I. M., & Manson, S. M. (1997). Domestic violence intervention in an urban Indian health center. *Community Mental Health Journal, 33*, 331–337.

O'Leary, K. D. (2000). Developmental and affective issues in assessing and treating partner aggression. *Clinical Psychology: Science and Practice, 6*, 400–414.

Phelan, M. B. (2007). Screening for intimate partner violence in medical settings. *Trauma, Violence & Abuse: A Review Journal, 8*(2), 199–213.

Rhodes, K. V., & Levinson, W. (2003). Interventions for intimate partner violence against women: Clinical applications. *Journal of the American Medical Association, 289*, 601–606.

Rosenbaum, A., Gearan, P. J., & Ondovic, C. (2002). Completion and recidivism among court and self-referred batterers in a psychoeducational group treatment program: Implications for intervention and public policy. *Journal of Aggression, Maltreatment and Trauma, 5*, 199–220.

Rothman, E. F., Gupta, J., Pavlos, C., Dang, Q., & Coutinho, P. (2007). Batterer intervention program enrollment and completion among immigrant men in Massachusetts. *Violence Against Women, 13*(5), 527–543.

Scott, K., & Straus, M. (2007). Denial, minimization, partner blaming and intimate aggression in dating partners. *Journal of Interpersonal Violence, 22*, 7.

Shadigian, E. M., & Bauer, S. T. (2004). Screening for partner violence during pregnancy. *International Journal of Gynecology and Obstetrics, 84*, 273–280.

Sharma, S. (1997). Domestic violence against minority women: Interventions, preventions and health implications. *Equal Opportunities International, 16*, 1–14.

Shattuck, S. R. (2002). An IPV screening program in a public health department. *Journal of Community Health Nursing, 19*, 121–132.

Shepard, M., & Campbell, J. (1992). The abusive behavior inventory: A measure of psychological and physical abuse. *Journal of Interpersonal Violence, 7*(3), 291–305.

Short, L. M., McMahon, P. M., Davis-Chervin, D., Shelley, G. A., Lezin, N., Sloop, K. S., et al. (2000). Survivors' identification of protective factors and early warning signs for intimate partner violence. *Violence Against Women, 6*, 272–285.

Singh, R. N., & Unnithan, N. P. (1999). Wife burning: Cultural cues for lethal violence against women among Asian Indians in the United States. *Violence Against Women, 5*, 641–653.

Smedslund, G., Dalsbø, T. K., Steiro, A. K., Winsvold, A., & Clench-Aas, J. (2007). Cognitive behavioural therapy for men who physically abuse their female partner. *Campbell Collaboration Systematic Review*. Retrieved September 20, 2007, from http://www.campbellcollaboration.org/doc-pdf/070716_CBT_violence_final.pdf

Straus, M. (Ed.). (2005). *Current controversies on family violence* (2nd ed.). Newbury Park, CA: Sage.

Straus, M. A., & Gelles, R. J. (1990). *Physical violence in American families: Risk factors and adaptation to violence in 8,415 families*. New Brunswick, NJ: Transaction.

Straus, M. A., & Smith, C. (1990). Violence in Hispanic families in the United States: Incidence rates and structural interpretation. In M. G. Straus & R. J. Gelles (Eds.), *Physical violence in American families* (pp. 507–528). Garden City, NJ: Anchor Press.

Stuart, G. L., Moore, T. M., Ramsey, S. E., & Kahler, C. W. (2003). Relationship aggression and substance use among women court referred to domestic violence intervention programs. *Addictive Behaviors, 28*, 1603–1610.

Swogger, M. T., Walsh, Z., & Kosson, D. S. (2007). Domestic violence and psychopathic traits: Distinguishing the antisocial batterer from other antisocial offenders. *Aggressive Behavior, 33*, 253–260.

Taylor, P., Zaichkin, J., Pilkey, D., Leconte, J., Johnson, B. K., & Peterson, A. C. (2007). Prenatal screening for substance use and violence: Findings from physician focus groups. *Maternal and Child Health Journal, 11*, 241–247.

Thackeray, J., Seltzner, S., Downs, S. M., & Miller, C. (2007). Screening for intimate partner violence: The impact of screener and screening environment on victim comfort. *Journal of Interpersonal Violence, 22*(6), 659–670.

Thompson, M. P., Kaslow, N. J., & Kingree, J. B. (2002). Risk factors for suicide attempts among African American women experiencing recent intimate partner violence. *Violence and Victims, 17*, 283–295.

Tjaden, P. T., & Thoennes, N. (2000). *Full report of the prevalence, incidence, and consequences of violence against women.* Washington, DC: National Center of Justice.

Tjaden, P. T., & Thoennes, N. (1998). *Prevalence, incidence and consequences of violence against women: Findings from the National Violence Against Women Survey* (No. NCJ 172837). Washington, DC: National Institute of Justice and the Center for Disease Control and Prevention.

Tollestrup, K., Sklar, D., Frost, F. J., Olson, L., Weybright, J., Sandvig, J., et al. (1999). Health indicators and intimate partner violence among women who are members of a managed care organization. *Preventive Medicine, 29*, 431–440.

Tolman, R. M., & Raphael, J. (2000). A review of research on welfare and domestic violence. *Journal of Social Issues, 56*(4), 655–682.

Tomasulo, G., & McNamara, J. (2007). The relationship of abuse to women's health status and health habits. *Journal of Family Violence, 22*(4), 231–235.

Turmen, T. (1998). The health dimension. *United Nations Chronicle, 35,* 18–20.

Ulbrich, P. M., & Stockdale, J. (2002). Making family planning clinics an empowerment zone for rural battered women. *Women and Health, 35,* 83–100.

U.S. Government Printing Office. (2000). UNICEF says domestic violence against women and girls still a global epidemic. *Public Health Reports, 115,* 304.

Van Hightower, N. R., Gorton, J., & DeMoss, C. L. (2000). Predictive models of domestic violence and fear of intimate partners among migrant and seasonal farm worker women. *Journal of Family Violence, 15,* 137–154.

Vindhya, U. (2000). Dowry deaths in Andhra, Pradesh, India. *Violence Against Women, 6,* 1085–1109.

Wathen, C. N., & MacMillan, H. L. (2003). Interventions for violence against women: Scientific review. *Journal of the American Medical Association, 289,* 589–601.

Waul, M. (2000). Civil protection orders: An opportunity for intervention with domestic violence victims. *Georgetown Public Policy Review, 6,* 51–70.

Weber, J. (2000). Courts responding to communities: Domestic violence courts: Components and considerations. *Journal of the Center for Children & the Courts, 2,* 23–33.

Weisz, A. N., Tolman, R. M., & Bennett, L. (1998). An ecological study of nonresidential services for battered women within a comprehensive community protocol for domestic violence. *Journal of Family Violence, 13,* 395–397.

Westbrook, L. (2007). Digital information support for domestic violence victims. *Journal of the American Society for Information Science and Technology, 58*(3), 420–432.

Whitaker, D. J., Haileyesus, T., Swahn, M., & Saltzman, L. S. (2007). Differences in frequency of violence and reported injury between relationships with reciprocal and nonreciprocal intimate partner violence. *American Journal of Public Health, 97*(5), 941–947.

Wiist, W. H., & McFarlane, J. (1998). Severity of spousal and intimate partner abuse to pregnant Hispanic women. *Journal of Health Care for the Poor and Underserved, 9*(3), 248–261.

Wodarski, J. S., Rapp-Paglicci, L. A., Dulmus, C. N., & Jongsma, A. E. (2001). *The social work and human services treatment planner.* New York: Wiley.

Yarbrough, D. N., & Blanton, P. W. (2000). Socio-demographic indicators of intervention program completion with the male court referred perpetrator of partner abuse. *Journal of Criminal Justice, 28,* 517–526.

Yoshihama, M. (2000). Reinterpreting strength and safety in a socio-cultural context: Dynamics of domestic violence and experiences of women of Japanese descent. *Children and Youth Services Review, 22,* 207–229.

Zink, T., Klesges, L. M., Levin, L., & Putnam, F. (2007). Abuse Behavior Inventory: Cutpoint, validity, and characterization of discrepancies. *Journal of Interpersonal Violence, 22*(7), 921–931.

6

Sex Offender–Specific Treatment: Historical Foundations, Current Challenges, and Contemporary Approaches

LAURIE L. GUIDRY

For many, the term *sex offender treatment* may represent somewhat of an oxymoron, because the belief that criminal sex offenders or sexual deviants are untreatable is a pervasive one. This dominant public opinion can be seen to arise from a number of convergent and quite valid factors, including, but not necessarily limited to, the personally visceral reaction to, and the societal abhorrence of, sex offenders as a group; the notably narrow, often media-hyped understanding that the public has of the highly complex phenomenon that sexually deviant behavior represents; and the unfortunate failure to date of the sex offender treatment and research field to adequately demonstrate and convincingly communicate to a legitimately frightened but misguided public the effectiveness of sex offender treatment and risk management practices in decreasing the risk for sexual violence and making our communities safer.

Despite public perception, it should be appreciated that sex offender–specific treatment has a substantive historical foundation as well as a dynamic, responsive, and ongoing evolution. Importantly, contemporary thinking regarding the principles of effective treatment is being guided by and grounded in increasingly sound theory and research, both of which are based on advances in methodologies and a more complete appreciation of the significance of the high degree of heterogeneity found among the sex-offending population both in type and behavioral expression.

This chapter will briefly explore the historical underpinnings of the current efforts to understand and establish effective, evidence-based approaches to address criminal sexual behavior and sexual psychopathology. Current challenges facing the sex offender treatment field, including working within and responding to the definitional complexity and composition of the treatment population, capturing in meaningful ways the effectiveness of treatment and developing practices that are empirically based and theoretically valuable, will be highlighted.

HISTORICAL FOUNDATIONS

Early Evolution

Contemporary sex offender–specific treatment has been built upon the bedrock of the work of a number of essential historical figures and has been shaped by several critical theoretical bends in the river. Laws and Marshall (2003) and Marshall and Laws (2003), in parts 1 and 2 of *A Brief History of Behavioral and Cognitive Behavioral Approaches to Sexual Offenders,* offer a concise and informative overview of the evolution of the sex offender–specific treatment field, which informs, among others things, the following summary.

Of course, it would seem no account of the evolution of 21st-century thought regarding sex offender treatment can go without the mention of the pivotal pioneer Sigmund Freud (1856–1939). Freud's seminal contributions to the understanding of human sexuality as it develops along both normative as well as deviant trajectories is well known (Freud, 1957). In addition to his theory of psychosexual development and his tortured reversals on the reality of his seduction theory of sexual abuse, Freud also influenced the early focus of psychology on the study of the unconscious motivation of behavior. However, Laws and Marshall (2003) point out that, while Freud may be considered the founding father of the study of human sexuality, there were other influential figures who came before him and many who were concurrently "talking and writing about the vagaries of human sexuality"(p. 76). Of note was Richard von Krafft-Ebing (1840–1902), who preceded Freud and who published in 1886 the first, and still considered one of the foremost, scientific accounts of sexually aberrant behavior titled *Psychopathia Sexualia* (Psychopathy of

Sex) (Kraft-Ebing, 1886). Importantly, it was these early pioneers who laid the foundation for our present conceptualizations regarding sexual deviancy and criminal sexual behavior.

However, coinciding and increasingly contrasting with the rising prominence of Freud's theories of psychosexual development, his intriguing explanations of the unconscious derivatives of human behavior, and the dominant emphasis at the time on the psychoanalytic approach to treating psychopathology was the growing interest in an ultimately competing theory in the form of behaviorism in general, and its application to sexually deviant behavior more specifically. Early behaviorism, pursued as the alter ego of psychodynamic theory and serving as the field of psychology's foray into the scientific, as opposed to the intuitive, study of understanding human behavior through the use of objective methods, arises from the work of a pair of prominent researchers in the field of animal psychology. Ivan Pavlov's (1849–1936) meticulous, empirical studies of classical conditioning laid the groundwork for understanding conditioned reflexes and established objective means for analyzing behavioral responses (Leahy, 2000). Edward L. Thorndike's (1874–1949) animal research led him to develop a theory of learning based on the law of effect, which illuminated the fundamental principle behind operant conditioning and stated that, if a behavior is followed by a pleasurable stimulus, the behavior will reoccur (Leahy, 2000).

Standing on the shoulders of these giants in the early 1900s, John B. Watson (1878–1958) and ultimately his successor B. F. Skinner (1904–1990) led the charge to fully break away from the traditional view of psychology as the study of consciousness (Leahy, 2000). This "new" psychology, historically identified as radical behaviorism, recognized the prediction and control of human behavior as its goals; goals that were perfectly suited to the application of altering aberrant behavior, including the goal of altering what was considered to be conditioned sexually deviant behavior. For example, aversive conditioning techniques represent an early behavioral approach that was applied to the problem of eliminating what was at the time considered to be sexually abnormal behavior (including homosexuality). Classical or operant conditioning principles were utilized when a noxious stimulus (including electric shock, nausea-producing agents, foul odors, aversive images, and/or emotional shaming) was paired with either an image or the enactment of the identified aberrant behavior, respectively, in order to reduce or eliminate the targeted sexually deviant behavior (Quinsey & Earls, 1990). In addition, behavioral principles derived from conditioning led to the development of phallometric methods of assessing patterns of sexual arousal (Marshall, 1996). Kurt Freund (1914–1996) is the noted pioneer of this work and developed the procedure for objectively measuring observable changes in the circumference of the penis in response to sexual stimuli in a laboratory setting (Wilson & Mathon, 2007). Of note is the enduring relevance of this approach to assessing sexual deviancy and the continued treatment emphasis on altering sexually deviant arousal patterns, as contemporary research points to the presence of deviant sexual arousal to children as measured by phallometric testing as the single factor most strongly associated with sexual offense recidivism (Hanson & Bussière, 1998).

It should be noted as well, however, that strict behaviorism alone, as it arose as a momentum-changing challenge to the popularity of psychodynamic theory and compelled a significant directional shift in the study of psychology, would ultimately fall short in illuminating the complexity of human behavior, including both normative as well as deviant sexual behavior. For instance, despite the initial enthusiasm, the limited research regarding the use of purely behavioral techniques such as aversive conditioning suggests that it should be included only as part of a more comprehensive approach to altering aberrant sexual behavior (Dougher, 1995; Fernandez, Shingler, & Marshall, 2006). Laws and Marshall (2003) suggest that of equal importance to the revolutionary paradigm shift represented by radical behaviorism in psychology and its practical application to sexual aberrance was the groundbreaking work of Alfred Kinsey (1894–1956) published in *Sexual Behavior in the Human Male* (Kinsey, Pomeroy, & Martin, 1948) and *Sexual Behavior in the Human Female* (Kinsey, Pomeroy, Martin, & Gebhard, 1953). Not unlike Krafft-Ebing and Freud before him, the work of Kinsey and his colleagues was variably scorned and praised. Nonetheless, his findings represented a systematic effort to recognize the extensive variability across the human species relative to sexual behaviors and today "remains the largest body of empirical information on human sexual diversity ever compiled" (Laws & Marshall, 2003, p. 80).

It was also the influential concept of social learning theory, as initially articulated by E. C. Tollman in the 1932 *Purposive Behavior in Animals and Men* and subsequently expanded by Alfred Bandura (1977), that offered a bridge from what had come to be seen as the perceived reductionism and oversimplification of behaviorism to the variegated depths of examining behavior as it is informed by cognition (Ormrod, 1999). Social learning theory suggests that human behavior, including sexual behavior, goes beyond the stimulus–response purported by pure behaviorism and states rather that human behavior is socially contextualized and is the result of the interaction between behavioral, cognitive, and environmental factors. As applied to the dilemma of changing abnormal and problematic sexual behavior, social learning theory moved beyond the still important but limited behavioral understanding of the singular primacy of sexual aberrance as a conditioned response that leads to deviant sexual preferences that are the focus of change in treatment (McGuire, Carlisle, & Young, 1965) to a broader appreciation of the complexity and multidetermined nature of deviant sexual behavior that evoked a more comprehensive treatment response.

Cognitive-Behavioral Therapy

As a result, more fully considered and multifaceted approaches to behavioral change began to emerge as cognitive psychology, the essential focus of which is on the mental process that mediates a behavioral stimulus–response, gained popularity and infiltrated the behavioral field. Cognitive-behavioral treatment (CBT) approaches with sex offenders enjoyed ascendency at this time. Guided by broader conceptualizations of assessing and addressing factors beyond those identified in single-factor theories of sexual offending or the presence of deviant sexual arousal alone, additional factors hypothesized to be associated with abnormal and/or criminal sexual behavior came to be recognized as relevant targets of treatment.

It was William Marshall in 1971 in an article on the treatment of sexual deviance who was reportedly the "first behavior therapist to suggest the value of not simply reducing interest in deviant sexual acts [in sex offender–specific treatment], but also enhancing appropriate interest and providing the offender with the skills necessary to act on the changed interests" (Marshall, 1996, p. 179). Marshall (1996) in turn recognizes Gene Abel as the single most influential contributor to the development of treatment methods for sex offenders. This was attributable to Abel's groundbreaking research that allowed for the protection from further prosecution the criminal sex offenders who participated in his study in return for a true accounting of their deviant sexual interests and behavior (Abel, Blanchard, & Becker, 1978).

Early CBT approaches to treating sexual deviancy included not only modifying sexual arousal through a range of behavioral techniques such as covert sensitization and masturbatory satiation (Marshall, Anderson, & Fernandez, 1999), but also included enhancing social skills; improving self-esteem; promoting assertive communication styles; providing sex education; training in developing empathy for sexual abuse victims; cultivating intimacy and anger management skills; dealing with substance abuse issues; and utilizing cognitive restructuring techniques to identify and alter cognitive distortions associated with justifications for sexually abusive behavior (Marshall, 1996). At the time, the CBT approach was a broad-based one, offered in a manualized group format, under a one-size-fits-all, social-learning paradigm that reflected the working knowledge of the times about how to stop sex-offending behavior.

Hormonal Approaches

Psychopharmacological approaches to treating sex offenders were developing concurrent with psychosocial interventions. With the emphasis on reducing deviant sexual arousal, hormonal medications provided an alternative to the dramatic and unappealing surgical procedures of stereotaxic neurosurgery (which involves removal of sections of the hypothalamus to decrease testosterone production) and orchiectomy (surgical removal of the testes or castration) that had gained popularity in Germany in the 1930s as a response to pedophiles and homosexuals (L. B. Guttmacher, personal communication, 2006). The most common testosterone-lowering agents utilized in the United States to decrease sexual arousal in men are medroxyprogesterone (MPA) and more currently leuprolide (Lupron), both of which were initially developed for use in women with menstrual disorders and as a female oral contraceptive, but more recently have been employed and studied in the treatment of prostate cancer in men.

A complete review of the current understanding of the complex neurophysiological role of testosterone in sexual offending and sexually deviant behavior is beyond the scope of this chapter (see Bradford, 1990; Grubin, 2008; Hucker & Bain, 1990). However, evidence in the literature supports the substantively, but not necessarily exclusively, influential role of testosterone in the sexual drive of men (Studer, Aylwin, & Reddon, 2005). In addition, follow-up data from surgical castration procedures with sex offenders (which serve essentially to lower testosterone levels) points to significant reductions in sex offense recidivism rates in large numbers of offenders over long periods of time (Bradford, 1990). As such, to the degree that testosterone is implicated in sexually aggressive behavior, the application of hormonal medications to sexual offending can be understood as a pragmatic and reasonable treatment response. In terms that circumvent the actual complexity of their mechanisms of function, MPA is a hormonal agent that prevents the conversion of testosterone by accelerating its metabolism, while leuprolide is an antiandrogen that blocks testosterone production altogether. The effect of these medications has been described as including a decrease in sexual drive and fantasies with a concurrent reduction in sexual activity.

Contrary to popular belief, these kinds of medications are not necessarily prescribed in all cases to completely eliminate sexual arousal. The desired effect in many instances is rather to reduce sexual drive to levels that are manageable for the individual who is struggling to control problematic, deviant, and/or criminal sexual behavior. The side effects of hormonal medications can be serious and can include, but may not be limited to, weight gain, decrease in sperm production, headache, fatigue, hot and cold flashes, nightmares, hyperglycemia, and leg cramps. Leuprolide, however, is gaining in popularity in part because it offers a better side-effect profile. Once the medication has been discontinued, evidence suggests that the side effects resolve, and testosterone levels—and, by extension, problematic sexual arousal levels—revert to their premedication levels.

More recently, selective serotonin reuptake inhibitors (SSRIs) are being explored as another psychopharmacological possibility for medically managing the behavioral expression of deviant sexual arousal, and there is some early evidence to suggest their effectiveness in this regard in some applications (Greenberg, Bradford, & Curry, 1996; Kafka, 1994). However, the mechanisms for how these medications work to manage sexual arousal are unclear, and little evidence is available from controlled studies to empirically support their treatment efficacy.

Although a number of studies suggest that antiandrogen medication can be effective in reducing sexual offense recidivism (Bradford, 1997; Krueger & Kaplan, 2001; Maletzky, Tolan, & McFarland, 2006; Thibaut, Cordier, & Kuhn, 1993), most studies to date have small samples sizes, include heterogeneous populations, and/or lack control conditions. A consensus view in the field, however, tends to support the utility of using medical interventions such as antihormonal agents when an individual's sexual drive is overpoweringly intense and unable to be controlled and/or when he fails to respond to other treatment modalities (Saleh & Guidry, 2003). A recent meta-analysis lends support for the use of medical interventions with sex offenders in conjunction with psychological treatments that include a CBT approach (Lösel & Schmucker, 2005). These findings point to an independent positive treatment effect for psychosocial interventions that, when paired with hormonal interventions, reduce deviant sexual arousal and reduce the reoccurrence of sexual offending behavior.

Relapse Prevention

Returning to and continuing with the evolution of psychosocial interventions for individuals who sexually abuse, in the early 1980s, relapse prevention (RP) for sex offenders, adapted from a cognitive-behavioral approach to treat alcohol addiction designed by G. A. Marlatt (1982), was introduced into the sex offender treatment field (Pithers, Marques, Gibat, & Marlatt, 1983). This approach utilized behavioral, cognitive, educational, and skills training components designed to help an individual identify and then interrupt the pattern or chain of behaviors that could lead to a substance use relapse. In its application to the sex-offender population, the goal of RP was to intervene in the cycle of behaviors that preceded and led to sexually criminal behavior in order to prevent a sexual reoffense from occurring (Laws & Ward, 2006). In the RP approach, sex offender treatment participants are taught to identify high-risk situations and subconscious choices or decisions and pathways to offending behavior that might increase their potential to act on deviant sexual interests. Then, a relapse prevention plan is crafted to target potential barriers to abstinence and identify proactive strategies and interventions in situations that might trigger a relapse.

For a number of reasons, not the least of which was the face-valid, commonsense approach of RP and the relative ease of implementation, this model was initially widely embraced by the professional treatment community, becoming standard practice in many sex offender treatment programs (Knopp, Freeman-Longo, & Stevenson, 1992) with few questions about its efficacy. In addition, as the tenets of the published model of RP for sex offenders spread into the nomenclature of the sex offender treatment provider community, RP as an intervention model began to morph and became inclusive of anything and everything that was designed to prevent a relapse of sex-offending behavior (Laws, 2003). RP was also often implemented as a stand-alone treatment approach rather than as it was initially designed as an adjunctive element to the more widely practiced sex offender–specific CBT that was suppose to facilitate the maintenance of the long-term treatment gains (Laws, 2003). Pointed criticisms of the RP model began to emerge. Some critics felt that RP was furthering an overly simplified, one-size-fits-all approach to sex offender treatment with no recognition of the variability in an individual's motivation to avoid reoffense (Ward & Hudson, 2000). Others criticized RP's exclusive emphasis on avoiding risk alone rather than on the facilitation of healthy life choices and practices (Ward & Hudson, 2000). There were also problems noted with applying the construct of the abstinence violation effect (AVE) (which consists of the negative response to a lapse in abstinence from substance use that may serve to prohibit full relapse) to the sex-offending population; the data on which suggested that, unlike substance abusers, sex offenders do not recognize preoffending behavior as prohibitive and do not demonstrate commitment to abstaining from these forms of preoffending or lapse behaviors (Wheeler, George, & Marlatt, 2006). In addition, there was a lack of empirical evidence for the efficacy of RP (Marshall & Anderson, 2000; Marques, Wiederanders, Day, Nelson, & van Ommeren, 2005).

In 2000, the original model of RP for sex offenders was reconsidered and revised by a number of experts in the sex offender treatment field (Laws, Hudson, & Ward, 2000), and efforts to demonstrate the efficacy of the revised model are ongoing. RP continues to be implemented widely, and over 90% of treatment programs surveyed indicated the use of some form of RP (McGrath, Cumming, & Burchard, 2003). However, questions about RP's ongoing utility are being raised (Carich, Dobkowski, & Delehanty, 2008), and new iterations, like the self-regulation model proposed by Ward and Hudson (2000) that challenges RP's assumption of a single pathway to sex offense relapse, are gaining in popularity.

CURRENT CHALLENGES

As the sex offender–specific treatment field has advanced, a number of barriers to knowing, applying, and demonstrating what works for whom to stop criminal and deviant sexual behavior have been difficult to overcome, while new challenges have emerged. First, the task of establishing clinically useful definitions to adequately categorize the target treatment population has grown increasingly complex. Although there is currently keen awareness, and nearly constant notation in the literature, of the heterogeneous composition within and the diversity across the sex-offending population, this insight has largely outpaced the clinical research that would inform evidence-based practice models. And although comprehensive and initially innovative, the overly inclusive approach of the first-generation expression of CBT for sex offenders fails to take into account the extensive variability within the population and fails to recognize potentially cogent differences in the treatment and risk management needs among relevant and distinct subgroups of sex offenders.

Second, Kirsch and Becker (2005) offer a critique of current practices in the field of sex offender–specific treatment that highlights two additional dilemmas. Their *theory of problem* suggests that, as the result of the absence of a unifying and comprehensive etiological theory to explain sex-offending behavior, the somewhat enduring and currently dominant practice of a comprehensive, multicomponent and global CBT approach to treating sex offenders (Marshall & Anderson, 2000) that includes everything from decreasing deviant sexual arousal to improving social skills to challenging distorted thinking patterns that can serve to maintain offending behavior lacks substantive empirical validity (Kirsch & Becker, 2005). With the goal of treatment understood as preventing future sexual reoffense, intervention efforts should rather be precisely aimed at those specific, evidenced-based factors that have been empirically demonstrated to operate to maintain aberrant sexual behavior.

Next, problems with the *theory of change* (Kirsch & Becker, 2005) identifies confounds to sex offender–specific treatment related to the delivery of treatment, the process (versus the content) of treatment, and the effectiveness of current treatment practices designed to change sex-offending behavior. As noted earlier, recognizing the significant heterogeneity of the sex-offending population, but operating otherwise and continuing to provide treatment that dilutes relevant within- and between-treatment group variability, is problematic. Providing treatment in formats that assume that all sex offenders are created equal, present with the same risk for reoffense, and have equal treatment needs that can be addressed by treatment delivered in a manualized, predetermined way can have the effect of homogenizing treatment to the point of making it wholly ineffective and/or masking any efficacy that particular elements of the approach may have with particular types of sex offenders. In addition, while it is imperative to focus the content of treatment on factors most strongly related to sexual reoffending, it is also important to attend to those process variables, such as therapist–client alliance, group cohesion, stages of change, and other factors that may serve to either impede or facilitate an individual's progress in treatment. To date, there is relatively little research in this area of sex offender–specific treatment (Beech & Fordham, 1997).

Finally, capturing the effectiveness of sex offender–specific treatment in meaningful ways is significantly complicated by a number of methodological limitations to useful research, as well as all of the aforementioned issues, and presents a substantial challenge. Although most treatment outcome studies are aimed at identifying the primary treatment effect of reducing sex offense recidivism—a difficult undertaking in and of itself—it is also important to include an examination both of specific treatment components as well as the relationship of therapeutic process variables to outcome in order to significantly improve and inform the ongoing efforts at developing effective, targeted, and tailored treatment program design (Kirsch & Becker, 2005).

CONTEMPORARY APPROACHES

Emergent responses to the challenges to sex offender–specific treatment are being influenced by the work of Andrews and Bonta (2006) based on the non–sex offender–specific but highly relevant general criminal treatment principles they have articulated and that were presented in an invited plenary address by Karl Hanson at the 2006 Association for the Treatment of Sexual Abusers annual conference (Hanson, 2006). Briefly described below, the discriminating tenets of risk–needs–responsivity and professional discretion are held as essential to effective intervention with the criminal population and can help to refine and focus current considerations of and challenges to treatment and risk management planning with sex offenders as well.

> *Risk Principle:* states that the level of intensity of treatment should match the level of risk of the offender.
>
> *Need Principle:* posits that treatment should target criminogenic (or dynamic) needs.
>
> *Responsivity Principle:* affirms that treatment should be generally tailored to the learning style of the offender and specifically adapted to relevant individual variables.
>
> *Professional Discretion Principle:* directs that the other three principles may be modified, contingent upon professional judgment. (Andrews & Bonta, 2006)

These principles can be and are being woven into present thinking about efficacy with sex offenders, providing a blueprint for more efficient, more targeted, and ultimately more effective approaches to treatment.

Challenge 1: Defining the Treatment Population

Sex offenders as a group are understood to be highly heterogeneous, but the term itself collapses critical differences and defines the treatment population in very broad, overinclusive, and simple ways. Unfortunately, it also contributes to the public perception, or rather misperception, that all sex offenders are of equivalent ilk. The term *sex offender* is an elusive social construct, the variable definition of which in many ways reflects the heterogeneity of the population. If defined in criminal terms, a sex offender is understood as someone who commits a sexual crime. However, what is legally understood to constitute sexually criminal behavior has tremendous variance, as evidenced by the substantive differences among each of the 50 states in the extensive classification systems of legal statutes they have each crafted and employ to define sexual crimes. For instance, with age of consent for sexual intercourse ranging from 14 to 18 depending on the state, an individual could be convicted of statutory rape and identified as a sex offender in one state but would not be considered so in another. In another instance, one man's legal or tolerated public nudity (e.g., in Vermont or in New Orleans on Mardi Gras) is another state's law against indecent exposure. Comparatively, if defined in clinical terms, a sex offender may be understood to have a paraphilic disorder, which, according to the *Diagnostic and Statistical Manual of Mental Disorders* (*DSM-IV-TR*; American Psychiatric Association, 2002) is defined as:

> recurrent, intense sexually arousing fantasies, sexual urges, or behaviors generally involving 1) nonhuman objects, 2) the suffering or humiliation with oneself or one's partner, or 3) children or other nonconsenting persons that occur over a period of at least 6 months (Criterion A). (p. 566)

The *DSM-IV-TR* describes nine primary paraphilic disorders: exhibitionism, fetishism, frotteurism, pedophilia, sexual masochism, sexual sadism, transvestic fetishism, voyeurism, and paraphilia not otherwise specified. So, just as there are a wide-ranging number of ways to be sexually criminal, the psychiatric community has constructed multiple variations on the ways one can be considered sexually deviant as well. However, *DSM-IV-TR* paraphilic diagnoses have been criticized as being diagnostically unreliable, poorly applied in research contexts, and not particularly helpful in understanding what interventions may be most effective with individuals who display sexually deviant behavior (Marshall, 2006; O'Donohue, Regev, & Hagstrom, 2000). Marshall (2006) instead suggests that a clinically useful approach would be to employ more flexible and relevant behavioral descriptors and descriptions of related problems that reflect the degree to which a sexual behavior problem is present on a spectrum. In addition, while both the criminal and clinical constructs of how sexually aberrant behavior is expressed encompass a wide variety of quite distinct and concerning sexual activity, neither are mutually exclusive nor universally inclusive of each other. Unfortunately, however, they have often been understood and studied as such—an unhelpful practice that can conflate important distinctions. The task then becomes how to most adequately define and appropriately group individuals who engage in sexually deviant and criminal sexual behavior in a way that promotes the most effective treatment and risk management paradigm.

Typological Definitions

In addition to the legal and clinical constructs noted above, a number of other ways that sex offenders are described and categorized have emerged over time and reduce, rather than amplify, the inherent heterogeneity of the population so that meaningful subgroups can be discerned. Fortunately, as knowledge in the professional field of sex offender–specific assessment, treatment, and risk management has advanced, the effort to define salient characteristics of the treatment population, establish treatment-relevant categories, and delineate useful group composition features within the broader sex-offender population has also advanced.

As noted earlier, one of the first simple, yet important, differentiations to be made among those with aberrant sexual behavior was based on the type of victim that the sexual perpetrator targeted. Men who targeted children (child molesters) and those who targeted women (rapists) were and continue to be an early focus of typological study and research. While others preceded him (Laws, 2003), the influence of Groth's (1979) work on the typologies of child molesters and rapists is still felt today. Through meticulous clinical case examination, Groth identified two types of child molesters, who differed along the key dimensions of sexual interest and psychological need, and four types of rapists, the distinctions between which were based on their motivation for sexual aggression against women. In his child-molester typology, Groth identified the fixated child molester, who is primarily sexually oriented toward children, as contrasted with the regressed child molester, whose sexual interest in children is situationally determined and the result of stressful external factors that erode the child molesters' masculine identity. Groth further subcategorized these two types of child molesters relative to the degree of force used to achieve the intended purpose of the sexual act (Schwartz, 1995). Pressure offenses against children are understood as coercive and suggest a relational need is being fulfilled. Offenses using force, however, indicate either the use of the child victim as a sexual outlet or for the expression of sadistic violence.

Groth's rape typology, again clinically derived, presupposed rape as an act of anger rather than of sexual desire (hypothesized by some to be the result of the influence of the women's movement of the times) (Schwartz, 1995) and included categorizations of rape as an expression of anger and frustration; rape as a result of panic secondary to rejection; rape as motivated by the need for dominance; and rape that results from sexualized anger (Schwartz, 1995).

Empirically refining the existing typologies based on the earlier clinical observations of Groth and others, Knight and Prentky (1990) advanced the effort to identify a clinically useful categorization system of sex offenders by creating a statistically derived classification framework for child molesters and rapists based on a large sample population of adult male incarcerated sex offenders at the Massachusetts Treatment Center (MTC). The child-molester typology they proposed expanded the former dichotomous two-type to a spectrum of 24 types based on two axes. The first axis includes the degree (high or low) to which the individual is fixated on the child victim and the child molesters' level (high or low) of social competence. The second axis includes the degree of contact with the child victim (high or low), the meaning of that contact (relational or sexual), and the level of physical harm in that contact (high or low and sadistic or nonsadistic). The Knight and Prentky rapist typology identifies nine types of rapists based on the statistical analysis of their data from the empirical findings of their MTC research. These include rapists who are described as opportunistic with high social competence; opportunistic with low social competence; pervasively angry; overtly sexually sadistic; muted sexually sadistic with high social competence; nonsadistic with high social competence; nonsadistic with low social competence; vindictive with low social competence; and vindictive with moderate social competence (Knight & Prentky, 1990).

This exponential growth in the empirical identification of sex-offender typologies has validated the increasing consensus that very relevant distinctions among sex offenders exist that have important treatment implications. For example, differential outcomes relative to treatment effectiveness have been obtained from studies both across and within the distinct sex-offender typologies of rapist, incest offenders, and extrafamilial child molesters (Hanson, 2001; Hanson & Bussière, 1998; Quinsey, Lalumière, Rice, & Harris, 1995). These findings provide support for the argument that, in contrast to the generally accepted clinical practice of including rapists and child molesters in the same treatment group, a more exclusive and discriminating group format may result in better treatment outcomes (Hanson & Morton-Bourgon, 2004). Placing rapists, incest offenders, and extrafamilial child molesters in separate and distinct therapy groups allows for treatment that is better tailored to the more clearly delineated characteristics and treatment needs of the group members. Unfortunately, Knight and Prentky's (1990) more sophisticated and discriminating typology has not yet been widely used to develop more specialized treatment approaches nor to match specific subtypes of sex offenders with treatment adapted to their more apparently distinct need (Kirsch & Becker, 2005)

Offense Pathway Distinctions

Another way to subdivide the sex-offender population that is built upon the framework of improved typological understanding takes into account the multiple pathways that can lead an individual to sexually reoffend and has been articulated by Ward and Hudson's (2000) response to the one-size-fits-all flaws of RP in the form of the self-regulation model of sexual offending. In this comprehensive yet tailored approach, the relapse or sexual reoffense process involves nine phases. Phase 1 is a life event that occurs and results in a given appraisal that leads to phase 2, a desire for deviant sex or activity. This fosters phase 3, the establishment of an offense-related goal whose central aim is to either reoffend (approach goal) or avoid reoffending (avoidance goal). Once the offense-related goal has been determined, this prompts phase 4, the selection of a strategy to achieve the goal, which is either an active or a passive strategy. This choice, in turn, results in four potential offense pathways: avoidant-passive, avoidant-active, approach-passive, or approach-active. The chosen offense pathway then leads to phase 5, the relapser's entrance in to the high-risk situation, which activates one of four possible reoffense paradigms that involves: (a) covert planning and underegulation on the part of the avoidant-passive relapse; (b) misregulation and ineffective strategies on the part of the avoidant-active relapse; (c) impulsive underegulation by the approach-passive relapse; or (d) explicit planning and intact regulation by the approach-active relapse. In phase 6, a lapse occurs, and the previously avoidant relapsers adopt an approach goal (to reoffend), and the previous approach relapsers maintain an approach goal (to reoffend). The lapse progresses to phase 7, wherein the behavioral relapse or sexual reoffense occurs. The relapse is then followed by phase 8, which involves a postoffense evaluative process. In this aftermath assessment, the avoidant relapsers will demonstrate the abstinence violation effect (AVE) and experience negative feelings associated with their reoffense. The approach relapsers, however, will not experience the AVE and will feel positively because they have obtained their goals. These postoffense evaluations influence phase 9 and each of the relapser's attitudes, intentions, and expectations regarding future reoffending (see Ward & Hudson, 2000, for further details of their self-regulation model).

This contemporary, multidimensional model of the pathways toward sexual reoffense emphasizes rather than dilutes the critical distinctions between behavioral goals and motivations of reoffender subtypes that have previously operated to confound rather than inform treatment. Yates and Kingston (2006) found empirical support for both the self-regulation theory as well as the utility of the pathways sexual offense model of relapse that it defines. In a sample of 80 offenders, including subgroups identified as rapists, child molesters with boy victims, child molesters with girl victims, incest offenders, and mixed offenders (both adult and child victims), "it was found that the four pathways contained in the model were differentially associated with offender types" (p. 259) and that these distinctions represented a conceptually accurate and useful expansion beyond the narrow, singular pathway previously outlined by RP.

Classification Based on Risk

An imaginary comparison of the differential risk for reoffense that might be presented by an exclusive exhibitionist, a first-time cybersex offender who downloaded images of child pornography, and a sexual sadist (Laws & O'Donohue, 2008) makes the obvious point of the relevance of distinguishing among sex offenders based on the levels of risk they pose for sexual reoffense as it relates to the development of effective treatment and risk management strategies. It was Hanson and Bussière's (1998) seminal study on sex-offender recidivism that set the stage and the standard for the contemporary understanding of the factors associated with the risk for reoffense among sex offenders that are now used to inform risk management and guide treatment development. The study, entailing a meta-analytic review of 61 studies on the sex offense recidivism rates for over 23,000 convicted sex offenders, found that the rate for reoffense among this population was relatively low (13.4% over a 4- to 5-year follow-up period) and that the risk for reoffense was variable among different types of offenders (Hanson & Bussière, 1998). Further, the results indicated that the two factors most strongly associated with the long-term risk for sexual reoffense were found to be sexual deviancy (as indicated by deviant sexual interests, prior sexual offenses, boy victims, and stranger victims) and general criminal lifestyle factors. The findings also provided empirical evidence against a few long-held intuitive clinical assumptions thought to be related to sex offense recidivism and adhered to by many in the professional field (i.e., denial of the offense, lack of empathy for the victim) (Hanson & Bussière, 1998).

This study led to the development of the Static-99, which is an actuarially based measure of risk for sex offense recidivism derived from the static (or fixed, unchangeable, historical) factors determined to be related to risk for sexual offense recidivism (Hanson & Thornton, 1999). The factors for Static-99 include being between the ages of 18 and 24.99; never having lived with a lover for at least 2 years; any convictions for nonsexual violence at the time of the index offense; any prior conviction for nonsexual violence; four or more sentencing dates prior to index offense; any unrelated victims(s); any stranger victims; and any male victims. The Static-99 allows for the nomothetic categorization of an individual as low, moderate-low, moderate-high, and high risk to reoffend based on a statistical calculation of risk to reoffend over 5, 10, and 15 years (Phenix, Hanson, & Thornton, 2000).

Actuarial risk assessment is designed to, within a statistically acceptable level of error or certainty, classify offenders based on their level of risk to reoffend and informs considerations of detention, supervision, and risk management. However, because the types of factors measured are inherently unchangeable, the assessment of static risk adds little to the efforts to identify specifically how to intervene and reduce an individual's risk for sexual reoffense. In response to this quandary, and also influenced by the Hanson and Bussière (1998) study, measures of dynamic risk, or assessment methods that will identify and capture changes in risk-related factors that could be amenable to the change process, have been developed (see STEP, Beech, Friendship, Erikson, & Hanson, 2002; SONAR, Hanson & Harris, 2000; SRA, Thornton, 2002), and some have already been refined (STABLE-2007, Hanson, Harris, Scott, & Helmus, 2007).

A further exploration of the empirically derived dynamic factors associated with risk for sexual reoffense will follow in the next section. Of import here is the recognition that the present challenge of decreasing the heterogeneity within the larger sex-offender population and making clinically germane distinctions that adequately define relevant treatment groups may be best met by adhering to the risk principle (Andrews & Bonta, 2006) (which dictates that the intensity of treatment should match the risk of the offender), and using empirically validated measures of an individual's risk for sexual reoffense in order to do so.

The findings from the study by Yates and Kingston (2006) on the validity of the self-regulation model provide some support for this kind of application. First, they were able to further validate that different types of sex offenders present at different levels of risk for sexual reoffense. More specifically, however, on measures of both static and dynamic factors associated with the risk for sexual offense recidivism (including the Static-99), the two types of approach-goal offenders (approach-active and approach-passive) were identified as being at significantly higher risk for sexual reoffense as predicted (Yates & Kingston, 2006). As such, the risk principle would dictate that the higher-risk approach-goal offenders receive the highest intensity of treatment services and resources that would match their elevated risk for reoffense, and the avoidant-active offenders would receive treatment at lower levels of intensity as indicated by their lower risk for reoffense (Yates & Kingston, 2006). Aimed at making treatment more focused, efficient, as well as effective, applying the risk principle to sex offender–specific treatment finds further support relative to minimizing possible negative dosing effects. Data suggest that the more standardized comprehensive CBT approaches (where all group members participate in all components of treatment) that have dominated sex offender–specific treatment in the past have resulted in the overprescribing of treatment for lower-risk offenders (Mailloux et al., 2003). This overdosing may have inadvertently served to increase rather than decrease risk for reoffense among previously low-risk offenders. As such, utilization of the risk principle to prescribe the appropriate intensity of sex offender–specific treatment could go far in addressing these kinds of treatment dosing effect concerns.

Challenge 2: Empirically Valid Targets of Treatment

Key to any successful therapeutic endeavor designed to change behavior, much less those designed to stop sex offenders from reoffending, is being able to identify through assessment and then target in treatment those factors that appear to contribute most significantly to the problem behavior. As the sex offender treatment field has advanced, there has been a corresponding growth in the number and sophistication of etiological theories proposed to explain the development of sexually deviant behavior with the aim of informing treatment efforts to change it.

For instance, Freud (1957) explained sexual deviance in general as a result of an individual becoming fixated at a given stage of psychosexual development and prescribed psychoanalysis as the clinical intervention. Later, multifactored theories appeared that reflected a growing awareness of important distinctions among sex offenders. For example, in the consideration of the etiological factors associated specifically with child sexual abusers, Finkelhor (1984) proposed a four-factor theory of child molestation: (1) motivation based on an individual's overidentification with children; (2) disinhibition that allowed individuals to overcome barriers that would normally prohibit their acting on deviant interests; (3) environmental characteristics; and (4) victim characteristics that would facilitate an offense. Malamuth, Heavey, and Linz (1993) have offered the confluence model of rape that has acquired some empirical support and suggests when hostile masculinity and sexual promiscuity converge with opportunity, the potential for sexually aggressive behavior is high.

Contemporary theories suggest that a number of potential initiating factors are at play in the development of sexual offending behavior patterns. They further seek the integration of these essential factors in an inclusive etiological model that will drive comprehensive and multidimensional treatment. A good example of this can be seen in Marshall and Barbaree's (1990) biopsychosocial conceptualization of sexual deviancy that incorporates developmental, hormonal, psychological, and social factors into an understanding of the pathway to sexual offending behavior.

Although a detailed examination of the numerous theories that attempt to explain the origins of sexually deviant behavior falls outside the focus of this chapter (see Laws & O'Donohue, 2008; Ward, Polaschek, & Beech, 2006), it is important to note the significant role they have played in the historical conceptualization of sex offender–specific treatment. However, while an etiological understanding of the distal variables that serve to initiate sexual deviancy is important relative to therapeutic attempts to decrease sex-offending behavior, more currently the increasing emphasis has been on identifying those more proximal factors that act to maintain sex-offending behavior (Hanson & Morton-Bourgon, 2004).

Criminogenic Factors

The continued practice of targeting as primary and universally addressing treatment foci factors that have not been empirically supported by methodologically more sound research (i.e., denial, empathy deficits) (Hanson & Bussière, 1998) appears to have more complex functions relative to their impact on sexual reoffense than previously conceptualized (i.e., cognitive distortions; Ward, Hudson, & Marshall, 1995), has proven to be differentially relevant depending on sex offense and/or offender type (i.e., social skills, impulsivity, offense pathways) (Kirsch, Becker, & Figueredo, 2004; Knight & Prentky, 1990; Ward & Hudson, 2000), and would appear to impede the provision of effective treatment and further obfuscate efforts to capture the efficacy of a given approach.

As such, Andrews and Bonta's (2006) need principle states that the focus of treatment for offenders should be on criminogenic factors—dynamic factors or those that are amenable to change and have been shown to be directly associated with a reoccurrence in criminal behavior (Andrews & Bonta, 2006). Andrews and Bonta (2006) identify seven major criminogenic factors among the nonsexual, general criminal offender population: antisocial personality patterns, procriminal attitudes, antisocial social influences, substance use, problems in the family or marital relationship, performance problems, dissatisfaction in work or school, and a lack of prosocial recreational activities. Treatment for criminal offenders then focuses on goals such as building self-management skills and a prosocial identity, reducing substance use, and teaching prosocial hobbies.

As articulated, the need principle matches well with the sex offender treatment field's current move toward focusing on empirically identifying, assessing, and targeting in treatment the dynamic risk factors associated with sexual offending behavior. It has become a critical and challenging task to empirically identify changeable factors associated with sex offense recidivism and effectively assess the differential weight they may be adding to the equation that leads to a sexual reoffense in any given individual. Of relevance to an evidence-based clinical endeavor of altering the risk for sexual reoffense is focusing on the most salient and empirically supported dynamic factors that both have the capacity for change and may be responsive to intervention.

As noted previously, Hanson and colleagues (2007) have developed the STABLE-2007, which contains empirically supported criminogenic factors drawn from the literature that are associated with the dynamic risk for sex offense recidivism. The STABLE-2007 is designed to not only identify the weighted relevance of each factor for the individual offender, but it can also be used to capture within treatment change along five factorial dimensions: significant social influences, intimacy deficits, general self-regulation, sexual self-regulation, and cooperation with supervision (Hanson et al., 2007). These criminogenic factors are summarized below.

Significant Social Influences. The first factor identifies the relative impact of both positive and negative social influences in the offender's life on the risk to reoffend. It helps examine to what degree the individual is engaged and interacting with prosocial, positive, and supportive people, thereby potentially mitigating the individual's risk for reoffense. This is compared with the degree to which the offender may be associating with more antisocial elements that could undermine control and increase vulnerability to return to more maladaptive and antisocial behavior patterns, thereby increasing the risk for reoffense.

Intimacy Deficits. The second factor focuses on the deficits an individual may have in the area of interpersonal intimacy that can contribute to the potential to reoffend. Elements of this factor that can serve as targets for treatment include increasing the individual's capacity to sustain healthy intimate relationships with appropriate others; for child molesters, targeting their inappropriate emotional identification with children; interestingly, for both child molesters and rapists, decreasing hostility toward women as evidenced in part by their expressed distrust of women, sexist attitudes, and conflicted relationships with women; improving social integration and decreasing the individual's subjective sense of loneliness and isolation; and increasing an individual's concern for others.

General Self-Regulation. Identification of the third factor allows for interventions that address the increased risk for reoffense that arises from an individual's difficulty with monitoring and censoring antisocial thoughts and behavior. Relative to this factor, problematic general self-regulation is associated with impulsivity as demonstrated across several domains, not just sexual impulsivity, and can present in the form of being easily bored and/or an individual easily engaging in opportunistic behavior that has a high likelihood of a negative consequence. Concerns in the domain of self-regulation can also be seen in the individual's pattern of impaired problem solving, including difficulty identifying that something is a problem as well as generating and assessing alternative options or solutions. Finally, negative emotionality and/or hostility can contribute to general dysregulation and is reflected in an attitude of near constant malcontent and grievance. As such, general dysregulation itself may contribute to an overall decline in an individual's ability for effective and appropriate self-management, foster poor decision making, and once again increase an offender's risk for reoffense.

Sexual Self-Regulation. The fourth factor is associated with the increased risk for sexual reoffense that is related to an individual's inability for effective and adaptive sexual regulation. This can manifest as an increase in an individual's level of sexual drive and/or an increase in the degree to which the offender is sexually preoccupied as evidenced by recurrent problematic sexual thoughts or behavior, engaging in sexual activity that is impersonal and/or interferes with prosocial goals, or is seen as excessive. An individual's maladaptive dependence on using sex as a means of coping with stress and negative emotions can contribute to an elevation in risk to sexually recidivate. Finally, as has been noted, the presence of deviant sexual interests is highly associated with an individual's risk for sexual reoffense and continues to be an important element to assess and a central focus of treatment.

Cooperation With Supervision. The final factor is associated with the degree to which the individual is seen as cooperating with supervision and adhering to imposed restrictions. An offender who is being uncooperative, deceptive, and/or manipulative could be seen to be at increased risk for sexual reoffense. As such, addressing the barriers that may impede the offender's motivation or ability to reasonably comply with parole or probation demands should be incorporated into the individual's treatment plan.

This move toward an empirical grounding of the dynamic treatment variables associated with sexual reoffense and the effect that interventions targeting these factors may have on the long-term risk for sex offense recidivism represents the cutting edge of research regarding what works in stopping the reoccurrence of sex-offending behavior (Hanson et al., 2007). In addition, being able to capture within treatment change on measurable factors contributes to the evolution of a more focused and hopefully demonstrably effective approach in addressing sexual deviancy and stopping the reoccurrence of sex-offending behaviors.

Challenge 3: Recognizing and Responding to Diversity

Although we have examined the issue of the substantial heterogeneity that exists within the broadly conceived population of sex offenders, we have not yet addressed the presence of the significant diversity across the population and how that relates to effective treatment. Most of the extensive historical literature available on sex offenders is limited to men, but they are not, in fact, the only people who commit sexual offenses, experience sexually deviant interest, or require treatment to desist from doing so. The empirically valid recognition of the relevant differences among men sex offenders lends credence to the need for research and the development of informed responses to those subgroups of sex offenders that differ markedly from men.

Andrews and Bonta's (2006) responsivity principle dictates that treatment approaches, in addition to being based on social learning methods that match the offender's learning style and ability to internalize information (general responsivity), should also be responsive to relevant individual variables (specific responsivity). Both are significant factors that, although not directly associated with the risk for reoffense in the same way as criminogenic factors are, may act to interfere with treatment receptivity and indirectly influence risk (Andrews & Bonta, 2006). As such, to maximize positive treatment effects, interventions should be tailored to relevant individual variables such as gender, age, and intellectual capacity.

Female Sex Offenders

An important and emergent subgroup of sex offenders that presents with distinct treatment challenges compared to men are women sex offenders. Interest in the woman sex offender has grown. A survey published in 2003 (McGrath, Cumming, & Burchard, 2003) of North American sex offender treatment programs identified 740 community and residential treatment programs for female sex offenders (including women, adolescents, and girls). Previous surveys from 2000, which identified 284 programs for females, and the 1986 figures did not report gender-distinct services separately (Bear, 2000; Burton & Smith-Darden, 2001). Although research on female sex offenders is limited, it is growing. Logan (2008) notes that the study of sexual deviance in women in the form of paraphilic disorders is minimal, with the focus of research more on the harmful or abusive sexual behavior that females engage in. Early research on female sex offenders failed to capture the extent of the abuse due to significant underreporting from male victims (Ford, 2006). However, a 2004 report on crime by the Federal Bureau of Investigation noted that females were responsible for 8.5% of sexual crimes (Saleh, Dwyer, & Grudzinskas, 2006). Barclay and Lie (2005) found even higher rates in a self-report sample of over 17,000 subjects in a health maintenance organization, which indicated that, in 40% of the cases of male victims of sexual abuse and 6% of the female cases, the identified perpetrator was female. Cortini and Hanson (2005) contrasted sexual offense recidivism between female and male offenders and found a rate of 1% compared with 13% to 14%, respectively, with a follow-up period of 5 years.

Early typological research on female sex offenders suggests interesting variations among them that highlight the need for a different approach from males in targeting relevant treatment foci. In an exploratory study, Matthews, Matthews, and Speltz (1989) found three distinct types of female offenders. It was suggested that the *teacher/lover* type sexually abused prepubescent and adolescent boys who they perceived as peers. The *predisposed* offender was a victim of significant early and sustained sexual abuse who would sexually abuse against her own children in an attempt to obtain emotional intimacy that is not threatening to herself. A female offender who sexually perpetrates in collaboration with a male offender was identified as a *male-coerced* offender. This type of female offender was identified as both dependent and nonassertive and reportedly would perpetrate against familial as well as nonfamilial children.

Nathan and Ward (2001) expanded the earlier work of Matthews and colleagues and described two overarching types of female offenders: the *self-initiated* abuser and the *accompanied* abuser. The self-initiated abuser type is further subdivided into two types. The predisposed offender generally has a history of sexual abuse and perpetrates out of emotional dysregulation associated with anger, loneliness, a sense of powerlessness, and/or deviant, compulsive sexual urges. The teacher/lover, as described similarly in the earlier Matthews et al. model (1989), sees her victim as her intimate equal, romanticizes the interpersonal connection, and is generally understood to be motivated by a search for an overidealized intimate relationship. There are also two types of accompanied offenders: the male-coerced type, who is forced to engage in sexual offending behavior at the direction of an abusive male upon whom she is likely dependent, and the male-accompanied type, who is a cooperative and willing participant with the male abuser and perpetrates to satisfy sexual needs (Nathan & Ward, 2001).

The focus of treatment in the 16 female sex offender cases studied by Matthews et al. (1989) included having the participants gain insight into their own sexual abuse as well as the sexual abuse they perpetrated; increasing their empathy toward their victims; examining their dependency issues and their relationships with men; improving their sense of self-esteem and self-worth; and exploring parenting issues. Of particular note was the importance of the treatment group members' recognition that sexual abuse was not normative, along with increasing their understanding of the impact of intergenerational abuse. Based on this study's findings, relevant change occurred within a treatment group context of acceptance and support, with improvement for the participants noted along several dimensions: an increase in self-worth, the adoption of a positive identity, and an increased awareness of their own issues (Matthews et al., 1989.) More recently, Ford and Cortoni (2008) point to a number of authors who have outlined treatment models for female sex offenders despite the dearth of empirical data available. In large measure, the themes are similar and include improving emotional management, enhancing self-esteem and assertiveness, clarifying misperceptions of victims' needs, identifying and finding better ways to satisfy their own unmet or inappropriately met intimacy needs, addressing cognitive distortions, and improving coping skills.

The foundation of much of the work on understanding and developing treatment models for female sex offenders is based on what is known about men (Ford, 2006). Similarities have been hypothesized (i.e., sexual deviance and general criminality; Clark & Howden-Windall, 2000) and have been utilized to establish treatment programs for female sex offenders (Eldridge & Saradjian, 2000). However, expected gender differences may have important implications for positive treatment outcomes and call for gender-responsive approaches that are tailored specifically to the differences between females and males (Ford, 2006). In a comparative analysis, Allen (1991) found that female sex offenders lived under less stable conditions than male sex offenders, experienced harsher childhoods, and demonstrated higher needs for both emotional as well as sexual fulfillment—noncriminogenic factors, perhaps, but nonetheless potentially significant when identifying treatment responsivity factors in female sex offenders. Further, Schwartz and Cellini (1995) suggest that differences in communication and relational styles argue for a group treatment process for female sex offenders that recognizes the need for intimacy and connection demonstrated by women as compared to the need for independence and autonomy more often displayed by men in group treatment settings. To date, however, there are limited data available regarding specific responsivity factors among female sex offenders that have been identified and that would increase treatment efficacy (Ford, 2006).

Adolescent Sex Offenders

Adolescents with problematic sexual behaviors make up a subpopulation of sex offenders whose treatment needs differ in important ways from those of men as well. Interest in this subgroup has increased, and treatment programming has increased in the United States from 346 treatment programs in 1986 to 937 in 2002 (McGrath et al., 2003). While some research suggests that a large percentage of sexual crimes are perpetrated by adolescents (20% of rapes and 30% to 50% of child molestation; Murphy & Page, 2000), it is important to note that most adolescent sex offenders do not go on to become adult sex offenders (Abel, Osborn, and Twigg, 1993; Hunter, 2000).

Although juvenile sex offenders represent a heterogeneous group, there are some common characteristics among them, including: male sex, ages 13 to 17, poor impulse control, impaired judgment, as many as 80% have been diagnosed with a psychiatric disorder, 30% to 40% demonstrate learning disabilities and academic deficits, 20% to 50% have experienced physical abuse, and 40% to 80% have histories of sexual abuse (Center for Sex Offender Management, 1999). Typologies for juvenile sex offenders largely have been based on the distinction between those who offend against children and those who offend against adults and/or their peers. Those who offend against children usually show both self-esteem and social skills deficits and have difficulty establishing healthy interpersonal relationships. Those who offend against adults and peers are more likely to demonstrate antisocial behavior patterns in other domains as well as display more violence and may cause harm to their victims (Center for Sex Offender Management, 1999).

Relative to treatment, adolescent sex offenders should not be understood as merely junior versions of adult sex offenders. They have significant developmental needs that should be taken into any account of intervening in their presentation of problematic sexual behavior (Cellini, 1995). Although limited and plagued by similar methodological problems associated with the outcome research on adult sex offenders, research available to date on the effectiveness of adolescent sex offender treatment suggests that, as a group, juvenile sex offenders respond positively to early interventions and CBT programs tailored to their special needs (Alexander, 1999; Becker, 1990) and that recidivism rates of adolescent sex offenders who have received CBT range from 7% to 14% with a follow-up of 5 years (Becker, 1990).

Multisystemic therapy (MST) with adolescent sex offenders demonstrates promising findings (Borduin, Henggeler, Blaske, & Stein, 1990). MST was developed with the special treatment needs of adolescent sex offenders in mind. It is an intensive approach that involves both family and community-based treatment designed to target the convergence of factors that are hypothesized to contribute to sexually problematic behavior in juveniles. Treatment is individually tailored and includes a prescriptive combination of interventions that emphasizes "changing behavior and interpersonal relations within the offender's natural environment" (Borduin et al., p. 105). Therapy may involve the individual, his or her family, and/or social environment (i.e., peers, school) and is aimed at improving the parent–child relationship and engaging the adolescent in school, extracurricular activities, and healthy peer relations. Outcome results from this approach are highly encouraging. Borduin et al. (1990) found that, when MST for juvenile sex offenders was compared to individual therapy, recidivism rates at a 3-year follow-up were 12.5% compared to 75%, respectively. CBT offered within a continuum-of-care approach has also yielded small but positive treatment effects with juvenile sex offenders (Winokur, Rozen, Batchelder, & Valentine, 2006).

Developmentally Disabled Sex Offenders

Individuals with developmental disabilities who engage in criminal and deviant sexual behavior represent another important, expanding, and distinct treatment population with unique responsivity challenges, both intellectual and otherwise. Interest in the developmentally disabled sex-offending population has increased since the move in the 1980s toward deinstitutionalization of chronic care psychiatric patients and efforts to have the disabled live in communities rather than in institutional settings. In 2002, over 50% of sex offender treatment programs offered special services for sex offenders with developmental disabilities (McGrath et al., 2003).

There are increasing but still limited empirical data on this sex offender subgroup. It is clear, however, that deficits particular to sex offenders with developmental disabilities demand that effective treatment approaches be designed, with their special needs and limitations taken into consideration. Haaven and Coleman (2000) indicate that treatment for offenders with developmental disabilities should take into account the extent of the offender's compromised learning ability and cognitive processing speed and other factors associated with greater difficulties with criminogenic as well as noncriminogenic factors, such as low self-esteem, impaired coping styles, difficulties with emotional regulation, lack of appreciation for causal relationships and consequences, and an inability to recognize and adapt to behavioral subtleties.

It is also important to note that most individuals with developmental disabilities are part of a service provider system that has conflicted feelings about identifying a disabled person as either sexually deviant or sexually criminal. Some care providers will want to absolve the developmentally disabled offender of any wrong because of their disability, while others may amplify such an offender's risk for reoffense for the same reason. These conflicted systems issues can raise important clinical concerns and represent another responsivity variable that points to the fact that this subpopulation of sex offenders has unique treatment challenges that must be considered.

One comprehensive approach to the developmentally disabled sex offender population that has demonstrated some efficacy (Bird, Sperry, & Carreiro, 1998) includes the following treatment components that appear to address their special needs: goal setting; comprehensive case management; social skills training; positive reinforcement strategies; crisis intervention as needed; competency-based skills training; monitoring and managing medications; and community-based living. Haaven, Little, & Petre-Miller (1990) describe an intensive residential program model for developmentally disabled sex offenders that represents one part of a larger continuum-of-care system. This approach focuses on social skills building in the context of a modified therapeutic community, treatment that is tailored to the needs of the individual, and the implementation of self-help skills. The intensive phase of treatment focuses on five areas (social skills competency, medical/psychiatric, alcohol/drugs, personality disorders, and sexual deviancy) and includes the adaptation of more standard CBT interventions to the developmentally disabled population. This phase of treatment is followed by an after-care plan that helps the sex offender with developmental disabilities transition to a less restrictive environment and to more integrated community living. Outcome data with this population, again notably flawed, suggest that the longer a resident stayed in services, the lower the rate for recidivism (less than 90 days had a 65% recidivism rate; 545 days with aftercare had a 29% recidivism rate) (Haaven et al., 1990). Subjective data collected revealed that participants were able to demonstrate competencies in both basic life and treatment skills, understood that behavior was influenced by thought, and were able to identify primary thinking errors (Haaven et al., 1990).

Evaluating treatment outcomes with the developmentally disabled sex offender population is fraught with common (e.g., random assignment) and particular problems (e.g., the extended length of time needed to demonstrate behavioral change in the developmentally disabled population) that makes it difficult at best to determine treatment efficacy. However, promising methods are emerging as there is a move toward the increased use of more rigorous meta-analytic techniques to establish evidence-based practice in the developmentally disabled sex offender treatment field as well as efforts to capture positive, demonstrable behavioral changes (e.g., social skills acquisition, improvement in problem solving, self-management, and vocational skills) that can prevent a reoccurrence of sex-offending behavior (Sturmey, Taylor, & Lindsay, 2004).

Noncriminogenic and Process Variables Associated With Responsivity

In addition to the potential treatment-specific confounds raised by the diversity of the sex-offending population noted above, the responsivity principle also supports the benefits of targeting both offender-specific noncriminogenic factors in treatment as well as therapeutic process variables. In a broad but in-depth review of a neglected area of exploration, Looman, Dickie, and Abracen (2005) suggest that viable, noncriminogenic variables can be drawn from the sex offender literature and that, when effectively addressed, can impact the degree to which a given individual benefits from treatment. According to Looman et al. (2005), these responsivity factors can include psychopathy, motivation, denial/minimization, intellectual functioning, hostility, personality profile, deviant arousal (which also serves as a criminogenic factor), and sex offender type; the authors note that this is not an exhaustive list and that these more indirect, internal factors that appear to influence treatment engagement and thereby treatment efficacy in a more circuitous manner require further research. For instance, Looman et al. (2005) and others (Bruhn, 2006; Rothman, 2007) argue for the need to address therapeutic process variables, such as therapist and setting characteristics, therapist client alliance, readiness for change, and so forth, that can function to facilitate treatment engagement. Although current research in this area is limited, it is growing. For instance, Beech and Fordham (1997) examined the therapeutic climate of 12 sex offender treatment programs and found that:

> A successful group was highly cohesive, was well organized and led and encouraged the open expression of feelings, produced a sense of group responsibility, and instilled a sense of hope in its members. A helpful and supportive leadership style was found to be important in creating an atmosphere in which effective treatment could take place. Overcontrolling leaders were seen to have a detrimental effect upon group climate. (p. 219)

As such, the significance of further understanding the impact that therapeutic process variables may have on successful treatment outcomes ought not to be underestimated, because they may, in fact, have quite a powerful influence on the effective delivery of treatment.

Challenge 4: Knowing and Using What Works

The principle of professional discretion purports that, based on professional judgments, the other three principles may be modified (Andrews & Bonta, 2006). It could be argued further that professional judgments to alter elements of treatment should only be made with, or at the very least be primarily informed by, the best available data about what works with sex offenders. The difficulty lies in the empirical knowing of the answer to this complex question and the difficulty in determining whether, in fact, given treatment interventions are having the desired effect and are achieving the overarching goal of reducing or eliminating sexual offending behavior and/or whether elements of a particular treatment are even useful. On the surface, the question of whether sex offender–specific treatment is effective seems like a relatively straightforward and dichotomous one: Does participating in treatment stop someone from committing further sexual offenses or not? However, this legitimate and seemingly simple question is rife with a number of complications that plague and confound the efforts of sex offender–specific treatment outcome research (Grossman, Martis, & Fichtner, 1999).

It was a now well-known and oft-cited 1989 review of studies on sex offense recidivism (Furby, Weinrott, & Blackshaw, 1989) that not only sparked the ongoing debate about whether sex offender treatment works, but also fueled the groundswell movement to improve the methods of capturing treatment effects that continues today. In brief, based on a review of 55 studies that examined the impact of treatment on sex offense reoffense rates, Furby et al. concluded that there was no statistical evidence to indicate that treatment decreased sex offense recidivism rates. However, it was also acknowledged that the methodologies employed by the studies that were reviewed to calculate treatment effects were far less than ideal. Nonetheless, what came to be, and unfortunately continues to be, the prevailing idea that sex offenders cannot be treated was launched and believed by the public to be supported by the best research in the field. The ensuing debate among professionals has highlighted a number of serious challenges to the endeavor of trying to capture sex offender–specific treatment effects on sexual offense recidivism. Primary among them is the low base rate of known sex offense recidivism, which is estimated to be about 13% over 4 to 5 years (Hanson & Bussière, 1998). With the detected incidence of the reoccurrence of a sexual offense already relatively low and the inability to include in any statistical calculation the actual incidence of sexual offending because of recidivism behavior that goes undetected, it takes large numbers of study subjects to generate enough data to capture even a minimal statistically significant treatment effect.

In addition, most sex offender treatment programs have limited ability to implement well-designed, rigorous clinical research studies that include random assignment to treatment groups. Further complicating clinical research matters are the variable ways of operationally defining recidivism (i.e., Do we measure rearrest, reconviction, or reincarceration for any reoffense or a new sex offense or a new sex offense of the same type?) and differing lengths of follow-up time that are reported (i.e., Are we examining recidivism at 3, 5, or 10 years post release from incarceration?). Also, the lack of a standardized treatment approach that could be compared across samples and settings leaves us with little opportunity to identify an evidence-based understanding of what works best in the treatment of sex offenders.

These and other methodological challenges were noted in a special issue on treatment outcome research in *Sexual Abuse: A Journal of Research and Treatment* (Miner, 1997). These limits to the outcome research have contributed to inconsistent (read: "inconclusive-therefore-must-not-work") results in sex offender treatment outcome research. Additionally, outcome studies that do exist offer conflicting findings that it is difficult to make sense of. For instance, a number of studies and reviews suggest that cognitive-behavioral treatment approaches can be effective in reducing recidivism among sex offenders (Aytes, Olsen, Zakrjsek, Murray, & Ireson, 2001; Maletzky & Steinhauser, 2002), but a number of studies point to treatment failure (Barbaree, 1997; Marques et al., 2005; Quinsey, Harris, Rice, & Lalumière, 1993; Rice, Harris, & Quinsey, 1991).

A recent example of this conflict can be seen in the presentation of the final results from the longitudinal treatment outcome study at the Sex Offender Treatment and Evaluation Project (SOTEP; Marques et al., 2005) in California; the results were both highly anticipated from the start and highly disappointing in their conclusions. The SOTEP was understood to represent the gold standard in the design of a sex offender treatment efficacy study by its inclusion of random assignment to treatment groups, the standardization of the relapse prevention approach being studied, and the inclusion of a 5-year follow-up period with a thorough calculation of recidivism. The findings from the SOTEP, however, failed to provide empirical support that treatment—specifically, a cognitive-behavioral approach based on relapse prevention—was effective in reducing sexual offense recidivism in their sample comprised of 190 child abusers and adult rapists.

In stark contrast, however, Hanson and colleagues (2002) reported on the findings of a meta-analysis that included 43 studies and examined the impact of treatment on recidivism rates for over 9,000 sex offenders. They concluded that cognitive-behavioral treatment produced statistically significant reductions in sex offense recidivism (as much as 20% with a follow-up of 4 to 5 years) within a mixed sample of offenders convicted of child sexual crimes as well as adult sexual crimes. This type of positive outcome has been found in several other studies using meta-analytic statistical methodologies (Alexander, 1999; Hall, 1995; Lösel & Schmucker, 2005).

Despite the mixed and partial results offered in the literature, and while incisive criticisms of treatment outcome research methodologies and interpretation can be launched in both directions, the balance of the data, imperfect as all of it may be, appears to suggest that there is increasing support that cognitive-behavioral treatment, in conjunction with hormonal therapies as appropriate, can in general be effective in reducing recidivism among the sex-offending population. Individually tailoring treatment to an offender's needs, however, as proposed by the risk–needs–responsivity principles, may make it more difficult to capture treatment effects because of the lack of a standardized approach. However, Andrews and Bonta's (2006) principles of effective treatment for offenders should improve treatment outcomes by improving the aim of treatment; it will be up to the professional field to figure out how to demonstrate that these new approaches are working and that clinical decisions can and should be made accordingly.

Hanson (1997) offers some guidelines for improving efforts at both providing a defensible foundation for the empirically based efficacy of sex offender treatment as well as establishing support for the validity and effectiveness of applied cognitive-behavioral approaches in real-world clinical settings with sex offenders. These recommendations include implementing controlled, single-site research studies with large samples; using meta-analytic techniques to examine the collective data from numerous small studies on sex offender treatment outcome; and, as noted previously in the discussion of criminogenic factors, the analysis of within-treatment change on dynamic factors that have been increasingly demonstrated to be associated with recidivism risk among sex offenders (Hanson & Harris, 2001).

CONCLUSION

Increasingly, it seems, sex offender–specific interventionists are seeking to implement integrated approaches that are not only the most effective, but also the most efficient and parsimonious. They seek to employ the most appropriate, effective methods to successfully target and treat the factors that matter most with the highly heterogeneous sex-offending populations under their care and management. Two of the relatively newer treatment models being implemented and studied are the Containment Model (English, 1998), which is a risk management approach derived from a criminal justice perspective, and the Good Lives Model (Ward & Stewart, 2003), which is a rehabilitative, strength-based approach. These two treatment models could be said to represent the emergent, current best practices in the field of sex offender treatment and management, because they include an appreciation of the contemporary challenges previously outlined and attempt to attend to the evolving empirical knowledge about what works with sex offenders.

Interestingly, while both models incorporate concepts from the risk–needs–responsivity principles of Andrews and Bonta (2006), differences in their emphasis on different principles make for dramatically different formulations of what is identified as the best way to treat and manage sex offenders. Briefly, the Containment Model (English, 1998) represents an integrated and multidimensional approach to sex offender management that emphasizes the risk–need principles outlined earlier. In practice, the highest-risk offenders are provided with the most intensive services, and the therapeutic focus is on eliminating criminogenic factors in order to reduce the risk for sexual reoffense. The theory behind the Containment Model elegantly weaves together: (1) the externally enforcing element of the criminal justice system through community supervision; (2) with the cultivation of internal control through therapeutic intervention; (3) within the polygraph-reinforced context of offender accountability and responsibility. Described as an "an evolving social experiment that operationalizes the best of empirical data and human experience" (p. 220), the containment approach is gaining in popularity, and research regarding its efficacy looks promising.

In contrast, the Good Lives Model, derived from the self-regulation pathways approach by Ward and Hudson (2000), integrates both the risk–need principles articulated by Andrews and Bonta (2006). However, it holds as primary the importance of the responsivity principle and includes the relevance of addressing noncriminogenic needs as well as criminogenic needs (Ward & Stewart, 2003). The Good Lives approach emphasizes the importance of "the *enhancement* of offenders' capabilities" to secure the basic human goods that can improve the quality of their lives and thereby reduce criminal behavior as compared with the containment emphasis on risk management (Ward & Stewart, 2003, p. 353). This approach is based on an integration of the findings from multiple areas of research regarding what causes people to make sustained changes in their behavior; it is also gaining popularity and beginning to gather empirical support for its efficacy.

The sex offender–specific treatment field continues to evolve, and there are new and exciting ideas appearing on the horizon all the time. For instance, neuroscience technologies are exploring the biological substrates of both normative as well as deviant human sexuality in order to illuminate essential differences that can impact deviant sexual behavior (Hyde, 2005; Langevin, 1990). Efforts are ongoing regarding improving treatment delivery and the implementation of evidence-based service provision. As such, the notion of treatment provider accreditation is gaining popularity, and more states are requiring some demonstrated expertise to improve the quality and effectiveness of sex offender–specific treatment (Home Office, 2003). And new ideas about old intuitions continue to be challenged. For example, Ward, Hudson, and Marshal (1995) proffer an alternative view of the cognitive distortions that are usually adhered to by many sex offenders to rationalize their behavior that suggests a deconstructed cognitive state leading to impaired information processing. This new conceptualization informs a very different treatment approach to this troubling clinical issue in sex offender treatment. And finally, energy and interest are being generated to continue to find better ways to bring about, as well as measure, meaningful changes in sexual-offending behavior. In time, the presumption that treatment for sex offenders does not work can be replaced with evidence that says it can and does work, in lots of ways for many kinds of sex offenders through the dedicated effort by the professionals in the field who are committed to making our communities increasingly safe from sexual violence.

REFERENCES

Abel, G. G., Blanchard, E. B., & Becker, J. V. (1978). An integrated treatment program for rapists. In R. Rada (Ed.), *Clinical aspects of the rapist* (pp. 161–214). New York: Grune & Stratton.

Abel, G. G., Osborn, C. A., & Twigg, D. A. (1993). Sexual assault through the life span: Adult offenders with juvenile histories. In H. E. Barbaree, W. L. Marshall, & S. M. Hudson (Eds.), *The juvenile sex offender* (pp. 104–117). New York: Guilford Press.

Alexander, M. A. (1999). Sexual offender treatment efficacy revisited. *Sexual Abuse: A Journal of Research and Treatment, 11*(2), 101–116.

Allen, C. M. (1991). *Women and men who sexually abuse children: A comparative analysis.* Brandon, VT: Safer Society Press.

American Psychiatric Association. (2002). *Diagnostic and statistical manual of mental disorders* (4th ed., rev.). Washington, DC: Author.

Andrews, D. A., & Bonta, J. (2006). *The psychology of criminal conduct* (4th ed.). Newark, NJ: LexisNexis.

Aytes, K. E., Olsen, S. S., Zakrajsek, T., Murray, P., & Ireson, R. (2001). Cognitive/behavioral treatment for sexual offenders: An examination of recidivism. *Sexual Abuse: A Journal of Research and Treatment, 13*(4), 223–231.

Bandura, A. (1977). *Social learning theory.* Englewood Cliffs, NJ: Prentice Hall.

Barbaree, H. E. (1997). Evaluating treatment efficacy with sexual offenders: The insensitivity of recidivism studies to treatment effects. *Sexual Abuse: A Journal of Research and Treatment, 9*, 111–128.

Barclay, L., & Lie, D. (2005, July 25). Consequences of childhood sexual abuse similar for both sexes. Medscape Medical News. Retrieved June 14, 2008, from www.netscape.com/viewarticle/508115

Bear, E. (Ed.). (2000). *1996 nationwide survey: A survey of treatment programs and models serving children with sexual behavior problems, adolescent sex offenders, and adult sex offenders*. Brandon, VT: Safer Society Foundation.

Becker, J. V. (1990). Treating adolescent sexual offenders. *Professional Psychology: Research, and Practice, 21*, 362–365.

Beech, A., & Fordham, A. S. (1997). Therapeutic climate of sexual offender treatment programs. *Sexual Abuse: A Journal of Research and Treatment, 9*(3), 219–237.

Beech, A., Friendship, C., Erikson, M., & Hanson, R. K. (2002). Static and dynamic predictors of reconviction. *Sexual Abuse: A Journal of Research and Treatment, 14*(2), 156–167.

Bird, F., Sperry, J., & Carreiro, H. (1998). Community habilitation and integration of adults with psychiatric disorders and mental retardation: Development of a clinically responsive environment. *Journal of Developmental and Physical Disabilities, 10*(4), 331–348.

Borduin, C. M., Henggeler, S. W., Blaske, D. M., & Stein, R. J. (1990). Multisystemic treatment of adolescent sexual offenders. *International Journal of Offender Therapy and Comparative Criminology, 34*(2), 105–113.

Bradford, J. (1990). The antiandrogen and hormonal treatment of sex offenders. In W. L. Marshall, D. R. Laws, & H. E. Barbaree (Eds.), *Handbook of sexual assault: Issues, theories, and treatment of the offender* (pp. 297–310). New York: Plenum Press.

Bradford, J. (1997). Medical interventions in sexual deviance. In D. R. Laws & W. O'Donohue (Eds.), *Sexual deviance: Theory, assessment, and treatment* (pp. 449–464). New York: Guilford Press.

Bruhn, S. L. (2006). *To change or not to change?: An examination of factors related to willingness to change in sex offenders.* Unpublished doctoral dissertation, University of Nebraska, Lincoln.

Burton, D. L., & Smith-Darden, J. (2001). *North American survey of sexual abuser treatment and models summary data.* Brandon, VT: Safer Society Press.

Carich, M. S., Dobkowski, M. A., & Delehanty, N. (2008, July 17). Clinical concerns: Should relapse prevention be abandoned? *ATSA Forum*, 1–11.

Cellini, H. R. (1995). Assessment and treatment of the adolescent sexual offender. In B. K. Schwartz & H. R. Cellini (Eds.), *The sex offender: Corrections, treatment and legal practice* (pp. 6-6–6-12). Kingston, NJ: Civic Research Institute.

Center for Sex Offender Management. (1999, December). Washington, DC: A Project of the Office of Justice Programs, U.S. Department of Justice.

Clark, D., & Howden-Windall, J. (2000). *A retrospective study of criminogenic factors in the female prison population.* London: Her Majesty's Prison Service.

Cortoni, F., & Hanson, R. K. (2005). *A review of the recidivism rates of adult female sexual offenders* (Research Report No. R-169). Ottawa: Correctional Service Canada.

Dougher, M. J. (1995). Behavioral techniques to alter sexual arousal. In B. K. Schwartz & H. R. Cellini (Eds.), *The sex offender: Corrections, treatment and legal practice* (pp. 15-1–15-8). Kingston, NJ: Civic Research Institute.

Eldridge, H. J., & Saradjian, J. (2000). Replacing the function of abusive behaviors for the offender: Remaking relapse prevention in working with women who sexually abuse children. In D. R. Laws, S. M. Hudson, & T. Ward (Eds.), *Remaking relapse prevention with sex offenders: A sourcebook* (pp. 402–426). Thousand Oaks, CA: Sage.

English, K. (1998). The containment approach: An aggressive strategy for the community management of adult sex offenders. *Psychology, Public Policy, and Law, 4*(1/2), 218–235.

Fernandez, Y. M., Shingler, J., & Marshall, W. L. (2006). Putting "behavior" back into the cognitive-behavioral treatment of sexual offenders. In W. L. Marshall, Y. M. Fernandez, L. E. Marshall, & G. A. Serran (Eds.), *Sexual offender treatment: Controversial issues* (pp. 211–224). West Sussex, England: Wiley.

Finklehor, D. (1984). *Child sexual abuse: New theory and research.* New York: Free Press.

Ford, H. (2006). *Women who sexually abuse children.* West Sussex, England: Wiley.

Ford, H., & Cortoni, F. (2008). Sexual deviance in females. In D. R. Laws & W. T. O'Donohue (Eds.), *Sexual deviance: Theory, assessment, and treatment* (2nd ed., pp. 508–526). New York: Guilford Press.

Freud, S. (1957). Three essays on the theory of sexuality. In J. Strachey (Ed. and Trans.), *The standard edition of the complete psychological works of Sigmund Freud* (Vol. 7, pp. 123–243). London: Hogarth Press. (Original work published in 1905)

Furby, L., Weinrott, M. R., & Blackshaw, L. (1989). Sex offender recidivism: A review. *Psychological Bulletin, 105,* 3–30.

Greenberg, D. M., Bradford, J.M.W., Curry, S., & O'Rourke, A. (1996). A comparison of treatment of paraphilias with three serotonin reuptake inhibitors: A retrospective study. *Bulletin of the American Academy of Psychiatry & the Law, 24,* 525–532.

Grossman, L. S., Martis, B., & Fichtner, C. G. (1999). Are sex offenders treatable? A research overview. *Psychiatric Services, 50*(3), 349–361.

Groth, A. N. (1979). *Men who rape: The psychology of the offender.* New York: Plenum Press.

Grubin, D. (2008). Medical models and interventions in sexual deviance. In D. R. Laws & W. T. O'Donohue (Eds.), *Sexual deviance: Theory, assessment, and treatment* (2nd ed., pp. 594–610). New York: Guilford Press.

Haaven, J., & Coleman, E. M. (2000). Treatment of the developmentally disabled sex offender. In D. R. Laws, S. M. Hudson, & T. Ward (Eds.), *Remaking relapse prevention with sex offenders: A sourcebook* (pp. 369–388). Thousand Oaks, CA: Sage.

Haaven, J., Little, R., & Petre-Miller, D. (1990). *Treating intellectually disabled sex offenders: A model residential program.* Orwell, VT: Safer Society Press.

Hall, G.C.N. (1995). Sexual offender recidivism revisited: A meta-analysis of recent treatment studies. *Journal of Consulting and Clinical Psychology, 63,* 802–809.

Hanson, R. K. (1997). How to know what works with sexual offenders. *Sexual Abuse: A Journal of Research and Treatment, 9*(2), 129–145.

Hanson, R. K. (2001). *Age and sexual recidivism: A comparison of rapists and child molesters* (User Report 2001–01). Ottawa: Department of the Solicitor General of Canada.

Hanson, R. K. (2006, September). *The dynamic supervision of sexual offenders: Updated data 2006.* Plenary presentation at the Annual Treatment and Research Conference of the Association for the Treatment of Sexual Abusers, Chicago.

Hanson, R. K., & Bussière, M. T. (1998). Predicting relapse: A meta-analysis of sexual offender recidivism studies. *Journal of Consulting and Clinical Psychology, 66*(2), 348–362.

Hanson, R. K., Gordon, A., Harris, A.J.R., Marques, J. K., Murphy, W., Quinsey, V. L., et al. (2002). First report of the collaborative outcome data project on the effectiveness of psychological treatment for sex offenders. *Sexual Abuse: A Journal of Research and Treatment, 14*(2), 169–194.

Hanson, R. K., & Harris, A.J.R. (2000). *The Sex Offender Need Assessment Rating (SONAR): A method for measuring change in risk levels* (User Report 2000–01). Ottawa: Department of the Solicitor General of Canada.

Hanson, R. K., & Harris, A.J.R. (2001). A structured approach to evaluating change among sexual offenders. *Sexual Abuse: A Journal of Research and Treatment, 13*(2), 105–122.

Hanson, R. K., Harris, A.J.R., Scott, T., & Helmus, L. (2007). *Assessing the risk of sexual offenders on community supervision: The Dynamic Supervision Project* (Corrections User Report No 2007–05). Ottawa: Public Safety Canada.

Hanson, R. K., & Morton-Bourgon, K. (2004). *Predictors of sexual recidivism: An updated meta-analysis* (Research Report No. 2004–02). Ottawa: Public Safety and Emergency Preparedness Canada.

Hanson, R. K., & Thornton, D. (1999). *Static-99: Improving actuarial risk assessments for sex offenders* (User Report 99–02). Ottawa: Department of the Solicitor General of Canada.

Home Office. (2003). What works: Accreditation—a summary. Retrieved May 31, 2008, from www.crimereduction.gov.uk/workingoffenders13.htm

Hucker, S. J., & Bain, J. (1990). Androgenic hormones and sexual assault. In W. L. Marshall, D. R. Laws, & H. E. Barbaree (Eds.), *Handbook of sexual assault: Issues, theories, and treatment of the offender* (pp. 93–102). New York: Plenum Press.

Hunter, J. A. (2000). *Understanding juvenile sex offenders: Research findings & guidelines for effective management & treatment.* Juvenile Justice Fact Sheet. Charlottesville: Institute of Law, Psychiatry, & Public Policy, University of Virginia.

Hyde, J. S. (2005). *Biological substrates of human sexuality.* Washington, DC: American Psychological Association.

Kafka, M. P. (1994). Serraline pharmacotherapy for paraphilias and paraphilia-related disorders: An open trial. *Annuals of Clinical Psychiatry, 6,* 189–195.

Kinsey, A. C., Pomeroy, W. B., & Martin, C. E. (1948). *Sexual behavior in the human male.* Philadelphia: Saunders.

Kinsey, A. C., Pomeroy, W. B., Martin, C. E., & Gebhard, P. H. (1953). *Sexual behavior in the human female.* Philadelphia: Saunders.

Kirsch, L. G., & Becker, J. V. (2005). Sexual offending: Theory of problem, theory of change, and implications for treatment effectiveness. *Aggression and Violent Behavior, 11,* 208–224.

Kirsch, L. G., Becker, J. V., & Figueredo, A. J. (2004, March). *Offense escalation in a population of civilly committed sex offenders.* Paper presented at the annual meeting of the American Psychology-Law Society, Scottsdale, AZ.

Knight, R. A., & Prentky, R. A. (1990). Classifying sexual offenders the development and corroboration of taxonomic models. In W. L. Marshall, D. R. Laws, & H. E. Barbaree (Eds.), *Handbook of sexual assault: Issues, theories, and treatment of the offender* (pp. 23–52). New York: Plenum Press.

Knopp, F. H., Freeman-Longo, R., & Stevenson, W. F. (1992). *Nationwide survey of juvenile and adult sexual offender treatment programs and models.* Brandon, VT: Safer Society Foundation.

Krafft-Ebing, R. von. (1886). *Psychopathia sexualia.* Stuttgart, Germany: Ferdinand Enke.

Krueger, R. B., & Kaplan, M. S. (2001). Depot-leuprolide acetate for treatment of paraphilias: A report of twelve cases. *Archives of Sexual Behavior, 30,* 409–422.

Langevin, R. (1990). Sexual anomalies and the brain. In W. L. Marshall, D. R. Laws, & H. E. Barbaree (Eds.), *Handbook of sexual assault: Issues, theories, and treatment of the offender* (pp. 103–113). New York: Plenum Press.

Laws, D. R. (2003). The rise and fall of relapse prevention. *Australian Psychologist, 38*(1), 22–30.

Laws, D. R., Hudson, S. M, & Ward, T. (Eds.). (2000). *Remaking relapse prevention with sex offenders.* Thousand Oaks, CA: Sage.

Laws, D. R., & Marshall, W. L. (2003). A brief history of behavioral and cognitive behavioral approaches to sexual offenders: Part 1. Early developments. *Sexual Abuse: A Journal of Research and Treatment, 15*(2), 75–92.

Laws, D. R., & O'Donohue, W. T. (2008). *Sexual deviance: Theory, assessment, and treatment* (2nd ed.). New York: Guilford Press.

Laws, D. R., & Ward, T. (2006). When one size doesn't fit all: The reformulation of relapse prevention. In W. L. Marshall, Y. M. Fernandez, L. E. Marshall, & G. A. Serran (Eds.), *Sexual offender treatment: Controversial issues* (pp. 241–254). West Sussex, England: Wiley.

Leahy, T. H. (2000). *A history of modern psychology* (3rd ed.). Englewood Cliffs, NJ: Prentice Hall.

Logan, C. (2008). Sexual deviance in females. In D. R. Laws & W. T. O'Donohue (Eds.), *Sexual deviance: Theory, assessment, and treatment* (2nd ed., pp. 486–507). New York: Guilford Press.

Looman, J., Dickie, I., & Abracen, J. (2005). Responsivity issues in the treatment of sexual offenders. *Trauma, Violence, & Abuse, 6*(4), 330–353.

Lösel, F., & Schmucker, M. (2005). The effectiveness of treatment for sexual offenders: A comprehensive meta-analysis. *Journal of Experimental Criminology, 1,* 1–29.

Mailloux, D. L., Abracen, J., Serin, R., Cousineau, C., Malcolm, B., & Looman, J. (2003). Dosage of treatment to sexual offenders: Are we overprescribing? *International Journal of Offender Therapy and Comparative Criminology, 47*(2), 171–184.

Malamuth, N. M., Heavey, C. L., & Linz, D. (1993). Predicting men's antisocial behavior against women: The interactional model of sexual aggression. In G. Nagayama Hall, R. Hirschman, J. R. Graham, & M. S. Zaragozee (Eds.), *Sexual aggression: Issues in etiology, assessment and treatment* (pp. 63–99). Bristol, PA: Taylor & Francis.

Maletzky, B. M., & Steinhauser, C. (2002). A 25-year follow-up of cognitive/behavioral therapy with 7,275 sexual offenders. *Behavior Modification, 26*(2), 123–147.

Maletzky, B. M., Tolan, A., & McFarland, B. (2006). The Oregon depo-provera program: A five-year follow-up. *Sexual Abuse: A Journal of Research and Treatment, 18*(3), 303–316.

Marlatt, G. A. (1982). Relapse prevention: A self-control program for the treatment of addictive behaviours. In R. B. Stuart (Ed.), *Adherence, compliance and generalization in behavioral medicine* (pp. 329–378). New York: Brunner/Mazel.

Marques, J. K., Wiederanders, M., Day, D. M., Nelson, C., & van Ommeren, A. (2005). Effects of a relapse prevention program on sexual recidivism: Final results from California's Sex Offender Treatment and Evaluation Project (SOTEP). *Sexual Abuse: A Journal of Research and Treatment, 17*(1), 79–107.

Marshall, W. L. (1996). Assessment, treatment, and theorizing about sex offenders. *Criminal Justice and Behavior, 23*(1), 162–199.

Marshall, W. L. (2006). Diagnostic issues, multiple paraphilias, and comorbid disorders in sexual offenders: Their incidence and treatment. *Aggression and Violent Behavior, 12*, 16–35.

Marshall, W. L., & Anderson, D. (2000). Do relapse prevention components enhance treatment effectiveness? In D. R. Laws, S. M. Hudson, & T. Ward (Eds.), *Remaking relapse prevention with sex offenders: A sourcebook* (pp. 39–55). Thousand Oaks, CA: Sage.

Marshall, W. L., Anderson, D., & Fernandez, Y. (1999). *Cognitive behavioural treatment of sexual offenders.* Chichester, England: Wiley.

Marshall, W. L., & Barbaree, H. E. (1990). An integrated theory of the etiology of sexual offending. In W. L. Marshall, D. R. Laws, & H. E. Barbaree (Eds.), *Handbook of sexual assault: Issues, theories, and treatment of the offender* (pp. 257–275). New York: Plenum Press.

Marshall, W. L., & Laws, D. R. (2003). A brief history of behavioral and cognitive behavioral approaches to sexual offenders: Part 2. The modern era. *Sexual Abuse: A Journal of Research and Treatment, 15*(2), 93–120.

Mathews, R., Matthews, J. K., & Speltz, K. (1989). *Female sexual offenders.* Brandon, VT: Safer Society Press.

McGrath, R. J., Cumming, G. F., & Burchard, B. L. (2003). *Current practices and trends in sexual abuser management: The Safer Society 2002 nationwide survey.* Brandon, VT: Safer Society Press.

McGuire, R. J., Carlisle, J. M., & Young, B. G. (1965). Sexual deviations as conditioned behaviour: A hypothesis. *Behaviour Research and Therapy, 3*, 185–190.

Miner, M. H. (Ed.). (1997). Treatment outcome research [Special issue]. *Sexual Abuse: A Journal of Research and Treatment, 9*(2).

Murphy, W. D., & Page, I. J. (2000). Relapse prevention with adolescent sex offenders. In D. R. Laws, S. M. Hudson, & T. Ward (Eds.), *Remaking relapse prevention with sex offenders: A sourcebook* (pp. 353–368). Thousand Oaks, CA: Sage.

Nathan, P., & Ward, T. (2001). Females who sexually abuse children: Assessment and treatment issues. *Journal of Sexual Aggression, 8*, 44–55.

O'Donohue, W., Regev, L. G., & Hagstrom, A. (2000). Problems with the DSM-IV diagnosis of pedophilia. *Sexual Abuse: A Journal of Research and Treatment, 12*(2), 95–105.

Ormrod, J. E. (1999). *Human learning* (3rd ed.). Upper Saddle River, NJ: Prentice Hall.

Phenix, A., Hanson, R. K., & Thornton, D. (2000). *Coding rules for the Static-99. Corrections Research: Manuals and forms.* Ottawa: Department of the Solicitor General of Canada.

Pithers, W. D., Marques, J. K., Gibat, C. C., & Marlatt, G. A. (1983). Relapse prevention with sexual aggressives: A self-control model of treatment and the maintenance of change. In J. G. Greer & I. R. Stuart (Eds.), *The sexual aggressor* (pp. 214–234). New York: Van Nostrand Reinhold.

Quinsey, V. L., & Earls, C. M. (1990). The modification of sexual preferences. In W. L. Marshall, D. R. Laws, & H. E. Barbaree (Eds.), *Handbook of sexual assault: Issues, theories, and treatment of the offender* (pp. 279–295). New York: Plenum Press.

Quinsey, V. L., Harris, G. T., Rice, M. E., & Lalumière, M. L. (1993). Assessing treatment efficacy in outcome studies of sex offenders. *Journal of Interpersonal Violence, 8,* 512–523.

Quinsey, V. L., Lalumière, M. L., Rice, M. E., & Harris, G. T. (1995). Predicting sexual offenses. In J. C. Campbell (Ed.), *Assessing dangerousness: Violence by sexual offenders, batterers, and child abusers* (pp. 114–136). Thousand Oaks, CA: Sage.

Rice, M. E., Harris, G. T., & Quinsey, V. L. (1991). Evaluation of an institutional based treatment program for child molesters. *Canadian Journal of Program Evaluation, 11,* 111–129.

Rothman, D. B. (2007). *The role of the therapeutic alliance in psychotherapy with sexual offenders.* Unpublished doctoral dissertation abstract, University of Manitoba, Canada.

Saleh, F. M., Dwyer, R. G., & Grudzinskas, A. (2006). An integrated look at dually diagnosed female sex offenders. *Journal of Dual Diagnosis, 3*(1), 23–32.

Saleh, F. M., & Guidry, L. L. (2003). Psychosocial and biological treatment considerations for the paraphilic and nonparaphilic sex offender. *Journal of the American Academy of Psychiatry and the Law, 31,* 486–493.

Schwartz, B. K. (1995). Characteristics and typologies of sex offenders. In B. K. Schwartz & H. R. Cellini (Eds.), *The sex offender: Corrections, treatment and legal practice* (pp. 3-13–3-36). Kingston, NJ: Civic Research Institute.

Schwartz, B. K., & Cellini, H. R. (1995). Female sex offenders. In B. K. Schwartz & H. R. Cellini (Eds.), *The sex offender: Corrections, treatment and legal practice* (pp. 5-1–5-22). Kingston, NJ: Civic Research Institute.

Studer, L. H., Aylwin, A. S., & Reddon, J. R. (2005). Testosterone, sexual offense recidivism, and treatment effect among adult male sexual offenders. *Sexual Abuse: A Journal of Research and Treatment, 17,* 171–181.

Sturmey, P., Taylor, J. L., & Lindsay, W. R. (2004). Research and development. In W. R. Lindsay, J. L. Taylor & P. Sturmey (Eds.), *Offenders with developmental disabilities* (pp. 327–350). West Sussex, England: Wiley.

Thibaut, F., Cordier, B., & Kuhn, J. M. (1993). Effect of long-lasting gonadotropin hormone-releasing hormone agonist in sex cases of severe male paraphilia. *Academy of Psychiatry Scandinavia, 87,* 445–450.

Thornton, D. (2002). Construction and testing a framework for dynamic risk assessment. *Sexual Abuse: A Journal of Research and Treatment, 14*(2), 139–153.

Tolman, E. C. (1932). *Purposive behavior in animals and men.* New York: Century.

Ward, T., & Hudson, S. M. (2000). A self-regulation model of relapse prevention. In D. L. Laws, S. M. Hudson, & T. Ward (Eds.), *Remaking relapse prevention with sex offenders* (pp. 79–101). Thousand Oaks, CA: Sage.

Ward, T., Hudson, S. M., & Marshall, W. L. (1995). Cognitive distortions and affective deficits in sex offenders: A cognitive deconstructionist interpretation. *Sexual Abuse: A Journal of Research and Treatment, 7,* 67–83.

Ward, T., Polaschek, D.L.L., & Beech, A. R. (2006). *Theories of sexual offending.* West Sussex, England: Wiley.

Ward, T., & Stewart, C. A. (2003). The treatment of sex offenders: Risk management and good lives. *Professional Psychology: Research and Practice, 34*(4), 353wh–360.

Wheeler, J. G., George, W. H., & Marlatt, G. A. (2006). Relapse prevention for sexual offenders: considerations for the "abstinence violation effect." *Sexual Abuse: A Journal of Research and Treatment, 18*(3), 233wh–248.

Wilson, R. J., & Mathon, H. F. (2007). Looking backwards to find the future: Remembering Kurt Freund (1914–1996). In D. S. Prescott (Ed.), *Knowledge & practice: Challenges in the treatment and supervision of sexual abusers* (pp. 1–20). Oklahoma City, OK: Wood 'N' Barnes Publishing.

Winokur, M., Rozen, D., Batchelder, K., & Valentine, D. (2006). *Juvenile sexual offender treatment: A systematic review of evidence-based research*. Fort Collins: Colorado State University, Applied Research in Child Welfare Project, Social Work Research Center, School of Social Work, College of Applied Human Services.

Yates, P. M., & Kingston, D. A. (2006). The self-regulation model of sexual offending: The relationship between pathways and static and dynamic sexual offence risk. *Sex Abuse, 18,* 259–270.

7
Keeping Vigil: Neuropsychiatry in the Forensic Setting

JOSEPH H. BASKIN

Mr. M was a 38-year-old man with multiple assault convictions. The assaults were marked by a gross overreaction to perceived slights. During a routine screening by a prison internist, the patient began to demonstrate signs of agitation. Astutely, the physician ran routine tests and found the patient's blood sugar level to be extremely low. Subsequent blood tests found high levels of endogenous insulin (originating from inside the body, as opposed to surreptitious self-administered insulin for secondary gain). An abdominal computed tomography scan revealed a tumor in the pancreas. The mass was removed and found to be an insulin-producing tumor. After the surgery, the patient experienced no further similar rage attacks.[1]

Many factors affect an individual's behavior, including internal body states, developmental issues, and socioeconomic status. Our knowledge of how the brain produces and mediates behavior is increasing rapidly. Integrating this progressive knowledge into assessment and treatment is a constant challenge. Mental health care delivery requires a keen investigative mind. Psychiatric patients can be poor communicators of ongoing medical and

---

Some material from this chapter was previously published by this author in the *American Journal of Law & Medicine*, 13(2/3), Summer 2007. Clinical vignettes were used with permission.
The author would like to thank Bruce Price and Benjamin Baskin for their assistance in producing this chapter.

psychiatric issues. Appointments are missed, and patients are lost to follow-up. Forensic considerations add another layer of complexity to this task. In addition to the challenges faced in data and history collection, one has to be mindful of legal constraints and the possibility of feigned illness.

The purpose of this chapter is to provide information about neuropsychiatric syndromes that can complicate the treatment of patients in a forensic setting. The goal is to provide neurological correlates for behavior, not to discount other theories of behavior production. For simplification, the focus is entirely on the biological.

The chapter begins with a brief overview of relevant neuroanatomy to give a backdrop to the illnesses described. This is followed by a review of some medical and neurological conditions that can cause behavioral symptoms. Delirium is a dramatic alteration in mental status with prominent fluctuations in consciousness. Substance withdrawal fits in this category but will not be thoroughly reviewed, because it exceeds the scope of this chapter. (For a detailed description of these syndromes, we recommend the *Diagnostic and Statistical Manual of Mental Disorders [DSM-IV-TR];* American Psychiatric Association, 2000.) Other topics include traumatic brain injury (commonly seen in forensic populations), memory, movement, and seizure disorders.

This chapter provides accessible reference to more frequently seen illnesses. Some sections begin with clinical vignettes to describe real-world examples. The intent is to explore medical issues that may complicate assessment and treatment. It is not necessary to provide detailed medical information, but rather an overview of important diseases or conditions that may be encountered. Expertise is not essential. Rather, the aim is to assist nonmedical clinicians in recognizing the need for a more thorough medical work-up.

Situations that should alert clinicians to the need for further assessment include:

- Sudden onset of symptoms without previous personal or family history of mental illness.
- Clinical signs and symptoms that are not commensurate with history obtained.
- Clinical signs and symptoms that are not typical of a known disease process.
- Illness that does not respond to multiple adequate doses/trials of medication.
- Any presentation that has significant alterations in consciousness.

A discussion of symptomatology must also take into account those who feign illness for secondary gain. Malingering or feigning mental illness for specific secondary gain (e.g., financial or legal) is a significant factor in the field of forensic mental health care. It is not classified in the *DSM-IV-TR* under factitious disorder, but it is a V code. Factitious disorder is the production of physical or psychological symptoms for the purpose of assuming the sick role. Malingering is differentiated from factitious disorder by the external incentive motivating the production of symptoms. Incentives can include financial considerations, evading military service, and avoiding criminal prosecution. While malingering should always be in the differential diagnosis for every patient, it is imperative that one exhaust all other causes of symptoms prior to making the diagnosis. The designation is a powerful notation on a person's medical record. Once given, it is exceptionally difficult to rescind. Its false application can render a patient forever labeled and unable to receive the appropriate care. Neuropsychiatric syndromes often present in unusual ways. This raises the potential for failing to make an accurate diagnosis and leaving the individual inappropriately treated.

NEUROANATOMY

A brief overview of neuroanatomy is useful. The central nervous system (CNS) coordinates interaction with the outside world. It receives sensory input, organizes information, and directs responses. The CNS is comprised of the brain and the spinal cord. The primary cellular building block of the CNS is the neuron—a cell that receives chemical communication and converts it into an electrical impulse. That impulse then travels the length of the neuron to be reconverted to a chemical message that is delivered to the next neuron in the chain. To preserve the electrical impulse that travels along the neuron, it is covered in a sheath called myelin that performs a function similar to the insulation around telephone and cable wires. Much of what we know about brain function comes from either animal studies (ablating areas of the rodent or primate brain) or human lesions (either tumors or injuries).

The brain can be rudimentarily divided into the brain stem (responsible for basic functions of life such as respiration), the cerebellum (which primarily coordinates movement), the limbic system, and the cerebrum, which is further divided into frontal, parietal, temporal, and occipital lobes (see Figure 7.1).

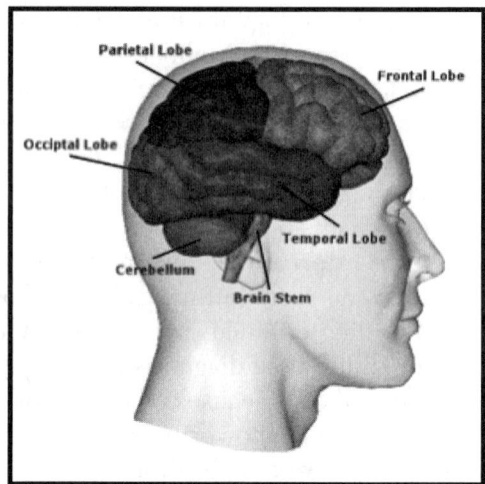

Figure 7.1 The human brain.

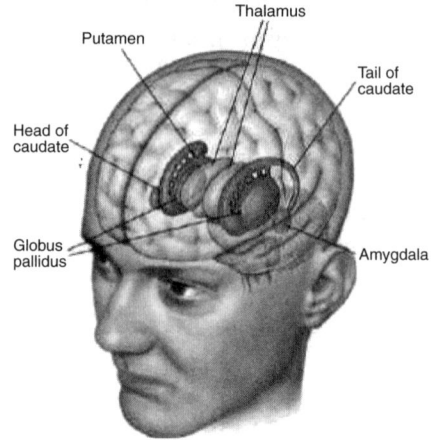

Figure 7.2 The basal ganglia.

Many of the brain structures, including the cerebellum, cerebrum, and deep brain structures, are lateralized—that is, they have left and right sides. The two hemispheres of the cerebrum are connected by a dense bridge known as the corpus callosum, allowing for communication between the two sides. Deeper portions of the brain play a particularly important role with regard to antipsychotic medications. One such important region of the brain is the basal ganglia, which modulates movement (see Figure 7.2). The basal ganglia will be discussed further in the section on movement disorders.

The frontal lobes, the temporal lobes, and the limbic region are most responsible for behavior production. The frontal lobes are the most recently developed and highly evolved portion of the human brain. The prefrontal cortices are a component of the frontal lobes and are responsible for the ability to reason, plan, and sequence ideas. These areas have been subdivided into five frontal-subcortical circuits, which subserve cognition, behavior, and movement. For our purposes, two of these circuits—the dorsolateral prefrontal circuit and the orbital frontal circuit—are the most relevant. The dorsolateral prefrontal circuit governs executive functions, including the ability to plan and maintain attention, problem solve, learn new information, retrieve memories, sequence the order of events, and adaptively change cognitive and behavioral sets. The orbital frontal circuit connects frontal monitoring functions to the limbic system. This circuit governs appropriate responses to social cues, empathy, social judgment, and interpersonal sensitivity. Dysfunction in this circuit can lead to aggression, irritability, disinhibition, and improper social behavior.

The limbic region is among the oldest and most primitive evolutionary parts of the CNS. It is intimately involved with regulation of emotion, memory, motivation, and autonomic and endocrine functions. It is a source for integrating primary sensations, emotions, and memories, and in this way has been implicated in evolutionary survival functions. There is debate about what comprises the limbic brain; for our purposes, we will consider it to include the amygdala, hypothalamus, cingulate gyrus, and temporal and prefrontal cortices. The amygdala infuses emotional valence to memories. The hypothalamus receives information concerning the internal state of the body and orchestrates endocrine (hormonal) responses through its control of the pituitary gland, known as the master gland of the body.

With this basic explanation of neuroanatomy, we will now describe the various conditions affecting behavior.

DELIRIUM

Delirium, also known as encephalopathy or confusional state, is a rapid deterioration of mental status. It is most significantly an alteration of consciousness. Delirium is always caused by an underlying condition. Some causes are internal metabolic derangements (such as changes in sodium and potassium), drugs (both illicit and prescription), infection, and medical illnesses such as kidney and liver disease. Individuals in a delirious state are generally disoriented to time and place. The most common reason for a delirium in a forensic setting is related to drug and alcohol withdrawal. If an encephalopathy is suspected, it should be considered a medical emergency. The treatment of delirium is the correction of the underlying cause, after which mental status changes can persist for several months. Delirium and dementia (to be described later) are frequently confused. In both cases, there can be disorientation to time and place. Further, the end stages of dementia also involve alteration in consciousness. However, delirium is rapid and reversible, while dementia is progressive and gradual.

Alcohol withdrawal can lead to a form of encephalopathy known as delirium tremens. Initial shakiness after cessation of drinking can be followed by delusions and hallucinations, known as alcohol hallucinosis. Visual hallucinations are more common than auditory hallucinations (which is important because visual hallucinations are more rare than auditory hallucinations in psychiatric syndromes) with alcohol withdrawal. If untreated, the condition can progress to delirium tremens. Seizures pose a significant risk to an untreated withdrawing alcoholic. Facilities that house newly arrested people must be mindful of the potential for withdrawal. Although other facilities may not contain individuals straight from the street, the presence of drugs and home brew in prisons makes vigilance for withdrawal imperative, as well. Visual hallucinations in an individual recently arrested should raise suspicions of acute alcohol withdrawal.

SUBSTANCE ABUSE

Substance abuse and its consequences are prominent in a forensic population. The Bureau of Justice Statistics (Karberg & James, 2005) reported a 68% rate of substance use among jail inmates in the year prior to their incarceration. Withdrawal symptoms can begin rapidly after cessation of drug or alcohol use. Often these individuals present without appropriate laboratory work or collateral information. In their intoxicated state, they may be treated with sedatives and antipsychotics. Aggressive treatment of intoxication confuses the diagnostic picture. Most street drugs are cleared from the body in the first days of incarceration.

Barring significant withdrawal symptoms, a person whose mental status might be stabilizing will now have antipsychotics (often in high doses) in his or her system, making an assessment of mental status difficult. It is a precarious balance between ensuring the inmate's safety from self-injury and assuring an accurate diagnostic picture.

It is not within the scope of this chapter to elaborate on the effects of different illicit drugs. However, one recreational drug is worth mentioning, given its proliferation in the youth culture and its neuropsychiatric effects. Ecstasy, or MDMA (3,4-methylene-dioxymethamphetamine), is a widely used stimulant/hallucinogen that acts by releasing neurotransmitters and preventing their rapid reuptake out of the synapse. Animal and human studies demonstrate its neurotoxicity. It can cause a myriad of neuropsychiatric symptoms including depression, anxiety, panic, and psychosis. Even after discontinuation of use, its effects can last for months. A thorough drug history should be taken, paying particular attention to unusual reactions to street drugs.

TRAUMATIC BRAIN INJURY

> Mr. H sustained a severe head injury as a teenager. He required surgery to his frontal lobe and was in a coma for 6 weeks. After his recovery, his family and friends noted a distinct change in his personality. As an adult, he had the mind of a 12-year-old. He would wander into homes uninvited, pester people on the street, and ride his bike on neighbors' lawns. Several years after the accident, egged on by friends, Mr. H lit a box of firecrackers in a crowded fireworks store. The ensuing fire killed 9 people and seriously injured 11. During his arraignment, Mr. H giggled like a delighted child and mugged for the cameras. As the charges were being read, he protested his innocence and yelled obscenities at the judge.

Traumatic brain injury (TBI) is an umbrella term describing significant injury to various regions of the brain. There are myriad neuropsychological and behavioral disturbances that can result from such an injury. Deb et al. (1999) studied TBI patients 1 year after the injury and found a rate of depression and anxiety significantly higher than the general population. A 30-year longitudinal study by Koponen et al. (2002) also reported significant percentages of patients with depression, substance abuse, and anxiety. TBI is particularly germane in a forensic population because the incidence of head injury in a forensic population is high. The frontal and temporal lobes are especially sensitive to the effects of trauma to the brain.

The frontal lobe of the brain houses the ability to reason, plan, and sequence ideas. The orbitofrontal portion of the frontal lobe governs appropriate responses to social cues, empathy, social judgment, and interpersonal sensitivity. Dysfunction in this area of the brain can lead to aggression, irritability, disinhibition, and improper social behavior. A famous example of this type of injury is that of Phineas Gage, a railroad foreman in the 1840s. A premature explosion while laying down dynamite caused a 3-foot spike to be propelled into his face and out the top of his head. Miraculously, Gage survived without deficits to his speech, language, and movement. However, he experienced a radical change in his personality. As described by his physician (detailed in *Descartes' Error* by Antonio Damasio), Gage was no longer responsible and industrious. His behavior became "fitful, irreverent, indulging at times in the grossest profanity which was not previously his custom" (Damasio, 1994, p. 8). The injury to Phineas Gage demonstrated that personality and behavior could be localized in the brain.

The temporal lobes also play a role in behavior. Heinrich Klüver and Paul Bucy (1939) produced a predicable behavioral syndrome in rhesus monkeys after surgically removing both temporal lobes. These monkeys were noted to explore items with their mouths, had impaired fear responses, and were excessively sexual. Their findings have been confirmed in humans with similar injuries to both temporal lobes. The syndrome that now bears their name, Klüver Bucy syndrome, involves excessive orality (eating, smoking, or drinking) and hypersexuality. The syndrome can be caused by trauma, herpes encephalitis (a brain infection caused by the herpes virus), and frontotemporal dementia.

Inmates should be screened for head injuries and early childhood illness of the brain, such as infections (meningitis, encephalitis). Antisocial behavior is obviously quite common in this population. Disregard for societal mores is inherent to the personality disorder. However, instances of unabashed indifference to the consequences of behavior coupled with a history of head injury warrant further investigation. Separating those who are just "bad" from those with comorbid brain injury is arduous. Further, there are limited treatment options once they are accurately diagnosed. However, the knowledge that such a diagnosis provides a treatment team is invaluable. Behavioral plans can be organized around individuals with head injury. It is also easier for clinicians to countenance behavior when it is known that there are neurological underpinnings that are not necessarily volitional.

DEMENTIA

> Mr. K, 58, had no previous psychiatric history. He was a highly educated, prominent member of his community. Over a 2-year period, his behavior deteriorated dramatically. He spat compulsively and urinated in public. At times he would masturbate publicly. This culminated in an arrest for open and gross lewdness for public urination. The charges elevated to child endangerment due to his proximity to a schoolyard. Neuropsychological testing demonstrated significant deficits on tests of executive functioning, suggesting pathology in the frontal lobes. Neuroimaging confirmed atrophy of the frontal lobes and the likelihood of frontotemporal dementia (also known as Pick's disease).

Dementia, defined as a disabling deterioration of previous intellectual function, is the result of brain diseases such as Alzheimer disease and cerebrovascular (brain blood vessels) disease. In general, dementia impairs memory, language, perception, and visual skills and, most notably, may also affect judgment, abstraction, and problem-solving skills. Common behavioral manifestations include agitation, aggression, dysphoria, disinhibition, paranoid delusions, hallucinations, and aberrant motor behavior, all of which can translate into violent behaviors. As the prison population ages, more and more institutions are obligated to deal with dementia among its inmates.

The most common form of dementia is Alzheimer dementia (AD). Although it is usually a disease of aging, it can occur in patients as young as their 40s. Some forms are genetic. Down's syndrome, a genetic disease that causes mental retardation, has a high incidence of early onset AD. The hallmark of AD is rapid forgetfulness. The disease progresses through three stages. In the initial stage, individuals have mild deficiencies in naming, performing visuospatial tasks, and short-term memory. Verbal skills remain fairly intact. During the second stage, cognitive and memory functions decline further. Specifically, memory for recent and remote items is diminished. A person in this state will have difficulty finding his or her way and may become lost. Verbal errors (use of incorrect words) increase. In the final stage, all intellectual functions are severely compromised. Motor functions fail, and the individual is susceptible to infections that lead to death. Medications have been shown to slow progression of the illness, but there remains no cure. The only way to make a definitive diagnosis is via post mortem examination of the brain.

Frontotemporal dementia (FTD), of which Pick's disease is a subset, is important in forensic contexts because of the behavioral changes that often signify the disorder's presenting symptoms. The disease impacts the frontal and temporal lobes, areas integral in the production and maintenance of behavior. Miller et al. (1997) have done extensive work on this disease and its implications on behavior. They compared 22 subjects with FTD with 22 subjects with AD and found a significant correlation between FTD and antisocial behavior. Diagnoses were made clinically and confirmed with single-photon emission computed tomography (SPECT) scans. Mendez and Shapira (2005) demonstrated that such patients suffered a loss of insight best described as a lack of concern. Positron emission tomography (PET) and SPECT scans (imaging modalities that utilize injected radioactive materials) confirmed the hypometabolism and hypoperfusion within these patients' prefrontal regions, the areas responsible for executive judgment. The effects of Pick's disease on judgment and insight have been designated as a form of acquired sociopathy.

Wernicke-Korsakoff syndrome, or alcohol-induced persisting dementia, is caused by deficiency of thiamine, or vitamin B_1. Characterized by short-term memory loss, it can be treated with thiamine replacement. It is misleading to attribute the dementia to alcohol because individuals with other illnesses (e.g., kidney disease) can also suffer from this type of dementia. Persons with Wernicke-Korsakoff syndrome confabulate. This is the process of filling in the blanks; individuals may use imagined or made-up statements to fill in memory gaps. This is not considered volitional lying; those afflicted with this type of dementia are not aware that they are confabulating. In the later stages, the dementia in chronic alcoholics can appear similar to Alzheimer dementia.

Pseudodementia is the label given to cognitive symptoms that are secondary to an underlying cause, rather than a true dementing process. Depression is a common precipitant of such symptoms. Treatment of the underlying condition should resolve the cognitive complaints. A good screening tool for cognitive deficits is the Mini-Mental State Exam (MMSE) developed by Folstein (Folstein, Folstein, & McHugh, 1975). With a maximum score of 30, it assesses different areas of cognitive functioning, including orientation, registration, recall, and concentration. Skills such as reading, writing, and copying address specific deficits that can occur with dementia or stroke. Those reporting memory problems should be assessed for their effort while performing the individual components of the MMSE. Depressed patients may shrug off the various tasks due to their illness. Scores obtained during a depressive episode are generally valuable for comparison with their posttreated results rather than a true assessment of their cognitive abilities. Those malingering tend to exaggerate deficiencies, thus generating low scores. In the initial study explaining the MMSE, Folstein et al. (1975) found the mean among demented patients to be around 12. Interestingly, schizophrenics generally scored in the normal range. Those malingering psychosis sometimes feign memory problems, believing that this bolsters their case. Developing comfort with the MMSE allows the clinician to gauge both the effort of the test taker and the need for further assessment.

SEIZURES

> Mr. R was a 25-year-old man charged with homicide in connection with a fire that he allegedly set in a warehouse. At the age of 2, he contracted herpes simplex virus encephalitis (a viral infection of the brain that has a predilection for frontal and temporal structures) that resulted in 4 hours of continuous seizure activity and subsequent coma. After his discharge from the hospital, Mr. R exhibited uncharacteristic behavioral disturbances, including random aggression and rage. His aggression continued throughout early childhood and adolescence and included violent outbursts, running away, and self-mutilation at home and at school.
>
> Between the ages of 2 and 12, Mr. R demonstrated symptoms of an ongoing seizure disorder. At age 13, his aggression began to decrease in severity and frequency, coincident with an increase in complex partial seizure activity and the beginning of fire-setting behaviors. Mr. R reported a consistent fascination and preoccupation with setting and watching fires. His seizures became more frequent and intense and included vomiting, dizziness, and agitation. Other components of the seizures included "lost time," fatigue, inability to concentrate, and mood swings with uncontrollable crying. He also exhibited automatisms or stereotyped involuntary movements, such as lip smacking. During the 4 years prior to his arrest, Mr. R's seizure disorder became intractable, resulting in up to eight seizures daily despite multiple anticonvulsant medications.

Seizures are a common cause of neurological illness. They involve an imbalance between excitation and inhibition in the brain. Epilepsy is the term used for recurrent seizures. Seizures are generalized if they globally affect the brain. They are partial or focal if they originate in a specific area of the cortex. In both cases, there can be impairment of consciousness. Although there are several types of seizures, we will discuss three: absence, grand mal, and complex partial seizures.

Absence seizures (known previously as petit mal epilepsy) are generalized seizures that manifest in childhood. The events are brief, no more than 30 seconds, and entail alteration in consciousness. They are characterized by a sudden change in activity accompanied by a blank stare. During the seizure, the individual may exhibit automatism, or semipurposeful behaviors of which the person is unaware, and will not remember afterward. Examples of automatisms include licking the lips, chewing, and grimacing to complex behaviors such as dealing cards or handling a toy. Absence seizure usually remit before puberty, but a small subset of individuals continues to suffer from seizures into adulthood.

When overexcitation in the brain occurs in a synchronized fashion, a grand mal seizure (GMS) may occur. These are also called generalized tonic-clonic seizures, referring to the stiffening and then jerking of limbs that is recognizable to the lay public. GMSs can be preceded by an aura, symptoms familiar to the individual as heralding the onset of a seizure. These can be unusual smells, lights, or bodily sensations. Individuals lose consciousness prior to the jerky limb movements. Subsequently, the person will be in a postictal (*ictus* being the Latin word for seizure) state marked by fatigue and confusion. Seizures are generally brief, lasting seconds, but in some cases can persist indefinitely. This condition is known as status epilepticus, and it is a medical emergency.

Complex partial seizures (CPSs, also known as temporal lobe epilepsy) are particularly important in psychiatry. These seizures include many neuropsychiatric symptoms that can appear similar to primary Axis I disorders. Frequently, individuals who suffer from these seizures had an early history of injury to their brains either by head trauma, infections of the central nervous system at a young age, or perinatal (around the time of birth) insults. Prior to a seizure, a person with CPS may experience a rising sensation in the stomach or chest. Feelings of déjà vu or *jamais vu* (French for "never seen"; situations that are familiar to the person are experienced as if for the first time) can accompany the physical sensations. There follows a period of altered consciousness, when automatisms such as lip smacking or swallowing may occur. Seizures can also include auditory hallucinations and visual distortions characterized by micropsia and macropsia, the illusion that images appear smaller or larger than usual, respectively. Olfactory hallucinations are also common, with most describing a foul smell such as burning rubber or rotten eggs. Following these episodes, which generally last less than a minute, there is a period of confusion. Memory of the seizures can be partial or nonexistent. An interesting but controversial subject is that of the interictal personality postulated by Waxman and Geschwind (1975), who described a personality distinct in the CPS population characterized by excessive writing, preoccupation with religious or philosophical issues, and diminished sexuality.

In a forensic population, some will attribute their behavior to seizure activity. More unsophisticated individuals may describe a grand mal seizure in great detail, including how it felt while shaking. Those in the throes of a GMS are unconscious and will have no recollection of the event. It may be more difficult to separate feigned seizure activity in those with knowledge of epilepsy. The most useful tool for assessing seizure activity is video-assisted electroencephalography (EEG). EEG measures the electrical activity of the brain similarly to how electrocardiography measures electrical activity of the heart. Those with suspected seizure disorders are admitted to a hospital for 96-hour video monitoring while EEG electrodes measure the activity of the brain. Any physical indication of seizure activity is correlated with EEG recordings to confirm the presence of a seizure.

The concept of epilepsy or seizures as the cause of violence has been debated. Marsh and Krauss (2000) presented several case examples of violence or aggression committed in the context of a seizure disorder. They subdivided the stages of seizures (preseizure, during the seizure, postseizure, between seizures) and describe the potential for aggression during each phase. Their findings did not demonstrate any tendency for directed aggression either during a seizure or between seizures. Although they noted some violent activity, it was random and not goal oriented.

Pseudoseizure is the designation for seizure-type symptoms that are not caused by physiological events in the brain. They can be classified as either factitious disorder, conversion disorder, and malingering, depending on the motivations of the individual and any obvious secondary gain. If the intent of the individual is to maintain the sick role, then it is seen as factitious disorder. Seizure symptoms produced with the intention of avoiding criminal prosecution would be considered malingering. If the individual is unaware of the motivations driving the production of symptoms and there is no discernable external incentive, it would be classified as a conversion disorder.

It can be difficult to differentiate between epileptic and pseudoseizures. Some differences notable in pseudoseizures are the lack of an aura, movements not characterized by the synchronous tonic-clonic aspects of epileptic seizures, and the ability of suggestions to impact the pseudoseizures. (A clinician might advise a patient to attempt nonpharmacological interventions to alleviate the condition.) Video-monitored EEG helps elucidate the diagnosis.

BRAIN TUMORS

> Mr. C was a 58-year-old man without a history of mental disorder. As a clearing officer for a brokerage house, it was his duty to receive funds and transfer or deposit them for the client companies. He performed this duty for many years successfully and was well respected in his field. This changed dramatically when he began collecting the checks, many of which were worth tens of thousands of dollars, and placing them in a drawer in his desk. He made no attempt to cash these checks nor to divert them to his own accounts. There is no evidence that Mr. C displayed any other significant psychiatric or behavioral changes. He finally sought medical attention at the urging of his regular squash partner, who noticed that if he hit a ball into the upper left corner of the court, Mr. C would consistently miss the return. This troubled Mr. C, and he sought a neurological evaluation.
>
> Magnetic resonance imaging revealed a craniopharyngioma, a tumor near the pituitary gland, situated in the deep brain close to the optic nerve. The tumor was pressing on the optic nerve, which accounted for the loss of vision that manifested in his squash game. Upon resection of the tumor, Mr. C's visual and behavioral abnormalities resolved. He was puzzled and embarrassed by his actions and sought to provide restitution for any financial damages caused by his failure to properly route the funds. No criminal charges were filed. However, he was sanctioned by the Securities Exchange Commission, and his securities license was permanently revoked.

Tumors, abnormal tissue that grows outside of the normal controls of the body, are another rare cause of dramatic behavior change. Because the skull is a limited space, a tumor growth will cause pressure to healthy parts of the brain. The symptoms associated with the tumor will coincide with the location in the brain where local pressure is applied. The above vignette describes a tumor that affects the frontal lobe as well as the optic nerve. Pressure in the frontal or temporal lobes can cause significant behavior changes.

The influence that a tumor has on behavior is controversial. The case of Charles Whitman is a famous example as described by Clayton (2001) in *It's Coming From the Tower*. In 1967, Whitman climbed the bell tower at the University of Texas and killed 11 people. The previous night, he had murdered his wife and mother. Shortly before his rampage, he saw a psychiatrist and described a desire to commit the very act he carried out. In a note composed prior to his rampage, Whitman wrote, "Lately, (I can't recall when it started) I have been the victim of many unusual and irrational thoughts." He complained of headaches and asked that a post mortem be performed to elucidate his "mental illness" (Clayton, 2001). The autopsy revealed a walnut-sized tumor in an area thought to affect behavior. Experts have continued to debate the potential role this tumor played in his actions.

A more recent example of aggression induced by a tumor was provided by Nakaji, Meltzer, Singel, and Alksne (2003). They presented two case reports of aggressive and antisocial behavior showing dramatic improvement after the successful resection of temporal lobe tumors. One of the patients was a 13-year-old boy with a seizure disorder since the age of 5. Magnetic resonance imaging (MRI) of the brain demonstrated a small right midline temporal lobe tumor that did not appear to be increasing the pressure inside the cranium. His treatment team made the decision to manage his seizures with medication rather than surgery. In addition to experiencing continued seizure activity, the boy was extremely aggressive and antisocial. He required frequent hospitalizations and was restrained for up to 6 hours per day. His behavior included bizarre suicide attempts (such as trying to ride his skateboard on the freeway) and violence against others. He was referred for neurosurgery and underwent a successful resection of the tumor. After the operation, he was successfully weaned off of the antiepileptic medication, and there was no resumption of the aggressive and violent behavior.

Definitive diagnosis of tumors is best made by MRI. These machines use powerful magnets and radio pulses to create a computer image of the tissue of interest. An MRI provides unprecedented detail of brain structures. It may not be feasible to obtain an MRI in a forensic setting because of the expense of the test and generally limited resources. Computed tomography scans, which employ computer-aided X-ray technology, are cheaper but do not provide the detail of an MRI. If standard treatments for behaviors fail and there are associated atypical symptoms, a tumor may be suspected. An MRI is the imaging test of choice to confirm the presence of an abnormal growth.

MOVEMENT DISORDERS

The basal ganglia are a group of deep brain structures that modulate movement. They do not control movement directly but act to select, accentuate, inhibit, or sequence the movements. As a group, diseases of the basal ganglia do not act on the spinal cord and thus do not cause paralysis. Instead, they cause involuntarily movements. Anxiety, fatigue, and stimulants can exacerbate these movements, while concentration can suppress them. Abnormal movements are generally absent during sleep. Diseases of the basal ganglia that we will describe are Parkinson disease, Huntington disease, Wilson disease, and progressive supranuclear palsy (PSP.) Because many psychotropics likewise affect the basal ganglia, side effects from medications can cause similar symptoms to primary movement disorders.

Parkinson disease (PD) is perhaps the best known of the involuntary movement disorders. Mohammed Ali and Michael J. Fox have drawn considerable attention to this disease. It is caused by a reduction in dopamine-producing neurons in a part of the basal ganglia called the substantia nigra (literally, "black substance" because of its coloration). There may a genetic component to PD. However, during the 1980s, groups of underground drug labs trying to make synthetic opiates created a toxic drug that caused a syndrome nearly identical to PD. Further research has discovered that certain toxins can cause PD.

Once dopamine neurons have been reduced by approximately 80%, individuals will experience symptoms of the illness. These include tremors, muscle rigidity, and a slowing of movement. Concomitant with the slowed movements is the profound flattening of affect that becomes noticeable in these individuals. The illness usually begins on one side of the body before manifesting in both sides. Depression has a high occurrence rate in patients with PD. Additionally, they may develop a dementia associated with PD. Patients with PD and dementia have a high incidence of neuropsychiatric symptoms. Aarsland and colleagues (2007) described a high rate of depression, apathy (a state of indifference distinct from depression because the latter involves dysphoria, an emotional state), anxiety, and hallucinations. Apathy is especially important because it can be prominent in dementing processes (both in PD and other types of dementia) and is often overlooked. Improved drug treatments as well as neurosurgical procedures are increasing the life expectancy of individuals with PD.

Huntington disease is genetic. It usually manifests in a person's 20s or 30s and dramatically reduces life expectancy. Persons who have a parent with the disease can have genetic testing to detect the presence of the faulty gene. Huntington chorea is characterized by random brisk movements that jerk the pelvis, trunk, and limbs. Chorea is the Greek word for dance, the defining appearance of the disease. If Parkinson disease represents the poverty of movement, Huntington disease is the overflowing of irregular and erratic movements. The faces of these individuals are afflicted by sporadic frowns, grimaces, and smirks. These patients have a high rate of depression and an increased prevalence of bipolar disorder. Dopamine blockers such as haldol treat some of the symptoms of Huntington disease. However, there is no known cure, and patients generally succumb to the disease in their 50s.

Wilson disease is noteworthy because of its appearance in a younger population. It is hereditary and caused by the failure of the body to properly metabolize copper. Deposits of copper build up in the brain and can cause abnormal movement. Cognitive and personality changes and conduct and mood disorders can all precede the onset of the abnormal movements and defy appropriate diagnosis. The abnormal copper deposits occur in the cornea, creating brownish rings (known as Kayser-Fleischer rings) that can alert a clinician to the correct diagnosis. Unlike the other conditions mentioned in this section, Wilson disease is treatable with a drug that binds copper allowing for its elimination. If caught early enough, the cognitive and behavioral effects of the disease can be reversed.

Progressive supranuclear palsy is a rare disease that causes rigidity of the trunk, dementia, and behavioral symptoms. These include apathy, depression, and disinhibition. Individuals with PSP experience frequent falls. As described on the Web site comedy-zone.net, British actor Dudley Moore (1935–2002) was afflicted with this disease. He had struggled with alcoholism, and his falls were incorrectly attributed to intoxication rather than PSP. The disease has limited treatment and no cure.

Current treatments for psychotic illness focus on the dopamine theory of psychosis. Dopamine, a neurotransmitter, mediates many neurological functions, including movement and reward, and plays a role in psychosis. Earlier antipsychotics (called typical antipsychotics or neuroleptics) target dopamine receptors for blockade. The medications are not selective for areas responsible for psychotic symptoms. They affect those involved in the modulation of movement, as well. This leads to the well known Parkinson-like side effects of treatment called extrapyramidal symptoms (EPS.) Newer antipsychotics (the atypicals) seek to modify various receptors, including dopamine and serotonin. They can cause similar side effects, but to a lesser degree than the older medications. While the reduction in extrapyramidal symptoms has been welcome, atypical antipsychotics have heralded new problems with metabolism, leading to increased risks of diabetes, obesity, and high cholesterol.

CONCLUSION

Treating patients in a forensic setting requires many considerations. Issues of secondary gain complicate the already difficult task of making accurate diagnoses of mental or neurological illness. The goal of this chapter was to provide a cursory overview of some of the neuropsychiatric illnesses that forensic mental health professionals may encounter in their work. It is an exciting time in the field of neuroscience. Improved imaging techniques are expanding our knowledge of the brain and how behavior is produced. The interconnectivity between regions known to be important in behavior production is emerging as a new area of interest. We are also discovering that the cerebellum is more involved with behavior than previously thought. Injury to these brain areas through trauma or disease can alter an individual's behavior.

The illnesses described in this chapter will not account for a majority of the individuals encountered in a forensic institution. The rarity of presentation increases the chance that the correct diagnosis may be missed. It is vital to remain alert for diseases that mimic or cause major mental illnesses. Misdiagnoses can lead to erroneous treatments and labels of malingering. Signs and symptoms that might indicate the presence of a neurological illness include alterations in consciousness, symptoms that are inconsistent with known disease entities, unusual presentations, and repeated failures to respond to adequate treatment trials.

The forensic setting harbors additional layers of complexity. In most forensic settings, it is difficult to obtain adequate records. Inmates and patients of forensic institutions may not be forthcoming with their histories. Collateral information, when available, becomes paramount. One is also constrained by what tests may be available in a particular institution. As clinical experience grows, the value of hunches commensurately increases. It is imperative that clinicians listen to intuition that alerts them to the possibility that something isn't right. Indiscriminate ordering of tests can be a nightmare for hospital administrators. However, when clinical experience dictates that something is awry, a good case can be made for ordering imaging or other studies for further assessment. Trusting those instincts can dramatically alter the trajectory of a forensic patient who may be laboring under an undiagnosed neurological illness.

NOTE

1. This vignette is from the clinical experience of the author. The frontotemporal dementia, seizure disorder, and tumor vignettes that appear later in the chapter were described to the author from the clinical practice of colleagues. The frontal lobe injury vignette is a matter of public record.

REFERENCES

Aarsland, D., Brønnick, K., Ehrt, U., De Deyn, P. P., Tekin, S., Emre, M., & Cummings, J. L. (2007). Neuropsychiatric symptoms in patients with Parkinson's disease and dementia: Frequency, profile, and associated care giver stress. *Journal of Neurology, Neurosurgery, and Psychiatry, 78,* 36–42.

American Psychiatric Association. (2000). *Diagnostic and statistical manual of mental disorders.* Washington, DC: Author.

Clayton, S. (2001). *It's coming from the tower.* Retrieved December 1, 2008, from http://www.whatwasthen.com/uttower.html

Damasio, A. (1994). *Descartes' error: Emotion, reason, and the human brain.* New York: Penguin Books.

Deb, S., Lyons, I., Koutzoukis, C., Ali, I., & McCarthy, G. (1999). Rate of psychiatric illness 1 year after traumatic brain injury. *American Journal of Psychiatry, 156,* 374–378.

Folstein, M. F., Folstein, S. E., & McHugh, P. R. (1975). "Mini-Mental State": A practical method for grading the cognitive state of patients for the clinician. *Journal of Psychiatric Research, 12,* 189–198.

Karberg, J. C., & James, D. J. (2005). *Substance dependence, abuse, and treatment of jail inmates, 2002* (Bureau of Justice Statistics Special Report, NCJ 209588). Washington, DC: U.S. Department of Justice.

Klüver, H., & Bucy, P. C. (1939). Preliminary analysis of functions of the temporal lobes in monkeys. *Archives of Neurological Psychiatry, 42,* 979–1000.

Koponen, S., Taiminen, T., Portin, R., Himanen, L., Isoniemi, H., Heinonen, H., et al. (2002). Axis I and II psychiatric disorders after traumatic brain injury: A 30-year follow-up study. *American Journal of Psychiatry, 159,* 1315–1321.

Marsh, L., & Krauss, G. L. (2000). Aggression and violence in patients with epilepsy. *Epilepsy & Behavior, 1,* 160–168.

Mendez, M. F., & Shapira, J. S. (2005). Loss of insight and functional neuroimaging in frontotemporal dementia. *Journal of Neuropsychiatry and Clinical Neurosciences, 17,* 413–416.

Miller, B. L., Darby, A., Benson, D. F., Cummings, J. L., & Miller, M. H. (1997). Aggressive, socially disruptive and antisocial behavior associated with fronto-temporal dementia. *British Journal of Psychiatry, 170,* 150–154.

Nakaji, P., Meltzer, H. S., Singel, S. A., & Alksne, J. F. (2003). Improvement of aggressive and antisocial behavior after resection of temporal lobe tumors. *Pediatrics, 112*(5), 430–433.

Waxman, S. G., & Geschwind, N. (1975). The interictal behavior syndrome of temporal lobe epilepsy. *Archives of General Psychiatry, 32*(12), 1580–1586.

8

Psychopathy: Assessment, Treatment, and Risk Management

JOEL T. ANDRADE

Psychopathy has been identified anecdotally for centuries, but the ability to accurately define this construct has challenged researchers and clinicians. Theoretical conceptualizations of psychopathy have changed over time. Some have stressed the interpersonal and affective aspects of this disorder (Cleckley, 1941), while others focus on characterological and behavioral traits equally (Hare, 1991, 2003). A significant amount of research has been conducted over the past 2 decades, since the standardization of several psychopathy measures, including: the Psychopathy Checklist–Revised (PCL-R; Hare, 1991, 2003); the Psychopathy Checklist: Screening Version (PCL:SV; Hart, Cox, & Hare, 1995); and the Psychopathy Checklist: Youth Version (PCL:YV; Forth, Kosson, & Hare, 2003). These measures provide the field of psychopathy research with a common heuristic and will be discussed at length throughout this chapter.

This chapter is divided into four sections. First, a historical overview of the psychopathy construct provides a context for the chapter. This section reviews psychopathy as quantified by the PCL measures and is followed by a review of the antisocial personality disorder diagnosis (ASPD) as defined in the *Diagnostic and Statistical Manual of Mental Disorders (DSM)*. Differences between the construct captured by the PCL measures and that captured by the *DSM* diagnosis of ASPD are discussed. Second, this chapter reviews the literature on the assessment of psychopathy and applies these assessment procedures to a clinical case. This is followed by a review of the prominent role psychopathy has played in the violence risk assessment literature. Third, this chapter discusses treatment options for psychopathic individuals, with a focus on incarcerated offenders. The treatment section uses various clinical examples and focuses on specific issues related to the treatment and risk management of psychopathic individuals. Finally, the chapter concludes with an overview of a program designed to treat psychopathic offenders in a correctional setting.

HISTORY OF THE PSYCHOPATHY CONSTRUCT

The construct of psychopathy has been identified throughout history in religious, literary, and political texts; however, the meaning of the term *psychopath* has changed significantly over time. In a historical overview, Walker and McCabe (1973) identified three meanings associated with psychopathy. The first encompassed all individuals who exhibit some form of psychopathology. The second included those who exhibit some form of psychopathology that was not attributed to psychosis. Finally, the term has been used to describe all individuals who display some form of antisocial behavior (Walker & McCabe, 1973).

The field of psychiatry struggled to articulate a specific definition of psychopathy, beginning in 1801 with Philippe Pinel (1962) in postrevolutionary France. Pinel was the first to describe a group of patients who were free from psychotic symptoms but presented as impulsive, violent, and lacking in remorse for their actions. He used the phrase *manie sans délire* to describe this constellation of symptoms, which translates literally to mean "insanity without delirium." In the early to mid-1800s, psychiatrists in the United States and Britain reported similar observations in their clinical work (Prichard, 1835; Rush, 1812). Prichard proposed the phrase *moral insanity* to describe a group of patients who he concluded knew the difference between right and wrong but were compelled to act aggressively due to an underlying deficit (Toch, 1998). Rush (1812) took this a step further and proposed that psychopathic individuals were not responsible for their criminal actions as he inferred this disorder to result from some type of birth defect or other disease. Rush concluded that psychopathic individuals were best treated in medical facilities as opposed to incarceration (Toch, 1998). Later conceptualizations described psychopathic individuals to lack guilt, remorse, and lasting bonds with others while possessing high levels of impulsivity (McCord & McCord, 1964).

In his groundbreaking work, *The Mask of Sanity*, Hervey Cleckley (1941) detailed the personality traits he believed comprised the psychopathic personality. This work is based on his clinical experience as a psychiatrist working with this population. Cleckley provides numerous case vignettes illustrating the psychopathic personality and catalogues 16 clinical criteria for psychopathy. Table 8.1 lists these criteria.

Cleckley stressed the personality dimensions of this disorder, which differs from other historical descriptions of psychopathy that incorporate violent and antisocial behavior into the criteria. It is clear that Cleckley believed that most psychopaths were not violent. According to Cleckley (1941), the psychopath

Table 8.1

CLECKLEY'S CRITERIA FOR PSYCHOPATHY

1. Superficial charm and good intelligence
2. Absence of delusions and other signs of irrational thinking
3. Absence of nervousness or psychoneurotic manifestations
4. Unreliability
5. Untruthfulness and insincerity
6. Lack of remorse or shame
7. Inadequately motivated antisocial behavior
8. Poor judgment and failure to learn by experience
9. Pathologic egocentricity and incapacity for love
10. General poverty in major affective reactions
11. Specific loss of insight
12. Unresponsiveness in general interpersonal relations
13. Fantastic and uninviting behavior with drink and sometimes without
14. Suicide rarely carried out
15. Sex life impersonal, trivial, and poorly integrated
16. Failure to follow any life plan

is not likely to commit major crimes that result in long prison terms. He is also distinguished by his ability to escape ordinary legal punishments and restraints. Though he regularly makes trouble for society, as well as for himself, and frequently is handled by the police, his characteristic behavior does not usually include committing felonies which would bring about permanent or adequate restrictions of his activities. He is often arrested, perhaps one hundred times or more. But he nearly always regains his freedom and returns to his old patterns of maladjustment. (p. 19)

The Hare Psychopath

Robert Hare attempted to quantify Cleckley's (1941) descriptive account of psychopathy, but Cleckley's 16 criteria were difficult to quantify due to their inherent subjectivity (Hare, 1980). Hare (1980) compiled a list of over 100 personality and behavioral traits found in the research literature related to the psychopathy construct. After analysis to refine these items, the list resulted in the 22 items of the original Psychopathy Checklist (PCL; Harpur, Hakstian, & Hare, 1988). Further analysis led to the deletion of 2 items and slight modification to the item names of 10 others, resulting in the Psychopathy Checklist–Revised (PCL-R; Hare, 1991, 2003). Table 8.2 lists the 20 items of the PCL-R.

Table 8.2

THE PSYCHOPATHY CHECKLIST–REVISED

1. Glibness/superficial charm
2. Grandiose sense of self-worth
3. Need for stimulation/proneness to boredom
4. Pathological lying
5. Conning/manipulative
6. Lack of remorse or guilt
7. Shallow affect
8. Callous/lack of empathy
9. Parasitic lifestyle
10. Poor behavioral controls
11. Promiscuous sexual behavior
12. Early behavioral problems
13. Lack of realistic, long-term goals
14. Impulsivity
15. Irresponsibility
16. Failure to accept responsibility for own actions
17. Many short-term marital relationships
18. Juvenile delinquent
19. Revocation of conditional release
20. Criminal versatility

Items are scored on a 3-point scale: 0 = does not apply; 1 = item applies to a certain extent; and 2 = item applies. Scores range from 0 to 40, and a cutoff score of 30 is used for the diagnosis of psychopathy. The PCL-R has been found to be valid and reliable in measuring the construct of psychopathy with good construct validity and very good interrater reliability (Harpur et al., 1988; Hare, 1991, 2003).

Exploratory factor analysis of the PCL-R resulted in a two-factor solution (Hare, 1980, 1991). Factor 1 measures affective and interpersonal deficits and includes: glib/superficial charm; grandiose sense of self-worth; pathological lying; conning/manipulative; lack of remorse or guilt; shallow affect; callous/lack of empathy; and failure to accept responsibility for own actions. Factor 2 measures behavioral manifestations and includes: need for stimulation/proneness to boredom; parasitic lifestyle; poor behavioral controls; early behavioral problems; lack of realistic long-term goals; impulsivity; irresponsibility; juvenile delinquency; and revocation of conditional release. The psychopathy construct captured by the two-factor model places as much importance on behavior as on personality traits.

Another assessment tool designed to measure psychopathy is the Psychopathy Checklist: Screening Version (PCL:SV; Hart et al., 1995). The PCL:SV is based on the PCL-R and was developed to assess psychopathy in civil psychiatric patients as part of the MacArthur Violence Risk Assessment study (Monahan et al., 2001). Several changes were made to the PCL-R to account for the lack of criminal history in a noncriminal sample, with the goal of maintaining good construct validity (Hart et al., 1995). The PCL:SV is a 12-item scale with very similar psychometric properties with the PCL-R (Hill, Neumann, & Rogers, 2004). Internal consistency, interrater reliability, test-retest reliability, concurrent validity, and convergent and discriminant validity have all been found to be satisfactory in research on the PCL:SV (Hart et al., 1995). Table 8.3 lists the 12 items that make up the PCL:SV.

Initial research of the factor structure of the PCL:SV supported the two-factor model (Hart et al., 1995), but questions have arisen about the validity of the original two-factor model. A study by Cooke and Michie (2001) proposed that, "although the two-factor-model has served as a useful heuristic device to guide research on psychopathy, it does not provide an adequate structural model for psychopathy" (p. 173). In this study, confirmatory factor analysis was used to test alternative factor structures, resulting in a three-factor solution. The first factor, "arrogant and deceitful interpersonal style," is composed of three PCL:SV items (superficial, grandiose, deceitful). The second factor, "deficient affective

Table 8.3

THE PSYCHOPATHY CHECKLIST: SCREENING VERSION

1. Superficial
2. Grandiose
3. Deceitful
4. Lacks remorse
5. Lacks empathy
6. Doesn't accept responsibility
7. Impulsive
8. Poor behavioral controls
9. Lacks goals
10. Irresponsible
11. Adolescent antisocial behavior
12. Adult antisocial behavior

experience," is composed of three items (lacks remorse, lacks empathy, doesn't accept responsibility). The third factor, "impulsive and irresponsible behavioral style," is also composed of three PCL:SV items (impulsive, lacks goals, irresponsible). The three-factor model places much less emphasis on behavior and more on character traits.

More recently, a four-factor solution has also been tested with good results (Hare & Neumann, 2006). This model includes the three personality-based factors in addition to a fourth factor that captures behavioral traits. The four factors are interpersonal, affective, lifestyle, and antisocial (Hare, 2003). The theoretical underpinning of this model is that behavioral characteristics, particularly antisocial and violent behavior, are necessary requirements. The authors conclude that "deceitful interpersonal behavior, deficient affect, and behavioral dysregulation in the context of violating critical social contracts, be they moral or legal, represent the manifestation of psychopathy proper" (Hare & Neumann, 2006, p. 84). The four factors are consistent with earlier findings from the two-factor model, with each of the original two factors being broken into two subfactors. The most recent PCL-R manual (Hare, 2003) suggests that, depending on the needs of a particular evaluation, the evaluator may choose to discuss psychopathy based on the PCL-R total score or in terms of the two-factor model or the four-factor model.

At the heart of the debate between the two-, three-, and four-factor models of psychopathy is whether to include the behavioral component or to include only character traits. Although there is debate as to the underlying factor structure of the PCL measures, since the validation of these tools (Hare, 1991, 2003), the concept of psychopathy has been reborn into the research literature.

To differentiate between the current construct of psychopathy based on the PCL measures and the clinical diagnosis of antisocial personality disorder (ASPD) found in the *DSM*, the following section will briefly review the history of the ASPD diagnosis.

Antisocial Personality Disorder

The *Diagnostic and Statistical Manual of Mental Disorders* is published by the American Psychiatric Association (APA) and categorizes mental disorders. The *DSM* is in its fourth edition, and the clinical diagnosis most closely resembling psychopathy has undergone several revisions in this manual over the years. The first edition of the *DSM* (APA, 1952) used the label "sociopathic personality disturbance" and based its diagnostic criteria of this disorder on Cleckley's (1941) description of psychopathy. Personality traits included lack of anxiety, lack of guilt, impulsivity, callousness, and a lack of accepting responsibility for actions. Because behavioral criteria were seen as overinclusive of general criminal behavior (McCord & McCord, 1964), the *DSM* diagnostic criteria did not include behavioral manifestations. The *DSM-II* (APA, 1968) retained the clinical descriptors of psychopathy and continued to lack a uniform listing of behavioral traits. Clinicians using the *DSM I* and *II* were guided by clinical descriptions but lacked specific guidelines or criteria. This focus on clinical tradition resulted in poor reliability between diagnostic raters.

The *DSM-III* (1980) and its revision *DSM-III-R* (APA, 1987) replaced sociopathic personality disturbance with a new label: antisocial personality disorder (ASPD). The diagnostic criteria for ASPD included a specific set of behavioral criteria as opposed to the more subjective clinical descriptors used in earlier editions. This transition resulted in increased reliability at the expense of validity (Hare, 1996), because the easy-to-assess behavioral traits result in an overinclusive, but reliably measured, construct. The updated set of criteria also increased the heterogeneity of those who met the criteria for this disorder, because the focus shifted to behaviors that violated social norms as opposed to focusing on personality traits.

The current nomenclature of the *DSM-IV* (APA, 1994) and its text revision (*DSM-IV-TR*; APA, 2000) continue to emphasize behavioral characteristics. The *DSM-IV-TR* defines ASPD as a pervasive pattern of disregard for and violation of the rights of others occurring since age 15 years, as indicated by three or more of the following:

1. Failure to conform to social norms with respect to lawful behaviors as indicated by repeatedly performing acts that are grounds for arrest
2. Deceitfulness, repeated lying, use of aliases, or conning others for personal profit or pleasure
3. Impulsivity or failure to plan ahead
4. Irritability and aggressiveness, as indicated by repeated physical fights or assaults
5. Reckless disregard for safety of self or others
6. Consistent irresponsibility, as indicated by repeated failure to sustain consistent work behavior or honor financial obligations
7. Lack of remorse, as indicated by being indifferent to or rationalizing having hurt, mistreated, or stolen from another

The term *psychopathy* was not included in the *DSM-III-R*, while the *DSM-IV* and the *DSM-IV-TR* include the following statement: "This pattern has also been referred to as psychopathy, sociopathy, or dissocial personality disorder" (p. 645 and p. 702, respectively). This increases diagnostic confusion, because the research literature discriminates between psychopathy and ASPD (Hare, 1991, 2003) while the *DSM-IV* and *DSM-IV-TR* indicate that these terms are synonymous.

The emphasis on behavior as opposed to personality traits results in limited clinical utility of the ASPD diagnosis. There are over 500,000 criterion combinations that could result in an individual being diagnosed with ASPD (Rogers, Duncan, Lynett, & Sewell, 1994). However, individuals who commit crime and break societal rules do so for a variety of reasons that are not captured by the diagnosis. An individual may be diagnosed with ASPD and exhibit only behavioral dysregulation, but not possess the character traits of psychopathy such as lack of remorse, guilt, and empathy.

A diagnosis of psychopathy, as defined by the PCL-R (Hare, 1991, 2003) in criminal populations or by the PCL:SV (Hart et al., 1995) in civil psychiatric and community populations, adds a great deal beyond a diagnosis of ASPD. Based on research on the PCL-R, the estimated prevalence of psychopathy in the community is approximately 1% (Hare, 1996), while among incarcerated populations in federal and state prison facilities, the rate of psychopathy is consistently found to be between 15% and 25% (Hare, 1991, 2003). Comparatively, in the general population, the base rate of ASPD is 3% in males and 1% in females (APA, 1994). Among incarcerated offenders, the base rate of APSD has consistently been found to be between 60% (Côté & Hodgins 1990) and 80% (Hare, 1991, 2003). Approximately 88% of those who meet the criteria for psychopathy also meet the criteria for ASPD (Hare & McPherson, 1984), while 33% of those diagnosed with ASPD meet the criteria for psychopathy based on the PCL-R (Cunningham & Reidy, 1998). Based on these data, psychopathy as quantified by the PCL-measures provides a more discriminating construct than the *DSM* diagnosis of ASPD to identify this particularly concerning subgroup of offenders.

THE CASE OF MR. Y

The case of Mr. Y will guide the discussion through the assessment section of this chapter.[1] This section is designed to illustrate the characterological and behavioral manifestations of psychopathy by briefly discussing Mr. Y's psychosocial history and current clinical presentation. The case of Mr. Y will also guide the discussion of psychopathy as a risk factor for violence and how this is communicated in a written report.

> Mr. Y is the youngest of six siblings. He was born addicted to heroin. His biological mother has an extensive history of substance abuse and prostitution. Mr. Y's biological father was killed in a motor vehicle accident before his birth. Mr. Y was removed from his home by the Department of Social Services at the age of 4 due to substantiated claims of physical abuse and neglect and placed in a temporary foster home with three other children. Mr. Y was removed from this home after 6 weeks because he was physically aggressive toward the other children. He was then placed in another foster home with no other children. Reports from his foster parents indicate that Mr. Y's aggressive behavior continued. At the age of 7, he was reportedly hitting, kicking, and biting other children at school. At the age of 11, he attempted to sexually force himself upon an 8-year-old girl at school. He was found by a teacher, and the police became involved. Mr. Y was hospitalized at that time and then placed in a residential treatment facility for sexually aggressive youth. He remained at this facility until the age of 15, at which time he returned to the home of his foster parents.
> At the age of 16, he was arrested for armed robbery. It was alleged that Mr. Y entered a liquor store with a gun along with a 16-year-old accomplice. Mr. Y held the loaded gun to the head of the store clerk and demanded money. He was given the money in the cash register. Mr. Y then shot the gun above the head of the clerk on his way out of the store. He was found within 2 hours by police and arrested. Mr. Y was later convicted and sentenced to a juvenile detention facility until the age of 19. Upon his

release, he moved in with his foster parents and sought employment at a grocery store. He was fired from this job within 2 weeks due to poor job performance and suspicion that he was stealing money and personal items from the employee break room.

Approximately 1 week later, he was arrested for assault and battery with a deadly weapon and attempted murder. Mr. Y was at a nightclub and made sexual advances toward a young woman. His advances were rebuffed, and a male friend of the woman confronted him. Mr. Y left the nightclub briefly and returned with a metal pipe. He searched for the man who confronted him earlier and found him in the bathroom, where he beat the man severely with the metal pipe. The man was rushed to the hospital and required 4 hours of emergency surgery to his left eye to prevent vision loss. Since the incident, the victim has required two reconstructive surgeries.

During pretrial proceedings, Mr. Y declined public representation and informed the court that he would represent himself. He was transferred to an inpatient forensic hospital for evaluation of his competence to represent himself. The evaluation indicated that Mr. Y had no history of mental illness and no current impairment that would interfere with his ability to act as his own attorney. It was recommended that he was competent to make legal decisions. During the trial, Mr. Y called several witnesses, including the young woman to whom he made sexual advances toward at the nightclub and the man who was the victim of the assault. Mr. Y was warned several times throughout the trial that his questioning was intimidating and threatening. The jury deliberated for 45 minutes prior to returning a guilty verdict on all counts. Mr. Y was sentenced to 10 years in state prison.

The case of Mr. Y is typical of the psychopathic offender who presents to the forensic practitioner with a tumultuous developmental history, an early history of antisocial behavior, and ongoing antisocial behavior through adulthood.

The Clinical Assessment of Psychopathy

At this point, Mr. Y has served 9 years of his 10 year sentence for assault and battery with a deadly weapon and attempted murder. During his incarceration, he has been a significant management problem, frequently engaging in fights with other offenders, assaulting staff, and being in possession of contraband, including weapons, drugs, and home brew. He is currently eligible for parole, and a formal violence risk assessment evaluation was requested by the parole department. As part of this evaluation, the PCL-R was scored to assess the presence of psychopathy. The following paragraphs illustrate how findings from the PCL-R were communicated to the parole department in a written report:

> The PCL-R is a 20-item scale devised to assess psychopathy. The PCL-R is a dimensional measure of the degree to which a given individual matches the prototypical psychopath. Items are scored on a 3-point scale: 0 = does not apply; 1 = item applies to a certain extent; and 2 = item applies. Scores range from 0 to 40, and a cutoff score of 30 is used for the diagnosis of psychopathy. As recommended by the PCL-R manual, the PCL-R was scored by two independent raters, and the scores were averaged to increase reliability.
>
> Mr. Y's total score of 34 places him in the 96th percentile among male offenders. He, therefore, is above the cutoff score of 30 and meets the criteria for a diagnosis of psychopathy. The PCL-R is made up of two factors. Factor 1 measures interpersonal and affective traits such as lack of remorse or guilt; lack of empathy; shallow affect; pathological lying; and a conning/manipulative interpersonal style. Factor 2 is comprised of behavioral traits such as impulsivity; irresponsibility; early behavioral problems; proneness to boredom; and revocation of conditional release. Mr. Y's Factor 1 score of 15 places him in the 99th percentile among male offenders, and his Factor 2 score of 14 places him in the 68th percentile among male offenders. Percentile ranks are based on normative data of 5,408 North American male offenders.

Psychopathy as a Risk Factor for Violent and Criminal Behavior

The relation between psychopathy and antisocial behavior has long been theorized, but, prior to the standardization and validation of the PCL measures, this research was plagued by poor construct validity when investigating this association. The greatest contribution the construct of psychopathy has made over the past 2 decades is its usefulness in violence risk assessment evaluations. Since the advent of the PCL measures, research has found a distinct difference between criminals who score higher on these measures and those who score lower. These individuals are found to be vastly more dangerous (Cornell et al., 1996), less amenable to treatment (Ogloff, Wong, & Greenwood, 1990), and more likely to recidivate (Hemphill, Hare, & Wong, 1998).

A retrospective analysis of the criminal histories of incarcerated offenders found that psychopathic offenders had significantly more convictions for assault, robbery, fraud, possession of weapons, and escapes from custody than nonpsychopathic offenders (Hare, McPherson, & Forth, 1988).

Psychopathic offenders also commit more violent crime than other offenders (Kosson, Smith, & Newman, 1990). A retrospective study of male inmates found that psychopathic inmates average more violent crimes than nonpsychopathic inmates (10.27 vs. 8.57, respectively; Porter, Birt, & Boer, 2001). When excluding sexual violence, psychopathic inmates average 7.32 violent crimes compared with 4.52 for nonpsychopathic inmates (Porter et al., 2001).

As the PCL-R was originally established among correctional samples, recidivism was most often employed as the criterion for antisocial behavior. A prospective study of 231 inmates released to the community found that psychopathic offenders were four times more likely than nonpsychopathic offenders to recidivate violently. Of those who scored 34 or higher on the PCL-R, 65% recidivated violently compared with 25% of those who scored below 24 (Hart, Kropp, & Hare, 1988).

Psychopathic offenders' rates of recidivism are significantly higher than nonpsychopathic offenders, and psychopathic offenders reoffend at faster rates than nonpsychopathic offenders. Psychopaths are between two and five times more likely than their nonpsychopathic counterparts to be reincarcerated for a violent offense (Serin & Amos, 1995). A meta-analytic review of the predictive ability of the PCL measures for general criminal recidivism and violent recidivism found moderate to strong effect sizes and concluded that the PCL-R is a good predictor of both general criminal recidivism and violent recidivism (Salekin, Rogers, & Sewell, 1996). These findings are consistent across international samples, such as Canadian (Porter et al., 2001) and Swedish offenders (Grann, Långström, Tengström, & Kullgren, 1999).

Psychopathy has also been found predictive of general criminal recidivism and violent recidivism in forensic psychiatric patients. For example, in a sample of 169 adult male offenders released from a forensic hospital setting, 77% of those diagnosed with psychopathy (based on PCL-R score) violently recidivated compared with 21% for those who were nonpsychopathic (Harris, Rice, & Cormier, 1991). Psychopathy was also found to be the single best predictor of postdischarge violence in a sample of civil psychiatric patients (Monohan et al., 2001). Also, institutional violence has been shown to correlate with psychopathy in both incarcerated samples (Hill, Rogers, & Bickford, 1996) and civil psychiatric samples (Heilbrun et al., 1998).

Understanding how each factor relates to violence has important clinical implications when considering intervention and risk management issues. Most studies using the original two-factor model find that Factor 2 (behavioral factor) is more predictive of future violence. This finding is consistent for incarcerated offenders and psychiatric inpatients (Heilbrun et al., 1998; Skeem, Mulvey, & Grisso, 2003). A meta-analysis examining the relation between factor scores and institutional misconduct (Walters, 2003) found a higher correlation between Factor 2 ($r = 0.21$) than for Factor 1 ($r = 0.14$).

Based on this research, the clinical construct of psychopathy is important to identify, because psychopathic individuals are responsible for an inordinate amount of crime and violence. Also, psychopathic individuals constitute a group that is at increased risk for ongoing criminal activity and future violence. Therefore, the PCL-R has been used widely among forensic populations and has shown predictive power in identifying which individuals are more likely to be violent in the future (Serin, & Amos, 1995; Sreenivasan, Kirkish, Eth, & Mintz, 1997).

Psychopathy as a Risk Factor

The following paragraphs illustrate the application of the PCL-R to the case of Mr. Y and how psychopathy increases his risk for future violence.[2] This example also demonstrates the communication of this risk in the form of a written report.

> Mr. Y's elevated total score indicates a combination of personality and behavioral traits consistent with a diagnosis of psychopathy. Mr. Y presents as a superficial and glib individual. He has an elevated opinion of himself and frequently refers to himself as "the man." He has indicated his desire to remain at the forensic hospital if he is not granted parole. When asked how he would benefit from treatment in a hospital setting he stated, "Really it's not how this place will help me, it's how I'll help this place. By the end of my six months, I'll be running this joint. I'll be telling the superintendent and the deputies what to do."
>
> Mr. Y lacks the capacity to experience genuine remorse for his actions. When asked to discuss issues that provoke feelings of guilt or remorse, he stated, "I don't feel guilty for anything. I've never done anything to intentionally hurt anyone. I'm a fun-loving guy, I'm not violent." When confronted on his history of violence and when specific incidents were discussed with him, Mr. Y stated, "It feels bad. It makes me feel bad. I feel remorse for things I did. I wish I could take it back—then I wouldn't be where I'm at right now."
>
> Mr. Y attempted to control the interview and dictate the topics that were discussed. He frequently evidenced his proneness to lie, and, when

confronted on these lies, he quickly attempted to refocus the interview. For example, when asked about his future plans, he stated, "My plan is to get out and go back with my foster mother until I get back on my feet. I talked to her the other day and she has some work lined up for me and a few job interviews. She can't wait to see me. She misses me a wicked lot and has big plans for me when I get home." Mr. Y was informed that I spoke with his foster mother and that it is not her intention to allow him back into her home. He then stated nonchalantly, "No, not my foster mother, my girlfriend's foster mother. I haven't been there in years, but that's my plan." Mr. Y was asked to provide the telephone number to his girlfriend's foster mother, but, when this number was attempted, it was out of service. After contacting his foster mother, she provided me with the number to his girlfriend's foster mother, who indicated that she has not had any contact with Mr. Y and that she has no plans to allow him into her home. She also informed me that her daughter, who resides in her home, has an active restraining order against Mr. Y. She stressed the fact that he would not be allowed anywhere in the vicinity of her home.

Another area that increases Mr. Y's risk for violence is related to impulsivity and general proneness to boredom. When asked about his history of unpredictable behavior, he stated, "I used to do things just to get the cops to chase me, just so I could run from them. It was a rush. If I had nothing to do or just got bored and I was walking around, I'd break a car window or something to see if the cops would come." Secondary to these traits, Mr. Y also has difficulty maintaining employment. When asked to describe his lack of any long-term employment, he reported, "I like to do carpentry and construction, but it doesn't last long. I get bored with it too easy, just like chicks. I get bored with them easy too, and move from one to another, to another—you know? If I get bored at work and want to go have some beers, I just leave. That's why I like jobs that pay you every Friday; that way, if I don't feel like coming back on Monday, I just don't."

Conclusions: In general, psychopathic offenders are at increased risk to engage in predatory violence, engage in criminal activity later in life, violate the terms of conditional release (i.e., parole/probation), and recidivate at a faster rate than nonpsychopathic offenders. Mr. Y's PCL-R total score of 34 and history of violence place him in this high-risk group of offenders. Mr. Y's high Factor 1 score is indicative of an individual with a conning and manipulative interpersonal style who lacks remorse for his actions, is unable to empathize with others, and lacks guilt for his wrongdoings. His high Factor 2 score highlights his history of antisocial behavior, impulsivity, and a generally antisocial lifestyle. This enduring pattern of personality and behavior traits coupled with his history of significant violence and antisocial behavior lead to my opinion that Mr. Y is at risk for general criminal recidivism, future violence, and failing to comply with the conditions of parole. Based on the available data, including reviewing Mr. Y's criminal history, correctional record, medical records, interviewing him, and scoring the PCL-R, it is my opinion that he is at risk for future violence and not a good candidate for parole.

TREATMENT

The study of the relation between psychopathy and treatment outcome is complicated for two reasons. First, prior to the standardization of the PCL measures, there was not a common method of quantifying this disorder. Therefore, studies used various assessment strategies resulting in poor construct validity between studies. Second, since the standardization of the PCL measures, which provides a valid and reliable measure of psychopathy, few studies have examined clearly defined and consistent treatment interventions across different samples. Due to these methodological issues, the available research literature reports inconsistent findings and disparate conclusions between studies.

One of the most often cited psychopathy/treatment studies was conducted retrospectively using a sample of 176 mentally disordered offenders. Participants in this study were treated for at least 2 years during a 10-year period from 1968 to 1978 in the social therapy unit (STU) at Penetanguishene maximum-security institution in Canada (Rice, Harris, & Cormier, 1992). Subjects in this study were matched with a control group of offenders who did not undergo treatment in the STU. The PCL-R was completed retrospectively, based on file information. Findings indicate that psychopathic offenders who were treated at the STU were more likely than nonpsychopathic offenders who were not treated to recidivate violently (77% vs. 55%, respectively). Based on findings from this study, it has been concluded by some that treating psychopathic individuals may *increase* their risk for future violence (Rice et al., 1992). However, the treatment interventions that were used in the STU raise significant questions about the validity of the results. The treatment groups were peer led as opposed to being led by mental health professionals. Treatment interventions included nontraditional therapies, including nude encounter sessions between group members and the use of drugs such as methedrine, LSD, and alcohol. This study continues to be cited as evidence that treatment increases psychopaths' risk for violence despite the obvious issues with the treatment interventions that were used.

Despite the belief that psychopathic individuals do not respond to treatment, or become more dangerous as a result of treatment, a meta-analysis found certain treatments to be effective (Salekin, 2002). This analysis included 42 treatment studies in which psychopathic individuals received some form of treatment. The findings indicate that psychopathic individuals responded well to intensive treatment interventions, such as long-term individual psychotherapy (Salekin, 2002). Residential treatment programs that did not include regular contact with mental health professionals were found to be the least effective. The most effective form of treatment combined cognitive-behavioral and insight-oriented techniques (Salekin, 2002).

D'Silva and colleagues reviewed 24 research studies on the treatment of psychopathy that used the PCL-R to measure psychopathy (D'Silva, Duggan, & McCarthy, 2004). The authors found that only 3 of the 24 studies had an appropriate research design to answer the question of whether psychopaths respond to treatment. They concluded that "the commonly held belief of an inverse relationship between high-scores on the PCL-R and treatment response has not been established" (D'Silva et al., 2004, p. 163).

This brief review raises an important question regarding the treatment of psychopathic individuals: If we haven't found an effective treatment approach, does that mean psychopathic individuals are untreatable, or have we not yet found effective interventions? For those who work with and treat psychopathic individuals, it is clear that, to this point, we have not been able to implement effective treatment strategies, but that does not mean that this group of offenders is untreatable.

Hurdles, Pitfalls, and Potential Landmines in Treatment

Limited empirical evidence is available regarding the effective treatment of psychopathic individuals. However, there are sound empirical and clinically derived areas of concern for practitioners working with this population. This section highlights six potentially problematic and challenging areas a practitioner faces when working with psychopathic individuals: (1) motivation and treatment goals, (2) treatment modality, (3) training and supervision, (4) boundaries, (5) empathy training, and (6) the use of incentive systems. Specific case examples will illustrate these areas.

As discussed earlier in this chapter, the prevalence of psychopathy is very low in the community but is between 15% and 25% in incarcerated populations (Hare, 1991, 2003). Therefore, practitioners who work in correctional facilities are responsible for nearly all the treatment of this population. The following discussion will focus on incarcerated offenders and case examples will be used to illustrate the characterological and behavioral manifestations of this disorder in this population with a focus on particular areas of concern for practitioners.

Motivation and Treatment Goals

Despite the obvious benefits for the offender, the institution in which he or she resides, and for society at large, the psychopathic offender is not likely to buy in to treatment. Psychopathic individuals are not inclined to desire change in their behavior, because their antisocial behavior is egosyntonic. The focus of treatment needs to be specific and address how the individual's antisocial behavior has led to specific consequences, particularly the loss of freedom. Psychopathic individuals frequently attempt to derail and refocus treatment. Therefore, the goal of any intervention must be clearly defined at the beginning of treatment and clearly articulated by the forensic practitioner. In correctional settings, the focus is often the management of violent and/or self-injurious behavior. This requires clear identification, and agreement between correctional administrators and practitioners, of the focus of treatment and specific interventions that will be employed.

The following case example illustrates how a psychopathic offender can refocus treatment and feign symptoms in order to convince treatment staff that he or she is in need of a particular type of treatment—in this case, inpatient psychiatric hospitalization.

Clinical Example

> Mr. A is a 24-year-old man serving a 2-year sentence for assault and battery. He was admitted to a maximum-security forensic hospital for evaluation due to his risk for suicide after he attempted to hang himself at the county jail where he was serving his sentence. Mr. A was in segregation at the time of the hanging attempt secondary to assaulting a correctional officer. Once at the forensic hospital, Mr. A was seen daily by the treatment team due to concerns about his risk for suicide. Over the course of his evaluation period, the treatment team noted Mr. A's depressive symptoms and risk for suicide if he returned to the county jail, but the team was also concerned that he was exaggerating his level of depression in order to remain at the hospital and avoid returning to jail. At the conclusion of

his evaluation period, Mr. A was committed to the hospital for long-term treatment and was transferred to a long-term treatment unit. After several weeks, Mr. A's new treatment team confronted him on the fact that he was not attending the treatment groups he was enrolled in. He gave several different reasons for his poor attendance but assured staff that he would be more dedicated to his treatment. A few weeks later, Mr. A was involved in a physical altercation with another patient in the visiting room. It was reported by correctional officers who observed this incident that Mr. A assaulted the other patient, who was allegedly staring at his girlfriend. Upon his transfer back to the unit, Mr. A was searched, as is the protocol after receiving a visit, and a small bag containing cocaine was found tucked into his pants. After the initial investigation, it was determined that Mr. A's girlfriend was bringing cocaine into the institution and giving it to him in the visiting room. Mr. A was informed that his visits would be suspended for 1 year. He then met with the treatment team, demanding to be discharged from the hospital. He stated, "Get me the hell out of here. I want to go back to my county jail. I'm not suicidal—you people are a bunch of idiots. I lost my visits up there so I took a trip down here and you guys committed me. I made all this crap up about being suicidal so I could come down here and get my visits." It was clear over the next several interviews that Mr. A was not suicidal and had successfully feigned symptoms of depression since his original evaluation period. Other patients were questioned as part of an overall investigation, and it was discovered that Mr. A had been bringing drugs into the institution since his admission.

This scenario could have been avoided if treatment staff at the forensic hospital contacted mental health staff at the county jail to determine whether Mr. A had any specific restrictions placed on him. If Mr. A was placed on the same restrictions at the forensic hospital, there would have been no secondary gain for feigning symptoms of depression.

Treatment Modality

The most consistently recommended treatment modalities for the treatment of psychopathy are behavior modification (Losel, 1998; Reid & Gacono, 2000) and cognitive-behavioral therapy (Meloy, 2001; Wong & Hare, 2005). Because psychopathic individuals do not form trusting relationships with treatment providers, incentives for good behavior and immediate consequences for poor behavior structure such programs. It is recommended that treatment programs remain very consistent in their approach and educate all staff involved of the expectations of the behavioral program (Reid & Gacono, 2000). Cognitive-behavioral treatment "works best when there are clear and unambiguous rules and consequences; skills that are taught are commensurate with developmental level; cognitive distortions and criminal lifestyle patterns are identified and modified" (Meloy, 2001, pp. 201–202). It is recommended that the treatment of psychopathy focus on the individual's risk factors for violent and criminal behavior. This will be discussed at length in a later section.

Training and Supervision

All practitioners providing treatment to psychopathic offenders, no matter their level of experience or comfort in working with such offenders, require training and ongoing supervision. Initial training requires an understanding of the empirical research in several areas, including psychopathy, violence risk assessment, behavior modification, cognitive-behavioral treatment, and relapse prevention. This training should be ongoing to allow practitioners to remain current with the rapidly expanding literature as they continue to work with this population. Ongoing supervision focuses on the process of delivering mental health services to this uniquely difficult population. Topics to be focused on in supervision include transference and counter-transference issues, ensuring that treatment goals remain specific and realistic, and ongoing discussion of whether the offender is appropriately using treatment. This supervision can be in the form of group supervision led by experienced staff or individual supervision.

Boundaries

In all forensic settings, strict boundaries between the client and the practitioner are necessary. Practitioners should be rigid in their roles when dealing with psychopathic offenders. The difference between evaluator and therapist must be clearly defined at the outset, and these boundaries must be strongly maintained (Meloy, 1988). McWilliams (1994) cautions clinicians not to become emotionally invested in the success of the psychopathic client, as is typical with other clinical populations, "because as soon as an antisocial person sees that need, he or she will sabotage psychotherapy to demonstrate the clinician's impotence" (p. 164). The following clinical example illustrates how boundary violations occur and the need for ongoing supervision for even the experienced clinician.

Clinical Example

Dr. Williams is a psychiatrist with 25 years of outpatient experience. He recently decided to work in a maximum-security prison with male offenders. Within weeks, Dr. Williams was sure he made the right decision, because he was fascinated by this work and found it extremely rewarding. He frequently worked late into the evening after other clinical staff had gone home. Initially, this was seen as positive by other staff, because the psychiatric need within the institution was significant.

Mr. B is a 34-year-old offender serving a 12- to 15-year sentence for masked armed robbery. Mr. B has a history of inconsistent mental health treatment since he began his current sentence. He has been diagnosed with antisocial personality disorder but was not seen regularly by mental health staff outside of his intermittent requests. Mr. B has an overall PCL-R score of 34, which places him in the 96th percentile among male offenders. His Factor 1 score of 14 places him in the 96th percentile, and his Factor 2 score of 17 places him in the 92nd percentile.

Mr. B has a history of attempting to engage female staff in inappropriate relationships, asking for their phone numbers and making sexual comments and propositions. Mr. B submitted a written request to be seen by mental health staff, stating, "I need to see someone from M.H. I'm feeling depressed and suicidal." Dr. Williams conducted the initial assessment. During this interview, Mr. B requested to be seen for individual therapy, and Dr. Williams agreed. As time went on, other staff began to notice Dr. Williams spending long periods of time with Mr. B. After therapy sessions, Dr. Williams would disclose to other staff his concern for Mr. B and his belief that Mr. B was being victimized by other offenders within the facility. Other staff members urged him to report these allegations to the investigative services unit. Initially, Dr. Williams reported these issues, but he became frustrated when investigative staff informed him that the allegations were unsubstantiated. Dr. Williams became particularly upset when an investigative officer insinuated that Mr. B was using his relationship with Dr. Williams for some kind of secondary gain. After that interaction, Dr. Williams began seeing Mr. B more frequently and stopped reporting Mr. B's allegations to the investigative services unit.

After seeing Dr. Williams for several months, Mr. B stated, "Hey doc. I just can't take it anymore in here. I've told you some stuff, but I haven't told you all of it. I don't really open up to people because I just don't trust them. I really feel like I can trust you though. I know that when they investigate things, they say I'm making it up, and I understand why. I'm having problems with a group of guys. I'm not sure whether they're an official gang or what, but they hang out in a group. A few years ago I was in a fight with one of them, and now they are threatening me. I have a little sister out there who is 17. You don't even want to know the things they say they're going to do to her if I don't get some drugs brought in for them. I know you have two daughters that went to college and they have good lives. I just want the same for my sister." At that point, Dr. Williams said, "Wow. I'm very glad that you trust me enough to be honest about your fears, but I am concerned for your safety here. I feel like I should do something. I should tell the investigators again, and maybe they can have you moved to another unit or another institution." Mr. B immediately said, "Oh, no. Please don't do that. Then they'd go after my sister on the street. I'd rather face them and hope they come after me and leave her alone. I wish there was something you could do, but just talking to me is enough, doc."

The therapeutic relationship continued for several months, and Mr. B reported feeling that he made gains in therapy. On one occasion, he stated, "I'm feeling better about myself. I really think that you've helped me see how I can be a more productive member of society when I get out. I really owe a lot to you, doc. Without your help, I don't know where I would be right now or what I'd do when I get out. Now I feel like I can make it out there."

After a few more months, Mr. B arrived to a therapy session and presented as very anxious and hypervigilant. He told Dr. Williams, "It's getting worse again, doc. One of the guys cornered me in the shower. He acted like he was going to attack me right there, but he didn't. He said that if I don't get some drugs in here, they will go after my sister. I know you could never bring something in here for me like that. Really that's probably not even the best way out of this. The best way would be to send money into my account. Then I could just pay them off." Dr. Williams thought long and hard and struggled internally with how he could help Mr. B. He was impressed with the progress Mr. B was making in therapy and felt compelled to help him in some way. He identified with Mr. B's struggle and was particularly concerned that correctional officials were not taking the threats from other offenders seriously. Finally, Dr. Williams said, "That's it—it seems like the only way. I'll see how I can get some money sent into your account." Initially, Dr. Williams mailed a small amount of cash in to Mr. B. Things went smoothly for 3 months or so, and Mr. B did not ask for anything more. In the interim, Dr. Williams became concerned about his actions and began seeing an independent clinician in the community for supervision who had a great deal of correctional experience. He informed his private supervisor of the situation. The supervisor recommended that Dr. Williams stop seeing Mr. B and inform the appropriate staff in the prison (both clinical and correctional administration). Dr. Williams heeded half of his supervisor's advice and planned on discontinuing treatment with Mr. B, but he did not plan to inform the administration.

In their next session, however, Mr. B presented as desperate and stated, "It's worse now, doc. I thought it went away because I gave them the money, but now they slipped a piece of paper into my cell with my mother's home address on it. They know where my sister lives. Now they're saying they want more. I don't know what to do." Dr. Williams was anxious but felt the best course of action at this point was to follow the advice of his supervisor. He informed Mr. B of his plan to terminate individual therapy and alert correctional staff of the situation. Mr. B's response was chilling, as he said, "Well, doc, I'm really surprised at your decision. You've been saying you were going to help me and you've done nothing. Now I'm really in a bind. I don't know exactly what I'm going to do. I guess I have a few options. I could tell the investigators that you're full of crap, and tell them about our late sessions and the money you sent me, or maybe give the other inmates your address. You know I know where you live, right? I would hate to see anything happen to those beautiful daughters of yours, doc." Dr. Williams immediately left the room frightened. He went to correctional officials and reported all that transpired. He informed them of the threats made against him and his family, as well as his overinvolvement with Mr. B and the fact that he mailed him money in the past. After a lengthy investigation, correction officials informed Dr. Williams, who no longer worked at the facility, that Mr. B was never being threatened by any group of offenders. In fact, he was attempting to extort money from other offenders as he had done with Dr. Williams. They also informed him that Mr. B has no sister and that his parents are both deceased.

Empathy Training

Empathy training focuses on improving offenders' understanding of how their behavior negatively impacts others, particularly the victims of their criminal behavior. The goal is to instill a sense of empathy in offenders in order to decrease the chances that they will engage in violent behavior in the future. Many treatment programs—particularly sex offender treatment programs—have a victim empathy component. Nonpsychopathic offenders in such programs may benefit from understanding the impact of their behavior on victims. However, this is not effective with psychopathic individuals and, in some cases, has shown to be harmful (Seto & Barbaree, 1999). Psychopathic individuals may actually apply lessons learned from such programs to feign empathy and become more adept at harming others. The following vignette illustrates how a psychopathic offender used what he learned in an empathy training program to lure new victims.

Clinical Example

Mr. D is a 37-year-old man with a history of serving two prior prison sentences for assault and battery and breaking and entering. He was recently convicted of rape and sentenced to 10 to 15 years in state prison. After his appeals were exhausted, he told his clinician, "I really tried to get out of this one. I've never had to do a lot of time before, but this sentence is a long one, 10 to 15 years. You know what is really funny about the whole thing is that the last time I was locked up I took one of those classes about understanding how other people feel. It was a real joke, but I did learn some stuff. I didn't realize what people are looking for in relationships and things like that. When I was out, I would go to those speed dating things where you talk to someone for 10 minutes, then switch to someone else, and at the end you would go talk to who you liked the most. Man, I was good at that. I was taking chicks home left and right. I was having sex with five different chicks a week and never calling any of them back. I liked going to their place so I could just get in, do what I went there to do, and then get out. Then this one pulled this stunt. She acted like she wasn't into it, but why else would she have me come to her place? She definitely enjoyed it the whole time, but then she pressed this bogus rape charge. I guess I just won't understand this one."

Incentive Systems

The primary providers of treatment to psychopathic individuals are mental health staff in correctional institutions. Therefore, correctional institutions require specialized treatment programs aimed at decreasing antisocial and violent behavior perpetrated by psychopathic offenders. The research literature on punishment and incentives is extensive and cannot be fully reviewed here (see Cornwell, 2006, for a full review). In short, punishment has not been found effective in the treatment of antisocial behavior. Treatment programs that use punishment as the sole treatment intervention have been found to be the least effective. Therefore, incentive systems are recommended. These incentive systems should be directly linked to clearly defined and consistently administered consequences. A detailed treatment program based on such an incentive and consequence system will conclude this chapter. The following clinical vignette illustrates the successful implementation of such an incentive system.

Clinical Example

Ms. C is serving a 15-year-to-life sentence for second-degree murder. Since her incarceration began 8 years ago, Ms. C has engaged in significant self-injurious behavior (cutting her forearms and ingesting foreign objects). After numerous evaluations at a forensic hospital, Ms. C has consistently been diagnosed as psychopathic. Her self-injurious behavior has been seen as a way to influence her housing placement—particularly so she can be transferred to the forensic hospital, where she is allowed to smoke, has access to male patients, and access to sedating medications. Prior to her incarceration, she did not engage in any self-injurious behavior. Ms. C has no history of significant relationships, no current relationships with family or friends, no connections with other offenders, and no connection with treatment staff. Ms. C's self-injurious behavior is infrequent but unpredictable. She is able to manage her behavior for lengthy periods of time, but, when in uncomfortable situations, particularly segregation, she engages in self-injurious behavior as a way to change her housing placement.

To break this cycle, Ms. C was enrolled in a treatment program in the maximum-security prison that used a cognitive-behavioral approach and a token economy system. She was involved in structured programming for 4 hours per day and semistructured recreational programming for 3 hours per day. Each day she completes her programming, Ms. C receives 0, 1, or 2 points (0 for not engaging, 1 for passive compliance, and 2 for active participation). She can exchange her points for privileges such as food items, keeping a television in her cell at night, sleeping in on the weekend, and longer periods of outdoor recreation. When an offender acts out, either violently or in a self-injurious manner, she is removed from the group and placed in an isolated area where she is segregated and monitored. This area is equipped with safety cells to ensure the safety of the offender. While on this status, the offender is seen regularly by mental health staff, but these meetings are very brief and focused on the assessment of risk to self or others.

Ms. C has participated in this program for nine months. She has required placement in isolation on two occasions, both in the first 2 months of her participation. The first was after an incident of self-injurious behavior, and she remained in the safety cell for 3 days. Her second incident occurred when she assaulted another offender with whom she was arguing. She was placed in the segregation unit for 3 days. Over the past 6 months, she has remained incident free in the program. Ms. C was asked to describe the benefits of remaining in this program, and she stated, "I like the programs we have every day. It's better than just wasting time. I have learned some stuff about myself and why I get so angry. I don't like many of the other people, but I get enough points to have my own room and can stay in my room on weekends and watch TV. That's good enough for me."

Criminogenic Need Focus of Treatment

The following section provides an overview of the criminogenic need focus of treatment for psychopathic individuals, followed by a proposed treatment program based on this approach. Research in the area of offender treatment finds that treatment interventions that address the risk–need–responsivity principles are more effective than treatments that do not (Andrews & Bonta, 2003; Andrews et al, 1990). The *risk* principle proposes that an offender's level of risk should be matched with intensity of intervention—meaning that high-risk offenders require the most intensive treatment interventions, followed by their medium-risk and low-risk counterparts. As discussed earlier in this chapter, psychopathy has consistently been shown to be one of the best predictors of recidivism (both general criminal recidivism and violent recidivism). Therefore, psychopathic offenders constitute a high-risk group. The *need* principle recognizes that each individual offender presents with different criminogenic needs that are related to his or her antisocial behavior. Criminogenic needs are defined as issues directly linked to the commission of violent behavior or other criminal activity and include antisocial attitudes, antisocial peer groups, and a pattern of criminal thinking. The risk–need–responsivity paradigm calls for specific intervention aimed at addressing these criminogenic needs that directly relate to target behaviors (Andrews, Bonta, & Wormith, 2006). The following criminogenic risk/need factors have been identified in the research literature and are referred to as the "big four." These factors are related to ongoing antisocial behavior and violence (Andrews & Bonta, 2003):

1. History of antisocial behavior—a pattern of rule-breaking behavior, beginning at an early age, and in various types of settings.
2. Antisocial personality pattern—sensation-seeking behavior, poor self-control, aggressive behavior.
3. Antisocial cognition—underlying attitudes and beliefs that advocate or justify the commission of criminal behavior and/or violence.
4. Antisocial peers—association with other individuals or groups that support an antisocial lifestyle.

These risk/need factors are prevalent in the general offender population and are highly concentrated among psychopathic offenders.

The *responsivity* principle focuses on individualizing treatment interventions to address the offender's unique deficits that may interfere with treatment. These may include cognitive ability, motivation for treatment, and other issues that are not directly related to recidivism but hinder treatment efforts.

THE CASE OF MR. E—INTERNAL PLACEMENT ISSUES

The following is a clinical example of an individual in a state correctional facility who presents as a severe management problem. Mr. E is representative of a group of offenders that often engage in predatory violence resulting in disciplinary sanctions—most often, placement in segregation. When in segregation, this group of offenders engages in significant, often life-threatening, self-injurious behavior.[3] Due to the high-risk nature of this population (i.e., at high-risk for unpredictable and significant violence when in the general population and at high-risk for suicide when in segregation), this small group of offenders frequently strains the relationship between correctional administrators, mental health administrators, and direct care staff. The case of Mr. E illustrates the personality and behavioral characteristics that make this group of offenders very difficult to manage. A description of a treatment program specifically designed to treat this group of offenders in a correctional facility follows the example.

> Mr. E. is a 35-year-old single man serving a 15-year sentence for attempted murder. Mr. E has served 8 years and has 7 years remaining to complete his sentence. He has a lengthy criminal history, primarily of violent and drug-related offenses (8 assault convictions; 10 assault and battery convictions; 2 attempted murder convictions; 4 convictions for possession of a deadly weapon; 12 convictions for possession of marijuana; and 9 convictions for possession of cocaine). Mr. E has an extensive substance abuse history beginning at the age of 12. He also has an extensive history of physical abuse by his stepfather and suspected sexual abuse, which he refuses to discuss. He has spent most of his life in institutions. At the age of 16, he was committed to a juvenile detention center and remained incarcerated there until his 21st birthday. Since that time, Mr. E has spent most of his adult life in prison, with the longest period of time in the community being 6 months. He was able to manage this period in the community with the help of a highly structured substance abuse treatment program.
>
> Mr. E's initial adjustment to incarceration was difficult, and these difficulties have persisted to the present. His institutional record is significant for the following incidents: 52 assaults on other offenders (4 of which included the use of a manufactured shank and stabbing other offenders); 3 assaults of correctional officers; 1 assault of a nurse; and 1 assault of a social worker.
>
> Throughout his incarceration, Mr. E has had very little support from family or friends, but he maintains a relationship with his older sister. She occasionally visits and speaks with him approximately twice per month on the telephone.

Mr. E also engages in significant self-injurious behavior, particularly cutting his forearms when he is frustrated and angry. He did not engage in this type of behavior prior to being incarcerated. These repeated self-injurious behaviors have resulted in 17 transfers to the state hospital for evaluation of his need for long-term care and treatment in a hospital setting. All of the evaluations from the state hospital indicate that he does not suffer from a major mental illness, but rather exhibits severe character pathology. He has consistently been diagnosed with a severe antisocial personality disorder in these evaluations. During his most recent evaluation, the PCL-R was completed. Mr. E's total score of 36 places him in the 99th percentile among incarcerated male offenders. His Factor 1 score of 14 places him in the 96th percentile, and his Factor 2 score of 18 places him in the 96th percentile.

Mr. E was most recently transferred to the state hospital for evaluation, because he wrote a letter to a state representative pleading his case for being treated "unfairly and inhumanely" due to his lengthy placement in segregation. He reported that, if there was not a decrease in his sanctions, he would commit suicide. When asked about this statement, he stated, "Look, it's not a threat. What can I do? I can't get my hands on someone else, so I'll go after the only person I can, and in this case it's myself. I've tried to get a correctional officer, but I haven't had a chance, and I know they don't want a suicide so I can only work with what I've got." Mr. E was asked to describe his aggressive behavior toward staff, and he stated, "You people keep harping on my violence against officers and other staff, and I'm the only one held liable. They are condescending to me and aggressive to me and nothing happens. I got one of them and I get locked up and he gets a nice, long vacation. He's probably drinking margaritas by his pool right now, and I'm locked up in this torture cell."

When at the state hospital, Mr. E has been housed on a maximum-security unit, cooperated with group therapy, and intermittently followed institutional rules. In this setting, Mr. E. is free to move around the unit with approximately 20 other patients. During his most recent hospitalization, he allegedly engaged in predatory violent behavior and was accused of sexually assaulting another patient. He spent the remainder of his 30-day evaluation period in seclusion due to his imminent risk of harm to others. When informed he would be transferred from the state hospital back to prison, he threw urine and feces in the face of a social worker. Mr. E was charged with rape of a disabled person and assault and battery of a correctional employee for the two incidents that occurred during this hospitalization.

At the completion of his 30-day evaluation, Mr. E. was transferred back to the maximum-security prison because he did not meet the clinical and statutory criteria for commitment. Upon his return to the correctional facility, he was again placed in isolation to serve the remainder of his allotted segregation time, and his frustration quickly returned. The result was violent outbursts, self-injurious behavior, destruction of property, and continued threats to engage in such behavior.

Correctional systems that lack resources to manage psychopathic offenders place forensic practitioners and correctional administrators in a difficult position. With few options, the forensic practitioner must choose among the following: (1) place the offender on some type of mental health or suicide watch; (2) allow the offender to live in the general population; or (3) allow the offender to be placed in segregation. To choose between these three options when a psychopathic offender is threatening to engage in or engaging in self-harm or violent behavior toward others inevitably results in placement on some type of mental health observation status. The result is a repeat of the cycle described in the case of Mr. E. To avoid this cycle, a systemic concerted effort is required. The following section details a program designed for psychopathic offenders in a correctional setting to avoid such poor outcomes. This program is designed for offenders similar to Mr. E.

TREATMENT PROGRAM OVERVIEW

The treatment of psychopathic offenders in correctional facilities is difficult for a variety of reasons. The most challenging aspect of implementing a treatment program for behaviorally problematic psychopathic offenders is establishing an agreed-upon treatment protocol that includes goals, interventions, and an incentive/consequence system. Without a well-defined and structured treatment protocol, correctional facilities are destined to repeat previous mistakes and continue to deal with the maladaptive behavior cycles of individuals such as Mr. E. The treatment program described below defines the program goals; inclusion criteria for offenders accepted into the program; an overview of treatment activities; an incentive and consequence system; and the ongoing evaluation and management of the program. This is a highly structured program based on the principles of behavior modification and cognitive-behavioral treatment. This protocol illustrates how such a program is implemented in a state department of correction, but it could be implemented in any type of correctional facility.

Program Goals

This treatment program for behaviorally disruptive psychopathic offenders has two main goals:

1. To provide meaningful programming for behaviorally problematic psychopathic offenders to facilitate reintegration from segregation into the general population in a safe and secure manner.
2. To decrease recidivism rates of this high-risk group of offenders when they complete their department of correction sentences and are reintegrated into society.

Procedures

A small work group of correctional administrators, mental health administrators, senior-level mental health staff, and experienced correctional staff in the department or facility will work collaboratively to establish a protocol for this program. The protocol provided here can be used as a guide and augmented to fit the specific needs of a given institution or department. This treatment program is not designed to provide acute psychiatric care. When an offender requires emergency psychiatric treatment, he or she should be transferred to an inpatient setting.

Staff Training

A specialized training program will be developed for treatment and correctional staff who work in this program. The training modules will cover the following areas:

1. Overview of the program design and goals
2. Overview of the incentive and consequence system
3. Clinical assessment of psychopathy
4. Treatment and risk management of psychopathic offenders
5. Behavior modification techniques
6. Cognitive-behavioral interventions
7. Overview of maladaptive behavior cycles of behaviorally disruptive psychopathic offenders
8. Relapse prevention

Admission Criteria

1. Admission and discharge decisions to and from this program are clinical decisions based on the admission criteria defined below. The prison warden or superintendent will approve placement of an offender into this program based on security needs, but acceptance into this program is clinically based.
2. Each offender enrolled in this program has a history of severe behavioral problems in the department of correction resulting in placement in segregation. While in segregation the offender continues to engage in problematic and concerning behavior including violence and/or self-injury.
3. Offenders voluntarily participate in the program as an alternative to segregation.

Ideally, offenders in each treatment unit should be serving similar-length sentences, because the goals set forth by the group who are serving shorter sentences will include reintegration into the community and would cause tension for those serving lengthier sentences, particularly those serving life sentences.

Location

Treatment units for psychopathic offenders should be available to offenders despite their classification level. To ensure that security is not compromised by transferring offenders to programs not consistent with their classification level, treatment units should be available across security levels (e.g., maximum-security and medium-security). The research literature indicates that psychopathic offenders are more likely to be violent and break institutional rules while incarcerated and are therefore concentrated in higher-security institutions. Therefore, these programs will likely be concentrated in the higher-security facilities within a correctional system.

Treatment Team

The treatment team will consist of a clinical director, an officer-in-charge, a psychiatrist, clinical staff members (master's level), rehabilitation therapists (bachelor's or master's level), and unit correctional officers. Clinical staff members will have other responsibilities in the prison and will conduct group sessions on a rotating basis. The rotation will decrease the likelihood of burnout that often occurs when working with such a challenging population. Hiring of clinical staff will be collaborative between the clinical director and the prison warden or superintendent.

Correctional Officers

Correctional officers are not forced to work in this setting, and their participation must be voluntary. Monetary and educational incentives are encouraged for correctional employees who opt to work in such a setting. All hiring will be collaborative between the clinical director and the prison warden or superintendent.

Treatment Activities

The following is a list of recommended treatment activities:

- Opening and closing meetings—The opening and closing meetings are held daily. The opening meeting provides an overview of the activities for the day. The closing meeting provides an opportunity to discuss the day's activities and highlight the next day's activities. It is likely that all staff who work in the unit will not be available each day for these two meetings. It is the responsibility of the clinical director and the officer-in-charge to be present and conduct the opening and closing meetings daily.
- Educational classes—Focus on the individualized needs of the offender. Such topics might include basic reading skills, reading comprehension, and math skills.
- Anger management—Focus on each individual's behavior cycle and the role anger plays in this cycle. The goal is to identify situations, cognitions, and emotions that lead to violent and other illegal behavior.
- Substance abuse—It is recommended that some substance abuse groups be led by volunteers, such as Alcoholics Anonymous and Narcotics Anonymous, while more formal substance abuse groups be led by trained clinicians.
- Life skills—Psychoeducational group focusing on job interviewing skills, money management, computer skills, and other skills necessary to function in society.

- Individual sessions (cognitive-behavioral focus)—Individual sessions will augment the work done in group sessions and focus on the individual's behavior cycle.
- Recreation—The amount of recreation time is built into the individualized treatment plan and will meet requirements of accreditation agencies.
- Visits—As with recreation, increasing the amount of visits should be built into the incentive system, outlined on the individualized treatment plan, and meet requirements of accreditation agencies.
- Treatment groups will not be conducted on a daily basis other than the opening and closing meetings. Groups can run 2 to 3 days per week, depending on the clinical need of the group.

Individualized Treatment Plan

Each participant in the treatment program will have an individualized treatment plan (ITP). The ITP is designed to reflect the individual's specific risk–need–responsivity issues.

The *risk* items include PCL-R total score and percentile rank, PCL-R factor scores and percentile ranks, and criminal history items.

The *need* items are the specific items that will be addressed in treatment that are directly related to violent and other criminal behavior. Treatment programs in correctional facilities should also include maladaptive and antisocial behavior specific to a correctional environment, such as self-injurious behavior and other institutional rule infractions. The ITP will identify problems that require intervention. Each problem will have a set of goals. For each goal achieved, the participant will receive a predetermined reward. The incentive system (described below) is directly linked to consequences (also described below) for breaking the conditions of the ITP.

Incorporated into this section of the ITP is the individual's behavior cycle. The initial step of establishing the offender's behavior cycle requires working with the offender to gain an understanding of the situations, cognitions, and emotions that result in problematic behavior. It also requires corroboration with official records and reports because the offender may be reluctant to accept responsibility for past behavior, may externalize blame for such actions onto others, or may flatly deny engaging in such behavior. The evaluation of the offender's understanding of this cycle is also useful to assess the motivation for treatment. The ITP and work done on the individual's behavior cycle will guide treatment and should be updated regularly as additional information becomes available.

The *responsivity* items are issues specific to the individual that may interfere with or hinder treatment efforts. These are identified on the ITP to alert staff of potential barriers to treatment.

The ITP will be updated every three months in a meeting with the offender, clinical director, psychiatrist, mental health practitioner, rehabilitation therapist, and officer-in-charge. Treatment plans can be reviewed by the warden or superintendent at his or her discretion. (See Appendix A for Mr. E's ITP. See Appendix B for Mr. E's individualized behavior cycle.)

Incentive System

The incentive system for this program will be based on a token economy. Each week, the offender will receive a predetermined amount of points for successfully achieving each target goal. Offenders will also earn 0, 1, or 2 points per group or individual session (0 for not engaging in treatment, 1 for passive compliance, and 2 for active participation). ITPs will include incentives unique to each offender and which the offender identifies. Such incentives may include television privileges, radio privileges, increased number of visits, additional recreation time, and so on. A list of general incentives must be agreed upon between the correctional and mental health administrators prior to the establishment of the program. (See Appendix A for Mr. E's incentive list.)

Consequences

Punishment has shown to be an ineffective intervention in decreasing antisocial behavior (Lipsey, 1992). Consequences for rule-breaking behavior should always be combined with some form of incentive system. Built into the incentive system are consequences for rule-breaking behavior. These rules must be clearly defined at the outset of the program. For consequences to have the desired effect of decreasing and eliminating rule-breaking behavior in the future, they must be immediately implemented when such behavior occurs. This is often problematic in correctional facilities, where consequences, frequently in the form of segregation, require lengthy hearings and appeals. Participation in this program is voluntary, and participants will be asked to waive lengthy hearings and appeals that are common for offenders in general population when they receive sanctions. It is recommended that these units have their own internal disciplinary process. Sanctions will typically include removal from the program and placement in segregation for a predetermined period of time based on the type of rule-breaking behavior.

For the effective administration of consequences, the following recommendations are made:

1. Rules should be clearly defined at the outset of the program or whenever an individual enters the program.
2. Consequences for specific rule-breaking behavior should be predetermined (e.g., the length of placement in segregation and removal from the program). Offenders should be informed of these time frames upon admission to the program. Unlimited or indefinite time in segregation is counterproductive and increases the risk for problematic behavior including aggression and self-injury.
3. When rule infractions occur, the consequences should be immediate.
4. Consequences should be intense, but short-term, to have the desired effect of extinguishing the rule-breaking behavior.
5. All incidents of rule-breaking behavior and resultant consequences should be integrated into the long-term treatment of the individual. The goal is to clearly define the cause-and-effect nature of the behavioral problem and the negative consequences that follow—therefore promoting prosocial behavior and modeling the internal controls that are necessary for prosocial behavior.

Phase System

The program will have a phase system that determines the level of privileges a participant receives as he or she moves through the program. The goal is for the offender to transition through the phase system and be reintegrated into the facility's general population. Typically, offenders who are identified to participate in this program will have significant sanctions and be housed in segregation prior to acceptance into the program. The phase system will begin with significant restrictions and slowly decrease these restrictions as appropriate. The phase system should be designed by the clinical director in conjunction with the officer-in-charge of the unit, mental health administrators, and the warden or superintendent of the facility. An example of a phase system is as follows:

- Observation level: Potential participants will be evaluated by the entire treatment team to determine acceptance into the program. During this phase, the motivation of the offender will be assessed. Also, the ITP will be established, and it will include goals for each identified problem.
- Phase 1: During this phase, the offender is restricted to group treatment interventions and individual sessions. Offenders in phase 1 attend group and individual programming with a physical barrier between them and other offenders and staff. Recreational privileges (out of the cell) will be alone and not with other offenders.
- Phase 2: An individual in phase 2 has demonstrated an ability to refrain from violent and self-injurious behavior. As the offender moves through the program, he or she is able to receive increased privileges as determined by the ITP. During this phase, the offender may request more recreation time, visits, and television or radio privileges. The addition of these privileges will be based on the point system described above. Offenders in phase 2 attend group and individual sessions unrestrained (without handcuffs and leg irons) and without a physical barrier between them and others.
- Phase 3: As offenders move from phase 2 to phase 3, they have demonstrated a lengthy period of behavioral control. They have no behavioral outbursts and are ready to reintegrate into the general population.

There are no predetermined time periods to transition from one phase to the next, or to transition from the program to general population. Some offenders may remain in the program throughout their entire incarceration, while others may move quickly through the phase system and return to general population. Time periods will vary from institution to institution based on appropriate housing alternatives and availability.

Evaluation of Outcomes

The objectives of a given program must be clearly defined prior to implementation. Measurable outcomes will allow for the evaluation of the program on an individual basis (each offender), an institutional basis (each institution), and a systemic basis (the entire department of correction).

Institutions will have different needs, and each institution or department should determine its needs prior to implementing such a program. A thorough needs assessment will aid in this process. This may be in the form of an outside consultant conducting an individualized needs assessment of the correctional system or a group of experienced staff convening to identify needs. For illustrative purposes, four general objectives will be used as examples to demonstrate the measurement of outcomes: (1) decrease the number of assaults on staff; (2) decrease the incidence of offender-on-offender assaults; (3) decrease the incidence of self-injurious behavior; and (4) decrease the number of disciplinary reports.

Institutional Objectives and Measures

- Objective 1—Decrease the number of assaults on staff.[4]
- Measure of objective 1—Statistics of assaults on staff will be reviewed on a quarterly basis and compared with the rate of assaults on staff prior to the initiation of the treatment program.
- Objective 2—Decrease the incidence of offender-on-offender assaults.
- Measure of objective 2—Statistics of offender-on-offender assaults will be reviewed on a quarterly basis and compared with the rate of offender-on-offender assaults prior to the initiation of the treatment program.
- Objective 3—Decrease the incidence of self-injurious behavior.
- Measure of objective 3—Statistics of self-injurious behavior will be reviewed on a quarterly basis and compared with the rate of self-injurious behavior prior to the initiation of the treatment program.
- Objective 4—Decrease the number of disciplinary reports or "tickets."
- Measure of objective 4—Statistics of disciplinary reports or "tickets" will be reviewed on a quarterly basis and compared with the rate of disciplinary reports or "tickets" prior to the initiation of the treatment program.

Recidivism Measures

Criminal recidivism should be tracked for all offenders who transition through the program and complete their correctional sentences. Because different locales have significantly different recidivism rates, recidivism rates of those who progress through this program should be compared with local rates. The offender's type of recidivism should be tracked and broken down into the following areas: property offenses; drug- and alcohol-related offenses; violent offenses; and sexual offenses. Such information will inform re-evaluation of the program and the implementation of new interventions that will increase the success of the program.

Continuous Improvement

The goal of implementing any new treatment program is to address a specific need. The implementation of such a program to treat psychopathic offenders requires the commitment to continuous improvement by correctional and mental health administrators as well as direct care staff.

The institutional treatment of psychopathic offenders with such targeted interventions will likely have immediate results. Some of these results will be positive, and some may be negative. Areas not considered prior to implementation may result in other issues that need to be addressed. To ensure ongoing improvement in the delivery of this service, it is recommended that an outside consultant, or group with institutional oversight, examine the results of the program on a regular basis. Because there is little empirical research on effective treatment strategies for this population, this consultation will aid in assessing effectiveness of current practices. Based on the analysis of these results, new strategies can be developed. When changes are implemented, they should be measured and assessed as described above.

DISCUSSION

Our understanding of the clinical construct of psychopathy has progressed significantly over the past 2 centuries. The progression from clinical lore to an empirically validated construct is due in large part to the standardization of the Psychopathy Checklist and its progeny. Although psychopathy has been researched extensively over the past 2 decades, the relation between psychopathy and violence remains complex. Recent empirical research indicates that psychopathy is a construct with various factors that impact behavioral manifestations as well as the practitioner's ability to use this construct in clinical settings. The most researched factor structure is the two-factor model, with Factor 1 measuring affective and interpersonal traits and Factor 2 measuring a chronically unstable and antisocial lifestyle

(Hare, 1991, 2003). Alternative models addressing only the characterological manifestations of this disorder have been proposed and have been found to have good psychometric properties (Cooke & Michie, 2001). Factor structures that address only personality traits may be informative regarding the underlying character pathology of psychopathic individuals, but they significantly decrease the predictive ability of this construct for future violence. Additional research on the antisocial behavior factor will further our understanding of how psychopathy relates to violence.

The treatment of psychopathy remains a significant challenge, but recent meta-analytic reviews and other research indicate that psychopathic individuals do respond to treatment. However, treatment strategies and interventions used with nonpsychopathic populations must be augmented for use with psychopathic individuals. Particular interventions, such as peer-led groups and empathy training, have been found to be counterproductive with psychopathic individuals. Interventions that show promise in the treatment of psychopathy include those that address criminogenic risks and needs.

A program for the institutional treatment of psychopathy was presented in this chapter. The goals of this program are to decrease the incidence of violence and self-injury in correctional facilities and to decrease recidivism by this high-risk group of offenders upon their return to the community. The program is based on principles found effective in the research literature to treat high-risk offenders.

NOTES

1. The case vignettes in this chapter are a not real cases, but are a conglomeration of clinical data based on the author's forensic experience.
2. It should be noted that the presence of psychopathy does not necessitate a finding of high risk. Likewise, the absence of psychopathy or psychopathic traits does not necessitate a finding of low risk. Psychopathy is one factor to be considered in an overall violence risk assessment evaluation. Because this chapter is dedicated to the assessment, treatment, and risk management of psychopathy, only risk factors related to psychopathy will be discussed. See chapters 1, 2, and 3 of this volume for detailed discussions of other risk factors that require consideration in a comprehensive violence risk assessment evaluation in adult populations.
3. Self-injury by psychopathic offenders is markedly different from the self-injury of offenders diagnosed with borderline personality disorder (BPD). Offenders diagnosed with BPD will likely have histories of such behavior prior to incarceration, while psychopathic offenders often times do not. The purpose of self-injury is often significantly different between these two groups; therefore, these groups should be treated separately in order to address each group's specific needs.

4. Statistics will be collected on an ongoing basis to allow for analysis of effective and ineffective program changes. Data will be entered weekly into a database. This will allow for queries to be run as needed. Quarterly reports will be reviewed by correctional and mental health administrators to discuss program progress and needs.

REFERENCES

American Psychiatric Association. (1952). *Diagnostic and statistical manual of mental disorders*. Washington, DC: Author.

American Psychiatric Association. (1968). *Diagnostic and statistical manual of mental disorders* (Rev. ed.). Washington, DC: Author.

American Psychiatric Association. (1980). *Diagnostic and statistical manual of mental disorders* (3rd ed.). Washington, DC: Author.

American Psychiatric Association. (1987). *Diagnostic and statistical manual of mental disorders* (Rev. ed.). Washington, DC: Author.

American Psychiatric Association. (1994). *Diagnostic and statistical manual of mental disorders* (4th ed.). Washington, DC: Author.

American Psychiatric Association. (2000). *Diagnostic and statistical manual of mental disorders* (4th ed., text revision). Washington, DC: Author.

Andrews, D. A., & Bonta, J. (2003). *The psychology of criminal conduct* (3rd ed.). Cincinnati, OH: Anderson Publishing.

Andrews, D. A., Bonta, J., & Wormith, S. J. (2006). The recent past and near future of risk and/or need assessment. *Crime and Delinquency, 52,* 7–27.

Andrews, D. A., Zinger, I., Hoge, R. D., Bonta, J., Gendreau, P., & Cullen, F. T. (1990). Does correctional treatment work? A clinically relevant and psychologically informed meta-analysis. *Criminology, 28,* 369–404.

Cleckley, H. (1941). *The mask of sanity* (1st ed.). St. Louis, MO: Mosby.

Cooke, D. J., & Michie, C. (2001). Refining the construct of psychopathy: Towards a hierarchical model. *Psychological Assessment, 13,* 171–188.

Cornell, D. G., Warren, J., Hawk, G., Stafford, E., Oram, G., & Pine, D. (1996). Psychopathy in instrumental and reactive violent offenders. *Journal of Consulting and Clinical Psychology, 64,* 783–790.

Cornwell, D. J. (2006). *Criminal punishment and restorative justice: Past, present, and future perspectives.* Winchester, England: Waterside Press.

Côté, G., & Hodgins, S. (1990). Co-occurring mental disorders among criminal offenders. *Bulletin of the American Academy of Psychiatry & the Law, 18*(3), 271–281.

Cunningham, M. D., & Reidy, T. J. (1998). Antisocial personality disorder and psychopathy: Diagnostic dilemmas in classifying patterns of antisocial behavior in sentencing evaluations. *Behavioral Sciences & the Law, 16,* 333–351.

D'Silva, K., Duggan, C., & McCarthy, L. (2004). Does treatment really make psychopaths worse? A review of the evidence. *Journal of Personality Disorders, 18*(2), 163–177.

Forth, A. E., Kosson, D. S., & Hare, R. D. (2003). *The Psychopathy Checklist: Youth Version (PCL:YV).* Toronto, Canada: Multi-Health Systems.

Grann, M., Långström, N., Tengström, A., & Kullgren, G. (1999). Psychopathy (PCL-R) predicts violent recidivism among criminal offenders with personality disorders in Sweden. *Law and Human Behavior, 23*(2), 205–217.

Hare, R. D. (1980). A research scale for the assessment of psychopathy in criminal populations. *Personality and Individual Differences, 1*(2), 111–119.

Hare, R. D. (1991). *The Hare Psychopathy Checklist–Revised.* Toronto, Canada: Multi-Health Systems.

Hare, R. D. (1996). Psychopathy: A clinical construct whose time has come. *Criminal Justice and Behavior, 23*(1), 25–54.

Hare, R. D. (2003). *The Hare Psychopathy Checklist–Revised* (2nd ed.). Toronto, Canada: Multi Health Systems.

Hare, R. D., & McPherson, L. M. (1984). Violent and aggressive behavior by criminal psychopaths. *International Journal of Law and Psychiatry. Special Issue: Empirical Approaches to Law and Psychiatry, 7*(1), 35–50.

Hare, R. D., McPherson, L. M., & Forth, A. E. (1988). Male psychopaths and their criminal careers. *Journal of Consulting and Clinical Psychology, 56*(5), 710–714.

Hare, R. D., & Neumann, C. S. (2006). The PCL-R assessment of psychopathy: Development, structural properties, and new directions. In C. J. Patrick (Ed.), *Handbook of psychopathy* (pp. 58–88). New York: Guilford Press.

Harpur, T. J., Hakstian, A. R., & Hare, R. D. (1988). Factor structure of the Psychopathy Checklist. *Journal of Consulting and Clinical Psychology, 56*(5), 741–747.

Harris, G. T., Rice, M. E., & Cormier, C. A. (1991). Psychopathy and violent recidivism. *Law and Human Behavior, 15*(6), 625–637.

Hart, S. D., Cox, D. N., & Hare, R. D. (1995). *Manual for the Psychopathy Checklist: Screening Version (PCL:SV).* Toronto, Canada: Multi-Health Systems.

Hart, S. D., Kropp, P. R., & Hare, R. D. (1988). Performance of psychopaths following conditional release from prison. *Journal of Consulting and Clinical Psychology, 56*, 227–232.

Heilbrun, K., Hart, S. D., Hare, R. D., Gustafson, D., Nunez, C., & White, A. (1998). Inpatient and post-discharge aggression in mentally disordered offenders: The role of psychopathy. *Journal of Interpersonal Violence, 13*, 514–527.

Hemphill, J. F., Hare, R. D., & Wong, S. (1998). Psychopathy and recidivism: A review. *Legal and Criminological Psychology, 3*, 141–172.

Hill, C. D., Neumann, C. S., & Rogers, R. (2004). Confirmatory factor analysis of the Psychopathy Checklist: Screening Version in offenders with axis I disorders. *Psychological Assessment, 16*(1), 90–95.

Hill, C. D., Rogers, R., Bickford, M. E. (1996). Predicting aggressive and socially disruptive behavior in a maximum security forensic psychiatric hospital. *Journal of Forensic Sciences, 41*(1), 56–59.

Kosson, D. S., Smith, S. S., & Newman, J. (1990). Evaluating the construct validity of psychopathy in black and white male inmates: Three preliminary studies. *Journal of Abnormal Psychology, 99*, 250–259.

Lipsey, M. W. (1992). The effect of treatment on juvenile delinquents: Results from meta-analysis. In F. Lösel, D. Bender, & T. Bliesener (Eds.), *Psychology and law: International perspectives* (pp. 131–143). Oxford, England: Walter De Gruyter.

Losel, F. (1998). Treatment and management of psychopaths. In D. C. Cooke, A. E. Forth, & R. D. Hare (Eds.), *Psychopathy: Theory, research and implications for society* (pp. 89–113). Dordrecht, The Netherlands: Kluwer Academic Publishers.

McCord, W., & McCord, J. (1964). *The psychopath: An essay on the criminal mind.* Oxford, England: D. Van Nostrand.

McWilliams, N. (1994). *Psychoanalytic diagnosis: Understanding personality structure in the clinical process.* New York: Guilford Press.

Meloy, J. R. (1988). *The psychopathic mind: Origins, dynamics, and treatment.* Northvale, NJ: Jason Aronson.

Meloy, J. R. (2001). *The mark of Cain: Psychoanalytic insights and the psychopath.* Hillside, NJ: Analytic Press.

Monahan, J., Steadman, H. J., Silver, E., Appelbaum, P. S., Clark Robbins, P., Mulvey, E. P., et al. (2001). *Rethinking risk assessment: The MacArthur study of mental disorder and violence.* New York: Oxford University Press.

Ogloff, J. R., Wong, S., & Greenwood, A. (1990). Treating criminal psychopaths in a therapeutic community program. *Behavioral Sciences & the Law, 8*(2), 181–190.

Pinel, P. (1962). *A treatise on insanity* (D. Davis, Trans.). New York: Hafner. (Original work published in 1801)

Porter, S., Birt, A. R., & Boer, D. P. (2001). Investigation of the criminal and conditional release profiles of Canadian federal offenders as a function of psychopathy and age. *Law and Human Behavior, 25*(6), 647–661.

Prichard, J. C. (1835). *A treatise on insanity and other disorders affecting the mind.* London: Sherwood, Gilber, & Piper.

Reid, W. H., & Gacono, C. B. (2000). Treatment of antisocial personality, psychopathy, and other characterologic antisocial syndromes. *Behavioral Sciences & the Law. Special Issue: International Perspectives on Psychopathic Disorders, 18*(5), 647–662.

Rice, M. E., Harris, G. T., & Cormier, C. A. (1992). Evaluation of a maximum security therapeutic community for psychopaths and other mentally disordered offenders. *Law and Human Behavior, 16,* 399–412.

Rogers, R., Duncan, J. D., Lynett, E., & Sewell, K. W. (1994). Prototypical analysis of antisocial personality disorder: DSM-IV and beyond. *Law and Human Behavior, 18*(4), 471–484.

Rush, B. (1812). *Medical inquiries and observations upon the diseases of the mind.* Philadelphia: Kimber & Richardson.

Salekin, R. T. (2002). Psychopathy and therapeutic pessimism: Clinical lore or clinical reality? *Clinical Psychology Review, 22*(1), 79–112.

Salekin, R., Rogers, R., & Sewell, K. W. (1996). A review and meta-analysis of the Psychopathy Checklist and Psychopathy Checklist–Revised: Predictive validity of dangerousness. *Clinical Psychology: Science and Practice, 3,* 203–215.

Serin, R. C., & Amos, N. L. (1995). The role of psychopathy in the assessment of dangerousness. *International Journal of Law and Psychiatry, 18,* 231–238.

Seto, M. C., & Barbaree, H. E. (1999). Psychopathy, treatment behavior, and sex offender recidivism. *Journal of Interpersonal Violence, 14*(12), 1235–1248.

Skeem, J. L., Mulvey, E. P., & Grisso, T. (2003). Applicability of traditional and revised models of psychopathy to the Psychopathy Checklist Screening Version. *Psychological Assessment, 15*(1), 41–55.

Sreenivasan, S., Kirkish, P., Eth, S., & Mintz, J. (1997). Predictors of recidivistic violence in criminally insane and civilly committed psychiatric inpatients. *International Journal of Law and Psychiatry, 20*(2), 279–291.

Toch, H. (1998). Psychopathy or antisocial personality disorder in forensic settings. In T. Millon, E. Simonsen, M. Birket-Smith, & R. D. Davis (Eds.), *Psychopathy: Antisocial, criminal, and violent behavior* (pp. 144–158). New York: Guilford Press.

Walker, N., & McCabe, S. (1973). *Crime and insanity in England* (Vol. 2). Edinburgh, Scotland: Edinburgh University Press.

Walters, G. D. (2003). Predicting institutional adjustment and recidivism with the Psychopathy Checklist factor scores: A meta-analysis. *Law and Human Behavior, 27,* 541–558.

Wong, S., & Hare, R. D. (2005). *Guidelines for a psychopathy treatment program.* Toronto, Canada: Multi-Health Systems.

APPENDIX A

Mr. E's Individualized Treatment Plan

Name: Mr. E

DOB: 12/6/73

Sentence structure: 15-year sentence for attempted murder. Sentence began: May 30, 2000. Sentence expires: May 30, 2015. Parole eligible: May 30, 2013.

HIGH-RISK OFFENDER ISSUES

Psychopathy

- PCL-R total score = 36
  - 99th percentile among male offenders
- Factor 1 = 14
  - 96th percentile among male offenders
- Factor 2 = 18
  - 96th percentile among male offenders

Criminal History

Criminal Convictions

- 8 assault convictions
- 10 assault and battery convictions
- 2 attempted murder convictions
- 4 convictions for possession of a deadly weapon
- 12 convictions for possession of marijuana
- 9 convictions for possession of cocaine

History of Incarceration

- Age 16 to 21—incarcerated at a juvenile detention facility
- Served two state prison sentences
- Served one county jail sentence
- Longest period in the community was 6 months

Awaiting Trial

- Rape of a disabled person
- Assault and battery of a correctional employee

TARGET BEHAVIORS

Target Behavior 1: Assaulting Staff

Brief history of behavior

- Three assaults of correctional officers
- One assault of a nurse
- One assault of a social worker

Previous consequences for this behavior

- Awaiting trial for assault and battery of a correctional employee

Goal

No assaultive behavior toward staff

Incentive

For each week of nonassaultive behavior toward staff, five points are awarded.

Consequences for engaging in assaultive behavior towards staff

1. Immediate removal from the group and transfer to segregation (a hearing will occur within 2 business days to determine length of segregation time, which will be between 10 and 30 days)
2. The local district attorney will review the case to determine whether criminal charges will be sought
3. Upon discharge from segregation, return to Phase 1 of the program
4. Loss of all privileges that have been accumulated
5. Upon return to the group, privileges will start from the beginning

Target Behavior 2: Assaulting Other Offenders

Brief history of behavior

- 52 assaults on other offenders (4 of which included the use of a manufactured shank and stabbing of other offenders)
- Alleged sexual assault of a patient while at the state hospital

Previous consequences for this behavior

- Of the 96 months Mr. E has been incarcerated, he has spent 54 months in segregation, 17 months at the state hospital, 18 months on suicide prevention watch, and 7 months in the general population.
- Awaiting trial for rape of a disabled person

Goal

No assaultive behavior toward other offenders

Incentive

For each week of nonassaultive behavior toward other offenders, five points are awarded.

Consequences for engaging in assaultive behavior toward other offenders

1. Immediate removal from the group and transfer to segregation (a hearing will occur within 2 business days to determine length of segregation time, which will be between 10 and 30 days)
2. The local district attorney will review the case to determine whether criminal charges will be sought
3. Upon discharge from segregation, return to Phase 1 of the program
4. Loss of all privileges that have been accumulated
5. Upon return to the group, privileges will start from the beginning

Target Behavior 3: Self-Injurious Behavior

Brief history of behavior

- Over 50 incidents of self-injurious behavior since incarcerated, including:
    - Cutting forearms (40+ incidents)
    - Cutting stomach (5 incidents)
    - Ingesting pieces of metal (10 incidents)
    - Inserting paperclip into penis (1 incident)

Previous consequences for this behavior

- Mr. E has required significant medical attention due to self-injury.
- By self-report, Mr. E does not benefit from this behavior other than short-term changes in housing.
- Mr. E has missed many visits from his sister because he has been on suicide prevention watch or at the state hospital.
- Mr. E has not been allowed property for months at a time due to concerns he will use items to harm himself.

Goal

No incidents of self-injurious behavior

Incentive

For each week of not engaging in self-injurious behavior, five points are awarded.

Consequences for engaging in self-injurious behavior

1. Immediate removal from the group and transfer to the safety cell without property or privileges
2. Staff will assess the continued need for monitoring on this status daily
3. Upon discontinuation of safety precautions, return to Phase 1 of the program
4. Lose all privileges that have been accumulated
5. Upon return to the group, privileges will start from the beginning

POTENTIAL BARRIERS TO TREATMENT

Potential Barrier 1: Below-Average Intellectual Functioning

As evidenced by

- Wechsler Adult Intelligence Scale—Full Scale IQ = 78
- Repeated inability to process information regarding institutional rules
- Inability to draw the connection between behavior and consequences

Intervention

- Thorough explanation of all information in basic terms
- Ensure that Mr. E is processing information correctly by frequently having him confirm his understanding

Individualized Incentives

In the left column are the incentives Mr. E chose to include in his Individualized Treatment Plan. In the right column is the cost of each item. Incentives can be added during treatment team meetings.

Incentives	*Point Cost*
Television in cell	2 points per day (14 for week)
Radio in cell	2 points per day (14 for week)
Law library access beyond the minimum that is allowed	4 points per additional hour
Additional recreation time	2 points per hour
Additional visits	2 points per hour

The following is an example of the individual point tracking sheet completed by Mr. E for the week of March 31 through April 6.

	Points for week
Target behavior 1. No assaultive behavior toward staff	5
Target behavior 2. No assaultive behavior toward other offenders	5
Target behavior 3. No incidents of self-injurious behavior	5
Life skills group	4
Anger management group	2
Alcoholics Anonymous	6
General equivalency diploma class	4
Total	31

Mr. E earned the privilege to choose the following incentives the subsequent week:

- Television in his cell every day—14 points
- Radio in his cell two nights—4 points
- 2 hours of additional recreation time—4 points
- 2 hours and 15 minutes of additional law library time—9 points

APPENDIX B

Mr. E's Individualized Behavior Cycle

Mr. E established the following behavior cycle (Figure 8.1) with clinical staff during his first month in the program.

Mr. E established an alternative behavior cycle with clinical staff during his third month in the program (Figure 8.2). He was encouraged to identify alternative ways of coping with situations as described above. Again, consequences to his actions are clearly defined and connected directly to his behavior.

The work on his alternative behavior cycle was accomplished by using the following worksheet to identify situations, cognitions, emotions, behaviors, and consequences (Figure 8.3). The cyclical pattern was discussed at length with Mr. E in individual and group sessions. The connection between cognition, emotion, behavior, and resultant consequence is diagramed repeatedly. This was done with alternative situations that begin the cycle. Also, alternative behaviors for the same situation were clearly reviewed in order to illustrate how such alterations in behavior result in different outcomes.

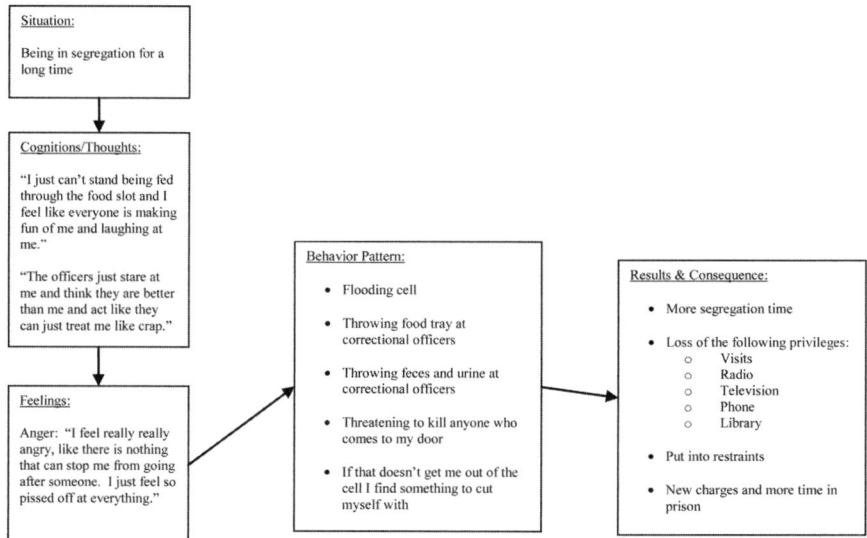

Figure 8.1 Mr. E's behavior cycle: First month in the program.

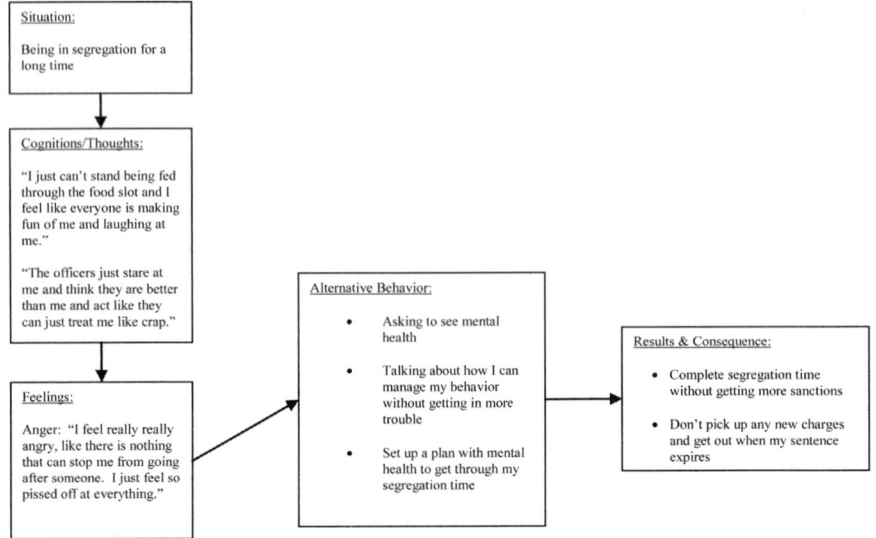

Figure 8.2 Mr. E's alternative behavior cycle: Third month in the program.

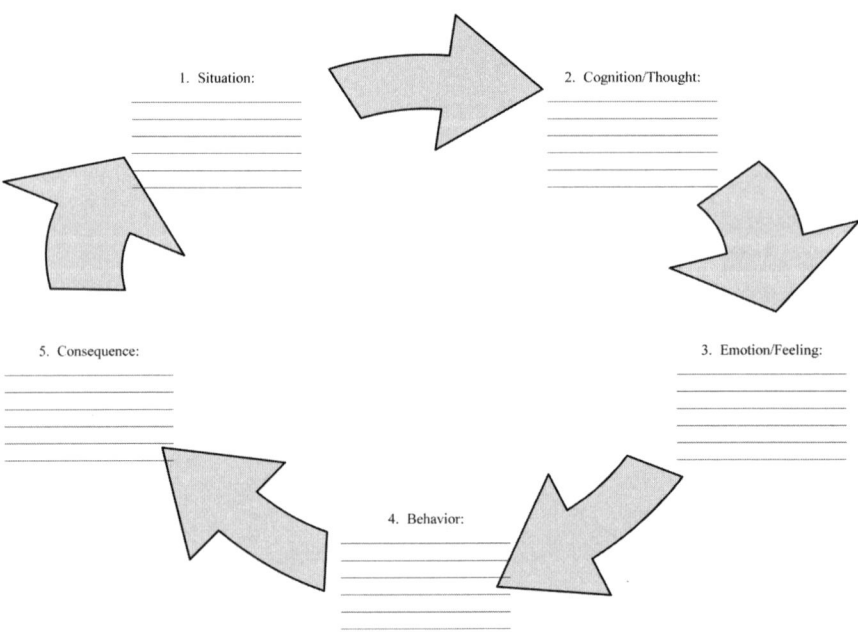

Figure 8.3 Behavior cycle worksheet.

9

Treatment and Management of Violence and Criminal Risk Among Mentally Ill Offenders

JOSÉ B. ASHFORD, KATHERINE O. STERNBACH, AND MAUREEN F. BALAAM

This chapter reviews an integrated approach to treating adult mentally ill offenders that included a generic cognitive intervention for reducing criminogenic needs. The cognitive intervention was a component of the treatment provided by a forensic assertive community treatment team and reinforced by a mental health court in Monterey County, California. It has shown promise not only in reducing recidivism, but also in reducing arrests for violent crimes in a sample of high-risk mentally ill offenders (Ashford, Wong, & Sternbach, 2008).

The chapter begins with an introduction of the issues surrounding the treatment of offenders diagnosed with serious mental disorders. This description of the problem is followed by an examination of the controversies surrounding the relationship between mental disorders and crime. We also provide a brief justification for why cognitive interventions need to be included in the treatment plans of offenders with serious mental disorders and a description of measures that are useful to assess their effectiveness. The Monterey County Supervised Treatment After Release (MCSTAR) research demonstration provided the cognitive skill program examined in this chapter. Following this discussion, we describe the characteristics of the cognitive intervention used to change the criminal attitudes of mentally ill offenders. The chapter concludes with a discussion of areas for future inquiry surrounding some unexpected findings in the research demonstration.

BACKGROUND OF THE PROBLEM

Lamb and Weinberger (1998, 2001) contend that most communities have inadequate mental health treatment, housing, and rehabilitation resources to serve the growing numbers of offenders with mental disorders in our communities. Moreover, when services are available, many service systems expect the offenders to voluntarily attend outpatient care when the real need for a large portion of this population is outreach services (Lamb & Weinberger, 1998, p. 483). Lovell, Gagliardi, and Peterson (2002) studied the use of mental health services among persons with serious mental disorders who were released from prison. Although 73% of the participants in their study received some form of postrelease mental health services, a sizeable proportion of these offenders (70%) were rearrested. However, Lovell and his colleagues also found that few of the offenders received clinically meaningful levels of services during the first year after release (Lovell et al., 2002, p. 1290). Clearly a major task confronting mental health providers is to increase access for mentally ill offenders to relevant clinical services for persons with criminal backgrounds (Nieto, 1999; Roskes & Feldman, 1999; Weisman, Lamberti, & Price, 2004).

One of the policy barriers to the treatment of offenders with serious mental disorders is that funding for services in many state and county systems is dependent upon Medicaid. Yet Medicaid does not pay for services when eligible individuals are incarcerated for more than 30 days. Upon release, it may take several months to establish Medicaid eligibility when the person is even eligible. State funding is usually targeted to adults with serious mental illness and co-occurring disorders (mental illness and substance abuse). Although some jurisdictions have targeted treatment of mentally ill offenders, many incarcerated individuals with a diagnosable mental illness have limited access to services while incarcerated or when released to the community. For example, persons with a diagnosis of a major depressive disorder are not considered the priority population for state-funded treatment in California except when the person is in a psychiatric crisis or psychosis is present.

One established solution for helping consumers to navigate systems of care is case management. Case management is a recognized intervention

Chapter 9 Treatment and Management of Violence and Criminal Risk

that focuses on the coordination in the community of services for persons with serious mental disorders (Ashford, Sales, & LeCroy, 2001; Ashford, Sternbach, & Balaam, in press; Lurigio, Fallon, & Dincin, 2000; Ventura, Cassel, Jacoby, & Huang, 1998). Yet many jurisdictions do not provide case management services to offenders diagnosed with serious mental disorders who are released from either jails or prisons (Lamb & Weinberger, 1998, 2001). Current research also demonstrates that very few communities employ assertive community treatment (ACT) teams in addressing the clinical needs of offenders with serious mental disorders (Lamberti, Weisman, & Faden, 2004; Morrissey, & Meyer, 2005). ACT teams are considered one of six evidence-based practices (Substance Abuse and Mental Health Services Administration, U.S. Department of Health and Human Services, 2008). ACT teams differ from other traditional service models of case management on several dimensions: (1) lower caseloads; (2) a team approach to the implementation of case management principles; (3) an emphasis on outreach; (4) and team provision of services in place of referring consumers to other providers for these services (Ashford et al., in press; Marshall & Lockwood, 2001; Ziguras & Stuart, 2000).

Research has shown that ACT, when compared with traditional brokered services models, significantly reduces psychiatric inpatient usage (Bond, Miller, Krumwied, & Ward, 1988; Borland, McRae, & Lycan, 1989; Lipton, Nutt, & Sabitini, 1988; Stein & Test, 1980). In addition, the results of meta-analytic studies have found ACT programs were superior to clinical case management in reducing hospitalization (Ziguras & Stuart, 2000). However, the results are equivocal as to whether ACT programs are effective in reducing arrests, improving symptoms, improving social functioning, and increasing client satisfaction with services (Cosden, Ellens, Schnell, Yamini-Diourf, & Wolfe, 2003; Marshall & Lockwood, 2001; Morrissey & Meyer, 2005).

Morrissey and Meyer (2005) have identified a number of ACT-like programs that communities are experimenting with to help keep individuals with serious mental illness out of jails and prisons. These hybrid programs are typically referred to as forensic assertive community treatment programs or FACT teams (Morrissey & Meyer, 2005). The research on these FACT teams with offenders with serious mental disorders remains small and methodologically limited (Lamberti et al., 2004). However, Solomon and Draine's (1995) randomized trial of case management approaches is a noteworthy exception. These researchers assigned 200 inmates released from a large urban jail system to one of four conditions: the assertive community treatment team, forensic specialist case managers, mental health agencies, and the usual referral to a community mental health center (Ashford et al., in press). The results showed that the participants who received the intensive case management services under an ACT team model were more likely than the other comparison groups to be returned to jail for nontreatment compliance. Offenders with serious mental disorders released under other case management conditions have also been at a much greater risk of experiencing difficulties in complying with the conditions of postrelease supervision (Feder, 1991; Heilbrun & Griffin, 1993; Jacoby & Kozie-Peak, 1997; Wilson, Tien, & Eaves, 1995). As a result, they are at a higher risk of having their probation or parole revoked. Given this unexpected consequence of increased supervision for mentally ill offenders, some jurisdictions have begun to experiment with the use of mental health courts in an effort to minimize the negative effects noted by Solomon and Draine (1995) in integrating ACT teams and other forms of intensive community supervision in the criminal justice process (Ashford et al., in press; Cosden, Ellens, Schnell, Yamini-Diouf, & Wolfe, 2003).

Judge Ginger Lerner-Wren presided over the first mental health court developed in Florida. Her problem-solving court provides the treatment that mentally ill offenders need to slow down "the revolving door of mentally ill patients who are repeatedly arrested and sent to prison when they really need treatment" (Marini, 2003, p. 59). Judges in this type of court use their authority to integrate treatment services and forge new responses to the treatment of mentally ill offenders (Berman & Feinblatt, 2003).

The State of California passed in 1998 Senate Bill 1485, the Mentally Ill Offender Crime Reduction grant program. This legislation authorized the California Board of Corrections to fund research demonstrations to reduce the crime, jail crowding, and criminal justice costs associated with mentally disordered offenders in California. No more than two of these demonstrations integrated ACT teams with mental health courts to address the crime cycle of mentally disordered offenders. However, most of these demonstrations did not include interventions that also targeted criminogenic needs (Lamberti et al., 2004). The following sections examine the utility of integrating cognitive interventions in targeting criminogenic needs in the treatment of offenders diagnosed with serious mental disorders. The MCSTAR research demonstration includes a cognitive intervention that targets criminogenic needs.

REVIEW OF THE LITERATURE

The relationship between mental disorders and crime is very complex (Ashford et al., 2008). This complexity can lead to unwanted consequences for the treatment of persons with serious mental disorders (Corrigan & Cooper, 2005). In particular, the public tends to stigmatize all persons with mental illness without identifying specific symptoms or disabilities resulting from mental illness that are associated with violence and crime (Corrigan & Cooper, 2005). Clearly, there are many individuals with a diagnosed mental disorder who do not commit crimes, but the evidence is becoming less equivocal "that people with mental illness are more likely to commit violent crimes than are comparable samples of people without mental illness in the general population" (Corrigan & Cooper, 2005, p. 169). However, we must be clear in our interpretations of the meaning and the significance of this observed relationship.

Most of the early research on the relationship between mental disorders and crime was based on persons in systems of care (Ashford, 1988; Link & Stueve, 1995). Most studies relied on persons involved in treatment, which introduced important selection biases in these studies. However, a growing body of research, based on probability samples (including individuals who may or may not receive treatment), shows that persons with a diagnosis of mental disorders are more likely to have a history of arrests and arrests for violent offenses (Hodgins & Janson, 2002). "Research of this kind completed in the United States show a two-to-six-fold increase in the rate of violence in samples of people with mental illness compared to samples of people without mental illness drawn from the general population"(Corrigan & Cooper, 2005, p. 169). Moreover, these rates tend to increase when the persons diagnosed with a major mental disorder also have a comorbid diagnosis of a substance abuse disorder.

Evidence from cohort studies also supports a similar conclusion concerning the relationship between mental disorders and crime. The Stockholm Project Metropolitan is an excellent example (see Hodgins & Janson, 2002). This study followed the entire cohort of persons born in Stockholm, Sweden, in 1953 for a period of 30 years. Although the project was not specifically designed to investigate the relationship between mental disorders and crime, the information collected for this longitudinal study has offered researchers excellent descriptive information about factors associated with the development of criminal behavior. Researchers involved with this study have investigated the criminal data for four groups of individuals in this birth cohort: (1) individuals with a diagnosis of major mental disorder (schizophrenia, bipolar disorder, and major depression); (2) individuals with alcohol- and/or drug-related disorders; (3) individuals with other disorders; and (4) individuals who were never admitted for psychiatric care or had a diagnosis of mental disorder (Hodgins & Janson, 2002). The results showed that 31.7% of the cohort without a diagnosis of any type of mental disorder had a registered record of a criminal offense by age 30; and 50.5% of the persons with a diagnosis of a major mental disorder (severe and chronic mental disorders) had a criminal offense by age 30 (Hodgins & Janson, 2002).

The Project Metropolitan cohort study also uncovered interesting findings regarding comparative risks for committing violent crimes. The results of this study showed that men with major mental disorders were at a greater relative risk of being convicted of a violent crime than men without a history of mental disorders. They were 4.75 times more likely to be convicted of a violent crime than the men without any type of mental disorder (Hodgins & Janson, 2002). In addition, 24.4% of the men with a diagnosis of a major mental disorder had a registered arrest for a violent crime compared to 6.4% of the individuals without a diagnosis of a major mental disorder. Similar differences were also found for women, but the relative risk for conviction of a violent crime was 11.8 times higher for women with a mental disorder than for women without a mental disorder. In addition, the women with mental disorders also had a higher percentage of registered arrests for violent crimes (6.3%) than the women without mental disorders (6%).

Further confirmation of an association between mental disorders and violence has been documented in other types of research (Ashford, 1989). Link, Andrews, and Cullen (1992) went beyond the examination of the connection between diagnoses and mental disorders. Their community-based study included measures of officially recorded arrests and self-reported arrests to further clarify the relationship between mental disorders and violent crime. Their results showed that the relationship remained when they controlled for respondents' sociodemographic and community residence characteristics—characteristics reflecting the level of homicide in the community where they lived. The relationship between mental disorders and crime also held when they controlled for individuals' social desirability biases in responding to the survey items (Link & Stueve, 1994). However, when they controlled for psychotic symptoms, the rates of violent arrests decreased, which suggested an alternative explanation for the higher rates of arrests and arrests for violence in persons with diagnoses of mental disorders. It is the type of psychotic symptoms that explains the relationship between diagnoses and violence.

Link and colleagues (1992) concluded from their epidemiological results that the higher rates of violence found in studies of arrests involving samples of persons in treatment is not due to criminalization, medicalization, or social selection processes. Instead, they concluded that there is an identifiable set of "threat-control override" symptoms that explain the observed relationships between diagnoses of mental disorders and violence. In essence, when the psychosis involves threats of harm or removal of self-control, then the person with a serious mental illness is more likely to engage in violence than are persons with a psychosis that involves other types of symptoms that are either nonthreatening or involve themes that are not consistent with a loss of self-control.

Based on the prior findings, Link and Steuve (1994) developed the "principle of rationality-within irrationality" to explain the relationship between mental disorders and violence. It is assumed in this principle that the nature and content of the psychotic experience are what is relevant to understanding the relationship between serious mental disorders and violent crime. Persons with mental disorders who do not have a psychosis involving a belief of potential harm or loss of control are less likely to commit a violent crime. It is implied in this principle that it is important to target the nature and content of the psychosis in order to reduce violence among offenders with a diagnosis of a serious mental disorder.

Evidence is mounting of an association between mental illness and crime, but Rice and Harris (1997) have argued that this association is better explained by the co-occurrence of personality disorders. Yet the treatment of personality disorders with cognitive interventions has had mixed results, especially for persons with a psychopathic personality diagnosis (Ashford, Sales, & Reid, 2001). Nonetheless, some investigators have questioned whether targeting the aspects of the mental illness associated with crime by itself is sufficient to reduce violence and aggression in persons with serious mental disorders (Ashford, Sales, & LeCroy, 2001; McMurran, Egan, Richardson, & Ahmadi, 1999). They ask: Do we also have to target other forms of criminogenic attitudes and beliefs that are also associated with criminal and violent forms of behavior?

Targeting Criminogenic Needs

The general literature in correctional rehabilitation has been influenced substantially by the risk–need–responsivity principles identified by Andrews and his colleagues (1990). These principles ushered in a major turn in correctional practices because they pushed correctional professionals to differentiate between static and dynamic risk factors in the prevention of criminal recidivism. The dynamic risk factors refer to criminogenic needs that are changeable and have established associations with criminal behavior (Andrews, Bonta, & Wormith, 2006). One of the key dynamic risk factors that is well documented in the criminological literature and supported by general personality and social psychology of crime theory is the construct of attitudes (Andrews et al., 2006; Simourd & Olver, 2002). In the social psychology literature, it is assumed that attitudes are causally linked to behavior that is mediated by the person's intention to commit the behavior. Criminal attitudes are considered one of the "big four" risk factors that plays a pivotal role in what has been termed the psychological moment of crime (Simourd & Olver, 2002). Moreover, research has shown that a composite measure of criminal attitudes and criminal peers predicts recidivism better than other more static or traditional predictor variables (Simourd & Olver, 2002).

The Options program, developed by Bush and Bilodeau (1993) for the National Institute of Corrections, is a manualized cognitive-behavioral program that was designed to change the criminal attitudes and social problem-solving abilities of offenders. Inasmuch as there is substantial support for the use of this type of manual-based intervention, few studies have focused on examining the use of similar models for treating mentally ill offenders (McMurran et al., 1999).

Duncan, Nicol, and Ager (2006) performed a systematic review of structured group interventions with mentally disordered offenders. This review included an examination of four types of interventions: (1) problem-solving skills, (2) anger/aggression management, (3) deliberate self-harm interventions, and (4) other types of interventions. Under the problem-solving category, the researchers were able to identify four published articles that employed evidence-based treatment manuals. The results for these four problem-solving interventions demonstrated some promising results in the treatment of offenders diagnosed with serious mental disorders (McMurran et al., 1999). However, none of these interventions indicated how the manualized treatments were modified to treat offenders diagnosed with serious mental disorders.

Attribution Biases

The research literature on aggression and violence is also demonstrating that violent offenders possess deviant ways of interpreting relevant social stimuli and social situations (Losel, Bliesener, & Bender, 2007). In fact, we now know that the cognitive deficits associated with violence and aggression in children and adolescents involve specific types of hostile attribution biases (Losel et al., 2007; McMurran et al., 1999). "A hostile attributional bias (i.e., the tendency to attribute hostile intent to others in ambiguous situations with a negative outcome) has consistently shown to be integral to aggressive behavior in children and adolescents" (Waldheter, Jones, Johnson, & Penn, 2005, p. 609). McNiel, Eisner, and Binder (2003) have identified the presence of similar biases in persons with psychiatric disturbances. Yet there are few interventions for mentally ill offenders that have focused on changing these attribution biases.

THE MCSTAR PROGRAM

An important aim of the Monterey County Supervised Treatment After Release program was to examine whether a cognitive intervention designed for changing problem-solving and other cognitive errors in ordinary offenders would be equally effective in changing the attitudes and attribution biases in a sample of mentally ill offenders. In addition, the program assumed that generic cognitive interventions designed for ordinary offenders would be effective in reducing recidivism in offenders with serious mental disorders if appropriate attention was devoted to the principle of offender responsivity (Ashford et al., 2008).

The principle of responsivity involves the matching of clinical interventions with the personality and other relevant capacities of the individual offender (Andrews et al., 2006). In keeping with this principle, the MCSTAR program modified the administration of the Options program to take into account the potential cognitive impairments possessed by offenders with a diagnosis of schizophrenia or other serious psychotic conditions (Green, 1998). The cognitive intervention used in MCSTAR was administered at a pace that did not exceed the cognitive capacities of the program's participants (Ashford et al., 2008). The traditional cognitive program for ordinary offenders consisted of 36 two-hour sessions that are administered from two to five times a week for about 8 weeks. Because this pace was too fast for mentally ill offenders, the average time for completing the curriculum increased and their average time in the cognitive program ranged from 4 to 6 months, instead of the prescribed 2 months. Participants with predominately negative symptoms of schizophrenia required more time to complete the cognitive intervention than offenders with a diagnosis of a bipolar mood disorder (Ashford et al., 2008).

Measures

Participants in the MCSTAR program were administered pre- and posttests to determine whether the program was effective in changing the attitudes and attribution biases of the program participants. The participants were administered the Pride in Delinquency (PID) Scale, the Criminal Sentiments Scale Modified (CSS-M), and the Hostile Interpretations Questionnaire (HIQ). The PID is a 10-item self-report instrument that assesses an individual's pride or shame about involvement in specific types of criminal behaviors (Shields & Whitehall, 1991). The CSS-M is a 41-item self-report instrument that contains five distinct subscales: attitudes toward the law, attitudes toward the court, attitudes toward the police, tolerance of law violations, and identification with criminal others (Simourd & Van de Ven, 1999). And the HIQ is a vignette-style inventory that assesses the individual's overall level of hostility, as well as his or her hostility in several different social contexts (Simourd & Mamuza, 2000).

The HIQ has roots in social information processing theory. Its design is predicated on the assumption that hostile individuals are likely to interpret ambiguous social situations as provocative. The questionnaire includes social situations that the designers observed in offender populations with whom they had worked. These situations were included in five types of vignettes involving authority, intimate/family, acquaintances, work, and anonymous sources of hostility (Simourd & Mamuza, 2000). The instrument also included vignettes that focused on hostile types of thinking errors, such as overgeneralization, attribution of hostility, personal responsibility, hostile reaction, and external blame (Simourd, 2000).

Outcomes

The results of the pre- and posttests for the participants in the MCSTAR program showed that the program was effective in changing a number of the offender's criminal attitudes and attribution biases (Ashford et al., 2008). Changes in expected directions were noted on all of the CSS-M subscales except the scale measuring identification with criminal others. However, no significant pre- and posttest differences were noted for the PID scale. For the HIQ, pre- and posttest differences were noted on the total score and on the authority, anonymous, overgeneralization, and attribution of hostility subscales (Ashford et al., 2008).

Inasmuch as the program was able to change some of the criminal attitudes and attribution biases in a sample of mentally ill offenders (n = 31), the only cognitive scale with pre- and posttest differences that was associated with measures of arrests (recidivism) that went in the hoped-for direction was the HIQ's overgeneralization subscale. Decreases in offender tendencies toward overgeneralization were associated with decreases in arrests during the study's 12-month criminal follow-up. In addition, other changes in the HIQ authority, attribution of hostility, personal responsibility, and hostile reaction subscales were associated with an offender's likelihood of having his or her probation violated on technical grounds (Ashford et al., 2008).

Ashford and colleagues (2008) also found that participants in the MCSTAR intervention had fewer arrests overall and fewer arrests for crimes of violence than the participants in a treatment-as-usual comparison group. These results also held when the researchers controlled for potential biases in responding to self-report instruments. In addition, the relationships remained when they controlled for the potential impact of the mental health court and FACT team. The findings provided preliminary support for an association between an important error in thinking—overgeneralization—and recidivism. In addition, the MCSTAR intervention identified several attribution biases that were associated with technical probation violations. In essence, the changes in cognition reported in this study indicate that cognitive interventions may be of value in reducing crime and violence in offenders diagnosed with serious mental disorders. We will describe the characteristics of the overall integrative treatment intervention used in MCSTAR as well as details of the cognitive intervention.

MCSTAR INTERVENTION

The MCSTAR program targeted mentally ill offenders who had a prior history of two or more arrests and a current diagnosis of a serious mental illness. This included individuals with diagnoses of schizophrenia, bipolar disorders, and other psychotic disorders as defined by the American Psychiatric Association's *Diagnostic and Statistical Manual of Mental Disorders*. Most of the participants had co-occurring disorders of serious mental illness and alcohol and/or substance abuse. The program focused on incarcerated mentally disordered adult offenders, ages 18 and older, in custody at the time of referral or released from jail following arrest.

Program eligibility was based on individuals' having met the criteria for serious mental illness as well as having been booked with a new charge, including a probation violation. Eligible individuals had to have a history of two or more arrests, including the current charge.[1] Essentially, the program targeted high-rate offenders with two or more arrests and with serious mental illnesses, including co-occurring substance abuse disorders. Individuals with violent felony convictions were also included in the program based on an assessment of their risk to the community by the probation officer on the FACT team, mental health staff, and the court team, which included the judge, public defender, and district attorney. This combined team assessed the prior violent and nonviolent crimes and determined whether the offender could benefit from the MCSTAR intervention.

The cognitive intervention was embedded in a systematic treatment and supervision program for serving mentally ill offenders. The key elements of the program included: (1) in-custody assessment and treatment services; (2) a FACT team; (3) a mental health court; (4) a cognitive skills training program; and (5) supervised and supportive community housing.

The program addressed the need for early identification of offenders with mental illness by placement of an in-custody social worker in the county jail. The social worker was responsible for assessing inmates for mental illness and providing an initial intervention to foster their engagement in treatment and entrance into the program. The FACT team provided 24-hour wraparound support, using a low staff-to-offender ratio, for a maximum of 45 offenders at any one time. Staffing included a clinical supervisor, two social workers, a peer specialist case manager, a psychiatrist, and a probation officer. The goals of the FACT team were to provide an intensive array of mental health services that engaged mentally ill offenders in their recovery and prevent their psychiatric symptoms from escalating, as well as to offer intensive supervision that provided a check on illegal behavior.

The mental health court provided judicial oversight and flexible sentencing that was used to enhance compliance with mental health treatment and probation requirements. The court had a special calendar that met weekly and a designated judge to provide oversight of the program participants. The availability of housing for this population also provided the opportunity for more structured supervision and improved community acceptance of the initiative.

Within this context, the cognitive intervention aimed to provide offenders with better decision-making skills to help them address their needs through noncriminal activity and to help them develop prosocial attitudes. Based on the Options program developed by Bush and Bilodeau (1993) and modified by the Maricopa County Adult Probation Department (Simourd, 2000), the program addressed: (1) critical thinking, problem solving, and decision making; (2) general strategies for recognizing problems, analyzing them, and conceiving and considering noncriminal alternatives; (3) ways to view frustrations as a problem-solving task and not a personal threat; (4) how to formulate plans; (5) ways to calculate the consequences of behavior—to stop and think before acting; (6) how to go beyond an egocentric view of the world and consider and comprehend the thoughts and feelings of other people; (7) ways to think logically, objectively, and rationally without overgeneralizing, distorting facts, and externalizing blame onto others; and (8) how to develop the abilities to regulate their own behaviors so that prosocial behavior is not dependent on external controls (i.e., prison and police).

The different cognitive skills needs of individuals pose distinct problems for the cognitive trainers. Individuals with more cognitive distortions (due to medication, psychosis, or other factors) required repeated sessions on the curriculum units. Individuals with less cognitive impairment were able to grasp the concepts more quickly. Interviews of the cognitive skill training participants about 12 months into the intervention revealed some impatience with repetitive classes for persons with a diagnosis of a bipolar disorder. As a result, staff began to tailor the classes to the different capabilities and expectations of the participants. Although there were drawbacks to having participants with different abilities, there were also benefits associated with combining individuals with different cognitive abilities. Those who were learning more quickly were able to support slower learners. This process also benefited the fast learners because they started sharing their knowledge with individuals who did not understand how to challenge their errors in thinking. Yet finding the correct balance was an ongoing challenge, because some participants were frustrated with the slow pace required for participants with severe cognitive impairments.

Transitioning to "treatment as usual" from the intense community treatment and probation supervision of the FACT team became an important area to address. Originally, the FACT team, mental health court, and cognitive skill training model was geared to an 18-month stay with staged periods of intervention. For some individuals, the length and intensity of the oversight was too long, and, for others, 18 months was not enough time. It was a challenge for the FACT team and the mental health court to determine when enough was enough, particularly because the participants had histories of serious mental illness and multiple arrests and most had co-occurring disorders of alcohol and substance abuse. Yet several participants had obtained jobs, others wanted to return to their family home after living in supported or supervised housing, and others desired more independence. Designing an exit strategy for the program was necessary to preserve the gains of the individual participants and to reinforce hope of recovery and change.

Initially, the program developed an advanced cognitive skill training segment for participants who had accomplished their priority goals and completed the core cognitive training units. Although this approach was successful, the peer specialist case manager on the FACT team emphasized the importance of moving on. Consequently, the advanced cognitive skill program began to emphasize transition planning and was renamed Moving On. Criteria to participate in this group included: (1) completion of all 36 core cognitive skill training courses; (2) 6 months of sobriety; and (3) 6 months of having stable housing. The initial sessions focused on clarifying the class rules (e.g., expectations about classroom behavior, attendance at every class to graduate, completion of assignments, and timeliness). Continued participation in Moving On required agreement to these rules. Assignments included continuation of "thinking reports" (documenting certain behaviors and thinking prior to the behavior) and exercises to help the participants plan for their transitions to more integrated community living. Response to the change was positive, and most participants reported appreciation of the recognition of their accomplishments and confirmation of their goal to graduate from the program.

An important component of the cognitive skill training was the reinforcement provided by the FACT team and the mental health court. Thinking reports were used as tools by the FACT team to help the participants understand the criminogenic aspects of their behavior and to apply the principles of the cognitive skill training. Furthermore, the mental health court judge could assign additional thinking reports as an alternative to a negative sanction, such as jail. Initially, remands to jail were frequent when individuals violated their terms of probation. As participants engaged and the FACT team and judge became more knowledgeable about the participants, a range of incentives and sanctions became available, such as the use of thinking reports.

Positive reinforcement by the FACT team and the judge tailored to the individual's gains influenced change in a positive direction. A survey of program participants revealed their appreciation of the judge's praise and support, which they saw as important to their recovery. Use of individualized incentives and sanctions also resulted in improved participant satisfaction with the program and better compliance with probation requirements. Pre- and posttests that were administered to participants verified positive changes in critical thinking skills. Reductions in criminal recidivism and violent crimes also occurred (Ashford et al., 2008).

SUMMARY AND FUTURE DIRECTIONS

The MCSTAR program is a research-supported program that indicates that offenders with mental illness can benefit from cognitive interventions that are designed to change their thinking deficits. In addition, the program was successful in changing attribution bias with links to recidivism rates. However, the results went in some unexpected directions. The program was much more successful in changing hostile attributions that affected rates of recidivism rather than the hypothesized criminal attitudes as measured by the CSS-M and PID. In other words, the initial program design was predicated on the risk–need–responsivity assumption that recidivism can be reduced by focusing on changing primary risk factors such as criminal attitudes (Andrews et al., 2006). However, it was found that changes in social problem-solving or information-processing skills as measured by the HIQ were more directly linked with reductions in recidivism.

The HIQ findings raise important questions about the relationships between mental disorders and violent crime because they point to some interesting interpretations of the nature of these relationships and their implications for treatment. The research for this program found that the overgeneralizations or the errors in thinking of offenders with mental illness were associated with their recidivism. This finding warrants closer scrutiny because it indicates that it might not be fruitful to just target changes in criminal attitudes. That is, future research needs to rule out whether the findings in this study were due to the nature of the intervention or to the appropriateness of targeting criminal attitudes or criminal thinking patterns. The intervention did not directly focus on changing attitudes, but rather focused on the development of appropriate social problem-solving skills. In essence, the findings raise important empirical questions about how the criminal attitudes construct is measured and how this construct is conceptually linked in treatment with appropriate program outcomes and with program designs.

Because criminal attitudes can be viewed as an outcome or as a mediating factor that affects criminal behavior, further research is needed on the nature of the relationship between criminal attitudes and thinking errors. The general body of research on attitudes has recognized for a long time that attitude changes involve important directionality considerations—whether changes in behavior influence attitudes or vice versus. For this reason, it would be useful for future researchers to control for this issue by examining whether errors in thinking are mediating factors in predicting variations in criminal attitudes. This type of research needs to be conducted before we prematurely eliminate criminal attitudes as either a measure or an outcome for designing programs for mentally disordered offenders. That is, the program was successful in changing the criminal attitudes of the offenders, but it was surprising that the changed attitudes did not show any association with subsequent measures of recidivism. For this reason, program designers cannot overlook current gaps in our knowledge about the causal ordering of the relationship between criminal attitudes and criminal behavior.

Regardless of the causal ordering concerns, the results of this integrative treatment program show that cognitive interventions may be of value in the design of integrative treatment approaches for offenders with mental illness. Clearly, the cognitive errors were associated with arrests, arrests for violent offences, and technical probation violations. These findings suggest that cognitive errors might represent even another dimension of an offender's illness that has not been previously examined in other research on the subject. Persons with paranoid delusions have attribution biases that the MCSTAR intervention could have influenced, and this might explain why the performance on the HIQ measures predicted rates of recidivism better than the CSS-M or the PID. Most of the subjects in the study had a diagnosis of schizophrenia. For this reason, future research should control better for types of disorders and their symptoms than the current research demonstration. However, we cannot ignore the potential validity of an alternative hypothesis that the HIQ is more effective than the CSS-M and PID in measuring criminal thinking abilities.

In sum, even though we cannot fully explain why the cognitive intervention improved on the rates of recidivism by the participants in the MCSTAR program, it is clear that the participants in this program's integrative treatment approach had fewer arrests and fewer arrests for violent offenses than the participants in the treatment-as-usual group. These positive results suggest a need for future studies on integrative treatment approaches that include cognitive interventions that have larger samples and administer pre- and posttests to an appropriate control group on the cognitive measures. Future studies also need to focus on monitoring how specific criminal attitudes are targeted by the intervention. Despite the many limitations contained in the research demonstration described in this chapter, the results of MCSTAR demonstration provide a preliminary justification for the pursuit of further investigations of the utility of treating criminogenic needs in offenders diagnosed with serious mental disorders.

NOTE

1. Individuals who met the prior criteria were automatically excluded if they: (a) were charged with a sex offense; (b) had a criminal history that posed a clear safety risk for the public; (c) were gang members; (d) were persons with a primary diagnosis of borderline personality disorder or other personality disorders; (e) were persons with a primary diagnosis of a major depressive disorder without psychosis; (f) were developmentally disabled persons with an IQ below 70; or (g) were found to have an organic disorder such as dementia.

REFERENCES

Andrews, D. A., Bonta, J., & Wormith, J. S. (2006). The recent past and near future of risk and/or need assessment. *Crime & Delinquency, 52*, 7–27.

Andrews, D. A., Zinger, I., Hoge, R. D., Bonta, J., Gendreau, P., & Cullen, F. T. (1990). Does correctional treatment work? A psychologically informed meta-analysis. *Criminology, 28*, 369–404.

Ashford, J. B. (1988). Offender characteristics of career criminals with severe mental disorders. *International Journal of Offender Therapy and Comparative Criminology, 32*, 143–151.

Ashford, J. B. (1989). Offense comparisons between mentally disordered and nonmentally disordered inmates. *Canadian Journal of Criminology, 31*, 45–48.

Ashford, J. B., Sales, B. D., & LeCroy, C. W. (2001). Aftercare and recidivism prevention. In J. B. Ashford, B. D. Sales, & W. H. Reid (Eds.), *Treating adult and juvenile offenders with special needs* (pp. 373–400). Washington, DC: American Psychological Association.

Ashford, J. B., Sales, B. D., & Reid, W. H. (2001). Political, legal, and professional challenges to treating offenders with special needs. In J. B. Ashford, B. D. Sales, & W. H. Reid (Eds.), *Treating adult and juvenile offenders with special needs* (pp. 31–49). Washington, DC: American Psychological Association.

Ashford, J. B., Sternbach, K., & Balaam, M. (in press). Offender re-entry and home based interventions. In S. Allen and E. Tracy (Eds.), *Delivering home based services: A social work perspective*. New York: Columbia University Press.

Ashford, J. B., Wong, K. W., & Sternbach, K. (2008). Generic correctional programming for mentally ill offenders: A pilot study. *Criminal Justice and Behavior, 35,* 457–473.

Berman, G., & Feinblatt, J. (2003). Problem solving courts: A brief primer. In B. J. Winick & D. B. Wexler (Eds.), *Judging in a therapeutic key: Therapeutic jurisprudence and the courts* (pp. 73–86). Durham, NC: Carolina Academic Press.

Bond, G., Miller, L., Krumwied, R., & Ward. R. (1988). Assertive case management in three CMHCs: A controlled study. *Hospital and Community Psychiatry, 39,* 411–418.

Borland, A., McRae, J., & Lycan, C. (1989). Outcomes of five years of continuous intensive case management. *Hospital and Community Psychiatry, 40,* 369–376.

Bush, J., & Bilodeau, B. (1993). *Options: A cognitive change program.* Longmont, CO: National Institute of Corrections.

Corrigan, P. W., & Cooper, A. E. (2005). Mental illness and dangerousness: Fact or misperception, and implications for stigma. In P. W. Corrigan (Ed.), *On the stigma of mental illness: Practical strategies for research and social change* (pp. 165–179). Washington, DC: American Psychological Association.

Cosden, M., Ellens, J. K., Schnell, J. L., Yamini-Diouf, Y., & Wolfe, M. M. (2003). Evaluation of a mental health treatment court with assertive community treatment. *Behavioral Sciences and the Law, 21*(4), 415–427.

Duncan, E., Nicol, M. M., & Ager, A. (2006). A systematic review of structured group interventions with mentally disordered offenders. *Criminal Behaviour and Mental Health, 16,* 217–241.

Feder, L. (1991). A profile of mentally ill offenders and their adjustment in the community. *Journal of Psychiatry and Law, 19,* 79–98.

Green, M. F. (1998). *Schizophrenia from a neurocognitive perspective: Probing the impenetrable darkness.* Boston: Allyn Bacon.

Heilbrun, K., & Griffin, P. A. (1993). Community-based forensic treatment of insanity acquittees. *International Journal of Law and Psychiatry, 16,* 133–150.

Hodgins, S., & Janson, C. G. (2002). *Criminality and violence among mentally disordered: The Stockholm Project Metropolitan.* Cambridge, England: Cambridge University Press.

Jacoby, J. E., & Kozie-Peak, B. (1997). The benefits of social support for mentally ill offenders: Prison to community transitions. *Behavioral Sciences and the Law, 15,* 483–501.

Lamb, H. R., & Weinberger, L. E. (1998). Persons with severe mental illness in jails and prisons: A review. *Psychiatric Services, 49,* 483–492.

Lamb, H. R., & Weinberger, L. E. (2001). Adult offenders and community settings: Some case examples. In J. B. Ashford, B. D. Sales, & W. H. Reid (Eds.), *Treating adult and juvenile offenders with special needs* (pp. 465–478). Washington, DC: American Psychological Association.

Lamberti, J. S., Weisman, R., & Faden, D. I. (2004). Forensic assertive community treatment: Preventing incarceration of adults with severe mental illness. *Psychiatric Services, 55,* 1285–1293.

Link, B. G., Andrews, H., & Cullen, F. (1992). Violent and illegal behavior of current and former mental patients compared to community controls. *American Sociological Review, 57,* 272–292.

Link, B. G., & Stueve, A. (1994). Psychotic symptoms and the violent/illegal behavior of mental patients compared to community controls. In J. Monahan & H. J. Steadman (Eds.), *Violence and mental disorders: Developments in risk assessment* (pp. 137–159). Chicago: University of Chicago Press.

Link, B. G., & Stueve, A. (1995). Evidence bearing on mental illness as a possible cause of violent behavior. *Epidemiological Review, 17,* 172–181.

Lipton, F., Nutt, S., & Sabitini, A. (1988). Housing and homeless mentally ill: A longitudinal study of a treatment approach. *Hospital and Community Psychiatry, 39,* 40–45.

Losel, F., Bliesener, T., & Bender, D. (2007). Social information processing, experiences of aggression in social contexts, and aggressive behavior in adolescents. *Criminal Justice and Behavior, 34,* 330–347.

Lovell, D., Gagliardi, G. J., & Peterson, P. D. (2002). Recidivism and use of services among persons with mental illness after release from prison. *Psychiatric Services, 53,* 1290–1296.

Lurigio, A. J., Fallon, J. R., & Dincin, J. (2000). Helping the mentally ill in jails adjust to community life: A description of post release ACT program and its clients. *International Journal of Offender Therapy and Comparative Criminology, 44,* 532–548.

Marini, R. A. (2003). Mental health courts focus on treatment: Criminals often overlooked in traditional system are sentenced to hospital care. In B. J. Winick & D. B. Wexler (Eds.), *Judging in a therapeutic key. Therapeutic jurisprudence and the courts* (pp. 59–62). Durham, NC: Carolina Academic Press.

Marshall, M., & Lockwood, A. (2001). The effectiveness of case management and assertive community treatment for people with severe mental disorders. In H. D. Brenner, W. Boker, & R. Genner (Eds.), *The treatment of schizophrenia: Status and emerging trends* (pp. 181–194). Kirkland, WA: Hogrefe and Huber.

McMurran, M., Egan, V., Richardson, C., & Ahmadi, S. (1999). Social problem solving in mentally disordered offenders: A brief report. *Criminal Behaviour and Mental Health, 9,* 315–322.

McNiel, D. E., Eisner, J. P., & Binder, R. L. (2003). The relationship between aggression attributional style and violence by psychiatric patients. *Journal of Consulting and Clinical psychology, 71,* 399–403.

Morrissey, J., & Meyer, P. (2005). *Extending assertive community treatment to criminal justice settings.* Delmar, NY: National GAINS Center.

Nieto, M. (1999, February). *Mentally ill offenders in California's criminal justice system.* Sacramento: California Research Bureau.

Rice, M. E., & Harris, G. T. (1997). Cross-validation and extension of the violence risk appraisal guide for child molesters and rapists. *Law and Human Behavior, 21,* 231–241.

Roskes, E., & Feldman, R. (1999). A collaborative community-based treatment program for offenders with mental illness. *Psychiatric Services, 50,* 1614–1619.

Shields, I. W., & Whitehall, G. C. (1991, December). *The Pride in Delinquency Scale.* Paper presented at the Eastern Ontario Correctional Psychologists' Winter Conference. Burritts Rapids, Canada.

Simourd D. J. (2000). *Evaluation of the Maricopa County Adult Probation Department Cognitive Intervention Program (CIP): The first follow-up.* Phoenix, AZ: Maricopa County Adult Probation Department.

Simourd, D. J., & Mamuza, J. M. (2000). The hostile interpretations questionnaire: Psychometric properties and construct validity. *Criminal Justice and Behavior, 27,* 645–663.

Simourd, D. J., & Olver, M. E. (2002). The future of criminal attitudes research and practice. *Criminal Justice and Behavior, 29,* 427–446.

Simourd, D. J., & Van de Ven, J. (1999). Assessment of criminal attitudes: Criterion-related validity of the Criminal Sentiments Scale–Modified and Pride in Delinquency Scale. *Criminal Justice and Behavior, 26,* 90–106.

Solomon, P., & Draine, J. (1995). One-year outcomes of a randomized trial of case-management with seriously mentally-ill clients leaving jail. *Evaluation Review, 19*(3), 256–273.

Stein, L. I., & Test, M. A. (1980). An alternative to hospital treatment: Conceptual model, treatment program, and clinical evaluation. *Archives of General Psychiatry, 37,* 30-2-397.

Substance Abuse and Mental Health Services Administration (SAMHSA), U.S. Department of Health and Human Services. (2008). Community support toolkits. Washington, D.C. Retrieved June 2008 from http://mentalhealth.samsha.gov/

Ventura, L. A., Cassel, C. A., Jacoby, J. E., & Huang, B. (1998). Case management and recidivism of mentally ill persons released from jail. *Psychiatric Services, 49,* 1330–1337.

Waldheter, E. J., Jones, N. T., Johnson, E. R., & Penn, D. L. (2005). Utility of social cognition and insight in the prediction of inpatient violence among individuals with a severe mental illness. *Journal of Nervous and Mental Disease, 193,* 609–618.

Weisman, R. L., Lamberti, J. S., & Price, N. (2004). Integrating criminal justice, community health care, and support services for adults with severe mental disorders. *Psychiatric Quarterly, 75*(1), 71–85.

Wilson, D., Tien, G., & Eaves, D. (1995). Increasing the community tenure of mentally disordered offenders: An assertive case management program. *International Journal of Law and Psychiatry, 18,* 61–69.

Ziguras, S. J., & Stuart, G. W. (2000). A meta-analysis of the effectiveness of mental health case management over 20 years. *Psychiatric Services, 51,* 1410–1421.

10 Treating the Morally Objectionable
JAMES KNOLL IV

> Did I request thee, Maker, from my clay to mould me Man? Did I solicit thee from darkness to promote me?
>
> —Shelley, 1831

Clinicians who treat offenders suffering primarily from psychopathic or antisocial traits commonly struggle with the tension between humanizing versus objectifying their clients (Friedrich & Leiper, 2006). On the one hand, there is the well-intended goal of helping the offender develop into a more functional human being. On the other, there are the common emotional reactions of anger, disgust, and even fear of predation (Meloy & Meloy, 2002).

The purpose of this chapter is to set forth a basic foundation for developing a more objective and, ultimately, a more therapeutic stance when treating offenders who arouse strong feelings of moral disgust in the clinician. For this purpose, important research and limitations in our current knowledge base regarding highly antisocial offenders will be covered, with an eye toward dispelling unfounded clinical lore. Next, common countertransference reactions observed in clinicians who treat the morally objectionable will be discussed. General treatment approaches and recently developed programs for this population will be covered. Finally, the important issue of compassion fatigue in clinicians will be touched upon.

For the purposes of this chapter, the term *morally objectionable* (MO) will be used to describe a subpopulation of highly antisocial or psychopathic individuals whose attitudes and behaviors cause most clinicians to find them morally objectionable. The MO have often been convicted of particularly heinous or callous offenses, thus increasing the tendency of the clinician to have very negative countertransferential reactions to them. Approximately 15% of prison inmates are likely to be psychopathic (Woodworth & Porter, 2002), with an even higher rate (31.4%) among homicide offenders (Laurell & Daderman, 2007). Thus, it is likely that forensic clinicians will encounter a small but significant population of MO offenders who are primarily psychopathic. Although general mental health clinicians are often taught to avoid treating antisocial patients, forensic clinicians frequently find themselves in circumstances that compel them to treat such individuals.

It is not uncommon for the MO to come to psychiatric attention in a correctional or forensic setting when they develop comorbid psychiatric symptomatology. Despite the presence of the comorbid and treatable psychiatric symptoms, it is possible that the disturbing nature of the MO offender's personality structure can make him or her not only difficult to treat, but objectionable. In these circumstances, there is little guidance to help clinicians competently and ethically carry out their treatment duties. Since Groves's (1978) classic article, "Taking Care of the Hateful Patient," was published, open acknowledgement and discussion of physicians' countertransference to very difficult patients became more widely accepted. In subsequent explorations, the challenges of maintaining empathy, considered the essence of the treatment relationship, in the face of a "hateful" patient's dysfunctional personality has been stressed (Strous, Ulman, & Moshe, 2006).

Yet in the realm of forensic mental health, nuances of the forensic and correctional setting add a particular twist that may invoke feelings of moral intolerance. After all, the MO offender's circumstances have been caused by his or her own actions. Or have they? Regardless, in no area of medicine do physicians reduce or eliminate care for victims of bad judgment (Levinsky, Friedman, & Levine, 1999). Indeed, refusal of care for those who have supposedly caused their own problems could arguably be applied to a very large percentage of the population. The issue of free will and truly autonomous behavior is exceedingly complex and beyond the scope of this chapter. However, in an effort to move toward objectivity, it may be helpful to review what is known about the development and substratum of the highly antisocial offender. This will provide some

DEVELOPMENT AND SUBSTRATUM

> I, the miserable and abandoned, am an abortion, to be spurned at, and kicked, and trampled on. Even now my blood boils at the recollection of this injustice.
>
> —Shelley, 1831

It should come as no surprise that many incarcerated offenders have developmental histories involving significant deprivation. For example, over one-third of jail inmates in 2002 grew up with a parent or guardian who abused substances, and almost half had a family member who had been incarcerated (James, 2004). Correctional populations also are less educated than the general population. Almost three-quarters of state prison inmates did not receive a high school diploma as of 1997 (Harlow, 2003). This is in contrast to 18% of the general population that did not finish the 12th grade. Already, we must question these distinct developmental differences and what they imply about how many offenders begin life at a significant disadvantage. It has been observed since the 1960s that crime flourishes where conditions of life are the worst (Currie, 2000). The economic deprivation–violence connection is yet another well-known factor operant in the lives of many antisocial offenders.

Low intelligence and low school attainment have been observed to predict juvenile violence. Further, the rate of serious juvenile violence increased dramatically between 1987 and 1994 (Farrington & Loeber, 2000). By way of extrapolation, this time period suggests that these juveniles have now become adult offenders who are the current recipients of treatment in the criminal justice system. Many offenders come from backgrounds of parental criminality, child maltreatment, and poverty, all of which increase the risk of juvenile violence. Childhood abuse or neglect has been observed to increase the risk for personality disorders during early adulthood (Johnson et al., 1999). Poor or abusive parenting has been theorized as playing a major role in the development of adult criminality (Lykken, 1998). These adverse conditions may be more profound than we currently understand, because preliminary neuroimaging techniques have documented structural changes that occur in the brains of individuals who suffer early maltreatment (McCollum, 2006).

These data are not cited with the intent to absolve MO offenders of their misdeeds. Rather, it is provided in a sincere and questioning manner regarding the true functionality of the MO offender's psychological makeup and how it came to be that way. For the clinician working with MO offenders, and who is in search of greater objectivity, it may be helpful to consider a psychiatric naturalist approach. From a naturalist point of view, Homo sapiens act the way they do "because of the various influences that shape them, whether these be biological or social, genetic or environmental" (Naturalism.org, 2007). Naturalism does not undermine the importance of responsibility or morality, but places them within the world as understood by science.

For example, whereas many offenders are commonly described as "predators" and "monsters," a judge and legal scholar has raised a question many would prefer to avoid: "Where do these monsters, predators, and punks come from? Did they parachute from another country? Did they emerge from a spaceship from another planet? . . . It is a rare predator indeed who has had a successful childhood" (Gill, 1994). Research has tended to support the concept that some forms of psychopathy are in fact, associated with childhood abuse or neglect. Poythress, Skeem, and Lilienfield (2006) found that a history of child abuse or neglect was related to the impulsive and irresponsible lifestyle or externalizing features of psychopathy. A study by Marshall and Cooke (1999) comparing 50 psychopaths and 55 nonpsychopaths found that negative familial and social experiences in childhood significantly increase the risk of adult psychopathy.

One integrated theory suggests that juveniles who experience developmentally adverse events (e.g., poor parenting, abuse) are likely to develop distorted internal models of interpersonal relationships and self-regulation (Marshall & Barbaree, 1990). A complementary theory posits an interplay of developmental trauma, childhood difficulties, and insecure attachment as leading to an increased risk of offending as an adult (Craissati & Beech, 2006). Thus, there may exist an interplay between biological predisposition and parental inadequacy that increases the likelihood of future psychopathy (Lykken, 1995).

Cognitive neuroscience studies and very preliminary genetic research on psychopathy have supported a developmental disorder theory (Viding, 2004). Other studies of criminal psychopaths have suggested impaired executive function, attention deficits, and a dissociation of emotional and cognitive processing (Birbaumer et al., 2005; Pham,

Vanderstukken, Philippot, & Vanderlinden, 2003). Many of the offenders that clinicians would consider MO may be thought of as psychopaths. Yet it is important to keep in mind how preliminary our current understanding of psychopathy is, despite the large amount literature devoted to the subject. This is largely due to the heterogeneous nature of psychopathy, which renders many conclusions speculative. In particular, data on treatment effectiveness with psychopaths are inconclusive at the present time.

PSYCHOPATHY AND CONTROVERSY

> The picture I present to you is peaceful and human. . . . Pitiless as you have been towards me, I now see compassion in your eyes; let me seize the favorable moment, and persuade you to promise what I so ardently desire.
>
> —Shelley, 1831

Well before either Cleckley or Hare, Pinel introduced the concept of the psychopathic personality at the turn of the 19th century (Pinel, 1801). He described general characteristics such as impulsive violence in the absence of appreciable deficits in intellect and cognition. In 1941, Cleckley's classic text, *The Mask of Sanity* (1976), provided more detailed clinical descriptions. Building upon the work of Cleckley, Hare approached the clinical construct by developing a research tool—the Psychopathy Checklist. The PCL-R takes a two-factor model approach to measuring psychopathy. Factor 1 measures core personality characteristics, and Factor 2 measures antisocial behavioral/lifestyle factors (Hare, 2006). It is important to note that Hare's model is still the subject of debate and revision, with alternative 3- and 4-factor models having been proposed (Hall, Benning, & Patrick, 2004; Hare, 2003).

As will be discussed later (and also in chapter 8), our current understanding of psychopathy remains limited. Nevertheless, it is not at all uncommon for some mental health staff, certain of their diagnosis of psychopathy, to proclaim an offender not only unamenable to treatment, but very likely to become a "better psychopath" from having gained a better understanding of the vicissitudes of human emotions. Such proclamations must be approached with more objectivity and less reflexive desire to adopt an attitude of therapeutic nihilism. When confronted with an assertion that a particular patient is a psychopath, and thus not a viable treatment candidate, the following considerations may be helpful to the clinician:

1. *Is the patient actually psychopathic, per the PCL-R?* Using the PCL-R to confirm the diagnosis is a time-consuming effort that requires sufficient training, record review, and hours of evaluation. The label *psychopath* may have been given, and perpetuated, in the absence of such painstaking efforts.
2. *Have all neuropsychiatric or other medical causes of psychopathic personality been ruled out?* (That is, is the offender a pseudopsychopath?) It is possible that a frontal lobe syndrome or other lesser-known brain lesion syndromes may produce a clinical picture characterized by impaired ability to plan, limited insight, unrealistic ambition, antisocial behavior, and poor judgment (Dewan & Pies, 2001). Given the lifestyles of many MO offenders, various forms of traumatic brain injury and/or substance-induced deficits must be excluded.
3. *What is the goal of treatment?* There is certainly little evidence to date that efforts to effect personality change will be successful. On the other hand, more modest goals of reducing specific problem behaviors are more realistic.
4. *What is the type of treatment being proposed?* Although certain therapeutic communities or insight-oriented therapies may be poor choices, behaviorally oriented programs may be reasonable choices.
5. *Has the patient's behavior/attitude/crime so repulsed staff that they have become unable to view the patient objectively?* This is a common clinical scenario, particularly in overburdened, undersupervised staff with limited resources. The issue of countertransference will be discussed later in greater detail.

Now let us turn to the well-worn clinical wisdom that psychopaths cannot be treated. In the past, it has been a widely accepted clinical axiom that psychopaths are untreatable in terms of psychotherapy. A study that is commonly cited to support this theory was done by Rice, Harris, and Cormier (1992) and suggested that treated psychopaths had higher recidivism rates than untreated psychopaths. On closer inspection, it becomes evident that any antitreatment conclusions based on this study are premature. The treatment used in this study was an unstructured, peer-oriented therapeutic community program with little input from professional staff. Offenders acted as therapists, and techniques included nude encounter groups and marathon therapy group sessions. While it may be concluded that this particular type of treatment approach is likely to be unhelpful, it cannot serve as evidence that psychopaths are globally untreatable.

Indeed, more recent studies have challenged this assumption. For example, Skeem and Monahan (2002) found that psychopathic patients appear as likely as nonpsychopathic patients to benefit from adequate doses of treatment, in terms of violence reduction. D'Silva (2004) performed a comprehensive analysis of existing research on the treatment of psychopaths and found that most studies did not have the appropriate research design. It was concluded that the commonly held belief of an inverse relationship between high scores on the PCL-R and treatment response has not been established. In a review of 42 treatment studies on psychopathy, Salekin (2002) found little scientific basis for the belief that all psychopathy is untreatable.

Other studies have similarly reported that there is insufficient evidence to conclude that psychopaths are either worsened by treatment or that they are untreatable (Barbaree, 2005; Kristiansson, 1995; Messina et al., 2002). Vien and Beech (2006) point out that there has been almost no empirical research on the issue of pharmacological approaches to treating psychopaths' behavioral symptoms, such as impulsivity and aggression. This point highlights some of the confusion surrounding psychopaths and treatment. The notion of untreatability is further confused when the goal of the treatment is not clearly understood. Having a clear treatment goal becomes paramount when engaging the psychopath in a clinical setting. For example, does the treatment set out to target recidivism, violence, impulse control, or other psychiatric symptoms? The distinction is critical for making realistic determinations about treatment efforts. The clinical forensic psychiatrist will undoubtedly encounter antisocial and/or psychopathic offenders who also happen to be suffering from legitimately treatable psychiatric illness (Goodwin & Hamilton, 2003).

Regarding substantially more ambitious goals such as reducing recidivism, the lack of clarity on this issue has not been helped by the fact that there is still considerable debate surrounding the nature and etiology of psychopathy. At the present time, it would seem reasonable to avoid considering all "psychopathic offenders as being uniform," and instead "look at differential responsivity among particular subgroups" (Looman, Abracen, Serin, & Marquis, 2005, p. 565). Given our current understanding, it is important to keep in mind that psychopathy, far from being a distinct and precisely defined disorder, is perhaps best described as a common set of behaviors and personality traits. While some researchers view psychopathy as a discrete taxon, others make a convincing argument that psychopathy is best understood as existing on a continuum (Marcus, John, & Edens, 2004). If this is the case, as it likely seems to be, future research will require a process for sorting out possible subtypes of psychopathy (Murphy & Vess, 2003). Once this has been reliably achieved, some of the neurobiological associations reported among psychopaths may begin to hold more relevance.

For example, some of the commonly cited deficits found in psychopaths include abnormal lexico-semantic processing (Kiehl et al., 2004), amygdala dysfunction (Blair et al., 1999), and impaired affective responses (Kiehl et al., 2001). (See Table 10.1.) The common clinical observation of attenuated emotional and fear response in psychopaths has undergone preliminary investigation by functional magnetic resonance imaging (Birbaumer et al., 2005). Whereas healthy controls showed enhanced activation of the limbic-prefrontal circuit in response to fear and emotion-arousing stimuli, psychopaths displayed no significant activity in this circuit. These findings have led researchers to conclude that emotional and cognitive processing of aversive stimuli may occur via different neural routes in psychopaths. To extend the speculation, psychopaths may process fear and emotions in a cerebral, as opposed to a limbic, manner.

What is interesting about studies showing impaired affective processing is to consider them in light of clinical observations describing

Table 10.1

NEUROPSYCHIATRIC DEFICITS IN PSYCHOPATHS

- Amygdala dysfunction
- Abnormal lexico-semantic processing, abnormal language lateralization
- Orbitofrontal cortex dysfunction
- Increased callosal white matter
- Attenuated fear response (limbic-prefrontal circuits)
- Increased neurological soft signs
- Increased risk of self-harm in prison

emotional *hypersensitivity* in some psychopaths (Martens, 2001). In other words, some psychopaths are capable of appearing emotionally normal, and even very sensitive to certain emotional cues in others. Whether this is the result of a "pantomiming" of emotions as suggested by Cleckley or neurodevelopmental abnormalities is unclear. It is also important to note that the lifestyle of some psychopathic persons may involve either substance misuse or head trauma, both of which may further influence any underlying neurobiological impairments (Blair, 2003).

The very challenging nature of treating MO offenders, many of whom may be psychopathic, induces many unpleasant and unhelpful emotions in treatment staff. One common barrier to an objective treatment approach is the tendency to view such individuals as evil, and thus beyond redemption or understanding. Before discussing putative treatment approaches and associated challenges, it is necessary to address this reaction to the MO offender, which often seriously corrupts treatment and management efforts.

EVIL

> Was I then a monster, a blot upon the Earth, from which all men fled, and whom all men disowned?
>
> —Shelley, 1831

Over the past several decades, an explicit emphasis on evil has been developed by a number of respected social psychologists (Baumeister, 1997; Darley, 1992; Miller, 1999; Miller, Gordon, & Buddie, 1999; Wilson, 2003). In the field of forensic psychiatry, there has even been some debate about whether forensic psychiatrists should define and testify about evil (Simon, 2003; Welner, 2003). Current sociological, political, and criminal justice trends have likely played a role in this development but will not be elaborated upon here. What is of immediate interest is that attempts by behavioral science to define evil as though it were an objective and quantifiable concept are inherently flawed. Because evil is a subjective moral concept with inextricable ties to religious thought, it cannot be measured by psychiatric science. Moreover, there does not appear to be any significant need to define or use the term *evil*, because forensic psychiatry already has working concepts describing deviant behavior that is harmful to others.

In addition to the potential for further stigmatization of mental illness, legitimizing evil as a psychiatric concept will have serious detrimental effects on forensic clinical practice. Mason, Richman, and Mercer (2002) conducted a study of forensic psychiatric nurses' approaches to treatment on a high-security psychiatric hospital in the United Kingdom. The nurses were given a series of vignettes describing themes such as child killing, serial rape, and interpersonal violence. The nurses' discourse in semistructured interviews was analyzed and compared to data collected from actual care plans of forensic patients on the nurses' wards. One critical, but not unexpected, finding was that, when a patient was judged to be evil, staff abandoned medical discourse and reverted to lay notions of badness.

Further, patients perceived as evil were viewed as being beyond help, which was then reflected in their care plans. The authors stressed that forensic psychiatry services may be actively limited in the face of socialized values and lay concepts of evil. The semantics of lay discourse proved to be of more than academic interest, particularly where forensic terminology is translated into practice and treatment. Those forensic patients who were labeled as evil by nursing staff were, in effect, excluded from the usual medical, symptom-centered approach (Mercer, Mason, & Richman, 1999). The implications of using the term *evil* as a form of punitive sanctions by the staff are being considered in future research.

The forces culminating in a punitive, condemning attitude toward MO offenders are often strong. The inherent tendency to find the offensive party evil and thus beyond the need for further exploration or understanding is both self-gratifying and self-preserving. In essence, the declaration is an expeditious substitute for thought (Masters, 1997). But the business of dismissing someone as evil is really too easy and "merely begs the question of how they became that way" in the first place (Watson, 1995, p. 215). Forensic clinical psychiatrists, who must follow general ethical guidelines for psychiatry, are instructed to avoid any policy that "excludes, segregates or demeans the dignity" of a patient (American Psychiatric Association, 2001, p. 4). When treating offenders, they must strike a balance between neutrality and beneficence, regardless of how heinous a crime the patient may have committed (Lally & Freeman, 2005).

Psychiatrists, who are often in clinical leadership roles, must set an example by eschewing the regressive pull to denounce an offender as evil. As Simon (1996) has observed, psychiatrists do not ordinarily apply the term evil, even to the apparent destructive acts they are called upon to understand and explain. Psychiatrists look at causes and effects in human behavior and try not to make moral judgments. What society labels evil behavior, the psychiatrist seeks to understand within the framework of the psychopathology of mental illness or even of everyday life. (p. 8)

That our species has a dark side should come as no surprise to the psychiatrist or other adequately trained mental health staff. When such dark impulses are seen as alien or evil, rational thought suffers and the way is paved for mistreatment or mismanagement of offenders. In lieu of evil, a more helpful way of conceptualizing the psychology of MO offenders is next suggested.

PERSECUTION, ENVY, AND NIHILISM

> Many times I considered Satan as the fitter emblem of my condition; for often, like him, when I viewed the bliss of my protectors, the bitter gall of envy rose within me.
> All men hate the wretched, how, then, must I be hated, who am miserable beyond all living things! Yet you, my creator, detest and spur me, thy creature, to whom thou art bound by ties only dissoluble by the annihilation of one of us.
>
> —Shelley, 1831

Those who have worked either around or directly with highly antisocial offenders rarely fail to notice certain commonly espoused themes. Offenders often adopt and cling to the position of the aggrieved "victim," who has been dealt with unjustly by authorities, "the system," or life in general. To the disdain and sometimes repulsion of staff, attitudes of personal responsibility and regret over past transgressions are conspicuously absent. Offenders may become stagnated in their own self-pity and persecutory ruminations. However, this is not surprising, because many highly antisocial offenders have had harsh early childhoods that may have resulted in an impaired ability to trust others as an adult (Kaylor, 1999).

Hyatt-Williams (1998) has conceptualized aggressive or violent offenders using the psychological theories of Klein and Bion. According to his theory, impediments to psychological development may cause the offender to become relatively fixed in a persecutory developmental stage, or what Klein has called the *paranoid-schizoid position*. In this stage, the individual's world view is based on feelings of mistreatment and frustration at what is perceived as intentional harm or unnecessary withholding of gratification. Increasing levels of distress may result in the offender assuming more paranoid cognitions, such as distrusting all authority, or unfounded beliefs that he or she is being singled out for especially punitive treatment. Fixation at this stage is associated with the use of more primitive defense mechanisms such as splitting, externalization, and projective identification.

Successful development necessitates the transition away from the persecutory position to a more mature stage, which Klein called the *depressive position*. In the depressive position, the offender will have developed fear or worry that he or she has injured or destroyed some aspect of society or otherwise, his fellow man. Cognitions associated with the depressive position include regret, victim empathy, and interests in making reconciliation with society. This developmental theory has been symbolized by P/S D, where P/S symbolizes the paranoid–schizoid position, and D represents the depressive position. A general overview of this concept of antisocial offender development is outlined in Table 10.2.

Thus, persecutory cognitions are felt as threatening, undeserved attacks upon the self. Offenders in this position feel a need to "look out for number one" at the expense of others. They are likely to have very sturdy, chronic defenses to protect against the expectation of being mistreated, "dissed," or otherwise abused. Consistent with their feelings of being persecuted, such offenders also suffer from strong feelings of destructive

Table 10.2

ANTISOCIAL OFFENDER DEVELOPMENT	
PERSECUTORY	**REALITY**
Persecution, mistreatment	Structure, organization
Frustration	Discipline, restraint, societal demands
COGNITIONS	
Victim, sufferer	Responsible citizen
"Screwed by the system" World is cruel, uncaring	Regret, victim empathy
Narcissistic inaccessibility	Personal accountability, reconciliation, reparation

envy. Via projection, they perceive society and others as persecutory also by withholding the goodness and happiness to which they feel entitled. These cognitions have been described by Mullen (2004) in his thorough analysis of five mass murderers who, by pure chance, were not killed and were incarcerated. The offenders were described as suspicious, resentful grudge holders who had strong feelings of persecution or mistreatment. They tended to ruminate over past humiliations and harbored resentment over old social rejections.

In contrast, the depressive position allows the individual to more smoothly confront reality. It involves feelings of responsibility, guilt, and concern over harm done to others. Some offenders may eventually take up pursuits that demonstrate a negotiation of the depressive phase. For example, a man sentenced to life for murder may become involved in running the prison lifers group. Others may take up creative pursuits such as art, music, or poetry, all examples of reparative activities.

Certainly, the successful transition out of the persecutory position is no simple task, and some offenders may not be capable, or only partially capable, of doing so. A stable continuity figure who is consistent, not overly judgmental, and able to withstand the emotional assaults associated with projective identification may assist the offender's transition. Of course, idealism in the clinician is to be avoided for the sake of both the clinician and the offender. Treatment failures and recidivism go with the territory, yet the clinician should not despair. As Hyatt-Williams (1998) notes, "Our task is to make the best of a bad job. This aim is not to be despised" (p. 167). Smooth progress is likely to be the rare exception, and clinicians should expect attacks on the treatment process as inevitable. By destroying the clinician's will to help, the MO offender is able to abdicate responsibility and comfortably ease back into a familiar sense of aggrievement.

One feature of a chronic, fixed persecutory position bears some discussion. Clinical observations suggest that some MO offenders struggle unsuccessfully in the persecutory position and ultimately develop an entrenched nihilistic attitude toward treatment, and life in general. Frankl (1959) was the first psychiatrist to emphasize the importance of studying meaning in life within a psychological context. Frankl's experience as a Nazi concentration camp prisoner led him to conclude that a primary motivation for humans is a "will to meaning," or a drive to find meaning and purpose in life. A failure to find meaning and purpose may result in feelings of hopelessness, suicidality, and other self-defeating actions (Edwards & Holden, 2001).

Based on the work of Frankl, the Purpose-in-Life (PIL) Test was constructed to assess or quantify the construct of meaning in life (Crumbaugh & Maholick, 1969). Unfortunately, there is little research on this subject as it relates to offenders. What research does exist was done primarily in the 1970s, and much about the correctional landscape has changed since then. A 1973 study found that recidivists scored significantly lower on the PIL (less purpose) than did first-sentence prisoners, who, in turn, scored significantly lower than normal control subjects (Black & Gregson, 1973). In a 1977 study, inmates were found to have scored significantly lower than normal subjects on meaning and purpose in life (Reker, 1977). Subsequent research has found an association between the development of substance abuse problems and a lack of purpose or meaning in life (Waisberg & Porter, 1994).

One might speculate that the current abandonment of rehabilitative programming in corrections has only served to reinforce the MO offender's diminished sense of self-worth and personal value. Ultimately, feelings of diminished personal worth lead to a questioning of purpose. Once an inmate reaches some individual-specific level of nihilism, he or she may demonstrate a greatly reduced ability to participate in and benefit from rehabilitative or treatment efforts. In essence, when there is no meaning for the offender, there is no purpose or reason to change. In addition, when an inmate has strong nihilistic beliefs, there is often little motivation to self-regulate behavior.

These empirical observations of the adverse effects of nihilistic beliefs in inmates are consistent with research findings in nonincarcerated populations. For example, social rejection has been found to increase feelings of meaninglessness and decrease self-awareness and the ability to self-regulate behavior (Baumeister et al., 2005; Twenge, Catanese, & Baumeister, 2005). Rejection by peers and staff of MO offenders is common due to unpleasant countertransference reactions. It has been speculated that, when the drive to avoid negative affect, meaning, and self-awareness becomes strong enough, there is a significantly increased risk of suicide and/or self-destructive behaviors (Baumeister, 1990).

This theory has been called the "escape theory" of suicide to denote the suicidal individual's motivation to escape from aversive self-awareness. The escape theory may have relevance to the psychology of suicidal MO offenders, particularly where the inescapable structure and discipline of a prison reduces their ability to avoid aversive affect and self-awareness. According to escape theory, when the individual is unable to avoid negative affect and aversive self-awareness, a process of "cognitive deconstruction" occurs in which there is a rejection of meaning, increased irrationality, and disinhibition. Suicide then becomes the ultimate step in the effort to escape from meaningful awareness and it's implications about the self. Table 10.3 provides an outline of how escape theory may explain some offenders' tendency to become nihilistic and, finally, suicidal.

If one conceives of punitive segregation as a rather severe form of social exclusion, escape theory may explain why some offenders are at increased risk of suicide and self-harm in prison units such as secure housing units and other forms of isolation (American Psychiatric Association, 2000). Single-cell disciplinary housing typically occurs without close observation or attentive mental health care presence. Enhanced observation of special housing inmates has been recommended, particularly in light of findings that most inmates who commit suicide in a secure housing

Table 10.3

THE DOWNWARD SPIRAL OF OFFENDER NIHILISM

SOCIETY

1. Fantasy of entitled gratification
2. Deficient self-regulation[a]: voluntary, involuntary, or mixed[b]
3. Conflict with societal demands = offending behaviors

PRISON

4. Societal exclusion: arrest, criminal adjudication, prison sentence
5. Feelings of persecution, mistreatment, rejection followed by hostility, anger, mistrust
6. Heavy reliance on defenses: externalization, projection, minimization, etc.
7. External reality of prison: discipline, structure, accountability resulting in reduced ability to externalize blame or avoid responsibility due to inescapable structure
8. Aversive self-awareness produces painful, negative affect
9. Cognitive deconstruction: rejection of meaning, impaired reality testing, cognitive rigidity, disinhibition
10. Desire to escape from the self: self-mutilation, hanging

[a] Self-regulation is defined as the mental ability to change oneself to meet external (societal) standards. From "Social Exclusion Impairs Self-Regulation," by R. Baumeister et al., 2005, *Journal of Personality and Social Psychology, 88*(4), pp. 589–604.
[b] It is common for offenders to possess *both* voluntary *and* involuntary deficiencies of self-regulation.

unit do so within the first 2 months of placement there (Way, Sawyer, Barboza, & Nash, 2007). Escape theory and offender nihilism remain consistent with previously observed research findings in correctional suicide. For example, strong feelings of hopelessness (whereby an inmate no longer perceives meaning or purpose in life) and suicidal behavior are significantly correlated in prison suicides (Gray et al., 2003; Ivanoff & Jang, 1991). In addition, poorer coping skills and more severe affective symptoms have been observed in inmates who harm themselves when compared with inmates who do not (Dear et al., 2001; Pen et al., 2003).

TREATMENT APPROACHES

> I thought, that as I could not sympathize upon him, I had no right to withhold from him the small portion of happiness which was yet in my power to bestow.
>
> —Shelley, 1831

As can be inferred from the previous sections, the lack of diagnostic and etiologic specificity with regard to antisocial offenders makes interpretations of various treatment approaches difficult, if not impossible. What research is currently available on the treatment of antisocial or psychopathic personality is often criticized in terms of methodology, inadequate follow-up, and poorly specified diagnostic criteria (Lee, 1999). Until distinct subtypes are reliably defined, this dilemma is likely to persist (Hodgins, 2007).

Despite these inherent problems and low expectations, some efforts have been made over the past decade to design and implement programs that "would have a reasonable chance of modifying the attitudes and behaviors" of psychopaths (Hare, 1998, p. 203). Rather than focusing on the development of empathy, super ego function, or personality change, experts have targeted the more modest goals of "convincing participants that they alone are responsible for their behavior and that they can learn more prosocial ways of using their strengths and abilities" (Hare, 1998, p. 203). In essence, the programs being utilized for psychopaths at the beginning of the 21st century all tend to share certain core features: assessment and reduction of risk, development of insight into antisocial behavior, acquiring cognitive skills, and relapse prevention.

Hare and others have been careful to state that programs such as the Psychopathy Treatment Program (PTP) should be viewed as guidelines rather than comprehensive treatment programs (Vien & Beech, 2006;

Wong & Hare, 2005). The main goal of the PTP is to reduce the offender's frequency and severity of violence, both in prison and after release. The PTP can be characterized as a behavioral self-management program and does not present itself as a "cure" for psychopathy. Offenders are taught that they will best maintain their societal freedoms by lifelong self-management of their behavior. The Violence Reduction Program (VRP) is a similar program and has as its target population "high-risk violent offenders, in particular those who are non-compliant, lacking in motivation, resistant to treatment, and have a history of institutional misconduct" (Wong & Gordon, 2000, p. 3).

The VRP consists of three phases of incremental learning and reinforcement. The tasks of each phase are listed in Table 10.4. Phase 1

Table 10.4

VIOLENCE REDUCTION PROGRAM

PHASE 1—OPENING THE DOOR TO CHANGE

- Admission, orientation
- Evaluation, risk assessment
- Identify treatment targets
- Increase insight into violence
- Increase motivation and engagement
- Develop therapeutic alliance and commitment

PHASE 2—SKILL ACQUISITION

- Examine and challenge destructive behavior patterns
- Cognitive restructuring, emotion and behavior management
- Learn and implement violence-reduction skills

PHASE 3—RELAPSE PREVENTION

- Relapse prevention planning
- Release planning
- Consolidating and reinforcing skills

Note. Adapted from "Assessment and Treatment of Violence-Prone Forensic Clients: An Integrated Approach," by S. Wong, A. Gordon, & D. Gu, 2007, *British Journal of Psychiatry, 190*(Suppl. 49), pp. s66–s74.

focuses on understanding the origins of violent behavior, developing insight, and therapeutic alliance building. Motivational interviewing techniques are a staple throughout the VRP. Phase 2 is the skill acquisition phase, in which offenders learn cognitive techniques for managing emotions and behaviors. Phase 3 focuses on relapse prevention and further reinforcement of acquired skills. Progression through the VRP does not depend on time, but on successful achievement of each phase's objectives. The program uses a group format but may be adapted for offenders who require individual programming. On average, the VRP program can take place over 12 to 18 months; however, highly resistant offenders may require treatment intermissions. Although the VRP may be adapted to a variety of institutional settings, effective implementation does require special staff training.

At present, most experts have acknowledged that the problem of poor motivation for change often remains a therapeutic dead end (Vien & Beech, 2006). Some offenders may not perceive themselves as needing to change, and Wong, Gordon, and Gu (2007) would refer to these individuals as being in the precontemplation stage. For these individuals, it is recommended that the therapist continue attempts to forge a treatment alliance, raise the issue of future goals, and employ a cost–benefit analysis of the offender's problem behaviors. In addition to the principles outlined by these newer programs, the individual clinician may also be guided by certain fundamental principles for treating difficult patients (Adler, 2006). These principles, listed in Table 10.5, could apply equally to the MO offender who is difficult to treat and/or manage. Several of these principles will be discussed in greater detail in the next section on countertransference issues.

Table 10.5

GUIDING PRINCIPLES FOR TREATING DIFFICULT PATIENTS

- Do no harm
- Treat recognizable psychiatric symptoms
- Protect self and patient
- Have realistic expectations
- Obtain support and consultation
- Know thyself; understand how you are perceived
- Maintain unswerving consistency, observance of policies and rules

COMMON COUNTERTRANSFERENCE ISSUES

> His words had a strange effect upon me. I compassionated him, and sometimes felt a wish to console him; but when I looked upon him . . . my heart sickened. And my feelings were altered to those of horror and hatred.
>
> You swear, I said, to be harmless; but have you not already shown a degree of malice that should reasonably make me distrust you? May not even this be a feint that will increase your triumph by affording a wider scope for your revenge?
>
> —Shelley, 1831

Clinicians working with MO offenders inevitably come to the realization that treatment simply cannot be a "dispassionate technical endeavour" (Freidrich & Leiper, 2006). Whether the therapeutic relationship involves psychotherapy or is limited to pharmacotherapy, the clinician must be able to experience, tolerate, and "hold the patient's feelings without retaliation" (Slowchower, 1991, p. 716). For many MO offenders, interpersonal conflict and destructive aggression may be primary symptoms that the clinician will encounter. Thus, there is the danger that the clinician may reflexively seek to avoid the resulting internal discomfort by responding in an attacking or rejecting manner. In addition, MO offenders with strong psychopathic traits may engender particularly corrosive countertransference emotions in the clinician such that they feel controlled or deceived by the offender.

Meloy (1988) has enumerated a number of interpersonal and intrapsychic features that he believes contraindicate any form of treatment. These features include a history of sadistic aggressive behavior, a complete absence of remorse for behaviors, absence of capacity for emotional attachment, and an experienced clinician's fear of predation in the patient's presence. These features appear to be derived from Meloy's clinical experience and certainly comprise sagacious and astute warning signs. However, the fact remains that these signs can and will be found among many MO offenders requiring treatment in a correctional or forensic setting. Forensic clinicians will find very little guidance in the literature about the particular countertransference reactions seen in the treatment of MO offenders. Table 10.6 lists some of the countertransference reactions that have been described by clinicians treating psychopaths and MO offenders. The term *countertransference* is used here in its broadest sense to mean the emotional reaction of the clinician to the patient (Ursano, Sonneberg, & Lazar, 1991).

Table 10.6

COUNTERTRANSFERENCE REACTIONS TO MORALLY OBJECTIONABLE OFFENDERS

- Therapeutic nihilism
- Malignant pseudo-identification
- Assumption of similarity
- Fear
- Disgust
- Absence of emotions
- Counter-phobic denial
- Self-devaluation
- Hatred, desire to punish/destroy

Note. Adapted from *The Psychopathic Mind*, by J. Meloy, 1988. New York: J. Aronson; "Countertransference Reactions in Therapeutic Work With Incestuous Sexual Abusers," by M. Friedrich and R. Leiper, 2006, *Journal of Child Sexual Abuse, 15*(1), pp. 51–68.

Friedrich and Leiper (2006) found that countertransference themes reported by clinicians who treat sex offenders can be grouped into three main domains: (1) negative and problematic reactions; (2) the clinician's experience of having something done to them; and (3) struggles to create a therapeutic relationship. Most of the reactions discussed here fall into the first and second domains.

Being intelligent, diligent workers, many clinicians will find themselves using isolation of affect to deal with unpleasant or difficult emotional reactions to their MO patients. Thus, an absence or lack of feelings about an MO offender will be a hallmark of this reaction. Consistent with this reaction, clinicians working with psychopathic offenders have described a process of engaging in detached, ritualistic task performance to avoid unpleasant countertransference feelings (Grounds et al., 1987). The problematic results of this reaction involve creating excessive distance from the patient, which may ultimately affect overall treatment progress.

Therapeutic nihilism is a common countertransference reaction experienced with MO or psychopathic offenders (Meloy, 1988). It involves the global assumption that all such individuals are similar in their lack of response to any treatment. The fallacy here is that, due

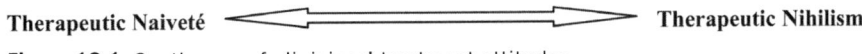

Figure 10.1 Continuum of clinicians' treatment attitudes.

to the heterogeneous nature of the clinical construct, it is untenable to conclude that all such individuals are immune to treatment efforts. As Meloy (1988) notes, therapeutic nihilism is often the result of oral tradition, passed down in the absence of objective data or experience. It is critical to have realistic expectations when working with MO offenders and not overestimate their treatment goals. The clinician must carefully navigate between the Scylla and Charybdis of therapeutic nihilism and therapeutic naiveté (see Figure 10.1). Balancing and finding the appropriate stance on this continuum is a difficult but fundamental task of the clinician working with MO offenders. It necessarily requires efforts to prohibit moral judgment from impinging upon an objective, professional approach to the patient.

Meloy (1988) has defined a reaction called malignant pseudoidentification, in which the psychopath consciously imitates, or unconsciously simulates, subtle narcissistic characteristics of the clinician. This process fosters the clinician's identification with the offender, which ultimately results in the clinician becoming vulnerable to manipulation. The process may involve the offender simulating mannerisms or beliefs of the clinician or otherwise creating the (false) impression of identification and alliance. The following vignette gives an example of malignant pseudoidentification.

Case Vignette: Mr. M

Mr. M was a 38-year-old man who was serving life without parole for several sexual murders that involved torturing of the victims. He was residing on a residential treatment unit of the prison due to his chronic threats of suicide and serious past suicide attempts. He was diagnosed with depression as well as posttraumatic stress disorder (PTSD), which he alleged to have developed as a result of his crimes. An experienced forensic psychologist scored his PCL-R at 37 (a cutoff score of 30 is used for psychopathy).

Dr. F was Mr. M's attending psychiatrist and was well known by staff and patients to be an academician interested in studying and understanding the psychology of psychopathy. In addition, he was a vigorous advocate for correctional mental health treatment. One day on teaching rounds, Mr. M observed that one of Dr. F's students was carrying a copy of Simon's book *Bad Men Do What Good Men Dream* along with her other notebooks. Mr. M subsequently ordered himself a copy of the text through the mail. Several weeks later, during a routine evaluation, Mr. M asked Dr. F, "Do you think I am a monster?" Fascinated, Dr. F began to listen as Mr. M told him that he had been reflecting on his crimes and wanted to understand what drove him to do such things.

Mr. M further garnered the interest of Dr. F with statements such as, "I think that everyone has a 'dark side' . . . the difference is that for some reason, I let mine come out." Mr. M told Dr. F that he would like to learn more about himself so that he might change for the better. However, Mr. M continued, "There are still things I have done that no one knows about. Really bad things. I need to talk about them with someone I can trust."

Dr. F began meeting with Mr. M on a more frequent basis. Eventually, Mr. M told Dr. F that it might help for him to make a journal of his thoughts about his crimes for Dr. F to study. Dr. F agreed to provide Mr. M with pencils and journaling books that were not on the prison canteen list. Mr. M later told Dr. F, "I think I am starting to see how messed up I was. You have been the only staff that listened and didn't judge me." Other prison staff began to notice how Dr. F paid special attention to Mr. M and began to subtly chide him about it. Mr. M seized this opportunity in a session with Dr. F, stating, "I can't believe they have the nerve to disrespect you. You have more knowledge than anyone here! You deserve a lot better staff than them."

In this example, Mr. M simulated the narcissistic characteristics of Dr. F and successfully developed a pseudoidentification with him. Mr. M made shrewd observations about what Dr. F valued and what held his interest. Mr. M carefully exploited the pseudoidentification such that Dr. F began to treat him as a special case. This ultimately made Dr. F vulnerable to Mr. M's strategy of creating a schism between Dr. F and other staff. This is a potentially dangerous position for Dr. F, because Mr. M could use this as the beginning stage of further manipulation. For Dr. F, it will be important that he develop a better understanding of how he is perceived by others, particularly patients and staff, so that he will be able to recognize when an offender is attempting to simulate aspects of his narcissism.

Somewhat related to pseudoidentification is the clinician's assumption that he and the offender share similar psychological processes and functioning. Meloy (1988) has termed this reaction the *assumption of psychological complexity*. However, the projective assumption on the part of the clinician may or may not be that the offender is psychologically complex. Rather, it may simply be that the offender generally "thinks like

I do," or shares the same general emotional responses that are familiar to the clinician. Thus, the term *assumption of similarity* is used here. The dangers involved in making an assumption of similarity include vulnerability to pseudoidentification, misjudgments of the offender's intentions or treatment responses, and misperception of risk.

Meloy and Meloy (2002) have hypothesized that clinicians' fearful responses to a psychopath are essentially a natural biological reaction of prey to a predator. In this sense, it is arguable whether or not fear, in its strictest sense, is truly a countertransference reaction as opposed to a normal physiological response. In either event, the clinician must not discount this signal. Thorough risk assessment, as described in chapters 1, 2, 3, and 8, will enable the clinician to make more objective estimates of the precautions necessary for patient interactions. It is helpful to view this process as ultimately protective of both oneself and the patient and should be a routine exercise for clinicians working with MO offenders. In contrast, some clinicians may respond in the opposite manner, with a counterphobic denial of potential danger. This may result from fantasies on the part of the clinician that he or she is physically invincible or otherwise too experienced to let something dangerous occur. The following vignette gives an example of counterphobic denial.

Case Vignette: Dr. T

> Dr. T was a psychiatrist who had served in the military and had worked in a correctional setting for many years. He prided himself on not only his clinical skills, but also his excellent physical condition. During his leisure time, Dr. T ran in marathons. During his military service, he had been a proficient amateur boxer. Dr. T never asked for correctional officers to be present when he met with patients, even when working in the secured housing units.
>
> One day, Dr. T was asked to evaluate an offender, Mr. U, who was serving a life sentence for killing another inmate in a racially motivated gang fight. Mr. U's reputation was well known throughout the prison. He was infamous for his aggressive behavior and for never backing down from a fight. Correctional officers told stories about how Mr. U took on five officers at once and was only subdued with the help of special defensive shields that could deliver electric stun shocks.
>
> Dr. T knew of Mr. U's reputation, yet told officers that he wished to meet alone with Mr. U in the evaluation room. When Dr. T began to address some of Mr. U's problem behaviors on the unit, Mr. U appeared only mildly annoyed. As Dr. T turned to reach for a blank progress note, Mr. U grabbed a pen off of the desk and stabbed Dr. T in the face.

Dr. T likely held the belief that he was too experienced and/or physically capable to be assaulted. In addition, the notion that he might require an officer's presence was likely to be experienced by Dr. T as a narcissistic insult. Mr. U's reputation of being particularly dangerous may have also added to Dr. T's unconscious sense of feeling challenged to not back down in any way from Mr. U. The clinician's work with the MO offender in no way involves tests or challenges to the clinician's physical capabilities. Thus, deliberations about how to interact with the MO offender should simply amount to an assessment of risk and prudent use of security staff. In such circumstances, it is critical for the clinician to make use of consultation with colleagues or supervision. These efforts to establish objectivity become especially important when the clinician must conduct a violence risk assessment of an MO offender. For example, de Vogel and de Ruiter (2004) found that clinicians who had subjective unpleasant feelings about their forensic patients gave them higher HCR-20 scores than clinicians who reported positive, relaxed feelings about their patients.

Some MO offenders will, in reality, always carry a rather poor prognosis. Such cases have the potential to induce subtle feelings of worthlessness and self-denigration in the clinician. Clinicians who derive their sense of professional satisfaction primarily through achieving treatment successes are particularly vulnerable to this reaction. Other similar self-devaluation reactions in the clinician include excessive questioning of one's abilities, feelings that one's work is insignificant, or reverting to an attitude of therapeutic nihilism. The following vignette gives an example of self-devaluation in the clinician.

Case Vignette: Mr. P

Mr. P was a 32-year-old man who had served multiple prison sentences since the age of 18 for a variety of crimes, including sexual assault, robbery, sale of narcotics, and involuntary manslaughter. Each time he was released from prison, he would quickly return due to another conviction. His psychiatrist, Dr. Q, treated him in prison for major depression. Mr. P responded extremely well to Dr. Q's pharmacotherapy and cognitive-behavioral therapy. When Mr. P was approaching the end of his current sentence, Dr. Q testified on Mr. P's behalf in front of the parole board. In addition, Dr. Q pled Mr. P's case to the local community mental health center, which was extremely reticent to accept Mr. P onto its case load due to his history of highly antisocial behaviors.

Dr. Q's efforts were ultimately successful, and Mr. P was granted parole. Approximately 2 weeks later, Mr. P was returned to the prison, having violated his parole by assaulting a man and stealing his car. When Dr. Q received the news, he felt a complex mixture of disappointment, humiliation, and anger. Over the next several months, Dr. Q began to wonder about the worth of his treatment efforts with other patients and developed a feeling that his work was trivial and insignificant.

Dr. Q put in tremendous effort in the case of Mr. P, and his reaction to Mr. P's relapse is not surprising. However, Dr. Q may have avoided feeling devalued had he considered Mr. P's long history of recidivism, which may be conceptualized as his fear of leaving prison. It may be that Dr. Q's goals for Mr. P were too lofty or otherwise unrealistic. Dr. Q made great strides with Mr. P in prison, which should be considered an accomplishment. It may be that, like Groves's (1978) self-destructive denier, Mr. P is "at base profoundly dependent" and has given up hope of ever living outside the prison.

Many MO offenders have grandiose fantasies, which conflict painfully with feelings of worthlessness. Offenders' fragile self-images involving high self-esteem are easily chaffed by perceived slights. MO offenders' arrogance, even after having been sentenced for a heinous crime, may arouse punitive feelings in the clinician. Feelings of hatred may be acted upon by the clinician in the form of inappropriate criticisms, hostile remarks, or premature withdrawal of care. The following vignette gives an example of countertransference hatred in the clinician.

Case Vignette: Mr. G

Mr. G was a 28-year-old man serving a life sentence for a particularly heinous sex offense that involved the abduction and rape of an 8-year-old girl. Mr. G had videotaped the rape, during which the victim had sustained severe internal injuries. Mr. G was a highly demanding and entitled person, in addition to having a remarkably annoying, attention-seeking quality to his personality. He had been banned from nearly every housing unit in the prison due to other inmates' persistent and severe harassment of him. After several inmates had used his bunk as a toilet and had threatened to kill him, Mr. G began stating that he would kill himself. He was found by correctional officers sitting on his bed with a sheet tied loosely around his neck. As a result, Mr. G was admitted to the prison psychiatric inpatient unit.

Dr. P was Mr. G's inpatient attending psychiatrist. Dr. P had worked for many years in a correctional setting where she had to carry a heavy case load. Dr. P found Mr. G's crimes particularly abhorrent and disgusting, as Dr. P had three children of her own and had originally trained as a child psychiatrist. When Dr. P admitted Mr. G to the inpatient unit, Mr. G had a litany of demands and requests. He appeared to take satisfaction from threatening staff with legal action and had memorized relevant prison policies. The inpatient staff were aghast at how Mr. G showed no appreciation for their efforts, nor for the fact that they were providing him a form of protection from inmate harassment.

Mr. G's crime and his repellent personality traits quickly became the focus of staff conversation. Eventually, inpatient staff began to make offhand comments that Mr. G "got what he deserved" from the other inmates and that "the world would be a better place" if Mr. G had committed suicide. Over several weeks, Mr. G's presence had severely disrupted the inpatient unit. Inpatient staff began to suggest to Dr. P that Mr. G was merely hiding out and needed to be promptly discharged. After a treatment team meeting in which Mr. G insulted Dr. P's clinical skills and knowledge, Dr. P made the decision to discharge Mr. G back into general population. Mr. G was then told by security staff that he would be discharged the next day. Later that evening, Mr. G committed suicide by hanging himself in his cell.

Dr. P would likely have benefited from a case consultation with a colleague or supervisor to gain better perspective on Mr. G. This may be particularly critical when the MO offender's crime "touches on a specific area of sensitivity for the therapist" (Hyatt-Williams, 1998, p. 258). Countertransference hatred is less likely to be acted upon when the clinician is conscious of it and can reevaluate clinical decisions more objectively. Dr. P's dilemma was worsened by the fact that the entire staff also had unconscious (as well as conscious) wishes to destroy Mr. G. Therefore, consultation with a colleague outside her unit would have been preferable. Ultimately, when a clinician finds, after appropriate consultation, that a particular MO offender engenders intractable, destructive countertransference, it may be necessary to transfer the patient to another colleague.

CONFRONTING COMPASSION FATIGUE

As I proceeded in my labor, it became everyday more horrible and irksome to me. Sometimes I could not prevail on myself to enter my laboratory for several days. . . . It was, indeed, a filthy process in which I was engaged.

I had before regarded my promise with a gloomy despair, as a thing that, with whatever consequences, must be fulfilled; but I now felt as if a film had been taken from before my eyes, and that I, for the first time, saw clearly.

—Shelley, 1831

Nietzsche's enduring line about staring into the abyss has likely been considered by many clinicians working with MO offenders. Continual work around offenders who have treated their fellow humans quite inhumanely has the potential to affect and even change the clinician in certain ways. In addition, there are the effects of the treatment environment to consider, particularly if it happens to be harsh, poorly resourced, or the staff suffer from low morale. Insufficient attention has been given to this subject, particularly as it relates to clinicians working in difficult forensic settings. Those who have given thoughtful consideration to the issue of working with challenging patients with personality disorders have stressed the importance of regular staff supervision and training to help counter therapeutic pessimism and encourage evidence-based practice (Kurtz, 2005).

Literature on the adverse emotional effects experienced by therapists was initiated in the field of trauma therapy. Therapists noted that engaging in therapeutic work with trauma survivors could have a negative impact on the therapist (Stamm, 1997). Subsequent literature has referred to this phenomenon by various names, including compassion fatigue, secondary traumatic stress, and vicarious traumatization. Compassion fatigue will be used in this chapter to describe the negative emotional and cognitive impact of the therapeutic engagement on therapists (Figley, 1995).

After the concept of vicarious traumatization was introduced by trauma therapists, it was next considered by therapists working with sex offenders. In a study of symptoms in a sample of 67 therapists working with sex offenders, Steed and Bicknell (2001) found that a variety of traumatic symptoms were reported by therapists. Further, a U-shaped relationship was found between years of experience and the PTSD-like symptom of avoidance, such that therapists with the least and most experience were most avoidant. The authors concluded that therapists, particularly new ones, would benefit from education and support on the phenomenon. Subsequent studies have confirmed that sex offender therapists do experience vicarious traumatization and that the severity may depend on professional experience, treatment setting, and coping strategies employed by the therapists (Moulden & Firestone, 2007; Way, VanDeusen, Martin, Applegate, & Jandle, 2004).

Following the lead of sex offender therapists, correctional mental health has begun to investigate the phenomenon of vicarious traumatization. DePass (2005) gathered qualitative data from 40 correctional mental health workers, both from a jail and a prison. The vicarious traumatization themes reported by participants were found to be related to the constructs of compassion fatigue, bystander guilt, and role ambiguity. Clinicians reported that, while they enjoyed the clinical experience and excitement of working in a correctional environment, they disliked the harsh environment and the negative attitudes and behaviors of coworkers. Again, the notion of better supervision, training, and debriefing were stressed as potential solutions.

Compounding the problem of the individual clinician's risk of compassion fatigue is the milieu and morale of the facility. Treatment facilities are commonly understaffed and short of necessary resources. These realities may ultimately affect overall staff morale and treatment attitudes. Depending on leadership style and other factors, a pervasive and malignant staff attitude may develop. This is a complex and sensitive issue that must nevertheless receive attention. It would seem to be common sense that toxic staff–inmate interactions will have a negative impact on the inmate's mental health. Nurse, Woodcock, and Ormsby (2003) performed a qualitative focus group study on correctional staff and inmates in an English prison. The authors described a "circle of stress" operative in the prison culture that had noxious effects on the prisoners' emotional states. The circle of stress was described as follows. Staff shortages create higher levels of staff stress and sickness. This, in turn, produces greater levels of tension and negative staff–inmate relationships. Participants believed that this ultimately had a negative impact on prisoners' mental health as well as their overall chances of successful rehabilitation.

Malignant staff attitudes may range from merely unempathetic to frankly hostile and punitive. Inmates with past histories of abuse, paranoia, or severe personality disorders are particularly susceptible to the effects of malignant staff attitudes. Their tendency to respond to adversity in a maladaptive way ensures that the vicious cycle of staff–inmate animosity is kept in motion. Therefore, this problem must be addressed on multiple levels. Administrative and clinical leaders should make it a priority to respond constructively to malignant staff attitudes.

Regular staff meetings, debriefings, and other activities help communicate to staff that they are both valued and expected to conduct themselves in a therapeutic manner. In a survey of 36 correctional psychiatrists, Knoll, Leonard, and Way (2007) found that, when psychiatrists felt their work was appreciated, they were less likely to feel pessimistic about humanity. Psychiatrists who felt appreciated were also less likely to regard their work as difficult or burdensome, despite the size of their case loads. This would suggest that administrative efforts at staff recognition would be worthwhile. The recommendation for special efforts to implement supportive management, education, and supervision has also been suggested for all staff working in the new dangerous and severe personality disorder units in the United Kingdom (Bowers et al., 2006).

Pross (2006) has noted that factors such as working in a position considered by the general mental health field to be an outsider position and having a relatively low level of social recognition for one's work may predispose the clinician to compassion fatigue. Certainly, the alienist position of the forensic clinician fits such a description. Clinical experience suggests that working therapeutically with personality disordered offenders is a demanding task that requires much of the clinician. The clinician must be able to maintain a healthy attitude toward the work and ensure a consistent and competent clinical presence. Therefore, it is imperative that the clinician make conscious efforts to recognize and avoid burnout or compassion fatigue. Table 10.7 lists some common warning signs of compassion fatigue in clinicians. In a survey of 133 forensic mental health professionals, Cacciacarne, Resnick, McArthur, and Althof (1986) found that feelings of apathy, frustration, and cynicism were highly correlated with a measure of professional burnout (see Table 10.7).

Table 10.7

COMPASSION FATIGUE WARNING SIGNS

- Apathy, rapid exhaustion
- Melancholy or irritability
- Inappropriate cynicism
- Experiencing work as a heavy burden
- Impersonal or uncaring attitude toward clients
- Feeling of failure or insignificance
- Social withdrawal or disconnection from loved ones
- Generalized despair and hopelessness
- Feeling disillusioned by humanity

Note. Adapted from "Burnout, Vicarious Traumatization and Its Prevention," by C. Pross, 2006, *Torture, 16*(1), pp. 1–9.

Table 10.8

PREVENTING COMPASSION FATIGUE

- Self-care—time for family, friends, hobbies
- Refresher training in psychotherapy principles
- Therapeutic self-awareness
- Regular self-examination (consultation with colleagues or external supervision)
- Limiting case load
- Continuing professional education
- Opportunities for research and training sabbaticals
- Careful balance between empathy and proper professional distance

Note. Adapted from "Burnout, Vicarious Traumatization and Its Prevention," by C. Pross, 2006, *Torture, 16*(1), pp. 1–9.

Because forensic clinicians cannot be inexhaustible suppliers of empathic care to MO offenders, it is advisable that they take a preventive stance regarding compassion fatigue. Table 10.8 lists suggested strategies for preventing compassion fatigue in forensic clinicians. A supportive administration will be of most help in arranging for adequate supervision, continuing education, and fostering a healthy, treatment-oriented milieu. The task of self-care is equally critical and is the responsibility of the individual clinician.

CONCLUSION

> It was a mystery; yet with how many things are we upon the brink of becoming acquainted, if cowardice or carelessness did not restrain our enquiries.
> There is something terribly appalling in our situation, yet my courage and hopes do not desert me. . . . If we are lost, my mad schemes are the cause.
>
> —Shelley, 1831

It is likely that forensic clinicians will encounter a small, but significant, population of patients who they will find not only difficult to treat, but objectionable. These patients may have been convicted of particularly deviant crimes. MO offenders are those who are highly antisocial or psychopathic and may arouse strong feelings of moral disgust in the clinician.

General clinicians are taught to avoid such patients in treatment; however, forensic clinicians are likely to find themselves tasked with the treatment of such individuals.

The purpose of this chapter has been to encourage objective thought regarding the origins, capacities, and treatability of these offenders. In particular, it should be acknowledged that the construct of psychopathy is not yet as distinct a disorder as would support globally drawn conclusions. In pursuit of objectivity and more efficient treatment efforts, clinicians should become familiar with the existing research on the development, neuropsychiatric impairment, and current treatment approaches for psychopathic individuals. Clinicians who are engaged in psychotherapy programs with these offenders will benefit from a sound knowledge of common countertransference reactions to MO offenders.

Many MO offenders have been previously rejected by society and are rather perceptive to the negative moral judgments of others. Clinicians should bear this fact in mind, as it is common for the clinician to struggle with conflicting views of the patient as either monster or human in need of treatment. Because the etiology and underpinnings of psychopathy are not well understood at present, clinicians venture into unknown scientific lands. It is important that they monitor their ambitions, countertransference, and risk of compassion fatigue. This is necessary for effective patient care as well as for maintaining the clinician's own humanity. Finally, clinicians will benefit from regular supervision and attention to impending signs of compassion fatigue when working with this very challenging population.

REFERENCES

Adler, D. (2006). Difficult patients: Within themselves and with caregivers. *Psychiatric Services, 57,* 767.

American Psychiatric Association. (2000). *Psychiatric services in jails and prisons* (2nd ed). Washington, DC: APA Press.

American Psychiatric Association. (2001). *The principles of medical ethics with annotation especially applicable to psychiatry.* Washington, DC: Author.

Barbaree, H. (2005). Psychopathy, treatment behavior, and recidivism: An extended follow-up of Seto and Barbaree. *Journal of Interpersonal Violence, 20*(9), 1115–1131.

Baumeister, R. (1990). Suicide as escape from self. *Psychological Review, 97*(1), 90–113.

Baumeister, R. (1997). *Evil: Inside human violence and cruelty.* New York: Henry Holt.

Baumeister, R., DeWall, C., Ciarocco, N., Twenge, J. (2005). Social exclusion impairs self-regulation. *Journal of Personality and Social Psychology, 88*(4), 589–604.

Birbaumer, N., Veit, R., Lotze, M., Erb, M., Hermann, C., Grodd, W., et al. (2005). Deficient fear conditioning in psychopathy: A functional magnetic resonance imaging study. *Archives of General Psychiatry, 2*(7), 799–805.

Black, W., & Gregson, R. (1973). Time perspective, purpose in life, extraversion and neuroticism in New Zealand prisoners. *British Journal of Social and Clinical Psychology, 12,* 50–60.

Blair, R. (2003). Neurobiological basis of psychopathy. *British Journal of Psychiatry, 182,* 5–7.

Blair, R., Morris, J., Frith, C., Perrett, D., & Dolan, R. (1999). Dissociable neural responses to facial expressions of sadness and anger. *Brain, 122,* 883–893.

Bowers, L., Carr-Walker, P., Allan, T., Callaghan, P., Nijman, H., & Paton, J. (2006). Attitude to personality disorder among prison officers working in a dangerous and severe personality disorder unit. *International Journal of Law and Psychiatry, 29,* 333–342.

Cacciacarne, M., Resnick, P., McArthur, C., & Althof, S. (1986). Burnout in forensic psychiatric staff. *Med Law, 5*(4), 303–308.

Cleckley, H. (1976). *The mask of sanity* (5th ed.). St. Louis, MO: Mosby.

Craissati, J., & Beech, A. (2006). The role of key developmental variables in identifying sex offenders likely to fail in the community: An enhanced risk prediction model. *Child Abuse & Neglect, 30,* 327–339.

Crumbaugh, J., & Maholick, L. (1969) *Manual for instructions for the Purpose-in-Life Test*. Saratoga, CA: Psychometric Affiliates.

Currie, E. (2000). Sociological perspectives on juvenile violence. *Child and Adolescent Psychiatric Clinics of North America, 9*(4), 749–754.

Darley, J. (1992). Social organization for the production of evil. *Psychological Inquiry, 3,* 199–218.

Dear, G., Slattery, J., & Hillan, R. (2001). Evaluations of the quality of coping reported by prisoners who have self-harmed and those who have not. *Suicide and Life Threatening Behavior, 31*(4), 442–450.

DePass, C. (2005). *Vicarious trauma in correctional mental health staff*. Unpublished doctoral thesis, Carlos Albizu University, Miami, FL.

de Vogel, V., & de Ruiter, C. (2004). Differences between clinicians and researchers in assessing risk of violence in forensic psychiatric patients. *Journal of Forensic Psychiatry and Psychology, 15*(1), 145–164.

Dewan, M., & Pies, R. (Eds.). (2001). *The difficult to treat psychiatric patient*. Washington, DC: American Psychiatric Publishing.

D'Silva, K. (2004). Does treatment really make psychopaths worse? A review of the evidence. *Journal of Personality Disorders, 18*(2), 163–177.

Edwards, M., & Holden, R. (2001). Coping, meaning in life, and suicidal manifestations: Examining gender differences. *Journal of Clinical Psychology, 57*(12), 1517–1534.

Farrington, D., & Loeber, R. (2000). Epidemiology of juvenile violence. *Child and Adolescent Psychiatric Clinics of North America, 9*(4), 733–748.

Figley, C. R. (Ed.). (1995). *Compassion fatigue: Coping with secondary traumatic stress disorder in those who treat the traumatised*. New York: Brunner/Mazel.

Frankl, V. (1959). *Man's search for meaning*. Boston: Beacon Press.

Friedrich, M., & Leiper, R. (2006). Countertransference reactions in therapeutic work with incestuous sexual abusers. *Journal of Child Sexual Abuse, 15*(1), 51–68.

Gill, C. (1994). Forward. In J. Westman, *Licensing parents*. New York: Insight Books.
Goodwin, R., & Hamilton, S. (2003). Lifetime comorbidity of antisocial personality disorder and anxiety disorders among adults in the community. *Psychiatry Research, 117*(2), 159–166.
Gray, N., Hill, C., McGleish, A., Timmons, D., MacCulloch, M., & Snowden, R. (2003). Prediction of violence and self-harm in mentally disordered offenders: A prospective study of the efficacy of HCR-20, PCL-R, and psychiatric symptomatology. *Journal of Consulting Clinical Psychology, 71*(3), 443–451.
Grounds, A., Quayle, M., France, J., Brett, T., Cox, M., & Hamilton, J. (1987). A unit for "psychopathic disorder" patients in Broadmoor Hospital. *Medicine, Science and the Law, 27*, 21–31.
Groves, J. (1978). Taking care of the hateful patient. *New England Journal of Medicine, 298*, 883–887.
Hall, J., Benning, S., & Patrick, C. (2004). Criterion-related validity of the three-factor model of psychopathic personality: Behavior and adaptive functioning. *Assessment, 11*, 4–16.
Hare, R. (1998). Psychopaths and their nature: Implications for the mental health and criminal justice systems. In T. Millon, E. Simonson, D. Burket-Smith, & R. Davis (Eds.), *Psychopathy: Antisocial, criminal and violent Behavior* (pp. 188–212). New York: Guilford Press.
Hare, R. (1999). Psychopaths: New trends in research. *Harvard Mental Health Letter, 12*, 4–5.
Hare, R. (2003). *The Hare Psychopathy Checklist–Revised* (2nd ed.). Toronto, Canada: Multi-Health Systems.
Hare, R. (2006). Psychopathy: A clinical and forensic overview. *Psychiatric Clinics of North America, 29*(3),709–724.
Harlow, C. (2003). *Education and correctional populations* (Bureau of Justice Statistics Special Report). Washington, DC: U.S. Department of Justice.
Hodgins, S. (2007). Persistent violent offending: What do we know? *British Journal of Psychiatry, 190*(Suppl. 49), s12–s14.
Hyatt-Williams, A. (1998). *Cruelty, violence and murder: Understanding the criminal mind*. New York: Jason Aronson.
Ivanoff, A., & Jang, S. (1991). The role of hopelessness and social desirability in predicting suicidal behavior: A study of prison inmates. *Journal of Consulting Clinical Psychology, 59*(3), 394–399.
James, D. (2004). *Profile of jail inmates, 2002* (Bureau of Justice Statistics Special Report). Washington, DC: U.S. Department of Justice.
Johnson, J., Cohen, P., Brown, J., Smailes, E., & Bernstein, D. (1999). Childhood maltreatment increases risk for personality disorders during early adulthood. *Archives of General Psychiatry, 56*(7), 600–606.
Kaylor, L. (1999). Antisocial personality disorder: Diagnostic, ethical and treatment issues. *Issues in Mental Health Nursing, 20*, 247–258.
Kiehl, K., Smith, A., Hare, R., Mendrek, A., Forster, B., Brink, J., et al. (2001). Limbic abnormalities in affective processing by criminal psychopaths as revealed by functional magnetic resonance imaging. *Biological Psychiatry, 50*, 677–684.
Kiehl, K., et al. (2004). Temporal lobe abnormalities in semantic processing by criminal psychopaths as revealed by functional magnetic resonance imaging. *Psychiatry Research-Neuroimaging, 130*, 297–312.

Knoll, J., Leonard, C., & Way, B. (2007). [Survey of work environment attitudes among correctional psychiatrists attending the 37th annual meeting of the American Academy of Psychiatry and the Law]. Unpublished data.
Kristiansson, M. (1995). Incurable psychopaths? *Bulletin of the American Academy of Psychiatry and the Law, 23*(4), 555–562.
Kurtz, A. (2005). The needs of staff who care for people with a diagnosis of personality disorder who are considered a risk to others. *Journal of Forensic Psychiatry and Psychology, 16*(2), 399–422.
Lally, M., & Freeman, S. (2005). The struggle to maintain neutrality in the treatment of a patient with pedophilia. *Ethics & Behavior, 15*(2), 182–190.
Laurell, J., & Daderman, A. (2007). Psychopathy (PCL-R) in a forensic psychiatric sample of homicide offenders: Some reliability issues. *International Journal of Law & Psychiatry, 30*(2), 127–135.
Lee, J. (1999). *The treatment of psychopathic and antisocial personality disorders: A review.* Retrieved January 25, 2009, from http://www.ramas.co.uk/report3.pdf
Levinsky, N., Friedman, E., & Levine, D. (1999). What is our duty to a "hateful" patient? Differing approaches to a disruptive dialysis patient. *American Journal of Kidney Diseases, 34*(4), 775–789.
Looman, J., Abracen, J., Serin, R., & Marquis, P. (2005). Psychopathy, treatment change, and recidivism in high-risk, high-need sexual offenders. *Journal of Interpersonal Violence, 20*(5), 549–568.
Lykken, D. (1995). *Antisocial personalities.* Hillsdale, NJ: Erlbaum.
Lykken, D. (1998). The case for parental licensure. In T. Millon, E. Simonson, M. Burket-Smith, & R. Davis (Eds.), *Psychopathy: Antisocial, criminal, and violent behavior* (pp. 122–143). New York: Guilford Press.
Marcus, D., John, S., & Edens, J. (2004). A taxometric analysis of psychopathic personality. *Journal of Abnormal Psychology, 113*(4), 626–635.
Marshall, L., & Cooke, D. (1999). The childhood experiences of psychopaths: A retrospective study of familial and societal factors. *Journal of Personality Disorders, 13*(3), 211–225.
Marshall, W., & Barbaree, H. (1990). An integrated theory of the etiology of sexual offending. In W. Marshall, D. Laws, & H. Barbaree (Eds.), *Handbook of sexual assault: Issues, theories, and treatment of the offender* (pp. 257–275). New York: Plenum.
Martens, W. (2001). Effects of antisocial and social attitudes on neurobiological functions. *Medical Hypotheses, 56*(6), 664–671.
Mason, T., Richman, J., & Mercer, D. (2002). The influence of evil on forensic clinical practice. *International Journal of Mental Health Nursing, 11,* 80–93.
Masters, B. (1997). *The evil that men do: From saints to serial killers.* London: Black Swan.
McCollum, D. (2006). Child maltreatment and brain development. *Minnesota Medicine, 89*(3), 48–50.
Meloy, J. (1988). *The psychopathic mind: Origins, dynamics, and treatment.* New York: J. Aronson.
Meloy, J., & Meloy, M. (2002). Autonomic arousal in the presence of psychopathy: A survey of mental health and criminal justice professionals. *Journal of Threat Assessment, 2*(2), 21–33.
Mercer, D., Mason, T., & Richman, J. (1999). Good & evil in the crusade of care: Social constructions of mental disorders. *Journal of Psychosocial Nursing, 37*(9), 13–17.

Messina, N., Wish, E., Hoffman, J., & Nemes, S. (2002). Antisocial personality disorder and TC treatment outcomes. *American Journal of Drug and Alcohol Abuse, 28*(2), 197–212.

Miller, A. (1999). Harming other people: Perspectives on evil and violence. *Personality and Social Psychology Review, 3,* 176–178.

Miller, A., Gordon, A., & Buddie, M. (1999). Accounting for evil and cruelty: Is to explain to condone? *Personality and Social Psychology Review, 3,* 254–268.

Moulden, H., & Firestone, P. (2007). Vicarious traumatization: The impact on therapists who work with sex offenders. *Trauma, Violence, & Abuse, 8*(1), 67–83.

Mullen, P. (2004). The autogenic (self-generated) massacre. *Behavioral Sciences & the Law, 22,* 311–323.

Murphy, C., & Vess, J. (2003). Subtypes of psychopathy: Proposed differences between narcissistic, borderline, sadistic, and antisocial psychopaths. *Psychiatric Quarterly, 74*(1), 11–29.

Naturalism.org. (2007). Retrieved July 9, 2007, from http://www.naturalism.org

Nurse, J., Woodcock, P., & Ormsby, J. (2003). Influence of environmental factors on mental health within prisons: Focus group study. *British Medical Journal, 30,* 1–5.

Penn, J., Esposito, C., Schaeffer, L., Fritz, G., & Spirito, A. (2003). Suicide attempts and self-mutilative behavior in a juvenile correctional facility. *Journal of the American Academy of Child and Adolescent Psychiatry, 42*(7), 762–769.

Pham, T., Vanderstukken, O., Philippot, P., & Vanderlinden, M. (2003). Selective attention and executive function deficits among criminal psychopaths. *Aggressive Behavior, 29,* 393–405.

Pinel, P. (1801). *Traite, medico—Philosophique sur l'alienation mental.* Paris: Richard, Caille et Ravier.

Poythress, N., Skeem, J., & Lilienfield, S. (2006). Associations among early abuse, dissociation, and psychopathy in an offender sample. *Journal of Abnormal Psychology, 115*(2), 288–297.

Pross, C. (2006). Burnout, vicarious traumatization and its prevention. *Torture, 16*(1), 1–9.

Reker, G. (1977). The Purpose-in-Life Test in an inmate population: An empirical investigation. *Journal of Clinical Psychology, 33*(3), 688–693.

Rice, M., Harris, G., & Cormier, C. (1992). An evaluation of a maximum security therapeutic community for psychopaths and other mentally disordered offenders. *Law and Human Behavior, 16,* 399–412.

Salekin, R. (2002). Psychopathy and therapeutic pessimism: Clinical lore or clinical reality? *Clinical Psychology Review, 22,* 79–112.

Shelley, M. (1831). *Frankenstein, or, the modern Prometheus.* London: Colburn & Bentley.

Simon, R. (1996). *Bad men do what good men dream.* Washington, DC: APA Press.

Simon, R. (2003). Should forensic psychiatrists testify about evil? *Journal of the American Academy of Psychiatry and the Law, 31*(4), 413–416.

Skeem, J., & Monahan, J. (2002). Psychopathy, treatment involvement, and subsequent violence among civil psychiatric patients. *Law and Human Behavior, 26*(6), 577–603.

Slowchower, J. (1991). Variations in the analytic holding environment. *International Journal of Psycho-Analysis, 72,* 709–718.

Stamm, B. H. (1997). Work-related secondary traumatic stress. *PTSD Research Quarterly, 8*(2). Retrieved January 23, 2009, from http://www.dartmouth.edu/dms/ptsd/RQ_Spring_1997.html

Steed, L., & Bicknell, J. (2001). Trauma and the therapist: The experience of therapists working with the perpetrators of sexual abuse. *Australasian Journal of Disaster and Trauma Studies, 1*. Retrieved November 20, 2008, from http://www.massey.ac.nz/~trauma/issues/2001-1/steed.htm

Strous, R., Ulman, A., & Moshe, K. (2006). The hateful patient revisited: Relevance for 21st century medicine. *European Journal of Internal Medicine, 17*, 387–393.

Twenge, J., Catanese, K., & Baumeister, R. (2005). Social exclusion and the deconstructed state: Time perception, meaninglessness, lethargy, lack of emotion, and self-awareness. *Journal of Personality and Social Psychology, 85*(3), 409–423.

Ursano, R., Sonnenberg, S., & Lazar, S. (1991). *Concise guide to psychodynamic psychotherapy*. Washington, DC: American Psychiatric Press.

Viding, E. (2004). Annotation: Understanding the development of psychopathy. *Journal of Child Psychology and Psychiatry, 45*(8), 1329–1337.

Vien, A., & Beech, A. (2006). Psychopathy: Theory, measurement, and treatment. *Trauma, Violence, & Abuse, 7*(3), 155–174.

Waisberg, J., & Porter, J. (1994). Purpose in life and outcome of treatment for alcohol dependence. *British Journal of Clinical Psychology, 33*, 49–63.

Watson, L. (1995). *Dark nature: A natural history of evil*. New York: Harper Collins.

Way, B., Sawyer, D., Barboza, S., & Nash, R. (2007). Inmate suicides and time spent in special disciplinary housing in New York State Prison. *Psychiatric Services, 58*, 558–560.

Way, I., VanDeusen, K., Martin, G., Applegate, B., & Jandle, D. (2004). Vicarious trauma: A comparison of clinicians who treat survivors of sexual abuse and sexual offenders. *Journal of Interpersonal Violence, 19*(1), 49–71.

Welner, M. (2003). Response to Simon: Legal relevance demands that evil be defined and standardized. *Journal of the American Academy of Psychiatry and the Law, 31*(4), 417–21.

Wilson, P. (2003). The concept of evil and the forensic psychologist. *International Journal of Forensic Psychology, 1*(1), 1–9.

Wong, S., & Gordon, A. (2000). *Violence reduction program: Program overview*. Department of Psychology, University of Saskatchewan. Retrieved November 20, 2008, from http://www.psynergy.ca/pdf/vrpuserguiderevisedwebsite_version.pdf

Wong, S., Gordon, A., & Gu, D. (2007). Assessment and treatment of violence-prone forensic clients: An integrated approach. *British Journal of Psychiatry, 190*(Suppl. 49), s66–s74.

Wong, S., & Hare, R. (2005). *Guidelines for a psychopathy treatment program*. Toronto, Canada: Multi-Health Systems.

Woodworth, M., & Porter, S. (2002). In cold blood: Characteristics of criminal homicides as a function of psychopathy. *Journal of Abnormal Psychology, 111*, 436–445.

Youth Violence

PART II

11

Youth Violence: Prevalence, Etiology, and Treatment

FRANK DICATALDO, MATT C. ZAITCHIK, AND KATE PROVENCHER

> The proportion of juvenile delinquents seems to be everywhere increasing and crime is more and more precocious. . . . The criminal adolescent is a victim of degenerate evolution.
>
> —G. Stanley Hall, 1907

> Violent juvenile crime is a national epidemic. Today's superpredators are feral, presocial beings with no sense of right and wrong.
>
> —U.S. Congressman Bill McCollum, Republican, Florida quoted in Ayers, 1997/1998

These statements, separated by nearly a century, one written by a late-19th-century academic psychologist, the founder and first president of Clark University and the American Psychological Association, the other uttered by a late-20th-century politician, a Republican congressman from Florida, could easily be exchanged, attributing one to the other without introducing a bit of confusion to the reader or listener. It is truly remarkable, even mind-boggling—a century's worth of distance between these statements, written at the dawn of the 20th century and uttered in its closing twilight, and not an iota of difference between them. The public discourse about juvenile offenders changed little over the course of the century. They are still generally regarded as careening too closely to some precipice of disaster, some pandemonium. Could it be possible that they have actually stood precariously perched on the edge of some abyss as we anxiously watched on these past 100 hundred years? Or is this image of impending crisis a product of our ways of seeing them; a more vital statement about our perennial view of adolescents as an omnipresent threat to a fragile social order? In the final analysis, it may be that the opening statements to this chapter say more about our enduring systems of thought about adolescents, particularly minority-status adolescents, than about the adolescents themselves.

The 1990s may come to be regarded as the hardest decade for the centenarian juvenile court system. This was the decade when, in the face of a surging escalation in the juvenile crime rate, particularly the murder rate, state legislatures across the county, in a dominolike effect, passed sets of legal changes that threatened to collapse the juvenile justice system back into the adult system from which it had emerged. Transfer laws—the substantive and procedural legal criteria and rules that govern the transformation of adolescent offenders into adult criminal defendants—were widened; the upward boundary for the age of juvenile jurisdiction was lowered, making 16- and 17-year-olds automatically adults instead of juveniles; and discretionary sentencing schemes were exchanged for more adultlike mandatory sentencing structures based on legal principles of proportionality and "just-deserts" rather than on the individual needs of the offender (Zimring & Fagan, 2000).

The collective fear driving these legal changes was the unfounded moral panic that the alarming rates of juvenile crime would continue to grow, maybe even geometrically grow, in future decades. To offset this coming catastrophe, something drastic needed to be done. But what was feared never came to pass. Instead of rising, the crime rates that had risen so steadily a decade before began to fall in the middle 1990s and continued to do so into the early part of the decade of 2000. For most categories of violent offending, the rates fell below where they were before the increase (Zimring, 1998, 2005). The tidal movement of crime rates is a topic of debate among academic criminologists. An academic career can be forged from such preoccupations. Whether the juvenile crime rate's abrupt reversal was an effect of the legal changes that followed it or merely coincidental to it, what was left in the wake of these legislative changes was a drastically altered landscape of juvenile justice. Over time, some states have retracted the changes, restoring the juvenile justice system to the state it was before the firestorm of the 1990s; but most states are still living within the legacy of this historical moment.

Many of the changes that occurred in the juvenile justice system across the county during this darkened decade were fueled by misinformed assumptions and projections by criminologists and public policy experts (DiIulio, 1995; Fox, 1996). Popular myths about juvenile offenders and the juvenile justice system abound (Glassner, 1999; Kappeler, Blumberg, & Potter, 2000). When the facts of juvenile violence are confronted, however, the conclusions are not as bleak as has been often portrayed in the past. This chapter sets out to review what knowledge social science can contribute to a more reasoned understanding of the prevalence, etiology, and prevention of youth violence. It is our view that juvenile offending, while a social problem deserving of attention and focus, is not an epidemic in need of quarantining strategies aimed at the eradication of some adolescent scourge. History informs that strategies such as this are doomed to fail and often end up causing more harm. It is our intention to communicate a more optimistic message than the conclusions reached by Professor Hall a hundred years ago and more recently by Congressman McCollum.

THE PREVALENCE OF YOUTH VIOLENCE IN THE UNITED STATES

The demonization of adolescent offenders that followed the sudden surge in violent offending in the late 1980s and 1990s did not give way to more balanced views when the storm subsided and crime rates ebbed to new, previously unrecorded lows. The "juvenile superpredators," "new breed of killers," "conscienceless psychopaths," and other dehumanizing monikers were not exchanged for more hagiographic descriptors when the violence rates let up. Nevertheless, when the smoke cleared, the rates of serious violent offending for youth were down significantly. Although recent reports indicate that they may be on the uptick again.

When it comes to the public perception of youth violence and the actual rates of known offending, there exist two separate realities—the perceptual and the actual. A recent Gallup poll, as reported by Borum and Verhaagen (2006), asked a representative sample of Americans about their perception of violent offending by juveniles and found that they believe that nearly half (43%) of all violent crime was caused by juveniles. In fact, the best available data supplied by the Office of Juvenile Justice and Delinquency Prevention estimate that the actual rates are significantly lower, about 13%. Borum and Verhaagen (2006) note, however, that the public concern about youth violence is not completely baseless, because the rates of violent crime committed by juvenile offenders did sharply rise from about 1987 to 1992, increasing by about 56%. Fortunately, what ballooned up eventually descended. Public perception has not kept pace with these ricocheting rates, however.

Official records about juvenile crime are an imprecise measure best conceived of as an approximation of the "dark statistic" of the actual rates of offending by juveniles (Best, 2001). Official statistics underrepresent juvenile offending because many crimes committed by juveniles are never reported, particularly juvenile-on-juvenile crime. Also, many juveniles who commit crimes are never arrested or are only arrested for a portion of the crimes that they commit. The exclusive reference to arrest rates can also inflate offense rates for particular types of crime (Zimring, 1998). A hallmark characteristic of juvenile offending is that adolescents tend to engage in delinquency as part of a peer group supportive of such conduct. A single incident of violent crime could result in multiple arrests of the members of a delinquent peer group who committed the act as a function of some group enterprise. Adults are less susceptible to such group-based forces. One crime with three participants can result in three arrests of juvenile offenders, inflating the arrest rate when it is compared to adult arrest rates.

A fuller, more accurate understanding of the rates of offending can be obtained from a combination of official crime statistics and self-report studies. Self-report studies can capture incidents of offending that escape official statistics. Overall, self-report studies provide a higher rate of juvenile offending than official reports (Snyder & Sickmund, 2006). Self-report methods, nonetheless, do come with their own set of limitations. Many juveniles, despite the anonymous and confidential manner in which such data are gathered, may be reluctant to disclose incidents of violence. Memory and recall of prior events may also be distorted or may decay over time. Finally, conducting a self-report study is methodologically complicated, time-consuming, and expensive, making the assembling of a large sample difficult. Victimization studies—another form of self-report study that examines the report of victims who indicate that they have been victimized by juveniles—is a third method that can aid in the approximation of the actual crime rate. But this method is limited by the same problems of other self-report methods. The best approach for determining the actual crime rates of juveniles will combine the three methods, thereby offsetting the limitations of each.

In 2003, the most recent year for which national crime statistics are available, the FBI's Uniform Crime Report indicated that law enforcement agencies across the country reported 2.2 million arrests of persons under the age of 18 (Snyder & Sickmund, 2006). Nearly 60% of these arrests were for simple assaults, property crimes, and other nonperson offenses. A little over 40% were in the FBI category of violent crime, comprised of murder and nonnegligent manslaughter, forcible rape, robbery, and aggravated assault. Two-thirds of these more serious violent offenses were committed by 16- and 17-year-old offenders and 45% by Black adolescents.

The most recent data about the rates of violent offending by juveniles indicate that violent crime by juveniles has steadily decreased since about 1993 or 1994 to rates lower than when the uptick began in the late 1980s. Between 2001 and 2003, the rate of decline began to plateau, with some evidence in 2002 that the rate as measured by violent victimization by juvenile offenders was edging up again. Between 1994 and 2003, juvenile arrests for violent crime decreased at a higher rate than for adults. The FBI's Violent Crime Index decreased by 32% for juveniles during this decade.

However, girls witnessed a substantially lower rate of decrease, about 10%. The crime rate among girls contrasts to the crime rate among boys. Between 1980 and 2003, the rate of arrest for girls for violent and property crimes increased. And while they, too, have demonstrated a decrease in their overall arrest rate in recent years, their rate of decline is much lower than is the case of boys. A parallel story has unfolded for young juvenile offenders below the age of 13. While the proportion of juvenile arrests involving young juveniles declined from 1980 to 2003, their proportional representation in the juvenile Violent Crime Index grew from 6% to 9%.

The murder rate for juvenile offenders has demonstrated a similar pattern of decline. In 2002, the number of murders by juveniles dropped to its lowest level since 1984, reversing the earlier increase (Snyder & Sickmund, 2006). A large share of the decline was likely due to the decrease in the murder of non–family members by boys with a firearm. In 2002, juveniles were involved in an estimated 1,300 murders or 8% of all murders. Nearly half (48%) of the total number of murders by juveniles were committed in the context of a group of codefendants.

DISRUPTIVE BEHAVIOR DISORDERS AND YOUTH VIOLENCE

Oppositional defiant disorder (ODD), conduct disorder (CD), and attention deficit hyperactivity disorder (ADHD) form a cluster of childhood disorders considered to be "disruptive behavior disorders" (American Psychiatric Association, 2004). Although most violent adolescents have more than one mental disorder (Borum & Verhaagen, 2006; Vermeiren, 2003; Wasserman, Ko, & McReynolds, 2004) and they may have internalizing disorders (e.g., depression) or substance abuse, substantially higher rates of physical aggression are found in adolescents with disruptive behavior disorders than for those with other mental disorders, with the exception of substance abuse disorders (Connor, 2002; Grisso, 2004; Teplin, Abram, McClelland, Dulcan, & Mericle, 2002). The fact that violent juvenile offenders are more likely to have these diagnoses is not surprising, because impulsive and/or aggressive behaviors are part of their diagnostic criteria. Additionally, there is relatively high comorbidity with substance abuse disorders, which are also associated with juvenile violence (Moeller, 2001).

The disruptive behavior disorders are clustered for good reason. Approximately 80% to 90% of adolescents with conduct disorder are diagnosed with ODD at an earlier age, and about 50% of children diagnosed with ADHD will be diagnosed with CD at some point during adolescence. In fact, more than two-thirds of adolescents with CD also are diagnosed with ADHD (Connor, 2002; Grisso, 2004). About 25% of children with ODD, however, will be diagnosed later with CD. These relationships are significant, because disruptive behavior disorders identify youths who are more likely to engage in criminal and aggressive behaviors as adults (Grisso, 2004; Kratzer & Hodgins, 1997). Some researchers think that the disruptive behavior disorders can be arranged on a continuum ranging from ADHD to ODD to CD (e.g., Barkley, 1998), and, although there are clearly other pathways to CD, research findings suggest that these three disorders are "distinct but related" (Borum & Verhaagen, 2006, p. 55).

Although most children have periods of negativism and mild defiance, those with ODD show a pattern of negative, hostile, and defiant behavior that results in significant family or school problems. ODD typically becomes evident between the ages of 8 and 12. Preadolescent boys are more likely to be diagnosed with ODD than girls, but the diagnosis is equally common in girls and boys after puberty. It has been suggested that sex differences found in the diagnosis of ODD may be due to biased sampling and/or biased assessment (Waschbusch & King, 2006). ODD involves a pattern of resistant, hostile, and irritable behaviors that interfere with home and/or school functioning, but children with ODD do not typically violate the rights of others. Behaviors associated with ODD may involve verbal aggression (e.g., yelling, making threats, or name calling) or physical aggression (e.g., hitting or kicking).

ADHD is a disorder involving inattentiveness and hyperactivity-impulsivity and is "more frequent and severe than is typically observed in individuals at a comparable level of development" (American Psychiatric Association, 1994, p. 78). ADHD is defined in terms of three behavioral criteria: attentional deficits, motor hyperactivity, and impulsivity. In order to meet diagnostic criteria for ADHD, a child must exhibit signs of the disorder prior to age seven. ADHD occurs in 2% to 7% percent of elementary school children in the United States (August, Realmuto, MacDonald, Nugent, & Crosby, 1996; Kashani, Orvaschel, Rosenberg, & Reid, 1989) and is more prevalent among boys than girls by a ratio between 4:1 and 9:1 (American Psychiatric Association, 1994). Children with ADHD are not necessarily aggressive, but the core symptom of impulsivity suggests lack of behavioral inhibition. Additionally, about 15% to 30% of children with ADHD have a learning disability (Barkley, DuPaul, & McMurray, 1990), and about half are placed in special education programs due to their problems in adapting to a typical classroom environment (Barkley et al., 1990). These factors can lead to poor educational achievement, a risk factor for adult aggression (Monahan, 1981). Children with ADHD who are also aggressive are more likely to have problems as adults. Andersson, Magnusson, and Wennberg (1997) found that 13-year-old boys who were rated by teachers to be unusually hyperactive and aggressive were more likely (28%) than their "normal" peers (3%) to develop alcoholism and criminality before the age of 25. Studies suggest, however, that ADHD alone does not predict adult criminality or violence; it is the combination of ADHD and aggression in childhood that predicts future criminality and violence (Vitelli, 1996).

CD is characterized by repetitive and persistent violation of societal rules and norms as well as the rights of others. Many of the behaviors associated with CD are illegal and are typically related to childhood aggression and violence. CD involves aggression toward people and/or animals, destruction of property, deceitfulness or theft, and serious violation of rules (American Psychiatric Association, 1994). The diagnosis is typically applied to youths under the age of 18. Prevalence rates range from 6% to 16% in boys under age 18 and 2% to 9% in girls (American Psychiatric Association, 1994). Some researchers have suggested that there are two subtypes of CD adolescents: delinquent and aggressive. The delinquent subtype is characterized by truancy, theft, running away, lying, and setting fires. The aggressive subtype is characterized by fighting, destruction of property, and cruelty to people or animals (Achenbach, 1993; Kazdin, 1995). This is consistent with earlier versions of the *DSM*, which defined two types of CD youths: socialized and undersocialized (American Psychiatric Association, 1980, 1987). Signs of CD can be observed as beginning either in childhood or adolescence, with child-onset CD having a greater likelihood of persistence of antisocial behavior into adulthood than adolescent-onset CD.

Evidence suggests that youths with disruptive behavior disorders are at risk for exhibiting antisocial and aggressive behavior as adults. This is especially true if they meet criteria for both ADHD and AD and showed signs of ODD earlier in childhood (Grisso, 2004). This does *not* mean that all, or even most, of these youths who are comorbid for these disorders will be criminal or violent adults. In fact, there may be other characteristics or disorders, when they co-occur with CD, that predict the subgroup of CD youth whose aggression and criminality will persist into adulthood. There is evidence, for example, that when CD is comorbid with substance abuse or depression, the risk of future violence is increased (Grisso, 2004; Loeber, Burke, & Lahey, 2002). Nonetheless, children with disruptive behavior disorders are more likely than their peers to be aggressive in adulthood.

PATTERNS OF JUVENILE OFFENDING

Juvenile offenders have been distinguished from nondelinquent youth on all sorts of variables and dimensions beginning in the late 19th century. Dawson (1896) measured and recorded the physical signs of degeneracy in 26 boys from the Lyman School for Boys, a juvenile reformatory in Westborough, Massachusetts, and 26 girls at the State Industrial School for Girls at Lancaster, Massachusetts, and compared them to a sample drawn from the Worcester Public Schools. Dawson found that the reformatory children bore many more of the physical stigmata of degeneracy—diminutive statures; lighter weight; decreased strength; more facial asymmetries; smaller and broader heads and faces; defective sensory functioning; and impairments in attention, memory, and association. He attributed these differences to an interaction between the degenerative process set off by the "drunken stock" of their parents and the "bad environments" in which they were reared. He left little doubt, however, about which of these causes is ascendant: "Their parents have undergone modifications in the direction of a less perfect physical structure and less highly developed psychical powers. They have deviated, morbidly, from the type of their race and civilization. In their unholy transmission of life, their diseased cells, potential for almost every moral and intellectual evil, have passed on to their children" (Dawson, 1896, pp. 256–257).

Later, William Sheldon (Sheldon, Hartl, & McDermott, 1949) examined the body types of delinquent boys referred to a social service agency in South Boston devoted to working with delinquent youth. He reported an overrepresentation of delinquents with mesomorphic body types—athletic-built, advanced muscular development, and body strength—possessing the temperamental characteristics of affinity for risk, inhibited fear response, and hypermasculinity.

The latter half of the 20th century brought the crossover from the delinquent body to the distinguishing psychological characteristics of delinquent youth. Nevertheless, biologically based, often genetically inherited temperamental and neurocognitive differences, have remained a central feature of many of these taxonomic systems. Terrie Moffitt (1993, 2003) proposed a binary taxonomic system that has received a significant amount of attention in the developmental psychopathology and juvenile delinquency literature. Moffitt divides juvenile offenders into two groups—adolescent-limited offenders and life-course persistent offenders—and posits separate lines of etiology and prognosis for them. Her schema is taxonomic, suggesting fundamental differences in the origin and outcomes of these phenomenologically different types of offenders, and moves beyond a simple behavioral description of them. Separate and distinct theories of origin govern the appearance and duration of these offender types. The life-course persistent offender is conceptualized as a form of chronic psychopathology, while the adolescent-limited offender is a temporary behavioral state that befalls the contemporary adolescent as he or she moves through the stormy high-risk developmental phase of adolescence before beaching onto the protective shoals of adulthood. This adolescent-limited offender is not necessarily a deviant trajectory and is described as often being a feature of normal adolescent development.

The dichotomous grouping of juvenile offenders based on cause and outcome has a long historical precedent beginning with Lombroso (1876), who described two general types of offenders: born criminals and passionate offenders. The first type has acquired deficits through disease, such as syphilis or some taint of mental illness, or some inherited organic degenerative defect. The second class of offenders has environmental causes, external to their constitutional makeup, at the root of their criminal acts. Morrison (1896) established a similar dichotomy for juvenile offenders, labeling them habitual and occasional offenders.

The life-course persistent offender is a relatively small subgroup of offenders, comprising between 5% and 10% of all delinquents who are likely responsible for a higher proportion of violent offending than their representative numbers would suggest. The age of onset of behavioral problems is one of the most distinguishing diagnostic features of this type of antisocial behavior. The offender's risk emerges early in life from inherited or acquired neuropsychological deficits or variation that may manifest differently over the course of development but is theoretically linked as part of the same deviant process—a characteristic often referred to as heterotypic continuity. In early childhood, the child may manifest delayed speech or other cognitive lags and hyperactivity. Later these problems may transmute into defiance and oppositionality, and later still into covert forms of offending, such as stealing, before switching over to overt aggression. Environmental risk factors come into play in the form of coercive parenting styles and disrupted bonding, which may exist as independent contributions or as evoked responses on the part of parents confronted with the challenge of rearing children with difficult temperaments or behavioral patterns. A transactional parent–child exchange is erected whereby a constitutionally difficult child produces harsh and coercive responses on the part of parents, which in turn spur increased problematic behavior in the child and so on—a case of people creating environments and environments creating people.

The environmental risk is expanded as the child matures beyond the family system and enters the social realm of the school and the peer world. Low academic achievement produces poor attachment to school and an eventual rejection of the acquisition of academic skills and advancement. School becomes a failed arena, setting the stage for a differential drift toward other low-achieving school rejecters. The offender initially experiences peer rejection and isolation as his or her aggressive and coercive behavior acts as a repellant among the early peer group. Later in early and middle adolescence, their aggressive behavioral patterns may act as attractors for other similar-styled aggressive children and even for more normally developing adolescents as some forms of delinquency temporarily become a more sought-after high-status activity in the social world of the adolescent.

The interaction of the individual and the environment may coalesce into the formation of a maladaptive and disordered personality style characterized by aggression and antisocial behavior. The well-worn track they have paved over the course of two decades of development often effaces other legitimate pathways, diminishing the opportunity and possibility for reform. As young adults, through a cumulative process, they find themselves educationally disadvantaged, vocationally unprepared, and without promising employment prospects or opportunities, differentially associated and attached to similarly placed peers who have also constructed similar antisocial identities. As a result, they are propelled into continued patterns of aggression and antisocial behavior that persist through adulthood, often dispersing into a lifestyle plagued by drug abuse, chronic unemployment, domestic violence, and various forms of violent and nonviolent criminality. The process is self-perpetuating and maintaining.

Moffitt describes a different life story for the adolescent-limited juvenile offender, with a separate origin and outcome, ending more happily in desistence from antisocial behavior through maturation. The adolescent-limited juvenile offender is contained within the cultural narrative of the wily "good kid" who gets temporarily mixed up with the "wrong crowd" but emerges, hopefully unscathed, as the wiser, better-controlled adult who assumes the role of the responsible grown-up with family, job, and a mortgage. Their youthful delinquent antics—though possibly serious and harmful at the time—recede as they settle into the path of a routine adult life, a Shakespearian Prince Hal phenomenon.

Unlike the life-course persistent juvenile offender, the adolescent-limited juvenile offender represents a much more prevalent form of antisocial behavior and comprises about 90% to 95% of all juvenile offenders. His or her antisocial behavior emerges later in life, in adolescence, when the modern adolescent experiences most profoundly what Moffitt describes as the "maturity gap"—the increasingly cavernous roleless period of development that has become the plight of the contemporary adolescent and society. Old enough to have undergone the maturation that makes them biologically similar to adults—although recent neuroscience has identified continued brain development and maturation into the early 20s (Giedd et al., 1999)—but too young to assume adult privileges and responsibilities, adolescents chafe at their still-dependent status and long for the independence and autonomy of adulthood. Within the spreading gap between these two opposing states of existence—biologically mature, socially dependent—it has become a normative rite of passage for them to become involved in some form of delinquent activity (Elliot, Huizinga, & Morse, 1986). For the modern adolescent boy, and it is increasingly the case for the girl as well, delinquency is normative. During adolescence, delinquency becomes socially enhancing and status elevating. Juvenile offending affords the appearance of maturity and autonomy from parents. It provides a forum for the acquisition of status among peers, social power, sexual conquests, monetary independence through drug trade and other illegal activities, and a rebellion against parental admonition and wider social rules and values.

During the adolescent passage, Moffitt argues, delinquency becomes the vanguard. The life-course persistent juvenile offender evokes a lifestyle that the adolescent-limited offender comes to emulate and mimic. During this phase, the behavioral differences between the two types of offenders are often indistinguishable. The adolescent-limited juvenile offenders can engage in forms of violent offending every bit as harmful as their life-course persistent counterparts. These types cannot be sorted out through a cross-sectional analysis of their offending behavior but only through the longitudinal examination of their life histories. It is age of onset and chronicity rather than severity of offending that sets them apart. The identification of life-course persistent juvenile offenders is most readily determined by their past functioning.

The story of the adolescent-limited juvenile offender most often ends happily in desistence as they emerge into adulthood. Their fortified early life is sustaining enough to allow them to cross over into adulthood and leave behind their limited run with delinquent behavior. They have established enough lifelines to pull themselves out, unlike their more determined counterparts, who find themselves increasingly entrenched on a pathway with fewer and fewer ways out. The journey out for the adolescent-limited juvenile offender often does not require heavy-handed legal and mental health intervention, because nothing has proved more curative for juvenile offending than the simple passage of time. Maturation alone and some protective cover along the way is often all that is needed. The major concern is that they do not encounter some type of snare—a serious charge that results in long-term incarceration, a serious record that limits opportunity, addiction, or a derailed education—that may inhibit their ability to transition successfully to adulthood.

DSM-IV capitalizes on this dichotomous system of classification within the conduct disorder diagnostic category. In many respects, conduct disorder is the psychiatric analogue to juvenile offending, or juvenile offending framed as a psychiatric disorder. Conduct disorder is a broad category that is likely to net both life-course persistent and adolescent-limited juvenile offenders. The distinction between these two types may be sorted out through the diagnostic subtyping of childhood onset and adolescent onset. The subtypes are distinguished by the appearance of any of the behavioral criteria prior to the age of 10. Conduct disorder, childhood-onset type bears close resemblance to the life-course persistent juvenile offender while conduct disorder, adolescent-onset represents the adolescent-limited juvenile offender.

A test of Moffitt's two-taxon schema was reported in the Dunedin Multidisciplinary Health and Development Study, a 30-year longitudinal study of a birth cohort of 1,000 New Zealand children (Moffitt & Caspi, 2001; Moffitt, Caspi, Dickson, Silva, & Stanton, 1996; Moffitt, Caspi, Harrington, & Milne, 2002). The study examined a set of childhood predictors from age 3 to 13 and found life-course persistent offending was differentially predicted by the status on neuropsychological and parenting risk factors at age 3. The neurodevelopmental factors included such variables as undercontrolled temperament, low intelligence, delayed motor development, hyperactivity, and reading difficulties. The parenting factors included having a teenage single parent, mother's poor mental health, harsh and neglectful parenting style, inconsistent parenting, low socioeconomic status, and peer rejection.

There is also accumulating evidence to support the conclusion that life-course persistent offending is more heritable than adolescent-limited offending and that aggressive behavior—a hallmark feature of the life-course persistent offender from as young as age 3—is more heritable than delinquency, a behavior pattern that adolescent-limited juvenile offenders share with their counterparts. Delinquency thus appears more rooted in ubiquitous social forces, while aggression seems to be a more exclusive individual difference. Furthermore, childhood-onset antisocial behavior appears to be strongly predictive of violent offending in early adulthood and other indicators of poor adult outcome such as low-level but chronic adult offending and other negative outcomes such as poor social relationships and isolation, poor job achievement, and problematic adult adjustment (Moffitt, 2003).

Mark: An Adolescent at Risk for Life-Course Persistent Offending

The following case describes a juvenile offender at risk for life-course persistent offending. He is referred to as at risk for this pattern of offending because, while he manifests many of the clinical characteristics described by Moffitt for this taxon, the category predicts or forecasts a prognosis, points ahead to a future outcome that has yet to be realized. Even though the predictive validity of the binary taxonomic system has been established to some degree, it is far from a guarantee that a particular youth identified as exhibiting characteristics consistent with life-course persistent offending will actually end up doing so. He could end up desisting because of some unaccounted-for "turning point" (Sampson & Laub, 1993) in his life, such as a marriage or some other life-altering relationship or an event that knocks him off course and brings about the unexpected process of desistance. The case of Mark could be the exception to the rule for life-course persistent offending.

Mark was the second of his mother's five children. His mother was described as having had a very traumatic childhood, sustaining a head injury in a serious car accident that killed a relative and left her in a coma for several months at the age of 5. She was also reportedly sexually abused as a child by her stepfather. She told her mother about the abuse, but she reportedly did nothing about it. She has an eighth-grade education, and was 15 years old when she became pregnant with her first child, a daughter. A year later, she had Mark; 2 years later, she had another son; and 2 years after that, she had her fourth child, a son, all with the same man. The couple never married and separated when Mark was 5. Mark's father was described as having had a serious alcohol abuse problem and was physically abusive toward Mark's mother. He had no contact with Mark or his siblings as they were growing up. Mark's mother had another child, her fifth, a boy, with another man with whom she had a 6-year on-again-off-again relationship. Mark's mother had a significant history of mental health problems. She attempted suicide via an overdose when he was age 5 that resulted in her children being taken into the custody of the child welfare system. She was admitted to a psychiatric hospital and attended outpatient psychotherapy for a period of time.

Mark's records contain little information about his early childhood. He reportedly was the product of an uncomplicated and unremarkable pregnancy. He reported in the past that he was not the victim of sexual abuse, but there was a report, made by his biological father, that his mother was physically abusive and neglectful of him. His early home environment was described as having been very chaotic. He was treated with various medications for various mental disorders (conduct disorder, oppositional defiant disorder, attention deficit hyperactivity disorder, and mood disorder) and for a variety of symptoms (impulsivity, anger, explosive behavior, and insomnia) beginning in early childhood. He was diagnosed with a severe expressive and receptive language learning problem, scoring many years below his age expectancy, and was provided special educational services early in his academic career. He was described as functionally illiterate. He began abusing marijuana and alcohol at age 14 or 15 and stated that he sometimes smoked every day.

He first became involved in the child welfare system when he was about 11 or 12, when his mother ingested medication in an apparent suicide attempt while in the care of her children. During the course of the investigation, she filed a child-in-need-of-supervision (CHINS) petition with the local juvenile court on behalf on Mark as a stubborn child. Later that year, another CHINS was filed against him when he was truant from school and missing for several days from home. The child welfare system was granted temporary custody, and he was placed in three different foster care placements because his mother did not want him back home. During this time, he was arraigned at the age of 11 for the first time in juvenile court for driving in a stolen car at a high speed. The case was later dismissed, and he was returned to foster care. After his mother failed to participate in the assessment, the child welfare agency plan changed from family reunification to long-tem substitute care.

Over the course of the next few years, Mark was placed in a variety of residential programs for at-risk youth, where he continued his pattern of noncompliance and running. At one placement, he picked up a delinquency complaint for threatening a staff member. He ran from the program on numerous occasions, picking up various delinquency complaints during his escapades while on the run from the program. Somewhere along the way, he reports having joined a street gang.

Mark has a significant history of delinquency adjudications beginning at the age of 14. His first adjudication was for breaking and entering into cars and stealing the contents with a codefendant. His second complaint was for larceny of a leather jacket from a peer-aged male victim. Mark later received a charge for threatening from an incident that involved a staff member at a residential placement. Mark allegedly told the staff member he was going to shoot him, stating, "I'm gonna bust a cap on you." He was detained for an incident of curfew violation and was found in possession of a screwdriver and shaved-down car keys the police believed he intended to use to break into cars. After his release from a treatment program, Mark was released to live with his mother but was detained again within a month following his involvement in a motor vehicle accident that narrowly missed hitting a police patrol car and crashed into a tree while attempting to elude the pursuing police. No one was significantly injured in the accident, but Mark and his four passengers were arrested for driving under the influence of narcotics (marijuana), operating a motor vehicle negligently, and knowingly receiving stolen property.

Throughout his residential placements, Mark was consistently described as stubborn, angry, and impulsive. He engaged in threats and violence toward other residents and staff. He was sanctioned repeatedly for smuggling contraband into his room, including sharp objects that he used to scratch his arm. He was also found in his room with a shirt tied around his neck and was discovered "cheeking" his medication. He bragged about being a member of a gang and taunted rival gang members. He threatened and was aggressive toward other residents and staff, yelling that he would throw feces at them. He urinated on his floor, smeared spit on his window, and threatened to throw a roll of toilet paper soaked in urine at staff. Returning from a community pass, he was discovered attempting to smuggle in a knife that he taped underneath his scrotum. He was sanctioned repeatedly for being at the center of a number of riots on his unit and, at one point, was placed in seclusion for his involvement in a fight with another resident, hitting him with a sock filled with two bars of soap. This was one of many instances of his having been in possession of self-made weapons.

He eventually worked his way to a discharge to a nonsecure residential program, but after a month he was arrested again for stealing a cache of firearms from a collector who lived next door to the program. Mark had observed that the neighbor was a collector of firearms and broke into his home while he was away. He hid the firearms in the woods nearby. He reported that he intended to run from the program and come back for the guns with some members of his gang.

Mark exhibits many of the early childhood markers defining a life-course persistent pattern of offending. He was born to a teenage mother with a history of a serious head injury and mental health problems who had five children with a man who was prone to domestic violence and substance abuse. Mark manifested early behavior and learning problems. He was diagnosed as having ADHD and a verbal learning disability early in childhood. His behavior is described as aggressive, undercontrolled, and impulsive. His behavior easily overwhelmed his mother's impaired parenting capacities, and he was removed from her care at the age of 11, when she attempted suicide. He entered the child welfare system, where he continued to be aggressive, noncompliant, and difficult to manage and graduated to the juvenile justice system after he joined a gang and engaged in a diverse array of delinquency that included reckless behavior, drug abuse, stealing, weapon possession, and violence. His problematic behavior never abated, even in the most secure settings. His threatening and aggressive behavior never stabilizes or becomes intermittent. Instead, it becomes more chronic and deeply entrenched over time and consistent across settings.

What makes his case such a compelling demonstration of the life-course persistent offender is that his problematic behavior has an early onset and is chronic, diverse, and persistent, but, up to this point, he never received a delinquency complaint for a serious offense. Seriousness of offense may be the least distinguishing offense-related characteristic between life-course persistent and adolescent-limited offenders. It does not indicate nearly as much as age of onset and chronicity. This characteristic is further demonstrated by the next case of an adolescent-limited offender who has a serious delinquent event but not the early-onset or chronic course.

John: A Case of an Adolescent-Limited Offender

The precipitating incident to the murder committed by John occurred several months earlier. An acquaintance, Michael, had committed an act of unthinkable cowardice—he abandoned a friend during a confrontation with a rival group of adolescents from another part of town. The friend was beaten up, but the beating was not as stinging as the humiliation of being left to face his fate alone. Now Michael was the target of revenge from his group for breaking a street code of conduct. Over the course of the next several weeks, he was jumped by the scorned friend and by a group of his other former friends. He was attacked at school and in the community, and the humiliation of the label "punk" and "chump" was infinitely more painful than the fists and the cane he was beaten with. Michael and his friend became bitter enemies, and a new rivalry splintered off from the first one.

Michael gathered a small group of friends and planned a confrontation to earn back his diminished status. Among the group that Michael assembled was John, a local 16-year-old boy whom he knew for only a few months. John barely knew the group of boys that Michael wanted to square off with.

The first confrontation between the two groups occurred on the platform of a subway train. The two groups passed each other, exchanging insults. Michael moved his hand across his front waistband where he hid a handgun as a threatening gesture of power. A member of the other group returned the gesture. However, there was no confrontation, just an exchange of words. Michael and his group felt ashamed about not taking action. It was another stinging humiliation, another sign of weakness. Michael took out his gun and pointed it in the air in a futile gesture of power, but the opportunity had passed. The group reassured each other that the next time would be different.

Up to this point, no adult has any knowledge of what is unfolding between these groups of adolescent boys; no adult is available to intervene. But news of the near-violent encounter spread throughout their adolescent network, where such events take on huge proportions of social significance. Not a word is communicated to a parent, teacher, counselor, law enforcement agent, or an interested adult who can read the dangerous signs in a social exchange that contains such insignificant stakes.

The groups pass each other on the street above the subway station the next day. Once again, they greet each other with the same threatening stares, the same exchange of socially diminishing epithets, and the same gestural displays signifying the hidden presence of a gun. And once again, they pass each other and nothing happens, until something spurs John into action. Maybe it is a laugh or a word or a particular look by the rival group; or maybe it was something said within Michael's group that tips John into action. Or maybe it was just an internally cued precipitant, a feeling that another humiliation from passivity was more than he could bear. Suddenly, John ran across the street, yelling, "I'll show these . . . I'm not playing," and he withdrew the gun hidden in his waistband as he chased after them down the stairs, with Michael yelling after him, "shoot 'em . . . shoot 'em." John fired two shots at a boy who dies. The next day, John remarks to a friend, "I shot the wrong guy." He shot another boy in his own group.

John was the eldest of seven children in his family. He lived with his parents in a housing project a block from the subway station where the murder took place. His father worked as an insurance salesman but later took a job as a maintenance worker when he lost his job. At the time of John's arrest, his father had been unemployed for about a year, and this had become a significant hardship for the family. His mother worked in a family planning clinic, counseling young pregnant women and adolescents at risk for prenatal problems. She described herself as a "community mom," visiting young girls and their families in the community, preaching the need for regular prenatal care and a healthy lifestyle for expecting mothers.

She had an unremarkable pregnancy with John with no complications or problems. He had no significant early childhood problems, achieving all major developmental milestones on time. She described him as an easygoing baby with a good temperament. There was no history of any major problems in the family history of either of his parents—no mental illness, substance abuse, or criminality. John was relative easy to rear. He had a close relationship with his parents and siblings, though he tended to be competitive with his next oldest brother. John's parents were active members of their church and attended services regularly with their children. Recently, John had become resistant to attending services, a shift they mark as coinciding with his association with a negative peer group. They tried to break his connection with the group, but the more they pushed, the more he dug in.

John was consistently an average student in school and was never identified as a behavior problem. His academic performance did precipitously decline, however, when he entered high school. The falloff coincided with a number of events in his life—the switch to a high school curricula and setting; a temporary break in his parents' marriage because of his father's infidelity, which resulted in his father moving out during John's sophomore year of high school; and his growing affiliation with a delinquent peer group. During the period when his father was out of the home, John insisted that his absence did not have an effect on him, but his parents recall him becoming withdrawn and angry. During the interview, John discussed his loss of idealization of his father and his disidentification with him. His father's infidelity and drop in status from white-collar to blue-collar to unemployed worker affected him and placed distance between them. John no longer looked up to his father.

With his father out of the house, the rules and disciplinary structure around him loosened up. His social identity came to revolve around his developing peer group, who were involved in delinquent activities. He drifted away from his family and school. He began to encounter gang members with "big street reps" who were able to buy expensive clothing and jewelry, drive new cars, and attract a lot of girls. He became increasingly frustrated that his parents could not afford to buy these things for him, and he began to aspire to the easy lifestyle and high street status many of the gang members who dealt drugs were able to afford. He wanted these things for himself.

Despite his growing involvement in an antisocial lifestyle, he did not completely break away from his prosocial connections. He remained at home with his family, and, although his relationship with his parents was tense, he still generally obeyed them and respected most of their wishes, keeping his delinquent associations and activities to himself. He continued to attend church periodically, stayed in school, and remained an active basketball player. He also had some nondelinquent peers with whom he maintained a relationship when he was not hanging out with his negative peer group. He also had a girlfriend who was not part of his negative peer group and who actively encouraged him to dissociate himself from them.

In the end, these prosocial connections were not enough to separate John from his delinquent peers and his fatal shooting of an adolescent boy much like himself. The act functioned as a means to stave off a fate that, in his immature adolescent mind, was worse than death—to be regarded by his peers as weak, passive, and ineffectual. His act of violence arrived with no precedent in his life. He had no prior delinquent arrests and no prior instances of serious violence. The act, as significant and horrifying as it was, stands alone. John was not transferred to adult court but was convicted of second-degree murder and sentenced to 10 to 15 years in prison. He was released from prison in 2003 after serving nearly 10 years. He is currently married, employed, and is deeply involved in his church.

John's history is strongly indicative of an adolescent-limited pattern of juvenile offending. The report of his initial adult adjustment in the community is further confirmation of this. It is unfortunate, yet all too common, that intervention did not arrive to address the problems that had so suddenly and startlingly emerged during his adolescence. Hopefully, his being snagged in the criminal justice system for 10 years will not foreclose upon his ability to make a safe adult adjustment over the long run. Only time can determine whether one is an adolescent-limited offender.

THE TREATMENT OF VIOLENT JUVENILE OFFENDERS

The deterrence of violent criminal behavior perpetrated by juvenile offenders has become an increasingly important concern of both national health care and social policy agendas, largely due to the associated social and economic expenses that juvenile offending imposes on society (Borduin et al., 1995; Henggeler, Brondino, Melton, Scherer, & Hanley, 1997). Chronic youth offenders are at increased risk for mental health problems, interpersonal difficulties, substance abuse, and poor academic performance. Additionally, economic expenditures associated with law enforcement, maintenance of correctional facilities, and victimization have reached an unanticipated high (Henggeler et al., 1997).

The research literature on the assessment of the risk factors for juvenile offending has progressed much further than it has for their treatment and rehabilitation. Kazdin (1994) identified over 230 different types of treatment programs across the country for youthful offenders, ranging from programs in secure correctional institutions to small residential programs to boot camps and various wilderness programs. Few residential treatment programs have demonstrated robust effectiveness at reducing delinquent and violent behavior (Tarolla, Wagner, Rabinowitz, & Tubman, 2002; Zigler, Taussig, & Black, 1992).

Despite the paucity of programs with demonstrable treatment results, some meta-analyses and reviews of juvenile treatment programs have carried the field beyond the previously held adage that "nothing works" (Andrews et al., 1990; Cottle, Lee, & Heilbrun, 2001; Cullen & Gendreau, 1989; Garrett, 1985; Lipsey, 1999; Tate, Reppucci, & Mulvey, 1995). Unfortunately, most of the examinations of treatment effectiveness report mild to modest effectiveness at best (Lipsey & Wilson, 1998). The most effective programs are those that focus on young offenders where the inventions target criminological risks and psychosocial needs, do not mix juveniles with different levels of risk, incorporate the family into the treatment, utilize social skill training and cognitive-behavioral interventions, and are conducted in the community.

Many of the most popular and politically cherished interventions for juvenile offenders may produce negative effects that increase future delinquency. Among these is the range of shock incarceration programs such as juvenile boot camps and peer-led programs (U.S. Department of Health and Human Services, 2001). Generally, treatment programs that aggregate high-risk juveniles in a residential program produce the most significant iatrogenic effects. Juveniles may be more likely to model antisocial behavior displayed to them within such settings than the targeted skills that are the intended intervention of the therapists. In a process labeled "deviance training" by Dishion, McCord, and Poulin (1999), juvenile offenders, particularly younger ones, may be differentially reinforced for increased delinquent behavior by older, more sophisticated peers who set the norm or the standard for what is considered status-enhancing behavior within the program.

Grounded by ecological and systems theories, multisystemic therapy (MST) conceptualizes antisocial youth behavior as multidetermined, the product of an interplay of interdependent social and psychological systems (Borduin et al., 1995). Bronfenbrenner's (1979) theory of social ecology provides the theoretical foundation from which multisystemic therapy is constructed (Swenson, Henggeler, Schoenwald, Kaufman, & Randall, 1998). From this perspective, individuals are viewed as members of interconnected systems (i.e., family, peer, community), and antisocial behavior is sustained by transactions within or between any combinations of these systems (Swenson et al., 1998). The fundamental principles of MST relate to the identification of problem behavior and the determination of its role within the juvenile's social ecology (Henggeler, Schoenwald, & Pickrel, 1995).

MST is implemented in a home-based service model, removing barriers to service access and increasing treatment engagement (Henggeler, Pickrel, Brondino, & Crouch, 1996; Swenson et al., 1998). Therapeutic interventions are most commonly provided by master's-level therapists in a school, home, church, or other community setting. Due to the therapeutic requirements of interventions (i.e., intense, frequent contact and around-the-clock availability), therapists are required to carry small caseloads (about four to six) at one time (Swenson et al., 1998). Services are time limited, averaging 60 hours of direct service over a 3- to 6-month period, a model successful at engaging and maintaining family involvement. Clinical examinations of MST discovered that 98% of juveniles and their families randomly assigned to MST conditions completed treatment (Henggeler et al., 1996).

The primary goal of MST is to empower families while simultaneously identifying and effectively resolving the problems presented by youths. The aim is to cultivate an environment in which primary caregivers are able to recognize potential problems (both current and impending) and act as a catalyst for change (Henggeler et al., 1995).

Initial therapy sessions identify the strengths and weaknesses of the offender, the family, and their interplay with other ecological systems (i.e., school, peers). The therapist and family collectively decide which problematic behaviors will be identified and the intended therapeutic goals (Swenson et al., 1998). To address each identified problem, an eclectic approach is embraced as modalities with substantiated empirical support are integrated as necessary. Ultimately, MST interventions are adapted from pragmatic, problem-focused treatments, including family therapy, cognitive-behavioral therapies, and behavioral parent training (Swenson et al., 1998). Additionally, psychopharmacological interventions are implemented if biological determinants are identified.

The evaluation of outcome studies has been an integral component in the development of MST (Curtis, Ronan, & Borduin, 2004). Currently, MST is recognized as one of the most well-validated interventions for juvenile delinquency by organizations such as the U.S. Department of Health and Human Services (2001) and the National Institute on Drug Abuse (1999). Such validation is based on the findings of six published outcome studies of youthful offenders and their families (Sheidow & Henggeler, 1995).

The first outcome study (Henggeler et al., 1986) implemented a quasi-experimental design to evaluate the short-term effectiveness of an MST intervention with juvenile offenders. MST was determined more effective than classic treatment at minimizing target problem behavior and association with deviant peers while concurrently increasing positive family relations. These encouraging findings led to three subsequent randomized trials of MST with both violent and chronic juvenile offenders (Borduin et al., 1995; Henggeler, Melton, & Smith, 1992; Henggeler, Melton, Smith, Schoenwald, & Hanley, 1993). Henggeler, Melton, and Smith (1992) discovered that MST interventions were more effective than typical juvenile justice services at increasing family and peer systems as well as reducing recidivism by 43% and out-of-home placement by 64% at a 59-week follow-up. Henggeler and colleagues (1993) determined that MST interventions doubled the survival rate (i.e., juveniles not rearrested) of serious offenders at a 2.4-year follow-up. Similarly, Borduin and colleagues (1995) discovered that MST, when compared to individual counseling, improved family functioning and decreased psychiatric symptomatology and recidivism at a 4-year follow-up. Henggeler et al. (1997) found that MST was more successful at decreasing juvenile psychiatric symptomatology at posttreatment than usual juvenile justice services, yielding a 50% reduction in incarceration rates at a 1.7-year follow-up. Interestingly, analyses showed significant associations between therapist adherence to MST treatment principles and reductions in recidivism rates. Finally, Henggeler, Pickrel, and Brondino (1999) examined the effectiveness of MST interventions on juvenile offenders meeting the diagnostic criteria for substance abuse or dependence. When compared to usual community services, MST showed decreased drug use at posttreatment as well as a 26% reduction in recidivism at 1-year follow-up.

Overall, outcomes studies have demonstrated reductions in rates of recidivism (from 26% to 69%) across studies of youthful offenders assigned to MST conditions when compared to treated control groups. These findings clearly demonstrate the ability of MST to identify and modify determinants of antisocial behavior embedded in an adolescent's social ecology as well as reduce rearrest and out-of-home placements for juvenile offenders.

REFERENCES

Achenbach, T. M. (1993). Taxonomy and comorbidity of conduct problems: Evidence from empirically based approaches. *Development and Psychopathology, 5*, 51–64.

American Psychiatric Association. (1980). *Diagnostic and statistical manual of mental disorders* (3rd ed.). Washington, DC: Author.

American Psychiatric Association. (1987). *Diagnostic and statistical manual of mental disorders* (3rd ed., rev.). Washington, DC: Author.

American Psychiatric Association. (1994). *Diagnostic and statistical manual of mental disorders* (4th ed.). Washington, DC: Author.

American Psychiatric Association. (2004). *Diagnostic and statistical manual of mental disorders* (4th ed., text revision). Washington, D.C: Author.

Andersson, T., Magnusson, D., & Wennberg, P. (1997). Early aggressiveness and hyperactivity as indicators of adult alcohol problems and criminality: A prospective longitudinal study of male subjects. *Studies on Crime and Crime Prevention, 6*, 7–20.

Andrews, D. A., Zinger, I., Hoge, R. D., Bonta, J., Gendreau., P., & Cullen, F. T. (1990). Does correctional treatment work? A clinically relevant and psychologically informed meta-analysis. *Criminology, 28*, 369–404.

August, G. J., Realmuto, G. M., MacDonald, A. W., Nugent, S. M., & Crosby, R. (1996). Prevalence of ADHD and comorbid disorders among elementary school children screened for disruptive behavior. *Journal of Abnormal Child Psychology, 24*, 555–569.

Ayers, W. (1997/1998). The criminalization of youth: Politicians promote "lock 'em up" mentality. *Rethinking Schools, 12*(2), 1–16.

Barkley, R. A. (1998). *Attention-deficit hyperactivity disorder: A handbook for diagnosis and treatment*. New York: Guilford Press.

Barkley, R. A., DuPaul, G. J., & McMurray, M. B. (1990). A comprehensive evaluation of attention deficit disorder with and without hyperactivity defined by research criteria. *Journal of Consulting and Clinical Psychology, 58*, 775–789.

Best, J. (2001). *Damned lies and statistics: Untangling numbers from the media, politicians, and activists*. Berkeley: University of California Press.

Borduin, C. M., Mann, J. J., Cone, L. T., Henggeler, S. W. Fucci, B. R., Blaske, D. M., et al. (1995). Multisystemic treatment of serious juvenile offenders: Long-term prevention of criminality and violence. *Journal of Consulting and Clinical Psychology, 63*, 569–578.

Borum, R., & Verhaagen, D. (2006). *Assessing and managing violence risk in juveniles.* New York: Guilford Press.

Bronfenbrenner, U. (1979). *The ecology of human development: Experiments by design and nature.* Cambridge, MA: Harvard University Press.

Connor, D. (2002). *Aggression and antisocial behavior in children and adolescents: Research and treatment.* New York: Guilford Press.

Cottle, C., Lee, R., & Heilbrun, K. (2001). The prediction of criminal recidivism in juveniles: A meta-analysis. *Criminal Justice and Behavior, 28,* 367–394.

Cullen, F. T., & Gendreau, P. (1989). The effectiveness of correctional rehabilitation: Reconsidering the "nothing works" debate. In L. Goodstein & D. MacKenzie (Eds.), *The American prison: Issues in research and policy* (pp. 23–44). New York: Plenum Press.

Curtis, N. M., Ronan, K. R., & Borduin, C. M. (2004). Multisystemic treatment: A meta-analysis of outcome studies. *Journal of Family Psychology, 18,* 411–419.

Dawson, G. E. (1896). A study of youthful degeneracy. *Pedagogical Seminary, 4,* 221–258.

DiIulio, J. (1995, November 27). The coming of the super-predators. *Weekly Standard,* p. 23.

Dishion, T. J., McCord, J., & Poulin, F. (1999). When interventions harm: Peer groups and problem behavior. *American Psychologist, 54,* 755–764.

Elliot, D., Huizinga, D., & Morse, B. (1986). Self-reported violent offending. *Journal of Interpersonal Violence, 1,* 141–155.

Fox, J. (1996). *Trends in juvenile violence: A report to the United States attorney general on current and future rates of juvenile offending.* Boston: Northeastern University Press.

Garrett, C. J. (1985). Effects of residential treatment of adjudicated delinquents: A meta-analysis. *Journal of Research in Crime and Delinquency, 22,* 287–308.

Giedd, J., Blumenthal, J., Jeffries, N., Castellanos, F., Liu, H., Zikdenbos, A., et al. (1999). Brain development during childhood and adolescence: A longitudinal MRI study. *Nature Neuroscience, 2,* 861–863.

Glassner, B. (1999). *The culture of fear: Why Americans are afraid of the wrong things.* New York: Basic Books.

Grisso, T. (2004). *Double jeopardy: Adolescent offenders with mental disorders.* Chicago: University of Chicago Press.

Hall, G. S. (1907). *Adolescence: Its psychology and its relations to physiology, anthropology, sociology, sex, crime, religion, and education* (Vols. 1–2). New York: D. Appleton.

Henggeler, S. W., Brondino, M. J., Melton, G. B., Scherer, D. G., & Hanley, J. H. (1997). Multisystemic therapy with violent and chronic juvenile offenders and their families: The role of treatment fidelity in successful dissemination. *Journal of Consulting and Clinical Psychology, 65,* 821–833.

Henggeler, S. W., Melton, G. B., & Smith, L. A. (1992). Family preservation using multisystemic therapy: An effective alternative to incarcerating serious juvenile offenders. *Journal of Consulting and Clinical Psychology, 60,* 953–961.

Henggeler, S. W., Melton, G. B., Smith, L. A., Schoenwald, S. K., & Hanley, J. (1993). Family preservation using multisystemic therapy: Long-term follow-up to a clinical trial with serious juvenile offenders. *Journal of Child and Family Services, 2,* 283–293.

Henggeler, S. W., Pickrel, S. G., & Brondino, M. J. (1999). Multisystemic treatment of substance abusing and dependent delinquents: Outcomes, treatment fidelity, and transportability. *Mental Health Services Research, 1,* 171–184.

Henggeler, S. W., Pickrel, S. G., Brondino, M. J., & Crouch, J. L. (1996). Eliminating (almost) treatment dropout of substance abusing or dependent delinquents through home-based Multisystemic Treatment. *American Journal of Psychiatry, 153,* 427–428.

Henggeler, S. W., Rodick, J. D., Borduin, C. M., Hanson, C. L., Watson, S. M., & Urey, J. R. (1986). Multisystemic treatment of juvenile offenders: Effects on adolescent behavior and family interaction. *Developmental Psychology, 22,* 132–141.

Henggeler, S. W., Schoenwald, S. K., & Pickrel, S. G. (1995). Multisystemic therapy: Bridging the gap between university and community-based treatment. *Journal of Consulting and Clinical Psychology, 63,* 709–717.

Kappeler, V. E., Blumberg, M., & Potter, G. W. (2000). *The mythology of crime and criminal justice* (3rd ed.). Prospect Heights, IL: Waveland Press.

Kashani, J. H., Orvaschel, H., Rosenberg, T. K., & Reid, J. C. (1989). Psychopathology in a community sample of children and adolescents: A developmental perspective. *Journal of the American Academy of Child and Adolescent Psychiatry, 28,* 701–706.

Kazdin, A. E. (1994). Psychotherapy for children and adolescents. In A. E. Bergin & S.O. Garfield (Eds.), *Handbook of psychotherapy and behavior change* (4th ed., pp. 543–594). New York: Wiley.

Kazdin, A. E. (1995). *Conduct disorders in childhood and adolescence* (2nd ed.). Thousand Oaks, CA: Sage.

Kratzer, L., & Hodgins, S. (1997). Adult outcomes of child conduct problems: A cohort study. *Journal of Abnormal Child Psychology, 25,* 65–81.

Lipsey, M. W. (1999). Can intervention rehabilitate serious delinquents? *Annals for the American Academy of Political and Social Science, 564,* 142–166.

Lipsey, M. W., & Wilson, D. B. (1998). Effective interventions with serious juvenile offenders: A synthesis of research. In R. Loeber & D. P. Farrington (Eds.), *Serious and violent juvenile offenders: Risk factors and successful intervention* (pp. 313–345). Thousand Oaks, CA: Sage.

Loeber, R., Burke, J., & Lahey, B. (2002). What are adolescent antecedents to antisocial personality disorder? *Criminal Behavior and Mental Health, 12,* 24–36.

Lombroso, C. (1876). *Criminal man.* Paris: F. Alcan.

Moeller, T. G. (2001). *Youth aggression and violence: A psychological approach.* Mahwah, NJ: Lawrence Erlbaum.

Moffitt, T. E. (1993). Adolescent-limited and life-course-persistent antisocial behavior: A developmental taxonomy. *Psychological Reviews, 100,* 674–701.

Moffitt, T. E. (2003). Life-course persistent and adolescent-limited antisocial behavior: A 10-year research review and a research agenda. In B. B. Lahey, T. E. Moffitt, & A. Caspi (Eds.), *Causes of conduct disorder and juvenile delinquency* (pp. 49–75). New York: Guilford Press.

Moffit, T. E., & Caspi, A. (2001). Childhood predictors differentiate life-course persistent and adolescent-limited pathways among males and females. *Development and Psychopathology, 13,* 355–375.

Moffitt, T. E., Caspi, A., Dickson, N., Silva, P. A., & Stanton, W. (1996). Childhood-onset versus adolescent-onset antisocial conduct in males: Natural history from ages 3 to 18. *Development and Psychopathology, 8,* 399–424.

Moffitt, T. E., Caspi, A., Harrington, H., & Milne, B. (2002). Males on the life-course persistent and adolescent-onset antisocial pathways: Follow-up at age 26. *Development and Psychopathology, 14,* 179–206.
Monahan, J. (1981). *Predicting violent behavior: An assessment of clinical techniques.* Troy, NY: Sage Press.
Morrison, W. D. (1896). *Juvenile offenders.* London: T. Fisher Unwin.
National Institute on Drug Abuse. (1999). *Principles of drug addiction treatment: A research-based guide* (NIH Publication No. 99–4180). Rockville, MD: U.S. Department of Health and Human Services, National Institutes of Health, Author.
Sampson, R. J., & Laub, J. H. (1993). *Crime in the making: Pathways and turning points through life.* Cambridge, MA: Harvard University Press.
Sheidow, A. J., & Henggeler, S. W. (2005). Community-based treatments. In K. Heilbrun, N. E. Sevin Goldstein, & R. E. Redding (Eds.), *Juvenile delinquency: Prevention, assessment, and intervention* (pp. 257–281). New York: Oxford University Press.
Sheldon, W. H., Hartl, E. M., & McDermott, E. (1949). *Varieties of delinquent youth: An introduction to constitutional psychiatry.* New York: Harper & Brothers.
Snyder, H. N., & Sickmund, M. (2006). *Juvenile offenders and victims: 2006 national report.* Washington, DC: U.S. Department of Justice, Office of Justice Programs, Office of Juvenile Justice and Delinquency Programs.
Swenson, C. C., Henggeler, S. W., Schoenwald, S. K., Kaufman, K. L., & Randall, J. (1998). Changing the social ecologies of adolescent sexual offenders: Implications of the success of multisystemic therapy in treating serious antisocial behavior in adolescents. *Child Maltreatment, 3,* 330–338.
Tarolla, S. M., Wagner, E. F., Rabinowitz, J., & Tubman, J. G. (2002). Understanding and treating juvenile offenders: A review of current knowledge and future directions. *Aggression and Violent Behavior, 7,* 125–143.
Tate, D. C., Reppucci, N. D., & Mulvey, E. (1995). Violent juvenile delinquents: Treatment, efficacy and implications for future action. *American Psychologist, 50,* 777–785.
Teplin, L., Abram, K., McClelland, G., Dulcan, M., & Mericle, A. (2002). Psychiatric disorders in youth in juvenile detention. *Archives of General Psychiatry, 59,* 1133–1143.
U.S. Department of Health and Human Services. (2001). *Youth violence: A report of the surgeon general.* Rockville, MD: U.S. Department of Health and Human Services, Substance Abuse and Mental Health Services Administration, Center for Mental Health Services, National Institutes of Health, National Institute of Mental Health.
Vermeiren, R. (2003). Psychopathology and delinquency in adolescents: A descriptive and developmental perspective. *Clinical Psychology Previews, 23,* 277–318.
Vitelli, R. (1996). Prevalence of childhood conduct and attention-deficit hyperactivity disorders in adult maximum-security inmates. *International Journal of Offender Therapy & Comparative Criminology, 40,* 263–271.
Waschbusch, D. A., & King, S. (2006). Should sex-specific norms be used to assess attention-deficit/hyperactivity disorder or oppositional defiant disorder? *Journal of Consulting Psychology, 74,* 179–185.
Wasserman, G. A., Ko, S. J., & McReynolds, L. S. (2004). *Assessing the mental health status of youth in juvenile justice settings* (Office of Juvenile Justice and Delinquency

Prevention Bulletin N. NCJ 202713). Washington, DC: Office of Juvenile Justice and Delinquency Prevention.

Zigler, E., Taussig, C., & Black, K. (1992). Early childhood intervention: A promising prevention for juvenile delinquency. *American Psychologist, 1,* 997–1006.

Zimring, F. (1998). *American youth violence.* New York: Oxford University Press.

Zimring, F. (2005). *American juvenile justice.* New York: Oxford University Press.

Zimring, F., & Fagan, J. (2000). Transfer policy and law reform. In J. Fagan & F. Zimring (Eds.), *The changing borders of juvenile justice* (pp. 407–424). Chicago: University of Chicago Press.

12

Risk/Needs Tools for Antisocial Behavior and Violence Among Youthful Populations

GINA M. VINCENT, ANNA M. TERRY,
AND SHANNON M. MANEY

RISK FOR RECIDIVISM SCREENING AND ASSESSMENT TOOLS FOR YOUTHFUL POPULATIONS

Assessments of the likelihood of future violence or serious delinquency are relevant for a variety of legal decisions in the juvenile justice system. Juvenile justice officials are routinely expected to make decisions involving the handling of youth who come into contact with the law at various points in the system. These decisions generally involve determinations of which youths pose a threat to public safety, which youths are likely to benefit from interventions, and which interventions are most likely to result in a positive change (Fagan & Zimring, 2000; Mulvey, 2005). Likewise, forensic clinicians often are asked to conduct specialized assessments of delinquents' likelihood of future harm to others (Grisso, 1998). For both clinicians and juvenile justice personnel, the need for performing some form of a risk assessment is a result of the juvenile justice system's obligation to protect public safety. As Grisso (2004) explained, this obligation functions to protect society from the immediate risk of harm from dangerous youth and functions to reduce recidivism by providing interventions to youths involved with the juvenile justice system. Arguably, the most dangerous youths should receive the most punitive sanctions and the most intensive interventions. To ensure treatment is done right, offenders must first be properly assessed to identify their risk level and treatment needs (Austin, 2006; Grisso, 2005a; Skowrya & Cocozza, 2007).

Aside from clinical assessments, in the past couple of decades there has been a push in juvenile justice for systems to adopt some form of structured decision making in an effort to increase the consistency and accuracy of risk assessments (e.g., Gottfredson & Tonry, 1988; Guarino-Ghezzi & Bryne, 1989). Structured decision making should incorporate findings from the social sciences about the factors that place youths at highest risk for reoffending. This is one of the factors that influenced the creation of a different class of risk assessment tools for youth—that is, tools that do not require psychological or social work training. These standardized risk assessment tools can be completed by nonclinical staff such as case managers, probation officers, and other juvenile justice personnel (Hoge, 2002). Such tools were designed to make recommendations to the court regarding appropriate sanctions and interventions in a structured, unbiased manner.

Although the notion of implementing risk for recidivism assessment tools on the surface seems like it would increase the consistency and validity of decision making, these tools could have deleterious effects if used improperly or if the tools themselves are invalid. Thus, it is important to understand some key issues related to youth risk assessment when making decisions about which tool (or tools) to use. To make informed decisions about the selection and use of risk assessment tools for youth, familiarity with the prominent issues in this area is critical, including approaches to decision making, developmental malleability and desistance, the nature of risk factors, reliability and validity, and the characteristics of instruments.

This chapter reviews the screening and assessment tools used to determine risk for recidivism among juveniles. The chapter begins by laying the foundation for the important concepts involved in selecting appropriate risk assessment tools. This is followed by a comprehensive review of the instruments available for assessing recidivism or violence risk among youth, including the details about reliability and validity. The chapter concludes with recommendations and cautions concerning the use of risk assessment tools with youth and a discussion of areas in dire need of further study.

DEFINING RISK ASSESSMENT WITH YOUTH

Consistent themes in many placement decisions in the juvenile justice system are risk for recidivism and treatment or service needs. The goal of risk assessment is to target those youth in greatest need of rehabilitation efforts and intensive risk management (Borum & Verhaagen, 2006; Mulvey, 2005). Thus, staff examiners and clinical evaluators require tools capable of assessing both the likelihood of a youth's risk to public safety in the future and the needs of youths that should be addressed in order to reduce a youth's risk. There is a distinction between *risk factors* (risk indicators that are likely to have a causal link to the antisocial behavior that, if changed, could reduce the likelihood of the negative outcome; Kraemer et al., 1997; Mulvey, 2005) and *risk markers* (risk indicators that are associated with later antisocial behavior but may not actually cause the antisocial behavior and do not guide treatment; such as age of first offense). Tools that contain actual risk factors are often referred to as *risk/needs instruments* in juvenile justice settings.

It is important to recognize that risk assessment tools differ in the way they define risk. Some were designed to identify risk for recidivism, meaning a rearrest for any type of offense. Other tools were designed to identify risk for violence specifically, which is commonly defined as the actual, attempted, or threatened physical harm of another person that is deliberate and nonconsensual (Webster, Douglas, Eaves, & Hart, 1997). Finally, some tools were designed to identify risk for antisocial behavior or conduct problems more generally. With respect to all of these areas of risk, some tools were intended to evaluate short-term risk or risk in the near future, whereas other tools were intended to evaluate longer-term risk. Staff or clinical examiners should pay particular attention to these differences when selecting a tool. However, as will be evident later in this chapter when we review the research evidence for specific tools, most tools designed to assess risk for violence also are able to predict recidivism generally. Likewise, tools designed to assess risk for antisocial behavior often are also good predictors of recidivism.

Relevance of the Decision Point

Risk assessments—or almost any screening and assessment methods, for that matter—should be tied to a particular decision point, meaning, in this case, a point in the juvenile justice decision-making process (Grisso, 2005b; Mulvey, 2005). The decision point should have a large impact on the type of assessment that is needed and the resources and amount of information that are available to conduct the assessment. There has been some variability in defining what these assessment points are. Grisso (2005b) elucidated five entry points to, or "doorways" through which youths pass in the juvenile justice process. Skowyra and Cocozza (2007) listed six critical decision points in their Blueprint for Change monograph (supported by the Office of Juvenile Justice and Delinquency Prevention). For our purposes, we categorize the relevant decision points as follows: (1) intake probation or juvenile court intake, (2) pretrial detention, (3) judicial processing, (4) disposition, (5) juvenile corrections assessment centers, and (6) community reentry.

Different decision points are associated with different questions. At intake, for example, the question may be whether the youth is appropriate for diversion from the juvenile justice system. At detention, the primary question is whether the youth needs secure pretrial detention in the short period between detention and adjudication in order to prevent recidivism and to ensure the youth appears in court. With respect to judicial processing, the question might regard waiver to adult court or transfer back to juvenile court. At disposition, several questions are relevant, including the appropriate placement (community or custody), security level, and subsequent treatment or service plans for the youth. Disposition decisions require the court to consider both the most appropriate sanctions and interventions with the best potential for reducing the likelihood of delinquent behaviors in the future (Grisso, 2005a). Community reentry or aftercare planning can benefit from risk assessment to determine the essential level of monitoring and interventions for the youth while in the community.

Another consideration is variability in the validation requirements of tools across decision points. As Mulvey (2005) noted, risk assessment instruments must be developed and validated with the requirements of a particular prediction task in mind. For example, the population of youths facing possible pretrial detention will be somewhat different than the population of youths facing a disposition decision, which are those recently found guilty of a crime. Different factors may have different associations with recidivism for these different groups of youth. However, this is probably more of an issue for tools designed specifically to sort youths into low- versus high-risk categories based on empirical associations between risk variables and recidivism. This may be less of an issue when using risk/needs assessments that contain actual risk/needs factors and that were designed to guide interventions regardless of the decision point.

Approaches or Frameworks to Risk Assessment

There is some variability across social science disciplines (i.e., psychology, criminology, social work) and across human service agencies (e.g., juvenile justice systems, child welfare systems, adult criminal justice system) in the terms used to categorize types of decision making. Nonetheless, the approaches to risk assessment generally will fall into one of three categories: clinical, actuarial, or structured professional judgment.

Clinical Judgment

Clinical or human judgment generally refers to unstructured assessments where risk variables are not necessarily explicit, may not be empirically validated, and demonstrate little value in the prediction of recidivism. Decision makers generally rely on intuition to make a decision about the likelihood of a youth reoffending. Similarly, they may rely on intuition yet follow some sort of semistructured system that identifies some variables to consider based on consensus judgments (Baird & Wagner, 2000). Reviews of the psychological research demonstrated that, when mental health professionals use either approach to make specific predictions about a client (the client will or will not be violent), they will likely be accurate in no more than one-third of cases (Grisso & Tomkins, 1996; Monahan, 1981, 1996; Rubin, 1972). Similarly, studies of child welfare workers also found little consistency in decisions related to need for foster care or hospitalization when using clinical judgment approaches (Rossi, Schuerman, & Budde, 1999). One of the reasons for the inconsistencies is the inherent biases that can be introduced in these subjective decision-making models (Schwalbe, 2004). Another reason, at least with respect to mental health professionals, was the tendency toward dichotomous (yes or no) decision making.

Actuarial Decision Making

Actuarial decision making is mechanical and "involves a formal, algorithmic, objective procedure (e.g., equation) to reach the decision" (Grove & Meehl, 1996, p. 293). Actuarial assessments generally contain items selected empirically, based on a known association with a given outcome (reoccurrence of violence), and are scored according to some algorithm to produce a judgment about the likelihood of violence or recidivism. Due to the consistency and predictive validity of actuarial tools, several researchers have argued persuasively for the superiority of actuarial decision making to estimate the likelihood of future violence or recidivism in the criminal justice system (Quinsey, Harris, Rice, & Cormier, 1998) and the likelihood of child abuse and neglect in the child protection system (Baird & Wagner, 2000).

Despite the ostensible statistical superiority of actuarial tools, several critics have pointed out the limitations of actuarial assessments and the dangers of over-reliance on actuarial decision making (Berlin, Galbreath, Geary, & McGlone, 2003; Borum, 1996; Dvoskin & Heilbrun, 2001; Grisso, 2000; Hart, 2003; Hart et al., 2003). First, actuarial tools have limited clinical utility. A consequence of the empirical test construction methods is that many risk factors make little sense theoretically or clinically. Consequently, assessment procedures are not tied to intervention strategies in a prescriptive manner. Second, actuarial measures are of little value when it comes to understanding the etiology of antisocial behavior and violence due to overemphasis on the effect of variables (the variable's statistical association with later offending), rather than the meaning of variables (Grubin & Wingate, 1996).

Another primary concern is that actuarial tools often make exclusive use of static variables, which, by definition, cannot measure changes in risk and provide little guidance for risk management. Grisso (2000) referred to this problem as the "tyranny of static variables," arguing that, if actuarial instruments are the sole clinical criterion for release decisions, then "examinees will be doomed to perpetual commitment because they will always achieve the same score." This is particularly problematic when assessing youth, a group for which we would expect risk to change over time. Finally, since only a few factors can be included in any one actuarial measure (Boer, Hart, Kropp, & Webster, 1997), factors that are idiosyncratic to an examinee do not enter assessments of risk regardless of their relevance to a specific case, a potential hindrance to generalizability.

Structured Professional Judgment

In light of the above concerns and in response to the limitations of current practices, scholars created a third approach to risk judgments, known as structured professional judgment (SPJ). Structured professional risk assessment tools are informed by the state of the discipline in clinical theory and empirical research to guide clinical decisions about risk and treatment planning. The intent was to improve human judgment by adding structure and improve actuarial decision making by adding some rater discretion. The SPJ model draws on the strengths of both the clinical and actuarial (formula-driven) approaches to decision making and attempts to minimize their respective drawbacks (Borum & Douglas, 2003). These instruments emphasize prevention rather than prediction. They typically contain both static and dynamic risk factors because they assume that risk is not entirely stable and can change as a result of various factors such as treatment quality and quantity, developmental factors, protective factors, and context. SPJ assessment tools are designed to guide examiners to determine what level of risk management is needed, in which contexts, and at what points in time. An increasing body of literature with adult populations suggests SPJ-based decisions about risk have incremental predictive validity to actuarial-based decisions (Douglas, Yeoman, & Boer, 2005).

Scholars have produced a few risk assessment schemes for youth using an SPJ approach, one such tool is the Structured Assessment of Violence Risk for Youth (SAVRY) (Borum, Bartel, & Forth, 2003). Based on their design, one would expect these tools to be capable of assessing increases and reductions in risk as long as evaluators conduct periodic reassessments; however, the ability to measure change has rarely been demonstrated empirically. Nonetheless, these tools provide a structured framework for evaluators to base their conclusions about a youth's risk for delinquency and the best practices for managing that risk.

SPECIAL CONSIDERATIONS WHEN ASSESSING RISK IN YOUTH

Generally, assessors will want to use risk assessment tools with known predictive validity that also are capable of guiding intervention and treatment planning as well as capturing changes in risk. Preference should be given to tools that are based on a developmental model and empirical evidence from the social science research about the factors that place youths at increased risk for antisocial behavior. This section briefly describes some of the prominent issues in this area.

Violent and Delinquent Behavior Will Desist for Most Youths

Several well-known longitudinal studies have mapped trajectories to serious delinquent offending (Farrington & West, 1993; Loeber,

Burke, & Lahey, 2002; Moffitt & Caspi, 2001; Moffitt, Caspi, Dickson, Silva, & Stanton, 1996; Roberts, Caspi, & Moffitt, 2001). These researchers, using large samples of young people, identified two relatively distinct pathways to serious adult offending: one group that begins criminal behavior during adolescence and desists around early adulthood (i.e., adolescent-limited or late-onset offenders) and another more deviant group that begins in childhood and persists throughout life (i.e., life-course persistent or early-onset offenders; Moffitt, 1993; Patterson, Forgatch, Yoerger, & Stoolmiller, 1998).[1] One of these studies was the Cambridge Study of Delinquent Development, which followed 411 boys from childhood to age 40 (Farrington, Barnes, & Lambert, 1996; West & Farrington, 1973). Almost 40% of these males were convicted of at least one criminal offense by age 32 (Farrington, 1992), but a mere 6% of them were responsible for half of all the officially reported crime (Farrington & West, 1993). Similarly, studies from the Dunedin sample in New Zealand found that 7% of males tracked from ages 3 to 18 appeared to be on the persistent or chronic offender trajectory, whereas 23% were on the adolescent-limited trajectory. Over the life span, the chronic offenders committed large numbers of offenses at high rates over long periods of time, tended to begin their criminal careers at the earliest ages, and were generally versatile and violent in their offending.

The point taken from this research is that, for the majority of adolescents who commit offenses, the behavior will desist in late adolescence or early adulthood. By desistance we mean the termination of offending. As noted by Farrington (2007), the policy implications include educating juvenile justice decision makers about desistance because it may be a waste of scarce prison resources to lock up these youths. Greenwood and Abrahamse (1982) suggested that secure custody be used selectively for only offenders that are predicted to be the most persistent and serious in their offending. The implication for risk assessment is that preference should be given to instruments that have been developed based on knowledge of the predictors of chronic and serious offending versus termination of offending (Farrington, 2007). The different pathways have different predictors. For example, early initiation of offending is strongly associated with impulsivity, attention deficit/hyperactivity symptoms (Loeber, Lahey, & Thomas, 1991), neuropsychological deficits, and difficult temperaments (Moffitt & Caspi, 2001). Late-onset, adolescent-limited offending is strongly associated with having delinquent peers, a personality trait referred to as social potency (Moffitt et al., 1996), and a tendency toward only nonviolent offending.

Risk Can Change Across Adolescence

Another crucial concept for assessments of risk for violence and serious offending among youth is the impact of developmental factors on the time frame for which predictions remain accurate. A significant limitation with attempts to identify those youth who will become chronic and violent offenders is the inevitable high false positive rate. Many youth who engage in violent behavior at one stage of development do not continue to do so as their development proceeds. Indeed, at least 50% of children who initiate pervasive and serious antisocial behavior between ages 6 and 12 do not develop into seriously antisocial adults (Patterson et al., 1998; Robins, 1974), and an even greater portion of serious offending adolescents do not develop into antisocial adults (Moffitt & Caspi, 2001). The National Youth Survey (Elliott, Huizinga, & Menard, 1989) found that, for about 50% of youths, violent behavior persisted into adulthood if their first violent acts occurred before age 11, about 30% persisted if their violence started between ages 11 and 13, and about 10% persisted if their first violent acts occurred in adolescence. Taken as a whole, the research indicates that even the most extreme youth who engage in violence or serious antisociality at a young age have only a 50–50 chance of persisting. A reasonable interpretation of these studies is that, if we simply use current violent behavior (regardless of the age of onset) as a predictor of violence in the future, we will be wrong more often than we are right. If we use the age of onset of this behavior as the sole criterion, our accuracy will be better, but still not dramatically better than chance.

As Mulvey (2005) noted, evaluating risk requires consideration of the developmental stage and social context. Different risk indicators at different ages mean different things (Odgers, Vincent, & Corrado, 2002). For example, smoking prior to age 12 is a significant risk factor, but smoking at age 15 when experimentation is a normal part of development is not a risk factor. Risk for violence/recidivism should be reassessed frequently, particularly for younger youth under age 16, and preference should be given to assessment tools that appear to be capable of measuring changes in risk. This means they should contain dynamic factors, and any policies for implementing risk assessments in a juvenile delinquency context should include procedures for reassessments.

Many Evidence-Based Risk Factors Exist

Many evidence-based risk factors for violence and recidivism exist. Some of these risk factors include: prior history of violence, early initiation of violence, school achievement problems, abuse, maltreatment and neglect, substance use problems, impulsivity, negative peer relationships, and community crime and violence (Borum & Verhaagen, 2006). These factors are discussed in more detail in other chapters, so they will not be covered here; however, two additional risk factors, mental disorder and history of self-harm, warrant further discussion.

Mental Disorder

Although many youth with mental disorders do not engage in violent behavior, it does appear that mental disorders can add to a youth's potential for violence (Borum & Verhaagen, 2006). Further, youth diagnosed with multiple disorders may be at greater risk for general criminal behavior than youth who are not diagnosed with comorbid disorders (Copeland, Miller-Johnson, Keeler, Angold, & Costello, 2007). The high rates of youth with one or more mental disorders in the juvenile justice system (approximately 60% of male and 70% of female juvenile detainees; Teplin, Abram, McClelland, Dulcan, & Mericle, 2002) imply that there is some relation between mental disorder and offending. Many of these youth have sequential or simultaneous involvement in mental health and juvenile justice systems (Cauffman, Scholle, Mulvey, & Kelleher, 2005).

There are many potential explanations for this relation between mental disorder and offending. A full discussion is outside of the scope of this chapter. But, briefly, some child and adolescent mental disorders may be causally connected to violence and antisocial behavior (see Vincent & Grisso, 2005, for a review): mainly, disruptive behavior disorders, psychopathic traits, and occasionally mood and psychotic disorders. In a complex analysis of longitudinal data, Copeland et al. (2007) reported that 19.5% of adult crime among women and 28.7% of crime among men was attributable to childhood psychiatric disorders. In other cases, however, child and adolescent disorders may not be connected to actual offending behavior. Instead, youths with mental health problems may simply have found themselves involved with the juvenile justice system because it was the only way to get mental health services. The youth literature in this area lags far behind the adult research. Research is needed to disentangle this relationship. In the meantime, however, in many cases it will be important to address the connection between psychopathology and risk as a component of youth risk assessment.

Histories of Self-Harm

Although the link between interpersonal violence and self-harm has long been recognized, organized and systematic efforts to understand the relationship between the two and to develop appropriate integrated interventions have not yet been undertaken (Lubell & Vetter, 2006). Research suggests that current perpetrators of interpersonal violence may be more likely to have a history of current and past suicidal behaviors rather than having a history of interpersonal violence (Lubell & Vetter, 2006). Delinquent adolescents are about five times as likely to seriously consider suicide, almost five times as likely to have a suicide plan, and about ten times as likely to have attempted suicide than their nondelinquent peers (Thompson, Kingree, & Ho, 2006). Suicidal ideation may even vary based on whether the juvenile is detained for a violent versus a nonviolent offense. One recent study found that detained juvenile males and females with current violent offenses were significantly more likely to report suicidal ideation than their peers with current nonviolent offenses (Maney, 2007).

Research suggests that interpersonal violence and suicide share some common antecedents (problem solving, coping skills, community environments, etc.). It is currently unknown whether suicidality causes violence, violence causes suicide, or whether they are "interchangeable outcomes of the same general process" (Lubell & Vetter, 2006, p. 172). Due to the apparent connection between violence and self-harm, clinicians should consider past and current suicidal ideation and suicide attempts in assessments of risk for violence. Additionally, due to the mounting evidence of the relationship between psychiatric comorbidity and risk for violence, if the youth are identified and treated for symptoms of mental disorder early on, this may reduce their risk of reoffending (Copeland et al., 2007).

Summary: Applying This Knowledge to Risk Assessment Tools

Taken as a whole, the social science evidence and decision-making approaches just reviewed can be translated into the selection of youth risk assessment tools in some important ways. Examiners will want to select tools with properties related to their usefulness for assessing risk for recidivism and later risk reduction (needs). Preference should go toward tools that:

- Contain dynamic risk factors that permit reassessment by providing a measure of change in risk level
- Contain dynamic risk factors that can be translated into needs or targets of intervention and services in order to direct service referrals or case/risk management efforts
- Contain protective factors or strengths
- Permits some rater or examiner discretion to account for idiosyncratic risk factors as opposed to a strict actuarial approach resulting in only score-based decisions

Other Factors Involved in the Selection of a Tool to Evaluate Risk for Recidivism or Violence

Before selecting an instrument designed to evaluate risk for recidivism or violence, it is important to be aware of some important characteristics of instruments generally. Several factors are involved in the selection of a risk assessment tool for use in a particular juvenile justice setting or facility. These factors were described in depth by Grisso, Vincent, and Seagrave (2005) and will be reviewed only briefly here. First, evaluators or juvenile justice administrators should determine whether the tool is relevant for answering the questions of interest or assisting with the decisions to be made. This relates to the decision point and whether a screening or assessment tool is needed. Different risk tools were designed for different purposes. Some are quick screening tools designed to assist with making a short-term decision (e.g., appropriateness for pretrial detention). Others are more comprehensive assessment tools designed for longer-term placement decisions (e.g., secure custody versus probation) or case management and service planning.

Screening Versus Assessment

Possibly the most important issue in tool selection is to understand the difference between screening and assessment. The differences between screening and assessment have been described in detail in several scholarly works (Grisso, 2005b; Grisso & Underwood, 2004; Vincent, Grisso, &

Terry, 2007), so we will only summarize briefly here. A screening tool is something that is conducted with every youth at intake or entry into some part of the juvenile justice system for the purpose of sifting youth into categories: one that is very unlikely to have the characteristic in question and one that is more likely to have the characteristic. Results of screening tools may lead to a few potential responses: (a) short-term in-custody placement decisions, (b) identification of youth who require some form of clinical referral to seek more information, or (c) identification of youth in need of a detailed assessment. Generally, a good screening tool will be relatively brief and will not require specialized training to complete. In the context of risk for recidivism or violence, one appropriate use of a screening tool may be to assist with decisions for short-term placement in pretrial detention versus the community while a youth is awaiting trial. A second appropriate use would be to target moderate- or high-risk youths in need of a more comprehensive risk assessment while ruling out low-risk youths who may not require the lengthy assessment process. Screening tools should not be used for long-term placement decisions or long-term service and case management planning. Screening tools generally do not contain dynamic variables and therefore do not lend themselves well to reassessment.

Assessment tools, on the other hand, are designed to gather a more comprehensive and individualized profile of a youth. The intent is to verify the presence or absence of the characteristic in question (e.g., risk of harm to others), determine the source or etiology of the characteristic for a particular youth, and develop an appropriate course of action for longer-range interventions. Interventions in the context of risk for recidivism or violence can include placement decisions, such as secure custody versus community placement, special programming, levels of monitoring or supervision, and services for the youth and family. Assessment tools, relative to screening tools, require a higher level of training in proper scoring and use of the assessment tool; more data gathering from several sources, including an interview with the youth, collateral information, and often an interview with the parents; and occasionally require the evaluator to have specialized credentials.

Properties of Instruments and Psychometrics

There are some critical details one should look for in a good test (see Grisso, 2005a). One important factor in the selection of a tool is *standardized assessment*. Tools that work best will be structured so that the same process is used for every youth; meaning the tool has some version of a manual with scoring rules and detailed item descriptions. Another factor in the selection of a tool is whether there is research evidence for *reliability*. In other words, will the tool produce consistent results across administration regardless of the trained individual rating the tool? Finally, an important attribute of a tool is evidence for *validity* for use with juvenile justice samples. Does the tool measure what it purports to measure? In this case, has it demonstrated that it predicts recidivism?

Other details that factor into the appropriate tool selection depend on the context and the setting. First, the tool should be relevant for the specific assessment question. Much of this relates to the setting and decision point as described previously. Second, administrators should consider the feasibility of completing the tool given the resources available and the skill set of their staff. Instruments vary in the level of expertise of the examiner and the amount of information required to complete the assessment. This is less of an issue for psychologists and qualified examiners who are expected to conduct comprehensive assessments with the most information.

To apply the concept of *evidence-based* to a screening or assessment tool, we must consider the evidence that the tool properly screens or assesses individuals. We propose a minimum standard for what should be considered an evidence-based risk assessment tool, based in part on Austin (2006). We further describe the criteria that should be used to determine if a tool has sufficient evidence and usefulness.

- A manual: A tool should have a test manual that contains scoring criteria and/or detailed item descriptions to structure the administration.
- Empirically based risk factors: A tool should contain youth risk factors that have been empirically demonstrated to have an association with future crime and violence.
- Known internal structure: The tool should have some reported scale analyses to justify the scoring of the instrument. Ideally, this would be a factor analysis; however, factor analyses will not apply to all types of risk assessment instruments. Risk for recidivism would not be conceptualized as a coherent construct, but, depending on the content of the instrument, we might expect a risk tool to contain several coherent subscales that could be tested with factor analyses. At the minimum, a tool should have reported evidence for internal consistency between items of subscales.

There should be some evidence of structural validity to justify the scoring of an instrument, if it is an instrument that is scored. Finally, for score-based, actuarial instruments, normative data that enable one to assess the relative standing of the examinee can also be important.

- Reliability: Risk assessment instruments should have some reported evidence for reliability. If the tool is self-report only (that is, the tool does not rely on examiner ratings), then the interest is in internal consistency and test–retest reliability. However, for tools that do rely on examiner ratings, evidence for interrater reliability is critical to provide confidence that the tool will be completed fairly consistently across examiners. The preferred measure of reliability in this case is intraclass correlation coefficients (ICCs). ICCs should be above 0.70 at least, and preferably above 0.90. An instrument should have at least one test, but preferably two, of reliability that was conducted in a juvenile justice setting by an independent party (not the test developer).
- Validity: A risk assessment tool must have evidence that it predicts recidivism and/or violence. When evaluating a tool, it is important to be familiar with this research, including the outcomes tested (e.g., institutional violence, community violence, official rearrests, self-reported delinquent behavior) and the methods used (e.g., prospective versus retrospective studies). At the minimum, we would want to see prospective studies of the tool's validity for predicting recidivism or antisocial behavior. There are many statistical procedures used to assess predictive validity. Preference goes to predictive models that take time at risk into account (e.g., Cox proportional hazards regression, survival analyses), and receiver operating characteristic (ROC) curves as a measure of predictive accuracy. The area under the ROC curve (AUC) is an index of the tool's overall accuracy—in this case, ability to correctly identify a youth who will reoffend. The AUC can range from 0 to 1.0, where 0.5 indicates chance-level accuracy, greater than 0.5 indicates above-chance accuracy, and less than 0.5 indicates below-chance accuracy. According to Swets (1988), AUCs for an acceptable screening tool would be between 0.70 and 0.90. There should be at least one study, preferably two, by an independent party demonstrating good predictive validity (medium to large effects) in a juvenile justice setting. Preferably, validity studies also will report differences by gender and race/ethnicity.

REVIEW OF THE INSTRUMENTS

This section reviews risk for recidivism or violence instruments available for youthful populations, including both juvenile justice and nonjuvenile justice populations. Each tool summary provides information relevant to the selection of an instrument, including its purpose and the population for which it was designed, content and summary scores, and evidence for reliability and validity. All the prominent tools in this area are covered in this chapter, yet it is not an exhaustive list. Preference went to tools that are in widespread use in adolescent service agencies (mainly juvenile justice) around the United States and/or appear in the mainstream professional journals.

Screening Tools

Homegrown or State-Based Risk Tools

Even though many risk tools are available, sometimes individual facilities decide that these instruments do not meet their specific needs, so they develop their own risk tool(s). Searches of the literature and the Internet indicated that some version of a homegrown tool exists in at least 50% of the U.S. states—for example, the Colorado Youthful Offender Level of Service Instrument, the Mississippi Delinquency Risk Assessment Scale, and the North Dakota Risk Assessment Instrument. The purpose of these tools varies (e.g., risk for recidivism, risk for institutional maladjustment) and so do the methods for developing them. Some states developed tools based on risk factors identified by research, some adapted an existing tool for their own use, and others created a tool based on what the facility considered to be risk factors. Many of these homegrown tools have not received an investigation of their psychometric properties, and only about half have any reported evidence of reliability or validity.

The purpose of most of these tools is to make decisions about placement in pretrial detention while awaiting trial. These are referred to as risk assessment instruments (RAI), and most were designed using the consensus-based approach described by the Anne E. Casey Foundation (Steinhart, 2006). We would consider these instruments to be homegrown because, although the Steinhart monograph provided a structure for the design of these tools including some items based on risk factors supported by the research, other items are created by individual facilities or are not supported by research. These items are based on value judgments about offense categories, with more serious offenses getting higher ratings. In effect, every RAI is different and is custom made for a particular site. Thus, the validity of one version cannot be assumed to generalize to other versions. States such as Utah, New York, and Virginia have begun systematic attempts at validating their RAIs; however, because each tool is unique, all other states using RAIs would need to conduct validation studies on their own tools.

We classify these tools as screening tools because they are designed to sort youths into categories of high versus low risk for short-term recidivism and failure to appear in court. They are not designed to assess needs factors or specific risk factors as described earlier in this chapter. They are based instead on value judgments and risk markers. The items typically do not address the causal factors of a youth's risk or needs. A more accurate title for these tools might be detention assessment instruments or detention screening instruments. The scores on these tools should be seen as having a limited shelf life because they generally do not contain dynamic factors or account for changes in risk according to a developmental model. One promising tool that was not developed using the RAI approach is the Arizona Risk/Needs Assessment Instrument (ARNA). This is a 10-item tool containing evidence-based risk factors that has some evidence for its predictive validity with a large sample of youth preadjudication (Schwalbe, 2008). On the surface, the items of this instrument appear to be generalizable to other jurisdictions, although research is needed to examine its validity in other states.

North Carolina Assessment of Risk (NCAR)

The North Carolina Assessment of Risk is a brief tool designed to evaluate risk for recidivism among juvenile offenders. There is no specified age range. The tool was developed by the North Carolina Department of Juvenile Justice with consultation from the National Council on Crime and Delinquency (NCCD). It consists of nine items that culminate into a total risk score that is translated into low-, medium-, or high-risk categories. This is an actuarial tool with few dynamic variables, and most items are based on the juvenile record. There is a brief manual that explains the scoring procedures and tells examiners to use the "best available information." The tool could be easily completed by juvenile justice personnel, and there do not appear to be any training requirements. The manual also contains a separate needs assessment, the North Carolina Assessment of Juvenile Needs, which contains 15 items related to the youth and family and results in a low-, medium-, or high-needs score. If examiners were to use the risk scale in isolation, we would refer to this as a screening tool given our previous definition. If examiners were to use both the risk and needs portions of this instrument, we would consider it to be more similar to an assessment.

There is good research evidence for the NCAR, but we were not able to find research related to the needs assessment portion at the time of this review. Schwalbe, Fraser, Day, and Cooley (2006) examined the predictive validity of the NCAR using a sizable sample of 9,534 delinquent offenders ($M = 13.7$ years) over an average 1-year follow-up. The NCAR was completed by court counselors. Cox regressions resulted in a hazard ratio of 1.08, which was significant due to the large sample size but is actually a very small effect. There were medium effects for individual items on the scale, such as number of runaways (1.24) and school behavior problems (1.27). The NCAR worked well for White and Black boys and Black girls, but, for White girls, it did not differentiate recidivists from nonrecidivists. To our knowledge, there are no rigorous studies of the tool's interrater agreement, but estimates have been produced to suggest the agreement is adequate (Schwalbe, Fraser, Day, & Arnold, 2004).

Risk/Needs Assessment Instruments for General or Violent Recidivism

Youth Level of Service/Case Management Inventory (YLS/CMI)

The YLS/CMI (Hoge & Andrews, 2006) is a standardized inventory for assessing risk for recidivism and need factors and assisting in case management for juvenile offenders aged 12 to 17. The authors designed the YLS/CMI primarily to assist with pre- and postadjudication case planning, but it also can assist with other decisions, such as preadjudication diversion and detention, waivers to adult court and the mental health system, and postadjudication dispositions. The YLS/CMI contains 42 items divided across eight subscales (e.g., prior and current offenses, parenting, education/employment, peer associations, substance abuse, personality, and attitudes), and it is divided into six sections (assessment of risks/needs, summary of risk/need factors, assessment of other needs/special considerations, assessment of the client's general risk/need level, contact level, case management plan, and case management review). It can be administered and scored by trained, front-line staff, based on an interview with the youth and collateral and file information. The scoring takes approximately 20 to 30 minutes after all relevant information is gathered.

The YLS/CMI was developed from the Youth Level of Supervision Inventory (Andrews, Robinson, & Hoge, 1984), the first youth version of the Level of Service Inventory–Revised (Andrews & Bonta, 1995). The YLS/CMI has undergone several revisions. It seems that the authors have not conducted a factor analysis of this instrument. The norm sample was comprised of 264 male (n = 173) and female (n = 91) adjudicated offenders, aged 12 to 17, who had received a probation or custody disposition (Hoge & Andrews, 2006). The manual includes norm tables that allow examiners to assess an examinee's relative standing. Items are scored using a checklist format, with the evaluator indicating whether risk factors and strengths are present. The instrument uses an "adjusted actuarial" approach using a total score derived by a sum of objective item ratings to designate the risk level as low, medium, high, or very high. Evaluators can consider additional risk factors not included in the checklist, and the actuarially derived risk level can by overridden based on clinical judgment. They recommend only about 10% of cases be suitable for an override.

There is a fair amount of research evidence for the YLS/CMI. Interrater reliability has been tested across researchers, mental health professionals, and probation officers. Comparing professionals and probation officers, Schmidt, Hoge, and Robertson (2005) reported intraclass correlation coefficients (ICCs) on the subscales from 0.71 to 0.85, with the exception of peer relations (0.61). Poluchowiz, Jung, and Rawana (2000) reported an ICC of 0.75 for the total risk score.

In terms of predictive validity, retrospective studies of the YLS/CMI's validity found that it postdicted any charges and convictions (AUC = 0.71; Marshall, Egan, & English, 2006) and correctly classified 75.38% of a young offender sample as recidivists or nonrecidivists (Jung, 1996). One study examined the YLS/CMI's ability to postdict community and institutional violence (instead of official juvenile charges), and the results were not significant (Marshall et al., 2006). However, it is not clear that this variable was recorded systematically, and the statistics did not factor in time to the event. In a prospective 3.5-year follow-up study of young offenders, Schmidt et al. (2005) found YLS/CMI total scores predicted serious reoffending (AUC = 0.67) and any reoffending (AUC = 0.61). In another prospective study of young offenders in Australia, YLS/CMI total scores completed by juvenile justice officers had an AUC with general recidivism of 0.75 given an average 16-month follow-up (Upperton & Thompson, 2007). The most significant predictor was the personality and behavior scale. The only nonsignificant predictor was peer relations. Another study of file-rated YLS scores from researchers with a 1-year follow-up reported the AUC's for general and violent recidivism around 0.74 (Catchpole & Gretton, 2003). Finally, a recent study of probation officer–rated YLS/CMI scores with an average 1.5-year follow-up reported an AUC of 0.60 with general recidivism (Welsh, Schmidt, McKinnon, Chattha, & Meyers, 2008). This is considerably lower than the Australian study, which also used probation officer–rated YLS scores.

The Washington State Juvenile Court Assessment (WSJCA)

The Washington State Juvenile Court Assessment (Barnoski, 2004b) is a tool to assess risk for reoffending for use with adolescents aged 12 through 18 who come into contact with the juvenile justice system. There is a paper-and-pencil version of the WSJCA with a manual, but most users utilize a computer-based program. The WSJCA (also known as Back on Track) helps to allocate resources in the juvenile justice system using a case management approach focused on reducing risk. Probation managers can identify the risk and protective factors specific to a case and can determine whether the court's intervention will have an impact on the targeted factors identified. The WSJCA has three parts: a prescreen, full assessment, and reassessment and can be administered by trained probation officers and other juvenile justice staff. Information for these assessments are gathered from an interview with the youth and collateral contacts.

The WSJCA prescreen contains 27 items that elicit factual information about the youth and takes approximately 45 minutes to administer. It produces two scores (criminal history and social history) that are combined to produce a rating of low, moderate, or high risk for recidivism. Those rated as moderate or high risk complete the full assessment, which includes a structured motivational interview with a youth and his or her family and a chart review. The full assessment includes 132 items, broken into 13 domains such as, criminal history, relationships, mental health, attitudes/behaviors, aggression, and employment. It requires 1 to 3 hours to complete.

The WSJCA dates back to 1997. Its development was based on a review of existing theoretical models and the risk prediction and juvenile delinquency literature (Barnoski, 2004b). The WSJCA Version 2.0 was implemented statewide in Washington in 1999, after many juvenile court professionals and international experts refined the first version of the instrument and it was tested with 150 youth from juvenile courts in the state of Washington. Factor analyses demonstrated that items from all but two domains (use of free time and alcohol/drug) loaded on more than one factor and confirmed the relative independence of the assessment domains (Barnoski, 2004b). Currently, there has not been any research reported on the interrater reliability of the WSJCA.

In terms of predictive validity, using a sample of 1,404 males and females placed on probation in Washington, Barnoski (1998) demonstrated that felony recidivism was linearly related to social history scores, independent of criminal history scores. The 6-month felony recidivism rates were 6.6% for the low-risk category, 19.4% for moderate risk, and 31.6% for high risk. Using another sample of 20,339 prescreen assessments and 12,187 full assessments for adjudicated youths placed on probation, Barnoski (2004b) found the felony recidivism rate of the low-risk group was 11.2% and 32.2% for the high-risk group after an 18-month follow-up. The rate of violent recidivism was 2.9% for the low-risk group and 11% for the high-risk group. Thus, the high-risk group had about three times the recidivism rate of the low-risk group. The AUC was 0.64 for both violent and nonviolent recidivism. The felony recidivism rate for high-risk males was 36% and 18% for high-risk females. The predictive validity is good for minority groups, but slightly lower than that for Whites (Barnoski, 2004a; Washington State Institute for Public Policy, 2004). The author recommends using a different item weighting system when scoring the instrument for girls or minorities.

A few companies have packaged the WSJCA for purchase by making slight modifications and developing software that requires their technical support. These modified versions are the Positive Achievement Change Tool (PACT) and the Youth Assessment and Screening Instrument (YASI). Both tools were expanded to include questions related to mental health. The YASI differs from the WSJCA in that it added a unique reporting format (the YASI Profile Wheel), more dynamic risk factors, and some questions related to past homicidal and suicidal attempts and ideation in order to signal potential mental health problems. Because the content of the YASI and the PACT is different from the

WSJCA, one cannot assume that findings pertaining to the reliability and validity of the WSJCA apply to the YASI. There is good evidence for the validity of both of these tools, but the YASI has only been tested by the creators in unpublished reports, and the PACT was tested in a dissertation (Baglivio, 2007). Interrater reliability has not been reported for either instrument.

The Structured Assessment of Violence Risk in Youth (SAVRY)

The SAVRY Version 2 (Borum et al., 2003) is a 30-item instrument using the structured professional judgment (SPJ) approach to assess violence risk in adolescents aged 12 to 18 years who have been detained or referred for an assessment of violence risk. Qualified trained evaluators conduct systematic assessments of predetermined risk factors that are empirically associated with violence, consider the applicability of each risk factor to a particular examinee, and classify each factor's severity. The instrument is coded based on record review and an interview with the youth examinee. The time required for assessments varies based on the complexity of each case.

The SAVRY protocol is composed of six items defining protective factors and 24 items defining risk factors. Risk items are divided into three categories: historical, individual, and social/contextual. Evaluators also can designate additional risk and protective factors because the SAVRY will not be exhaustive for any given individual. In the course of conducting a risk assessment or assessing patterns in past violent episodes, additional factors or situational variables may emerge that are important in understanding potential for future violence. In such situations, the additional factors should be documented and weighed in final decisions of risk. The ultimate determination of an examinee's overall level of violence risk (low, moderate, or high) is based on the examiner's professional judgment as informed by a systematic appraisal of relevant factors.

The first version of the SAVRY was developed in 2000, when two SPJ risk assessment tools were combined into a single instrument (Borum, Bartel, & Forth, 2005). Item selection was based on the empirical relationship to violence, identified through literature reviews and meta-analyses. The SAVRY has been translated into over a half dozen languages and is being used regularly in forensic institutions in Canada; detention facilities in Connecticut; and several locations in the United Kingdom, Sweden, Italy, Germany, and the Netherlands.

Interrater reliability has been tested between trained student raters and is acceptable. Catchpole and Gretton (2003) reported the ICC for SAVRY total scores at 0.81 and 0.77 for summary risk ratings. McEachran (2001) reported an ICC of 0.83 for SAVRY total scores and 0.72 for summary risk ratings. There is evidence for concurrent validity. Catchpole and Gretton (2003) found the SAVRY total risk index demonstrated significant correlations with both the Psychopathy Checklist: Youth Version (PCL:YV; 0.68; Forth, Kosson, & Hare, 2003) and the YLS/CMI (0.64; Hoge & Andrews, 2006). With respect to generalizability, using a detention sample, Chapman, Desai, Falzer, and Borum (2006) found that Black youth were significantly more likely than their White counterparts to be rated as low risk for violence. However, until these researchers relate these scores to offending, it is unclear whether this is due to a race bias in SAVRY scoring or whether the disparity in scores reflects real differences in risk between Blacks and Whites.

With respect to validity, although the instrument was designed for violence specifically, research indicates that the SAVRY also predicts general reoffending and other aspects of antisocial behavior. The Individual/Clinical Scale predicted institutional aggression and the number of aggressive conduct disorder symptoms (Bartel, Forth, & Borum, 2003). The SAVRY showed substantial incremental validity above the PCL:YV and the YLS/CMI for its relation to conduct disorder symptoms. In a retrospective follow-up study of adolescent male offenders who committed crimes after reaching adulthood, McEachran (2001) reported an AUC of 0.70 for SAVRY total scores and 0.89 for SAVRY summary risk ratings for violent reoffending using SAVRY scores calculated from files.

Prospective studies of clinical SAVRY ratings have shown a significant association with future violence and general reoffending. In a 1-year follow-up study, Catchpole and Gretton (2003) found that adolescent offenders classified as low risk had a violence recidivism rate of 6%, moderate-risk youth had a violence recidivism rate of 14%, and high-risk youth had a rate of 40%. In another 1-year follow-up study of 176 young offenders, Gretton and Abramowitz (2002) reported an AUC for general reoffending of 0.66 for SAVRY risk ratings and 0.68 for SAVRY total scores. For violent reoffending, the AUCs were 0.74 for the summary risk rating and 0.67 for the total score. The low-risk group had a 5.7% violence recidivism rate, the moderate-risk group had a rate of 13.1%, and the high-risk group had a rate of 40.4%. An unpublished prospective study of adolescent offenders found that both total scores and summary risk ratings on the SAVRY predicted nonviolent and violent reoffending after a 2-year follow-up (Penney, Lee, Moretti, & Bartel, 2007) for both boys and girls. This was regardless of using official charges or self-reported offending. Finally, the protective factors scale of the SAVRY alone is negatively related to rearrest (Dolan & Rennie, 2008), meaning the more protective factors a youth has, the less likely he or she is to be rearrested. A recent study compared the SAVRY to the YLS/CMI in the ability to predict general and violence recidivism. When comparing the two instruments, the SAVRY outperformed the YLS/CMI (Welsh et al., 2008) in the prediction of both types of recidivism with an AUC = 0.77 for general recidivism and 0.81 for violence recidivism. However, the SAVRY was rated by psychology graduate students, and the YLS was rated by probation officers. It is possible that rater qualifications led to the disparity in predictive validity.

The Early Assessment Risk Lists (EARL-20B and EARL-21G)

The Early Assessment Risk List for Boys (EARL-20B), Version 2 (Augimeri, Koegl, Webster, & Levene, 2001), and the Early Assessment Risk List for Girls, (EARL-21G) Version 1 (Levene et al., 2001), are SPJ risk assessment devices for use with children under 12 years of age with disruptive behavior problems. The purpose of these instruments is to increase general understanding of early childhood risk factors for violence and antisociality, provide a structure for developing risk assessment schemas for individual children, and to assist with risk management planning.

The EARL-20B and EARL-21G contain 20 or 21 items, respectively, divided across three categories: family, child, and responsivity (the ability and willingness of the child and family to engage in and benefit from interventions). These checklists are coded based on all available collateral information and interviews with examinees where possible. Each item is rated on a three-point scale, with higher scores indicating greater risk. Evaluators provide an overall decision about one's level of risk (low, medium, or high) and appropriate interventions commensurate with the level of risk. In addition, evaluators can also identify critical risk items that are particularly concerning and may represent high risk for a youth.

The EARL-20B was developed from an informal risk assessment list called "Risk Factors Associated with Possible Conduct Disorders and Non-Responders" (Augimeri & Levene, 1994) as well as an extensive review of the child development literature to identify the risk factors associated with aggressive and violent behavior. While the EARL-20B has been revised and is currently in Version 2, the EARL-21G, Version 1, is still being evaluated (Augimeri, Koegl, Levene, & Webster, 2005).

Interrater reliability of the EARL-20B, Version 1, total score was tested across three raters and demonstrated a highly acceptable level of agreement (ICC = 0.80; Augimeri et al., 2001). Enebrink, Langrstrom, Neij, Grann, and Gumpert (2001) reported ICCs for the EARL-20B, Version 2, for total, child items, and family item subscale scores ranging from 0.90 to 0.92. Levene et al. (2001) reported ICCs of 0.64 to 0.84 for the EARL-21G across three raters. A retrospective follow-up study that tracked youth behavior for approximately 7.8 years after age 12 found that the EARL-20B predicted subsequent official adolescent and adult criminal contact for both boys and girls (Augimeri et al., 2001). In a prospective study, Enebrink, Langstrom, and Gumpert (2006) found EARL-20B baseline assessments were positively correlated with aggressive and conduct-disordered behavior among males at both a 6-month and a 30-month follow-up.

Jesness Inventory–Revised (JI-R)

The Jesness Inventory–Revised (Jesness, 2003) is a brief, self-report, true/false item personality classification system that was designed to assess functioning across a variety of areas for youth and adults beginning at age 8. The JI-R takes approximately 30 to 45 minutes to administer, requires only a fourth-grade reading level to complete, and can be given in group or individual paper-and-pencil administrations. It is recommended that evaluators have a master's degree, experience with delinquent populations, and training on the instrument.

The JI-R contains 11 scales that measure key traits and attitudes (e.g., social maladjustment, manifest aggression, social anxiety, repression, denial, value orientation), two validity scales, and two new scales that relate directly to the *DSM-IV* diagnostic categories for conduct disorder and oppositional defiant disorder. The JI-R can be scored manually or via a software program, which produces a detailed report including all responses, raw scores, *T* scores, and the subtype classification for the youth. There are nine potential subtypes (undersocialized–active, undersocialized–passive, conformist, cultural conformist, manipulator, neurotic–acting out, neurotic–anxious, situational, and cultural identifier) that are designed to classify youth according to their level of developmental maturity and provide specific suggestions about treatment and risk. The norm sample for the JI-R was derived from over 20 sites and included 4,380 men and women and nondelinquent and delinquent youths.

Jesness (2003) tested the internal consistency of the revised version with the new standardization sample and found alpha values ranging from 0.61 to 0.91 for the nondelinquent sample and subtype scales ranging from 0.66 to 0.92 for the delinquent sample. Indices of test–retest reliability for the original JI after approximately 1 year resulted in a median correlation of 0.65 for subtype scale scores, with 48% obtaining the same primary classification (Jesness, 1986). Studies have indicated that JI-R scale scores differentiate groups of adolescents (e.g., nondelinquents versus delinquents) in the expected direction (e.g., Martin, 1981; Munson & Revers, 1986). Kunce and Hemphill (1983) found that four subscales (values orientation, social maladjustment, manifest anger, and autism) of the JI correlated with the frequency of prior and previous institutional stays among a sample of 1,122 male delinquents. In a 10-year follow-up study of 2,582 juvenile offenders, Haapanen and Jesness (1982) found that chronic offenders (defined as 10 subsequent arrests or more) obtained significantly higher scores on the social maladjustment and asocial index scales than those who had no or few arrests for minor violations. However, over 75% of youths in this study were chronic offenders.

The Risk & Resiliency Checkup (RRC)

The Risk & Resiliency Checkup (RRC) Justice System Assessment and Training (J-SAT; 1998) is a semistructured interview designed to initially assess behaviors that may place a youth at risk for recidivism. It is a risk/needs classification tool that also can assist agencies in making informed disposition recommendations and decisions about the services that youth may need. The RRC contains 60 standard questions divided across six scales (delinquency, education, family, peers, substance use, and individual). Each scale is further divided into two sections—risk factors and protective factors—for a total of 12 sections. J-SAT allows juvenile justice agencies to adapt the tool to meet the needs of the agency; however, the 60 base items remain the same. Both San Diego and Los Angeles have versions of the RRC that they adapted to meet their needs.

The RRC can be administered and scored by trained front-line staff (probation officers) conducting a semistructured interview with the youth and collaterals using motivational interviewing techniques and supplemented with file information. To score all of the items, the RRC administrator must have access to the youth's current history (over the previous 6 months), the past year, entire life history, and 6 months prior to institutional confinement, because each item will ask the administrator to rate the item according to one of these time categories. There are also guidelines for conducting reassessments. Items are scored on a three-point scale according to whether the behavior is present. All of the risk factors are summed to produce a total risk score (a negative sign is put in front of the sum), and all of the protective factors are summed to produce a total protective score. The total protective score (a positive number) is then added to the total risk score (a negative number) to produce the total resiliency score. The eight additional protective factors are also summed. There are no predetermined cutoffs for these scores. The agencies decide where they want to place the cutoffs depending on the risks they want to identify and the resources for interventions.

To date, no studies have evaluated the interrater reliability or the internal consistency of the RRC, but there has been one published study of its predictive validity by an independent party. In this prospective study, probation officers gave the RRC to 1,165 youth, and arrest data for the next 12 months were obtained from four probation departments in the San Diego area (Turner, Fain, & Sehgal, 2005). Since J-SAT has not established cutoffs for the RRC, the researchers divided the total resiliency score into three categories: low (score of 12 or less), medium (score of 13–33), and high (score of 34 or higher). The study found that 8% of those in the high-resiliency group had been rearrested during the 12-month follow-up compared to 36% of those in the low-resiliency group. Logistic regression analyses indicated the RRC predicted recidivism equally well for girls and boys and racial groups; however, the resiliency total score was not as good a predictor of recidivism for Hispanic youth.

Risk Assessments for Juvenile Sexual Offenders

The Estimate of Risk of Adolescent Sexual Offense Recidivism (ERASOR)

The Estimate of Risk of Adolescent Sexual Offense Recidivism (Worling & Curwen, 2001) is an empirically guided checklist designed to estimate the short-term risk of sexual recidivism for individuals between the ages of 12 and 18 who have previously committed a sexual offense.

The ERASOR consists of five scales (sexual interests, attitudes, and behaviors; historical sexual assaults; psychosocial functioning; family/environmental functioning; and treatment) and contains 25 items for males and 24 items for females (item 12, ever sexually assaulted a male victim, is not scored for females). Each item is scored based on the degree to which the item is present in the youth (present, possibly or partially present, not present, and unknown). Items can be scored based on psychological testing, observation, collateral reports, and clinical interviews with the youth and the youth's family (Worling, 2004). Examiners should be master's- or doctoral-level clinicians due to the clinical judgment required to rate the items and final risk estimate.

The ERASOR was modeled after the HCR-20 (Webster et al., 1997) and the Sexual Violence Risk-20 tool (Boer et al., 1997) in that it follows the SPJ framework. Risk factors in the ERASOR were identified by reviewing the juvenile and adult literature as well as other risk tools, checklists, and guidelines (Worling, 2004). Worling developed a pilot version with 23 risk factors in 2000 and circulated it to other clinicians and researchers for feedback and a field test. Based on the feedback, the final version contained 25 items (16 dynamic and 9 static) and included the option of listing a case-specific factor that the evaluator feels should be calculated into the clinical judgment of risk. Examiners assign a final risk estimate (low, moderate, or high) based on all available evidence and clinical judgment. There should be a relation between the number of risk factors present and the final risk estimate; however, the authors caution users that if a juvenile professes his or her intent to reoffend, then this one factor could also result in a high risk score.

Worling (2004) conducted a preliminary study of the ERASOR's psychometric properties using a sample of 136 male adolescents, ranging from 12 to 18 years of age, from two settings: community-based agencies in Toronto and a residential treatment center in Minnesota. The adolescents had either been convicted of or admitted to a sexual offense. ERASOR ratings were completed upon intake, part way through treatment, and upon discharge by clinicians (usually pairs of clincians). Interrater agreement was acceptable for item ratings (average ICC = 0.60 or higher) and excellent for the overall clinical risk estimate (ICC = 0.92). Total scores had acceptable internal consistency (α = 0.75), and the correlation between the overall risk rating and the number of factors coded as present was significant (r = 0.68). Total scores were significantly higher for youth in residential treatment than in the community settings, and they were significantly lower at discharge than at intake on average for both samples. Worling tested the ERASOR's predictive efficiency by using scores to classify youths as past repeat offenders or non–repeat offenders. The postdictive efficiency did not differ significantly between total scores (AUC = 0.72) and overall risk ratings (AUC = 0.66). There is tentative support for reliability and validity of the ERASOR, but predictive validity will have to be examined using prospective recidivism data.

The Juvenile Sex Offender Assessment Protocol–II (J-SOAP-II)

The Juvenile Sex Offender Assessment Protocol–II (Prentky & Righthand, 2003) is an empirically based checklist designed to estimate the risk of engaging in a contact sexual reoffense in males between the ages of 12 and 18 who previously committed a sexual offense (Righthand et al., 2005). The J-SOAP-II contains 28 items comprising four scales, two of which focus on static risk factors (sexual drive/preoccupation and impulsive/antisocial behavior) and two that are more dynamic in nature (intervention and community stability/adjustment). Each item is scored on a three-point scale. The tool results in four scale scores and an overall J-SOAP-II score. Examiners calculate the proportion of risk for each scale score and for the overall score by dividing raw scores by the highest possible scores. Examiners are required to have experience and training in assessing juvenile sex offenders, but no formal education criteria are listed by the authors of the tool. Because there are no cutoff scores, a large degree of clinical judgment must be used to determine which risk management and treatment options are best suited for a particular youth. It is recommended that clinicians use multiple sources of information in their assessments and look at each case carefully to determine individual risk (Prentky & Righthand, 2003).

The J-SOAP-II began in 1994 as a nameless risk assessment scale for juvenile sexual offenders (Prentky & Righthand, 2003). The construction and validation sample included 96 juvenile sex offenders from 9 to 20 years old who were referred to an institute in Philadelphia. After the tool's first revision in 1998, it became known as the J-SOAP (Prentky & Righthand, 2003). This version revised a few of the original items and added a couple of items. It was tested on a sample of 153 male juveniles. Adequate interrater reliability (ICCs from 0.80 to 0.91) and high to moderate internal consistency was found for all four scales. Principal components analysis lent support for the four J-SOAP scales. Concurrent validity was investigated against the YLS/CMI total score, which was highly correlated with J-SOAP total ($r = 0.91$) and individual scale scores in the expected direction (sexual drive/preoccupation $r = 0.37$, impulsive/antisocial behavior $r = 0.81$, intervention $r = 0.88$, and community stability/adjustment $r = 0.91$).

In 2003, the J-SOAP was revised and became the J-SOAP-II; changes from the earlier version involved the addition of four items, the deletion of one item, and the extensive revision of another item (Prentky & Righthand, 2003). Until recently, the psychometric properties of the J-SOAP-II had yet to be reported; however, two studies have now assessed the predictive validity of the instrument. The first validity study used adolescent males ($n = 60$) between the ages of 12 and 18 who were admitted to a community-based sex offender treatment program (Martinez, Flores, & Rosenfeld, 2007). The follow-up period is unknown. There was adequate interrater reliability for the total score (ICC = 0.70) and for all of the scales (ICC range 0.63 to 0.88) except one (community stability, ICC = 0.42). There was strong internal consistency for the total score ($\alpha = 0.87$) but less consistency within individual scales ($\alpha = 0.69$ to 0.90). There was good predictive validity of the total score for both sexual (AUC = 0.78) and nonsexual reoffending (AUC = 0.76). Interestingly, the dynamic scales taken together performed better than the total score for predicting sexual reoffending (AUC = 0.86), whereas the static scales taken together performed worse (AUC = 0.63).

In contrast, a second validity study (Viljoen et al., 2008) compared the J-SOAP-II to the Juvenile Sex Offender Assessment Protocol-II (Epperson, Ralston, Fowers, & DeWitt, 2005) and the SAVRY using a sample of males in a residential treatment program for sexually abusive adolescents ($n = 169$) who had been discharged for at least 250 days. Recidivism data were collected by reviewing treatment, law enforcement, and probation records. Youth were followed for an average of 6.58 years (ranging from 2.80 to 12.01 years). The study found high interrater reliability for the total score (ICC = 0.84) and large correlations with SAVRY total scores ($r = 0.88$). Surprisingly, J-SOAP-II total scores at admission were neither significantly predictive of sexual aggression during treatment nor significantly predictive of sexual reoffending after treatment; however, the total score did significantly predict nonsexual aggression during treatment. The J-SOAP-II was better at predicting outcomes for older youth (ages 16 to 18) than younger youth (ages 12 to 15). Overall, this study could not provide evidence of the J-SOAP-II's predictive validity for sexual reoffending, but it was predictive of nonsexual recidivism.

The Juvenile Sexual Offense Recidivism Risk Assessment Tool–II (J-SORRAT-II)

The Juvenile Sexual Offense Recidivism Risk Assessment Tool–II (Epperson et al., 2005) is a 12-item actuarial risk assessment tool designed to estimate the risk of sexual recidivism for males between the ages of 12 and 18 who have previously committed a sexual offense. The J-SORRAT- II was validated by the authors but did not have any independent studies of its validity until recently. Viljoen et al. (2008) found that the total score on the J-SORRAT-II did not predict any type of reoffending. Further research is needed to assess whether the J-SORRAT-II is predictive of any form of recidivism.

Web- and Computer-Based Tools for Evaluating Risk for General Recidivism

Juvenile Assessment and Intervention System (JAIS)

The Juvenile Assessment and Intervention System was developed and is made available by the National Council on Crime and Delinquency (NCCD) and has substantial support from organizations such as the Office of Juvenile Justice and Delinquency Prevention. It is described as a combination of a risk assessment, a needs assessment, and strategies for juvenile supervision for use with youth aged 12 to 18 who have been arrested for or convicted of a delinquency. There is a different version for girls and boys. This is a Web-based program that collects data for 74 items across 11 risk/needs domains (e.g., mental health, family relationships, social skills, peer relationships, vocational skills) using a semistructured interview and file review form. The ratings of the items are entered into a computer program, which combines the scores algorithmically to achieve summary scores for various scales, and then prints out interpretive information for the examiner's consideration. There is no manual that describes the scoring algorithm procedure, so this cannot be evaluated.

The JAIS results in a total risk assessment score indicating "the degree of potential for the offender to commit subsequent offenses," a recommended strategy for case supervision (including supervision level and services), and ratings in 11 areas related to risk/needs. The risk assessment piece is actuarial and results in a rating of low, moderate, or high risk and a probability estimate (such as, 5%–10% of low-risk offenders nationwide are either revoked or experience a new felony conviction within 24 months of placement on probation or parole supervision).

There is very little information on the JAIS in the mainstream professional journals that publish research on child, adolescent, or delinquency assessment tools. Instead, NCCD has written some validation reports based on data from a few states that have implemented the JAIS (Wiebush, Wagner, & Ehrlich, 1999; National Council on Crime and Delinquency, 2004). Although the validity looks promising on the surface, there are two inherent limitations. First, none of the validation reports uses the same version of the JAIS risk assessment. They all use different numbers of items, suggesting the states are either able to customize the instrument, or the validation studies were not for the final version of the JAIS, but instead were for past derivatives. Second, we are aware of only one of these studies in which the validity of the risk assessment tool was tested against a sample of youth that is different from the sample on which the local tool was developed. In other words, all the other studies only reported the predictive validity for the items they selected to be in the tool based on an empirical association with recidivism in the development sample. To our knowledge, there are no studies of the tool's reliability; it seems to be based primarily on self-report information, and we are unaware of any justification in the literature for the probability estimates provided by the tool.

Youth Correctional Officer Management Profiling for Alternative Sanctions Risk and Needs Assessment (Youth COMPAS)

The Youth COMPAS is an automated 171-item, semistructured assessment instrument that yields 32 criminogenic and need scales organized into eight domains: youth criminal history, usual behavior and peers, personality/attitudes, substance abuse and sexual behavior, school and education, family and socialization, primary socializing family, and recent family living situation. It is designed to be easy to use and accessible for workers with high case loads. There are no specifications about who is able to use the tool or whether training is necessary to administer it. It appears to be intended for use by probation officers and front-line staff. Software is available and appears to be necessary. The length of the assessment can be adjusted by having various combinations of the 31 scales, depending on the workload, treatment goals, and needs of the agency. Information for the Youth COMPAS is taken from an interview with the youth and file review. The software program generates a report that provides recommendations for case planning, treatment, and placement decisions, a general delinquency risk score, and estimates of low, medium, or high risk on each of the 31 scales. Youth are also categorized into one of the seven typologies (e.g., internalizing youth–abused and rejected, conformists or socialized delinquents, undercontrolled serious delinquents, accidental/situational delinquents—Moffitt's normal adolescent limited youth).

Brennan (2003) studied the internal consistency of the Youth COMPAS on a sample of 2,393 youth assessed in juvenile justice agencies over a period of 2 years. Most of the Youth COMPAS scales exceeded $\alpha = 0.80$. Similarly, Dieterich and Brennan (2004) found that 24 of the 31 Youth COMPAS scales had alpha coefficients well above 0.70 in a sample of 558 youth (78% male) on probation. The scales with the lowest internal consistency were academic failure, hard drugs, and promiscuity ($\alpha = 0.42, 0.51, 0.61$, respectively). At the time of this writing, we could not find any published evidence for interrater reliability.

We also were unable to find any evidence of the Youth COMPAS's predictive validity or evidence to support the validity of the Youth COMPAS youth typologies. There is an association between some scale scores with age at first offense and history of violent offending. Dietrich and Brennan (2004) found that age at first adjudication correlated negatively with the personality scales of impulsivity, low empathy, low remorse, manipulative, aggression and violence tolerance; and some scales were consistent with longitudinal delinquency research studies (e.g., family discontinuity, socioeconomic, family crime/drugs, inconsistent discipline, and neighborhood). The number of past violent felony adjudications correlated as expected with the scale scores for impulsivity, manipulative, and aggression and violence tolerance.

Global Risk Assessment Device (GRADcis™)

The GRADcis™ (Gavazzi, Lim, Yarcheck, & Eyre, 2003) is an assessment tool that was developed to collect standardized information about families of at-risk youth or court-involved youth. There is no manual for this tool that specifies an age group, but the GRADcis™ has been studied with youths age 10 to 19. The Web-based tool tracks referrals to service providers, provides effectiveness data on services delivered, and provides juvenile justice professionals a tool that offers comprehensive information about a youth's risk and needs. The GRADcis™

takes approximately 20 minutes to administer and has a youth version and a parent version. An interview with either the youth or parent is required. Evaluators are encouraged to collect information from the youth, family members, and other collateral contacts if possible. Training is not required to administer the GRADcis™. The GRADcis™ contains 40 demographic questions and 132 items that the computer program calculates into high-, moderate-, or low-risk scores within 11 different domains (e.g., prior offenses, family/parenting, education/vocation, accountability, traumatic events, and health services). There is *not* an overall risk score. The computer generates a report that creates treatment recommendations corresponding to individual risk levels. It also provides an examinee's relative standing on the GRADcis™ after the user selects the appropriate norm group: diversion/status offenders, probation, detention, or community/outpatient setting.

Gavazzi and colleagues (2003) studied the factor structure and item reliability of the GRADcis™ in a sample of 248 youth and their families (130 males, 118 females) who were part of a family-based diversion initiative. Inter-item reliability coefficients for the eight subscales indicate high internal consistency (α = 0.87 to 0.97). Confirmatory factor analyses indicated good model fit for the 11 independent scales (root mean square error of approximation = 0.07). Interrater reliability has not been reported for this instrument. However, because there is no instrument manual, it is unclear whether interrater agreement is applicable to this tool. The tool may be based on self-report information only, in which case rater agreement is not relevant.

With respect to validity, there is some evidence that high scores on the GRADcis™ are associated with mental health referrals and recidivism. In a sample of adolescents (age 10 to 17) assessed by intake workers in a juvenile court, youth who they referred for mental health services had significantly higher scores on every GRADcis™ domain than youth who were referred to less intensive services (Gavazzi et al., 2003). Discriminant function analysis indicated 72% were classified correctly as needing a mental health referral, the false negative rate was 22%, and the false positive rate was 6%. Other studies have reported differences between minorities and differences between status offenders and delinquents (Gavazzi, Yarcheck, & Lim, 2005) in GRADcis™ domain scores in the expected direction.

We found one study that evaluated the GRADcis™'s predictive validity for recidivism. This study used the parent interview only (no youth interview or collateral information) with a sample of 711 youth first-time, misdemeanant offenders (Gavazzi, Yarcheck, Sullivan, Jones, & Khurana, 2008). Of the 12.5% of youth that were adjudicated on a subsequent delinquency charge, three GRADcis™ domain scores combined (accountability, education, and family) correctly classified 74% of the reoffenders as high risk (with a 26% false negative rate) and 63% of offenders as low risk (with a 37% false positive rate). For Black youths, a higher proportion of those scoring high-risk on the GRADcis™ recidivated (29%) than did high-risk youths in the sample as a whole. Thus, it appears the GRADcis™ not only has predictive validity for Black youths, but it performs better for this group than for Whites.

The GRADcis™ is a promising tool with wide utility and a growing body of research. An advantage of the GRADcis™ is that it can be used with both status offenders and delinquent youths and has specific norms for each group. Potential limitations are the lack of a manual to evaluate scoring procedures, the lack of a requirement for collateral information (it appears to be mostly self-report), and it is unclear whether there is an evidence-based association between the treatment recommendations and risk scores. The content of the GRADcis™ is consistent with research and it contains both dynamic and static variables, but it is unclear whether it permits rater discretion. To date, no research is available from an independent party.

Tools for Evaluating the Risk of Harm for Non–Juvenile Justice Populations

Adolescent and Child Urgent Threat Evaluation (ACUTE)

The Adolescent and Child Urgent Threat Evaluation (Copelan & Ashley, 2005) is a 27-item assessment tool designed to measure risk of near future harm to self or others (within hours to days) in youth aged 8 to 18 in a variety of settings, including inpatient and outpatient clinics, schools, emergency rooms, and juvenile justice facilities. The ACUTE can be administered by psychiatric, psychological, or social worker staff and requires approximately 10 to 20 minutes to complete. Information is gathered through an interview with the youth and family, chart review, and collateral contacts. Items are rated yes or no and are summed to provide a total score, an overall threat classification (extreme, high, moderate, and low clinical risk factors), and a threat cluster score. The threat cluster score allows an examiner to focus more narrowly on specific risk factors. The total risk score considers a youth's overall violence risk factors. There are six possible threat score clusters: threat (items reflect the expectation of death or violence within 72 hours); precipitating factors (items are related to near future violence); early precipitating factors (items reflect interpersonal instability, actual or perceived tensions, or severe threat to self-esteem and/or humiliation); late precipitating factors (items are related to cognitive distortions, obsessive thoughts, anxiety, and motor restlessness); predisposing factors (items related to antecedent historical and clinical information); and an impulsivity factors cluster (items reflect pattern of aggression, hostility, and antisocial behavior).

The ACUTE was developed over a 9-year period using three pilot samples between 1985 and 1994 (Copelan & Ashley, 2005). The standardization sample included 542 males and females aged 8 to 18 in four classification groups (nonthreat, suicide threat, homicide threat, and homicide–suicide threat). For the standardization sample, Copelan and Ashley reported alpha coefficients in the moderate to high range for the cluster scores and coefficients ranging from 0.70 to 0.85 for total scores. Test–retest was examined over a period of 24 to 48 hours with a subset of the combined threat (homicide and suicide threat) group ($n = 77$) resulting in correlations ranging from 0.71 to 0.97. Among trained raters, the clusters had interrater reliability ranging from 0.74 to 0.99, and the total score was 0.94.

Evidence for validity is sparse. Copelan and Ashley (2005) compared scores on the ACUTE to the Clinical Assessment of Depression (CAD), the Children's Depression Inventory (CDI), and the Suicide Ideation Questionnaire (SIQ). They found low to moderate correlations between the ACUTE clusters and the CAD and CDI scales and moderate correlations with the SIQ. To date, there is no published evidence for the ACUTE's predictive validity.

Psychosocial Evaluation and Threat Risk Assessment (PETRA)

The Psychosocial Evaluation and Threat Risk Assessment (Schneller, 2005) is a brief 60-item self-report instrument intended to assess the risk of violence threat for middle school and high school students aged 11 to 18. It is used with students who express a threat of violence to themselves or to others. The purpose is to quickly gather and summarize threat-related data, guide interventions, and determine whether further evaluation is required. Thus, we would define the PETRA as a screening tool.

Formal training is not required to administer or score the instrument but is recommended for interpreting the scores. The PETRA is written at a third-grade reading level and can be completed in approximately 10 to 15 minutes in individual or group settings. Students answer questions on a four-point scale. Scores are summed to produce a total score, three additional domain scores (psychosocial, resiliency problems, and ecological), and eight cluster scores (depressed mood, alienation, egocentricism, aggression, family/home, school, stress, and coping problems). There are also two items measuring response style (inconsistency and social desirability). Relative standing is assessed using conversion tables grouped by age and gender for the domain scores, cluster scores, and response style items. The PETRA includes an additional eight critical items identifying known threat risk factors, which evaluators use to score the PETRA Threat Assessment Matrix to classify the content of the threat as low, medium, or high. PETRA scores are interpreted through a five-step process, including a brief follow-up interview with the youth and consideration of other relevant clinical data.

The PETRA was developed from a comprehensive review of school violence and other relevant literature to make items for clinically and theoretically relevant scales (Schneller, 2005). The normative sample was approximately 1,770 male and female students aged 11 to 18 from a range of ethnic/racial backgrounds drawn from 10 schools. Test–retest reliability was assessed for a period of 7 to 10 days following the first administration, with correlations ranging from 0.63 (coping problems) to 0.88 (aggression) on PETRA domain and cluster scores. To test the concurrent validity, Schneller compared PETRA scores of 89 individuals to scores on the Behavior Assessment System for Children Self-Report of Personality, the Child Behavior Checklist (CBCL), the CAD, the CDI, and the SIQ. For the CBCL total score, PETRA total scores correlated 0.77, but there was a low correlation for the ecological domain score ($r = 0.31$). For the threat assessment group, total scores had moderate correlations with the CAD ($r = 0.46$), and the depressed mood cluster correlated highly with the CAD depressed mood scale ($r = 0.71$). For the SIQ total score, the PETRA total score correlated moderately ($r = 0.38$), but it correlated strongly with the PETRA depressed mood cluster ($r = 0.74$) and the PETRA stress cluster ($r = 0.51$). We were unable to find any published studies that examined the predictive validity of the PETRA.

CONCLUSIONS AND RECOMMENDATIONS

This chapter outlined a number of the important concepts related to assessing risk for antisocial behavior, violence, and recidivism in youth as well as concepts related to the selection of risk screening and assessment tools. We described a minimum standard for an evidence-based tool, including presence of a manual with scoring criteria, analyses of the structure of the instrument, evidence for reliability from independent parties, and evidence of validity from independent parties. This was followed by a review of the most prominent risk assessment tools available today with special consideration of the important factors in the selection of instruments. In light of the standard for instruments and the needs to address developmental issues in these assessment tools, the only tools that achieve our proposed criteria at this time are the YLS/CMI and the SAVRY. With respect to screening tools, we would consider the NCAR to be evidence-based because it has two published studies of its predictive validity by an independent party and some evidence for interrater reliability. A few other tools came close to meeting the standard, and, therefore, we would consider these to be promising. These were the WSJCA/YASI, EARL-20B, RRC, ERASOR, and J-SOAP-II. The J-SOAP-II would have met all criteria, but one study found it did not predict sexual violence, and one study found it did predict sexual violence.

For the most part, very few of the tools available to assess youth risk for recidivism have reported interrater reliability. This is problematic because the item scoring rules are not always straightforward. Very few tools contain dynamic factors that would lend themselves to reassessment and even those tools designed to measure change lack evidence with respect to their ability to do this. This issue is critical given the potential detrimental effects of labeling a youth as high risk without a method for measuring his or her reduction in risk in the near future. We make an appeal to researchers and test developers to investigate the ability of these tools to measure changes in risk. We should be particularly cautious of the use of instruments that are based entirely on historical, static variables, where scores can go up but they cannot go down.

The class of tools that are entirely computer or Web-based require some further discussion. On the surface, these tools are very attractive to probation officers and case managers because they generate case management plans, thereby making one's job easier. The problem is that there is no research-based evidence about the value of matching particular youth with particular services based on assessment data at this time.

Another problem is what happens when the resources recommended by the tool are not available in the particular community. There does not seem to be much latitude for examiner discretion, and these tools are not transparent in that the scoring algorithms are not available. The GRADcis™ shows the most promise in this regard given the generated norms and the growing research evidence. Hopefully, we will see some evidence for the GRADcis™'s reliability and some studies by an independent party in the near future. The limitations with these tools are critical in light of the financial burden some of them can impose to the states that implement them.

The concept of *evidence-based* as applied to the social sciences generally refers to shaping governmental policies based on scientific evidence that shows the policy has some cause and effect (Austin, 2006). An evidence-based practice commonly refers to a treatment or intervention that scientists have demonstrated to show some effect. At this point, there have not been any randomized studies showing that implementing risk assessment tools in juvenile justice has an impact on recidivism or appropriate intervention planning. On a positive note, one close approximation was a pre–post study conducted in the state of Maryland. Researchers examined the potential impact of implementation of a standardized risk assessment tool on service referrals and out-of-home placement decisions (Young, Moline, Farrell, & Biere, 2006). There were some shifts in referrals and placement decisions post-implementation; however, probation officers and judges did not entirely base decisions on assessment data. Research for the youth juvenile justice system lags far behind that for adults, where studies of the LSI-R have indicated a reduction in recidivism after implementation of the instrument (Flores, Lowenkamp, Holsinger, & Latessa, 2006). In conclusion, in the strict definition of the term, we cannot consider implementation of risk assessment tools in juvenile justice agencies to be an evidence-based practice at this time, but evidence is near. Conventional wisdom dictates that this would have a positive impact on the lives of youth involved in the juvenile justice system, but only if the tool is relevant, reliable, and valid. This is another area in need of research.

NOTE

1. The two-trajectory theory seems to oversimplify the nature of youth offending. More recent analyses using growth curve modeling indicate the existence of four antisocial behavior trajectories (Odgers et al., 2008). It will take several years before this research is translated into risk assessment frameworks.

REFERENCES

Andrews, D. A., & Bonta, J. (1995). *Level of Service Inventory–Revised.* North Tonawanda, NY: Multi-Health Systems.

Andrews, D. A., Robinson, D., & Hoge, R. D. (1984). *Manual for the Youth Level of Service Inventory.* Ottawa, Canada: Department of Psychology, Carleton University.

Augimeri, L. K., Koegl, C. J., Levene, K. S., & Webster, C. D. (2005). Early assessment risk lists for boys and girls. In T. Grisso, G. Vincent, & D. Seagrave (Eds.), *Mental health screening and assessment in juvenile justice* (pp. 295–310). New York: Guilford Press.

Augimeri, L. K., Koegl, C. J., Webster, C. D., & Levene, K. S. (2001). *Early Assessment Risk List for Boys: EARL-20B, Version 2.* Toronto, Canada: Earlscourt Child and Family Centre.

Augimeri, L. K., & Levene, K. S. (1994). *Risk factors associated with possible conduct disorders and non-responders.* Toronto, Canada: Earlscourt Child and Family Centre.

Austin, J. (2006). How much risk can we take? The misuse of risk assessment in corrections. *Federal Probation, 70*(2), 58–63.

Baglivio, M. (2007). *The prediction of risk to recidivate among a juvenile offending population.* Unpublished doctoral dissertation, University of Florida, Gainesville.

Baird, C., & Wagner, D. (2000). The relative validity of actuarial- and consensus-based risk assessment systems. *Children and Youth Services Review, 22,* 839–871.

Barnoski, R. (1998). *Validation of the Washington State Juvenile Court Assessment* (Report No. 98–11–1201). Olympia: Washington State Institute for Public Policy.

Barnoski, R. (2004a). *Assessing risk for re-offense: Validating the Washington State Juvenile Court Assessment* (Report No. 04–03–1201). Olympia: Washington State Institute for Public Policy.

Barnoski, R. (2004b). *Washington State Juvenile Court Assessment manual, Version 2.1* (Report No. 04–03–1203). Olympia: Washington State Institute for Public Policy.

Bartel, P., Forth, A., & Borum, R. (2003). *Development and concurrent validation of the Structured Assessment for Violence Risk in Youth (SAVRY).* Manuscript under review.

Berlin, F. S., Galbreath, N. W., Geary, B., & McGlone, G. (2003). The use of actuarials at civil commitment hearings to predict the likelihood of future sexual violence. *Sexual Abuse: A Journal of Research and Treatment, 15*(4), 377–382.

Boer, D. P., Hart, S. D., Kropp, P. R., & Webster, C. D. (1997). *Manual for the Sexual Violence Risk–20: Professional guidelines for assessing risk of sexual violence.* Vancouver, Canada: British Columbia Institute Against Family Violence and the Mental Health, Law, and Policy Institute, Simon Fraser University.

Borum, R. (1996). Improving the clinical practice of violence risk assessment: Technology, guidelines, and training. *American Psychologist, 51,* 945–956.

Borum, R., Bartel, P., & Forth, A. (2003). *Manual for the Structured Assessment for Violence Risk in Youth (SAVRY): Version 1.1.* Tampa: Louis de la Parte Florida Mental Health Institute, University of South Florida.

Borum, R., Bartel, P., & Forth, A. (2005). Structured Assessment of Violence Risk in Youth. In T. Grisso, G. Vincent, & D. Seagrave (Eds.), *Mental health screening and assessment in juvenile justice* (pp. 311–323). New York: Guilford Press.

Borum R., & Douglas, K. (2003). New directions in violence risk assessment. *Psychiatric Times, 20*, 102–103.

Borum, R., & Verhaagen, D. (2006). *Assessing and managing violence risk in juveniles.* New York: Guilford Press.

Brennan, T. (2003). *Youth COMPAS psychometrics report.* Traverse City, MI: Northpointe Institute for Public Management.

Catchpole, R., & Gretton, H. (2003). The predictive validity of risk assessment with violent young offenders: A 1-year examination of criminal outcome. *Criminal Justice and Behavior, 30*, 688–708.

Cauffman, E., Scholle, S. H., Mulvey, E., & Kelleher, K. J. (2005). Predicting first time involvement in the juvenile justice system among emotionally disturbed youth receiving mental health services. *Psychological Services, 2*(1), 28.

Chapman, J., Desai, R., Falzer, P., & Borum, R. (2006) Violence risk and race in a sample of youth in juvenile detention: The potential to reduce disproportionate minority confinement. *Youth Violence and Juvenile Justice, 4*, 170–184.

Copelan, R., & Ashley, D. (2005). *Adolescent and child urgent threat evaluation: Professional manual.* Lutz, FL: Psychological Assessment Resources.

Copeland, W. E., Miller-Johnson, S., Keeler, G., Angold, A., & Costello, E. J. (2007). Childhood psychiatric disorders and young adult crime: A prospective, population-based study. *American Journal of Psychiatry, 164*, 1668–1675.

Dieterich, W., & Brennan, T. (2004). *Youth COMPAS data for Ventura County Probation Agency: Descriptive statistics and basic psychometric properties.* Traverse City, MI: Northpointe Institute for Public Management.

Dolan, M. C., & Rennie, C. E. (2008). The structured assessment of violence risk in youth as a predictor of recidivism in a United Kingdom cohort of adolescent offenders with conduct disorder. *Psychological Assessment, 20*(1), 35–46.

Douglas, K. S., Yeoman, M., & Boer, D. P. (2005). Comparative validity analysis of multiple measures of violence risk in a sample of criminal offenders. *Criminal Justice and Behavior, 32*, 479–510.

Dvoskin, J. A., & Heilbrun, K. (2001). Risk assessment: Release decision-making toward resolving the great debate. *Journal of the American Academy of Psychiatry and the Law, 29*(1), 6–10.

Elliott, D. S., Huizinga, D., & Menard, S. (1989). *Multiple problem youth: Delinquency, substance use and mental health problems.* New York: Springer-Verlag.

Enebrink, P., Langstrom, N., & Gumpert, C. H. (2006). Predicting aggressive and disruptive behavior in referred 6- to 12-year-old boys: Prospective validation of the EARL-20B Risk/Needs Checklist. *Assessment, 13*, 356–367.

Enebrink, P., Langstrom, N., Neij, J., Grann, M., & Gumpert, C. H. (2001). *Brief report: Interrater reliability of the Early Assessment Risk List: EARL-20B: A new guide for clinical evaluation of conduct-disordered boys.* Huddinge, Sweden: Karolinska Institute.

Epperson, D. L., Ralston, C. A., Fowers, D., & DeWitt, J. (2005). *Development of a sexual offense recidivism risk assessment tool–II (JSORRAT-II).* Unpublished manuscript, University of Iowa, Iowa City.

Fagan, J., & Zimring, F. E. (Eds.). (2000). *The changing borders of juvenile justice: Transfer of adolescents to the criminal court.* Chicago: University of Chicago Press.

Farrington, D. P. (1992). Explaining the beginning, progress, and ending of antisocial behavior from birth to adulthood. In J. McCord (Ed.), *Facts, frameworks, and forecasts: Advances in criminological theory* (pp. 253–286). New Brunswick, NJ: Transaction Publishers.

Farrington, D. P. (2007). Advancing knowledge about desistance. *Journal of Contemporary Criminal Justice, 23,* 125–134.

Farrington, D. P., Barnes, G. C., & Lambert, S. (1996). The concentration of offending in families. *Legal and Criminological Psychology, 1*(1), 47–63.

Farrington, D. P., & West, D. J. (1993). Criminal, penal, and life histories of chronic offenders: Risk and protective factors and early identification. *Criminal Behaviour and Mental Health, 3,* 492–523.

Flores, A. W., Lowenkamp, C. T., Holsinger, A. M., & Latessa, E. J. (2006). Predicting outcome with the Level of Service Inventory–Revised: The importance of implementation integrity. *Journal of Criminal Justice, 34,* 523–529.

Forth, A. E., Kosson, D. S., & Hare, R. D. (2003). *Hare Psychopathy Checklist–Revised: Youth Version.* Toronto, Canada: Multi-Health Systems.

Gavazzi, S., Lim, J., Yarcheck, C., & Eyre, E. (2003). Brief report on predictive validity evidence of global risk indicators in the lives of court-involved youth. *Psychological Reports, 93,* 1239–1242.

Gavazzi, S., Yarcheck, C. M., & Lim, J. (2005). Ethnicity, gender, and global risk indicators in the lives of status offenders coming to the attention of the juvenile court. *International Journal of Offender Therapy and Comparative Criminology, 49*(6), 696–710.

Gavazzi, S., Yarcheck, C., Sullivan, J., Jones, S., & Khurana, A. (2008). Global risk factors and the prediction of recidivism rates in a sample of first-time misdemeanant offenders. *International Journal of Offender Therapy and Comparative Criminology, 52*(3), 330–345.

Gottfredson, D., & Tonry, M. (1988). *Prediction and classification: Criminal justice decision-making.* Chicago: Chicago University Press.

Greenwood, P., & Abrahamse, A. (1982). *Selective incapacitation* (R-2815-NIJ). Santa Monica, CA: Rand Corporation.

Gretton, H., & Abramowitz, C. (2002, March). *SAVRY: Contribution of items and scales to clinical risk judgments and criminal outcomes.* Paper presented at the biennial conference of the American Psychology-Law Society, Austin, TX.

Grisso, T. (1998). *Forensic evaluation of juveniles.* Sarasota, FL: Professional Resource Press.

Grisso, T. (2000, March). *Ethical issues in evaluations for sex offender re-offending.* Paper presented at the Sex Offender Re-Offence Risk Prediction Training, Sinclair Seminars, Madison, WI.

Grisso T. (2004). *Double jeopardy: Adolescent offenders with mental disorders.* New York: Guilford Press.

Grisso, T. (2005a). Evaluating the properties of instruments for screening and assessment. In T. Grisso, G. Vincent, & D. Seagrave (Eds.), *Mental health screening and assessment in juvenile justice* (pp. 71–93). New York: Guilford Press.

Grisso, T. (2005b). Why we need mental health screening and assessment in juvenile justice programs. In T. Grisso, G. Vincent, & D. Seagrave (Eds.), *Mental health screening and assessment in juvenile justice* (pp. 3–21). New York: Guilford Press.

Grisso, T., & Tomkins, A. J. (1996). Communicating violence risk assessments. *American Psychologist, 51,* 928–930.

Grisso, T., & Underwood, L. (2004). *Screening and assessing mental health and substance use disorders among youth in the juvenile justice system: A resource guide for practitioners* (Document #204956). Washington, DC: Office of Juvenile Justice and Delinquency Prevention.

Grisso, T., Vincent, G. M., & Seagrave, D. (2005). *Mental health screening and assessment in juvenile justice.* New York: Guilford Press.

Grove, W. M., & Meehl, P. E. (1996). Comparative efficiency of informal (subjective, impressionistic) and formal (mechanical, algorithmic) prediction procedures: The clinical-statistical controversy. *Psychology, Public Policy, and Law, 2*(2), 293–323.

Grubin, D., & Wingate S. (1996). Sexual offence recidivism: Prediction versus understanding. *Criminal Behavior and Mental Health, 6,* 349–359.

Guarino-Ghezzi, S., & Byrne, J. M. (1989). Developing a model of structured decision making in juvenile corrections: The Massachusetts experience. *Crime & Delinquency, 35,* 270–302.

Haapanen, R., & Jesness, C. F. (1982). *Early identification of the chronic offender.* Sacramento: California Youth Authority.

Hart, S. D. (2003). Actuarial risk assessment: Commentary on Berlin et al. *Sexual Abuse: A Journal of Research and Treatment, 15*(4), 383–388.

Hart, S. D., Kropp, R., Laws, D. R., Klaver, J., Logan, C., & Watt, K. A. (2003). *The risk for sexual violence protocol (RSVP): Structured professional guidelines for assessing risk of sexual violence.* Burnaby, Canada: Simon Fraser University.

Hoge, R. D. (2002). Standardized instruments for assessing risk and need in youthful offenders. *Criminal Justice and Behavior, 29,* 380–396.

Hoge, R. D., & Andrews, D. A. (2006). *Youth Level of Service/Case Management Inventory: User's manual.* North Tonawanda, NY: Multi-Health Systems.

Jesness, C. F. (1986). Validity of the Jesness Inventory Classification with nondelinquents. *Educational and Psychological Measurement, 46,* 947–961.

Jesness, C. F. (2003). *Jesness Inventory Revised–Technical manual.* North Tonawanda, NY: Multi-Health Systems.

Jung, S. (1996). *Critical evaluation of the validity of the risk/need assessment with Aboriginal young offenders in northwestern Ontario.* Unpublished master's thesis, Lakehead University, Thunder Bay, Canada.

Justice System Assessment and Training. (1998). *Risk & Resiliency Checkup manual.* Boulder, CO: Justice System Assessment and Training.

Kraemer, H. C., Kazdin, A. E., Offord, D. R., Kessler, R. C., Jensen, P. S., & Kupfer, D. J. (1997). Coming to terms with the terms of risk. *Archives of General Psychiatry, 54*(4), 337–343.

Kunce, J. T., & Hemphill, H. (1983). Delinquency and Jesness Inventory scores. *Journal of Personality Assessment, 47,* 632–634.

Levene, K. S., Augimeri, L. K., Pepler, D., Walsh, M., Webster, C. D., & Koegl, C. J. (2001). *Early Assessment Risk List for Girls: EARL-21G, Version 1, consultation edition.* Toronto, Canada: Earlscourt Child and Family Centre.

Loeber, R., Burke, J. D., & Lahey, B. B. (2002). What are adolescent antecedents to antisocial personality disorder. *Criminal Behaviour and Mental Health, 12,* 24–36.

Loeber, R., Lahey, B. B., & Thomas, C. (1991). Diagnostic conundrum of oppositional defiant disorder and conduct disorder. *Journal of Abnormal Psychology, 100*(3), 379–390.

Lubell, K. M., & Vetter, J. B. (2006). Suicide and youth violence prevention: The promise of an integrated approach. *Aggression and Violent Behavior, 11*(2), 167.

Maney, S. M. (2007). *Gender, offense type, and caution scores on MAYSI-2 scales: Implications for MAYSI-2 users in the juvenile justice system.* Unpublished master's thesis, Suffolk University, Boston.

Marshall, J., Egan, V., & English, M. (2006). The relative validity of psychopathy versus risk/needs-based assessments in the prediction of adolescent offending behaviour. *Legal and Criminological Psychology, 11,* 197–210.

Martin, R. D. (1981). Cross-validation of the Jesness Inventory with delinquents and nondelinquents. *Journal of Consulting and Clinical Psychology, 49,* 10–14.

Martinez, R., Flores, J., & Rosenfeld, B. (2007). Validity of the juvenile sex offender assessment protocol-II (J-SOAP-II) in a sample of urban minority youth. *Criminal Justice and Behavior, 34*(10), 1284–1295.

McEachran, A. (2001). *The predictive validity of the PCL:YV and the SAVRY in a population of adolescent offenders.* Unpublished master's thesis, Simon Fraser University, Burnaby, Canada.

Moffitt, T. E. (1993). Adolescence-limited and life-course-persistent antisocial behavior: A developmental taxonomy. *Psychological Review, 100*(4), 674–701.

Moffitt, T. E., & Caspi, A. (2001). Childhood predictors differentiate life-course persistent and adolescence-limited antisocial pathways among males and females. *Development and Psychopathology, 13*(2), 355–375.

Moffitt, T. E., Caspi, A., Dickson, N., Silva, P., & Stanton, W. (1996). Childhood-onset versus adolescent-onset antisocial conduct problems in males: Natural history from ages 3 to 18 years. *Development and Psychopathology, 8,* 399–424.

Monahan, J. (1981). *Predicting violent behavior: An assessment of clinical techniques.* Beverly Hills, CA: Sage.

Monahan, J. (1996). Violence prediction: The last 20 years and the next 20 years. *Criminal Justice and Behavior, 23,* 107–120.

Mulvey, E. P. (2005). Risk assessment in juvenile justice policy and practice. In K. Heilbrun, N. E. Sevin Goldstein, & R. E. Redding (Eds.), *Juvenile delinquency: Prevention, assessment, and intervention* (pp. 209–231). New York: Oxford University Press.

Munson, R. F., & Revers, M. P. (1986). Program effectiveness of a residential treatment center for emotionally disturbed females as measured by exit personality tests. *Adolescence, 21,* 305–310.

National Council on Crime and Delinquency & New Mexico Children, Youth and Families Department, Juvenile Justice Division. (2004). *Structured decision-making for adjudicated juvenile delinquents.* Madison, WI: National Council on Crime and Delinquency.

Odgers, C. L., Moffitt, T. E., Broadbent, J. M., Dickson, N., Hancox, R. J., Harrington, H., et al. (2008). Female and male antisocial trajectories: From childhood origins to adult outcomes. *Development and Psychopathology, 20*(2), 673–716.

Odgers, C., Vincent, G. M., & Corrado, R. R. (2002). A preliminary conceptual framework for the prevention and management of multi-problem youth. In R. R. Corrado, R. Roesch, S. D. Hart, & J. K. Gierowski (Eds.), *Multi-problem violent* youth: *A foundation for comparative research on needs, interventions and outcomes* (pp. 302–329). Amsterdam: IOS Press.

Patterson G. R., Forgatch M. S., Yoerger K. L., & Stoolmiller M. (1998). Variables that initiate and maintain an early-onset trajectory of offending. *Developmental Psychopathology, 10,* 531–547.

Penney, S., Lee, Z., Moretti, M., & Bartel, P. (2007, March). *The predictive validity of the Structured Assessment of Violence Risk in Youth (SAVRY).* Poster presented at the Annual Forensic Psychiatry Conference, Vancouver, Canada.

Poluchowicz, S., Jung, S., & Rawana, E. P. (2000, June). *The interrater reliability of the Ministry Risk/Needs Assessment Form for juvenile offenders.* Presentation at the annual conference of the Canadian Psychological Association, Montreal, Canada.

Prentky, R. A., & Righthand, S. (2003). *Juvenile Sex Offender Assessment Protocol: Manual.* Bridgewater, MA: Justice Resource Institute.

Quinsey, V. L., Harris, G. T., Rice, M. E., & Cormier, C. A. (1998). *Violent offenders appraising and managing risk.* Washington, DC: American Psychological Association.

Righthand, S., Prentky, R., Knight, R., Carpenter, E., Hecker, J. E., & Nangle, D. (2005). Factor structure and validation of the Juvenile Sex Offender Assessment Protocol (J-SOAP). *Sexual Abuse: A Journal of Research and Treatment, 17*(1), 13–30.

Roberts, B. W., Caspi, A., & Moffitt, T. E. (2001). The kids are alright: Growth and stability in personality development from adolescence to adulthood. *Journal of Personality and Social Psychology, 81*(4), 670–683.

Robins L. N. (1974). Antisocial behavior disturbances of childhood: Prevalence, prognosis, and prospects. In E. J. Anthony & C. Koupernik (Eds.), *The child in his family: Children at psychiatric risk.* Oxford, England: Wiley.

Rossi, P. H., Schuerman, J., & Budde, S. (1999). Understanding decisions about child maltreatment. *Evaluation Review, 23*(6), 579–598.

Rubin, B. (1972). Prediction of dangerousness in mentally ill criminals. *Archives of General Psychiatry, 27,* 397–407.

Schmidt, F., Hoge, R., & Robertson, L. (2005). Reliability and validity analyses of the Youth Level of Services/Case Management Inventory. *Criminal Justice and Behavior, 32*(3), 329–344.

Schneller, J. (2005). *Psychosocial evaluation and threat risk assessment: Professional manual.* Lutz, FL: Psychological Assessment Resources.

Schwalbe, C. (2004). Re-visioning risk assessment for human service decision making. *Children and Youth Services Review, 26,* 561–576.

Schwalbe, C. (2008). Risk assessment stability: A revalidation study of the Arizona Risk/Needs Assessment Instrument. *Research on Social Work Practice Online, 1,* 1–9.

Schwalbe, C., Fraser, M., Day, S., & Arnold, E. (2004). North Carolina Assessment of Risk (NCAR): Reliability and predictive validity with juvenile offenders. *Journal of Offender Rehabilitation, 40,* 1–22.

Schwalbe, C. S., Fraser, M. W., Day, S. H., & Cooley, V. (2006). Classifying juvenile offenders according to risk of recidivism: Predictive validity, race/ethnicity, and gender. *Criminal Justice and Behavior, 33,* 305–324.

Skowyra, K. R., & Cocozza, J. J. (2007). *Blueprint for change: A comprehensive model for the identification and treatment of youth with mental health needs in contact with the juvenile justice system.* Delmar, NY: National Center for Mental Health and Juvenile Justice.

Steinhart, D. (2006). *Juvenile detention risk assessment: A practice guide to juvenile detention reform* (Vol. 1). Baltimore: Annie E. Casey Foundation.

Swets, J. A. (1988). Measuring the accuracy of diagnostic systems. *Science, 240*, 1285–1293.

Teplin, L. A., Abram, K. M., McClelland, G. M., Dulcan, M. K., & Mericle, A. A. (2002). Psychiatric disorders in youth in juvenile detention. *Archives of General Psychiatry, 59*(12), 1133–1143.

Thompson, M. P., Kingree, J. B., & Ho, C. (2006). Associations between delinquency and suicidal behaviors in a nationally representative sample of adolescents. *Suicide and Life-Threatening Behavior, 36*(1), 57–64.

Turner, S., Fain, T., & Sehgal, A. (2005). *Validation of the risk and resiliency assessment tool for juveniles in the Los Angeles county probation system.* Santa Monica, CA: Rand Corporation.

Upperton, R. A., & Thompson, A. P. (2007). Predicting juvenile offenders recidivism: Risk-need assessment and juvenile justice officers. *Psychiatry, Psychology and Law, 14*(1), 138–146.

Viljoen, J. L., Scalora, M., Cuadra, L., Bader, S., Chavez, V., Ullman, D., et al. (2008). Assessing risk for violence in adolescents who have sexually offended: A comparison of the J-SOAP-II, J-SORRAT-II, and SAVRY. *Criminal Justice and Behavior, 35*(1), 5–23.

Vincent, G. M., & Grisso, T. (2005). A developmental perspective on adolescent personality, psychopathology, and delinquency. In T. Grisso, G. Vincent, & D. Seagrave (Eds.), *Mental health screening and assessment in juvenile justice* (pp. 3–21). New York: Guilford Press.

Vincent, G. M., Grisso, T., & Terry, A. (2007). Mental health screening and assessment in juvenile justice. In C. L. Kessler & L. Kraus (Eds.), *Mental health needs of young offenders: Forging paths toward reintegration and rehabilitation* (pp. 270–287). Cambridge, England: Cambridge University Press.

Washington State Institute for Public Policy. (2004). *Assessing risk for re-offense: Validating the Washington State Juvenile Court Assessment* (Document No. 04–03–1201). Seattle, WA: Author.

Webster, C., Douglas, K., Eaves, D., & Hart, S. (1997). *HCR-20: Assessing risk for violence* (Version 2). Burnaby, Canada: Mental Health, Law, and Policy Institute, Simon Fraser University.

Welsh, J., Schmidt, F., McKinnon, L., Chattha, H., & Meyers J. (2008). A comparative study of adolescent risk assessment instruments: Predictive and incremental validity. *Assessment, 15*, 104–115.

West, D. J., & Farrington, D. P. (1973). *Who becomes delinquent?: Second report of the Cambridge Study in Delinquent Development.* Oxford, England: Heinemann Educational Publishers.

Wiebush, R. G., Wagner, D., & Ehrlich, J. (1999). *Development of an empirically-based risk assessment instrument for the Virginia Department of Juvenile Justice.* Oakland, CA: National Council on Crime and Delinquency.

Worling, J. R. (2004). The Estimate of Risk of Adolescent Sexual Offense Recidivism (ERASOR): Preliminary psychometric data. *Sexual Abuse: A Journal of Research and Treatment, 16*(3), 235–254.

Worling, J. R., & Curwen, T. (2001). Estimate of Risk of Adolescent Sexual Offense Recidivism (ERASOR; Version 2.0). In M. C. Calder, H. Hanks, & K. J. Epps (Eds.), *Juveniles and children who sexually abuse: Frameworks for assessment* (pp. 372–397). Dorset, England: Russell House.

Young, D., Moline, K., Farrell, J., & Biere, D. (2006). Best implementation practices: Disseminating new assessment technologies in a juvenile justice agency. *Crime & Delinquency, 52*, 135–158.

13

Reducing Risk for Violence and Aggression in Youth

CRAIG S. SCHWALBE

Richard is a 13-year-old boy who was adjudicated for misdemeanor simple assault. His offense was beating up another boy during an argument in the playground located on the grounds of his apartment complex. Because Richard has a reputation of being a neighborhood "tough" and has associated with known gang members for the past 2 years, the parents of the boy insisted that charges be brought against Richard. Based partly on Richard's prior record of assault, the juvenile court judge ordered Richard to probation and placement in a group home.

In nearly every respect, Richard can be considered a high-risk adolescent. He is known to have a quick temper and to engage in frequent verbal and physical altercations. He has variously been described as hyperactive, impulsive, and having a propensity toward risk taking. At school, he performs below grade level and has been frequently suspended since entering middle school. As mentioned above, he associates with known gang members, and many of his peers engage in delinquent behaviors. During the intake assessment with the probation officer, Richard divulged that his mother and older brother both abuse alcohol; for his part, Richard has been known to consume alcohol and marijuana with increasing frequency during the past year. Richard's parents have a history of domestic violence, and their relationship remains strained. In terms of parenting, both his mother and father express a desire to help Richard but express deep frustration over his unwillingness to comply with their rules and expectations regarding curfew, school performance, peer associations, and household chores.

During the initial assessment interview with the probation officer, Richard's mother acknowledged that their parenting had been rough, not abusive, but maybe a bit inconsistent.

Complex cases like Richard's are the norm rather than the exception among youths involved in forensic settings. Among youths who appear before the juvenile court, not only is the prevalence of psychosocial problems like mental health disorders and school-related problems high, but the co-occurrence of these problems is more common than not. Indeed, psychosocial problems tend to bundle in youths to create subgroups of youths with complex, seemingly insurmountable obstacles to resilience.

Compounding this situation is a forensic service system that is fragmented at every level. Fragmentation across the service system is well documented (MacKinnon-Lewis, Kaufman, & Frabutt, 2002). Less well documented is the fragmentation that can exist within the processing of individual cases. It is perhaps more the norm than the exception that assessment and intervention planning procedures are less coordinated and more disjointed than we would like. Moreover, despite a chorus of expert advice imploring forensic practitioners to individualize services, intervention plans, and even assessments, often are geared toward the availability of interventions in the community rather than toward the circumstances of individual youths like Richard.

This chapter explores strategies aimed at reducing fragmentation and increasing coherence within cases by emphasizing risk reduction and asset promotion. The target of this exploration is the use of risk assessment instruments as clinical case planning tools. Risk assessment instruments are research-based assessment tools originally designed to predict the likelihood of delinquency and violence. They are often called "actuarial" tools because of the statistical methods that are used in their development. Usually, a set of risk factors such as parental supervision and history of aggression is chosen for an instrument based on their ability to predict an outcome like violence or delinquency. Ratings of individual risk factors are added together in some fashion to describe the overall risk of violence or delinquency posed by individual youths. Then, the risk assessment instrument is tested in a longitudinal study to estimate its ability to classify risk for the chosen outcome.

Not surprisingly, the risk assessment instrument used by Richard's probation officer, the Joint Risk Matrix (Schwalbe, Fraser, & Day, 2007), classified him as high risk. To achieve this level of risk, he had elevated scores on 10 of 14 risk factors; Table 13.1 shows the risk factors included

Table 13.1

RISK FACTORS INCLUDED IN THE JOINT RISK MATRIX

1. Early age at first complaint of delinquency to the juvenile court
2. **Number of prior referrals to the juvenile court**
3. **History of running away from home or placement**
4. **Known use of alcohol or illegal drugs during the past 12 months**
5. **School behavior problems during the past 12 months**
6. **Delinquent peer associations**
7. **Parental supervision**
8. **Problems with hyperactivity/impulsivity/attention**
9. Hostility toward others
10. Juvenile cooperation with court interventions
11. **Juvenile's attitude toward the most recent offense**
12. Parental cooperation with court interventions
13. **Mental health problems**
14. Family criminality

Note. Elevated risk factors for Richard are indicated in bold type.

on the Joint Risk Matrix and shows risk factors with elevated scores in Richard's case. Importantly, both he and his parents were both cooperative with the court intervention, and Richard's problems with the law appear to have a later onset.

To date, little has been written about the clinical utility of risk assessment instruments for case planning. The meager literature on the utilization of risk assessment instruments suggests that, despite their widespread use in forensic settings, these assessment instruments are as often ignored by practitioners as they are carefully considered (Hilton & Simmons, 2001; Krysik & LeCroy, 2002; Lyle & Graham, 2000; Schwalbe, 2004). In part, this may happen because risk assessment instruments tend to reveal little that is new for forensic social workers who complete them. For instance, by the time Richard's probation officer sat at his desk to complete the risk assessment instrument, he already knew about the risks and probably already had a sense about the complexity of Richard's case. In effect, completing the instrument contributed little to the probation officer's clinical thinking about Richard. Risk assessment instruments may be ignored by practitioners for other reasons as well. In the United States, several leading scholars have carefully circumscribed the purpose of risk assessment instruments to limit its use to disposition restrictiveness rather than case planning per se (Baird, 1984; Howell, 2003; Shlonsky & Wagner, 2005).

However, others see a wider potential for the integration of risk assessment instruments with case planning (Hoge & Andrews, 2003; Schwalbe, 2004). As may seem obvious in Richard's case, well-constructed risk assessment instruments can play a pivotal role in clinical case planning in addition to providing information about risk of future aggression and violence. This chapter takes the latter view and provides specific and detailed guidelines for the use of risk assessment instruments by forensic social workers.

The chapter begins by discussing recent advances in risk and resilience and offers this perspective as a conceptual framework for the integration of risk assessment and case planning. Next, it provides a brief overview of the literature on risk and protective factors for violence and aggression and follows with a review of the literature on risk assessment instruments. Then, it outlines a general approach for integrating risk assessment instruments with traditional case planning approaches. Finally, it describes a comprehensive case planning system that may be implemented by individual practitioners or by agencies that provide forensic services. When implemented, the case planning protocol described in this chapter will support the efforts of forensic social workers to reduce risk and increase protective factors for aggression and violence among individual youths seen in forensic settings.

RISK, RESILIENCE, AND YOUTHFUL AGGRESSION

Risk assessment is founded on the growing risk and resilience literature. Risk and resilience is an ecological approach to understanding the development of problematic and risky behaviors such as aggression and violence and, alternatively, to understanding the capacity of youths to achieve successful developmental milestones despite adversity (Fraser, 2004). Research into resilience can be traced to seminal studies by Garmezy (1971), Rutter (1979), and Werner and Smith (1982). These scholars established the study of resilience and adaptive functioning as a counterpoint to traditional research, which emphasizes developmental problems and deficits. Using the risk and resilience framework, researchers and practitioners are guided to consider the many influences on youth development that increase the likelihood of aggression and violence, *risk factors,* and to identify the keystone *protective factors* that make resilient functioning more likely.

Risk factors can be classified in different ways. In general, a risk factor is anything that increases the probability of poor developmental outcomes—aggression or violence in the present case. Hoge (2002), writing for criminal justice and juvenile justice scholars, defined three types of risk factors: static factors, criminogenic needs, and responsivity factors. Static risk factors are historical in nature and, as such, tend to remain fixed or indicate greater risk over time. Assaults to fetal development through maternal alcohol or tobacco consumption and history of aggression in early childhood are two examples. Criminogenic needs are dynamic risk factors that are potentially malleable and may be altered through changing circumstances and interventions. Common examples include parenting problems and peer associations. Responsivity factors, on the other hand, are correlates of successful intervention like motivation and beliefs about the reasons that justify formal intervention. These would not be expected to activate risk of aggression or violence except in the presence of other static risk factors or criminogenic needs.

Protective factors operate in the presence of risk to reduce the probability of aggression and violence and to promote more resilient functioning. Pioneering work on youth development and resilience by Masten, Rutter, Luther, and others (Masten & Coatsworth, 1998; Masten et al., 1999; Rutter, 2005) have isolated three common sources of protection. The first is cognitive capacity. The second is the capacity for emotional regulation and social problem solving. The third is a strong attachment to primary caretakers whose caretaking strategies balance warmth with age-appropriate control. Importantly, these protective systems are not independent and are, in fact, mutually reinforcing. Research indicates, for instance, that the effects of parenting and youth behavior are reciprocal—that is, that they influence each other (Jang & Smith, 1997; Stern & Smith, 1998; Thornberry, Lizotte, Krohn, Farnworth, & Jang, 1991). For example, aggressive parenting strategies in early childhood inhibit the development of emotional regulation in children, resulting in aggression and explosive behaviors. In turn, aggressive and explosive behaviors in children tend to erode positive parenting approaches, leading to an escalating cycle of negative parenting practices and aggressive childhood behaviors.

Fraser, Kirby, and Smokowski (2004) outline four mechanisms through which these and other protective systems might influence youth resilience. (1) Some protective factors alter exposure to risk conditions. Strong parenting may shield youths from the effects of neighborhood violence and disorder, for example. (2) Other protective factors disrupt a sequence of risk that would otherwise lead to poor outcomes. For instance, in some communities, youth programs are specifically targeted to increase adult supervision during periods in which they would otherwise be vulnerable to delinquent peer associations. (3) Still other protective factors buffer youths by increasing their sense of self-esteem and self-efficacy, as when mentoring programs enhance prosocial skills (Rhodes, Grossman, & Resch, 2000). (4) Finally, some protective factors operate at the neighborhood and community levels to open opportunities for youths, as when adults hire and pay neighborhood children to complete chores.

Importantly, the risk and resilience framework, like all ecological perspectives, does not on its own identify the causes of aggression and violence. Indeed, research consistently shows that the cumulative effect of risk and protection is more predictive of aggression and violence than the presence of any given risk factor (Burchinal, Roberts, Hooper, & Zeisel, 2000; Pollard, Hawkins, & Arthur, 1999; Stouthamer-Loeber, Loeber, Homish, & Wei, 2001). That is, children with more risk factors and fewer protective factors are more likely to engage in violent behavior than children with fewer risk factors and more protective factors. Ultimately, an underlying assumption of the risk and resilience framework is the presence of multiple pathways leading to aggression and violence. At the individual level, these pathways, or risk chains, can only be known through careful assessment in individual cases.

As a practice model, risk and resilience provides a flexible framework for assessment, case planning, and intervention. In general, interventions should be aimed at reduction of cumulative risk and the increase of protective factors. In terms of risk reduction, a careful assessment of criminogenic needs and responsivity factors is required to identify potential intervention targets. Because risk factors are interrelated, it may be possible to identify keystone risk factors that, if changed, may result in a cascading effect and reduce risk in multiple areas. For example, successful truancy reduction for some youths may (a) reduce the role of negative peer influence on their behavior and may (b) reduce the strain on parents that tends to erode parenting capacity. In terms of protective processes, intervention may emphasize the three protective processes (cognitive capacity, emotional regulation, effective primary caretakers) or four protective mechanisms (reduce exposure to risk, disrupt risk effects, buffer risk, open compensatory opportunities) identified above. Which should we focus on first? Although decisions like this must be made in collaboration with clients, the research suggests that, although it can be beneficial to focus resources toward protective processes, active efforts toward risk reduction are also necessary for lasting change among high-risk youths (Pollard et al., 1999).

Common Risk and Protective Factors

Empirical research on risk and protective factors for aggression and violence predates the emergence of risk and resilience as a framework for research and practice. For example, William Healy, who organized and directed the first psychiatric institute dedicated to the assessment of delinquent youths in 1909, conducted a landmark study of risk factors for chronic delinquency (Healy, 1927). Using an individual case study approach, he examined 1,000 youths to uncover the various "causes" of repeated delinquency among youths referred to the psychiatric study center. He reported results for 823 case studies and concluded that mental abnormalities like "feeblemindedness" and mental health problems were causally related to delinquency among 72% of youths, that defective home conditions were causally related to delinquency for 68% of youths, and that hereditary problems such as criminally involved and mentally ill parents and grandparents were causally related to delinquency for 61% of youths. "Bad companions" were noted as a causative factor for 34% of youths studied. Like contemporary risk and resilience scholars, Healy resisted the temptation to derive a generalized theory of aggression and violence. Rather, he held that different risk and protective factors operate within individual cases to increase their propensity toward chronic offending.

More recent research on risk factors for aggression and violence has been summarized in two comprehensive meta-analyses by Lipsey and Derzon (1998) and by Cottle, Lee, and Heilbrun (2001). Lipsey and Derzon summarized the findings of 34 longitudinal studies of the correlates of serious criminal or violent behavior, defined as any index offense, while Cottle et al. focused on 22 studies of the risk factors associated with rearrest, readjudication, probation violation, and recommitment among youths referred to the juvenile justice system. Both studies found risk factors with strong effects in the domains of offense history, psychological factors, family factors, and peer factors. Specifically, Lipsey and Derzon reported five strong predictors: aggressive behavior before age 12, history of general offenses (e.g., property crimes, status offenses), psychological traits (e.g., impulsiveness, risk-taking behavior), antisocial parents, and delinquent peer associations. Similarly, Cottle, Lee, and Heilbrun identified what might be called four keystone risk factors: age at first offense, psychological problems (nonsevere psychopathology and conduct problems), family problems (parenting problems), and delinquent peer associations. Considering the sample differences of the two studies, the correspondence of their findings is striking.

Research into protective processes generally shows that attachment to parents, schools, and other conventional social institutions protects youths from aggression and violence (Franke, 2000). And, as research evidence accumulates, it is becoming clear that exposure to multiple protective processes is required to neutralize the effects of risk factors on aggression and violence (Herrenkohl, Huang, Tajima, & Whitney, 2003; Herrenkohl, Tajima, Whitney, & Huang, 2005; Pollard et al., 1999). For instance, Herrenkohl et al. (2003) examined the risk and protective processes of 154 aggressive 10-year-old children and followed them until they were 18 years old. They showed that community factors (e.g., prosocial neighborhood opportunities and attendance at religious services), family factors (e.g., bonding to family, positive family involvement, good family management), school-related factors (e.g., bonding to school, positive school involvement, high academic achievement), peer-related factors (e.g., prosocial peer involvement), and individual-level factors (e.g., prosocial beliefs) all protected against aggression and violence. Moreover, Herrenkohl et al. found that, at every level of risk (no risk, low risk, medium risk, high risk), having more protective factors reduced the likelihood of aggression. That is, the cumulative effect of having more protective factors reduced the chances of aggression and violence among youth.

Of interest to juvenile justice scholars and practitioners are gender differences in risk and protective processes that may justify the need for gender-specific interventions and services. As might be expected, many studies suggest greater similarity across gender than differences. In a large-scale longitudinal study of a birth cohort in New Zealand, Moffitt, Caspi, Rutter, & Silva (2001) reported on the role of gender in the relationship between risk factors and antisocial behavior. Over the course of childhood and adolescence, males in this study were exposed to greater levels of harsh discipline, neurological problems, and peer delinquency then females. These differences, in turn, accounted for gender differences in the rates of antisocial behavior. However, these risk factors functioned similarly for females and males. That is, members of both genders who had neurological impairments had higher rates of involvement in conduct problems than their nonexposed peers. This study, in concert with others, suggests that a risk factor is a risk factor regardless of gender (Silverthorn, Frick, & Reynolds, 2001; Simourd & Andrews, 1994).

Still, some researchers have identified subtle patterns suggesting meaningful differences between males and females. For instance, girls may be less influenced by peers toward delinquency than boys. Mears, Ploeger, and Warr (1998) examined the influence of delinquent peer relationships on the antisocial behavior of boys and girls and found that girls were more heavily influenced by their own internal moral compass than boys. In other words, in the face of peer pressure, boys were more likely to conform with peer expectations regardless of their moral evaluation of behavior, whereas girls were more likely to conform their behavior to their own moral standards. In addition to variation in peer influences over behavior, at least two studies suggest that poor school attachment might predict aggression more strongly for boys than girls and that family-related problems may be a more salient risk factor for girls than boys (Ayers, Hawkins, Peterson, Catalano, & Abbott, 1999; Blum, Ireland, & Blum, 2003).

Complicating the research findings is the effect of developmental time on the salience of risk and protective factors on aggression and violence. A common hypothesis suggests that family-related risk and protective processes are of critical importance in the development of chronic conduct problems beginning in early childhood but that peer-related risk processes are salient for youths whose conduct problems have a later onset (Frick, 2004; Harachi et al., 2006; Moffitt, Caspi, Harrington, & Milne, 2002). Depending on the time frame, some research bears this out, though not always as expected. For instance, Sameroff, Peck, and Eccles (2004) examined the effects of peer-, school-, and family-related influences on conduct problems in a longitudinal study from the period beginning in middle school and ending in young adulthood. They showed that the influence of positive parental control and discipline harshness was consistent across periods and that the effects of negative peer influence was similarly constant but that the effects of positive peer influences increased across these periods. In other words, parenting quality mattered throughout development, but the influence of peers changed over developmental stages.

Of course, risk and protective factors do not operate in isolation from one another. Indeed, research confirms what practitioners know well—that risk and protective factors interact in complex ways. For instance, the joint effects of parenting and peer deviance have been frequently examined (Knoester, Haynie, & Stephens, 2006). The work of Simons and colleagues stands out in this regard (Simons, Chao, Conger, & Elder, 2001; Simons, Simons, Burt, Brody, & Cutrona, 2005). In a longitudinal study of oppositional behaviors, parenting, community supports, and deviant peer associations, Simons et al. (2001) showed that, over time, oppositional behavior by youths tended to erode parental controls, which in turn promoted involvement with deviant peers. Moreover, data from the same longitudinal study indicated that the effects of authoritative parenting on deviant peer associations and on conduct problems are amplified when families reside in communities characterized by high degrees of cohesion and support. These studies, along with a newly developing literature on gene–environment interactions, provide strong evidence for the complex interplay of risk and protective factors.

CLINICALLY USEFUL RISK ASSESSMENT INSTRUMENTS

Actuarial risk assessment instruments can ground forensic practice in several ways. First, actuarial risk assessment instruments align forensic practice with empirical research into risk factors that act individually and cumulatively to increase the likelihood of aggression and violence. Across actuarial instruments, most include common risk factors in the domains of offending history, substance abuse, family-related problems, and school-related problems, among others (Howell, 1995). To the extent that forensic practice emphasizes interventions into empirically supported risk and protective processes, actuarial risk assessment instruments can inform those efforts. Second, actuarial risk assessment instruments help forensic social workers organize their assessments. Several risk assessment packages include semistructured interview schedules, for instance. In other cases, probation officers have reported that the administrative requirement of completing risk assessment instruments has increased the range of risk and protective factors they commonly assess. Finally, actuarial risk assessment instruments can help forensic social workers sharpen their case planning practices by honing in on the keystone risk and protective factors that were described in previous sections.

But not all risk assessment instruments are designed to increase clinical utility (Bonta, 1996). Early risk assessment instruments were composed of primarily static risk factors such as history of delinquent behaviors, and they emphasized the predictive function of risk assessment. Offending history variables add value to the predictive capacity of an actuarial risk assessment instrument but indicate little by way of malleable intervention targets. More recently, risk assessment instruments that incorporate criminogenic needs and responsivity factors have been developed. These instruments aim to maximize both the predictive validity and clinical utility of risk assessment instruments. These assessment instruments, grounded in the empirical literature on risk and resilience reviewed above, identify malleable risk factors that, if changed through intervention, might lead to risk reduction and the eventual prevention of future aggressive and violent behaviors. Further, if administered periodically, such risk assessments may provide an estimate of changing risk during the course of intervention and therefore may serve evaluation purposes as well.

Among risk assessment instruments, two stand out for their potential for clinical utility and for the depth of their empirical support: the Structured Assessment of Violence Risk in Youths (SAVRY) and the Youth Level of Service/Case Management Inventory (YLS/CMI) (Grisso, Vincent, & Seagrave, 2005; Hoge & Andrews, 2003). The YLS/CMI provides an empirical assessment of risk and identifies potential intervention targets in seven categories of criminogenic needs and responsivity factors: family circumstances/parenting, education/employment, peer relations, substance abuse, leisure/recreation, personality/behavior, and attitudes/orientations. These are measured using multiple indicators, 42 items in all, each contributing a single point to the total risk score. The SAVRY is a 30-item instrument that provides a guide for the clinical assessment of risk for violence in youths. It is comprised of 24 risk factors in three categories (historical, social or contextual, individual) and 6 protective factors. Examples of risk factors include history of violence, peer delinquency, poor parental management, risk taking/impulsivity, and low interest in or commitment to school. Examples of protective factors include prosocial involvements and strong commitment to school. Each item is rated low, medium, or high using clinical judgment. Like the YLS/CMI, items on the SAVRY point to potential intervention targets.

The design and empirical support underlying the YLS/CMI and the SAVRY recommend them for consideration in many forensic settings (Grisso et al., 2005). Both were designed with clinical utility in mind.

For instance, the YLS/CMI includes a semistructured interview guide and case planning protocol with the manual. And, compared to other risk assessment instruments, the YLS/CMI and the SAVRY have comparably deep research support. Both have been tested for their ability to predict violence and general delinquency and have been shown to be reliable measures of risk for violence and delinquency (Schwalbe, 2007).

BLENDING RISK ASSESSMENT INSTRUMENTS WITH CASE PLANNING

To be clinically useful, the findings of any risk assessment instrument must be translated into the case planning process. In many instances, case planning and risk assessment are nonoverlapping processes. Rather than directly informing case plan development, some forensic social workers and probation officers use risk assessment instruments strategically as a way to justify case plans in some instances but then ignore risk assessment instruments in other instances. Unfortunately, this approach underutilizes risk assessment instruments and eliminates the potential benefits of risk assessment instruments for the case planning process.

The gap between risk assessment instruments on the one hand and case planning procedures on the other is partially sustained by a discrepancy in how statistical judgments and clinical judgments are made (Dawes, Faust, & Meehl, 1989). Risk assessment instruments rely on mechanistic statistical tests to demonstrate their effectiveness. Grounded in findings on the effects of cumulative risk, risk assessment instruments simply count risk factors, weight them in some fashion, and add scores to identify the relative likelihood of future behaviors such as aggression and violence. The strengths of the statistical approach include consistency and accuracy. Because the process is standardized, estimates of risk for future aggression and violence should be less prone to vary across social workers when risk assessment instruments are used. Moreover, well-developed risk assessment instruments have been shown to be as accurate, or more accurate, than unaided clinical judgment for making forecasts about future events (Grove & Meehl, 1996). The weakness of the statistical approach is that, on their face, risk assessment instruments do not answer questions that are of paramount importance to clients. For instance, risk assessment instruments do not show how risk factors interact, which risk factors are causally related to the future behavior in question, and what might be the effect of unmeasured protective factors on the true likelihood of aggression and violence. Answers to these questions are necessary to develop case plan goals and intervention plans.

In contrast to the statistical judgments, case planning processes are built on more impressionistic decision-making strategies and pattern-matching approaches (Klein, 1998; Lipshitz, Klein, Orasanu, & Salas, 2001; Meehl, 1954). Whether obvious or hidden, nearly all case plans for aggressive or violent youths derive from hypotheses about either (a) how juveniles became aggressive in the first place or (b) the conditions under which aggression and violence are manifest and sustained. Implicit in the answer to these questions are estimates of risk for future aggression and assumptions about how specific interventions provide hope for changing risk. In the impressionistic approach, answers to these questions are made through the development of a story, or theory, that explains the case (Dawes, 1999). In Richard's case, the clinical manager responsible for establishing his care plan for the group home may develop a story about how Richard, who struggles in school and experiences disorder and instability in his home, may be seeking companionship and validation in a street culture that is characterized by gang activity, drug and alcohol use, and physical violence. Such a story helps forensic social workers make sense of a case. Research involving the direct observation of decision makers across a wide spectrum of professions and settings indicates that these case-based stories are created through carefully conducted assessments. Once created, case-based stories are compared against known prototypes, which subsequently suggest goals and intervention strategies that are grounded in common sense and generalized knowledge. When confronted with novel situations for which known prototypes do not exist, decision makers select among interventions by using mental simulation to play out their likely results. These two processes, comparison against known prototypes and mental simulation, form the basis of clinical case planning.

While the impressionistic approach captures well the most common planning strategies employed by forensic social workers, it is not without weaknesses. For example, habits of mind, called heuristics by psychologists, can interfere with the case planning process by biasing the case-based stories that practitioners develop (Tversky & Kahneman, 1974, 2002). One well-documented heuristic is the tendency to ignore disconfirming evidence in favor of first impressions once a case-based story is developed. Another heuristic is the tendency to create case-based stories around highly provocative information without regard for its overall relationship to aggression and violence. Thus, it is possible to base case plans on case-based stories or hypotheses that, in the end, ignore or disregard key information and consequently are not related to the problem of aggression and violence.

Transcending the divide between statistical and impressionistic decision making is the creative, and disciplined, act of the forensic social worker. Forensic social workers should not seek to abandon the impressionistic approach to case planning in favor of the more accurate statistical approach, nor should they simply disregard the statistical approach. Instead, forensic social workers should strive to maximize the benefits of both. Moreover, the key is not to conform either approach to the other but rather to shift nimbly between them to avoid making mistakes in judgment. This can be done by structuring the case planning process to take advantage of the complementary strengths of both approaches. For instance, the benefits of the actuarial approach should be highly prized by forensic social workers. These include the consistency of actuarial risk assessment instruments and their grounding in empirical research on risk and protective factors. Alternatively, the impressionistic approach offers the benefit of explaining how a planned intervention, if implemented properly, can succeed. The relative advantages of both approaches should be combined to reduce the potential for error and critical omissions in the case planning process.

To accomplish this integration, case planning procedures should be structured to maximize the benefits of statistical and impressionistic approaches. Moreover, specific strategies may be employed to discipline case planning procedures to reduce the potential for error. Needed is a case planning protocol that will help forensic social workers incorporate risk assessment instruments with impressionistic strategies. A sequence of stages that will accomplish this objective is described below. In each stage, forensic social workers are advised to ask critical questions that will strengthen case plans. Individual case planning protocol stages include case assessment, selection of priority risk and protective factors, developing case-based hypotheses, identifying intervention goals, and specifying intervention plans.

Case Assessment

Although they are not the direct focus of this chapter, assessment procedures involving both risk assessment and more general needs assessment underlie the case planning process. Clinically useful risk assessment instruments strengthen assessment and case planning processes, but they are, nevertheless, limited. Many risk assessment instruments incorporate simple measures of mental health problems and substance abuse but do not provide detailed information about these conditions, for instance. Rather, items on most risk assessment instruments summarize critical case information and indicate the need for more detailed assessment, which should be provided through competent clinical interviews and supplemented by other psychometric tests. Nevertheless, risk assessment instruments increase the consistency of assessment practices and ensure that critical criminogenic needs and responsivity factors are considered for all youths.

To complete the translation of the statistical approach and the impressionistic approach at the assessment stage, the forensic social worker should persistently pose and answer the following question: Assuming that the assessment has missed a critical piece of information, what information is required to complete this assessment? Occasionally, assessment interviews can attend to vivid content and develop great depth in a small number of areas at the expense of more seemingly mundane concerns that would increase the breadth and scope of the assessment. Yet mundane concerns may hold keys to fruitful intervention opportunities. Forensic social workers should resist the temptation to conclude that their assessments are complete and instead should strive toward greater comprehensiveness.

Select Priority Risk and Protective Factors

The next stage in an integrated case planning process is to explicitly identify priority risk and protective factors. These factors will become the basis for all subsequent stages of the case planning process. Many candidate risk factors are included in clinically useful actuarial risk assessment instruments such as the YLS/CMI and the SAVRY. Care should be taken to select factors that, in the judgment of the social worker and client, contribute substantially to the development and maintenance of aggression and violent behavior. Additionally, factors should be selected to take advantage of a potential cascading effect whereby change in one factor leads to beneficial changes in multiple risk and protective factors. Finally, restraint at this stage is warranted. Best practices in case planning strongly recommend limiting the number of priority risk and protective factors to three or fewer (Griffin & Torbet, 2002). Moreover, best practices in case planning support a collaborative stance with youths and their families on the selection of priority risk and protective factors.

In Richard's case, the clinical care manager chose two priority risk factors: hostility/anger toward others and parental supervision. The care manager reasoned that, if Richard could develop less aggressive strategies for engaging others and if his parents could provide more consistent and effective monitoring of his behavior, Richard would be less prone to aggression and violence.

How is one to know that these are the most fruitful intervention targets? One strategy is to conduct a mental simulation exercise called the premortem strategy (Klein, 1998). The premortem strategy is an exercise in critical thinking in which an unexpectedly poor outcome such as continued aggression or violence is assumed or imagined in the future despite efforts toward changing the priority risk factors. The task of the premortem strategy is to explain the poor outcome. In Richard's case, several reasons for ongoing aggression despite changes to the priority risk factors may be developed. For instance, the effects of changes to Richard's level of hostility and level of supervision may have been washed out by other powerful risk factors like gang involvement. Or alcohol abuse by other family members may interfere with parental efforts toward skillful supervision and monitoring of their children. The premortem strategy provides a check on the decision to select specific priority risk and protective factors and provides a rationale for revising or maintaining that choice. In Richard's case, the exercise may suggest replacing hostility with a focus on peer relationships or may alert the clinical care manager to the relationship between parental supervision and alcohol abuse in the family.

Identify Case-Based Causal Hypotheses

Having selected priority risk and protective factors, causal hypotheses should be identified to explain how each of the priority risk and protective factors are created and sustained. The subject of these hypotheses is less about the relationship between risk factors and aggression and violence; rather, the focus is on the risk and protective factors per se. In the end, the objective of this approach is to reduce the risk for aggression and violence by intervening with youths to change their profile of risk and protective factors. Thus, hypotheses should reflect this effort. Hypotheses take the form "A contributes to priority risk factor B for person C under X conditions" (Henggeler, Borduin, Schoenwald,

Rowland, & Cunningham, 1998). For example, Richard's clinical care manager may hypothesize:

1. Poor modeling by parents and peers contributes to Richard's hostile approach to others when adults attempt to set limits on his behaviors.
2. Concern for his reputation contributes to Richard's hostile approach to others when he feels challenged or threatened.

From this example, it is clear that A is a condition that may or may not be included in the actuarial risk assessment instrument but that is believed to cause or maintain the priority risk factor in some way; B is the priority risk factor about which multiple hypotheses may be developed; C represents the target client system and could include an individual or a family; X refers to the conditions under which the relations between A and B are thought to exist—for instance, in the absence of certain protective factors or in the presence of some other risk process as was illustrated by Richard's example.

To translate statistical and impressionistic processes at this stage, forensic social workers should resist the temptation to hold hypotheses in too high esteem. Indeed, a key feature of all hypotheses is that they can be disproved. Moreover, hypotheses will in all likelihood be revised as more information about a case comes to light. Forensic social workers should evaluate the strength and durability of their hypotheses by answering the question: What evidence do we have that suggests an alternative explanation for B? To answer this question, the forensic social worker may consider the mechanisms of action for other risk and protective factors identified on the actuarial risk assessment instrument or may consider information obtained during follow-up assessments of priority risk and protective factors. The answer to this question may initiate an iterative process of hypothesis revision or, in an extreme case, may culminate in the rejection of a favored hypothesis in favor of a competing hypothesis.

Identify Intervention Goals

With explicit hypotheses grounded in empirically supported risk and protective factors in hand, the development of intervention goals should be straightforward. Intervention goals should be aimed at eliminating or reducing B through a risk reduction approach, reducing exposure of the client to A by expanding related protective factors, by reducing the influence of A on B by developing other compensatory strengths, or by altering the context of A and B by intervening into X. In general, goals should be precise, be aimed at an active change rather than the absence of a condition, be achievable, and be measurable to the greatest extent possible. The following goal statements might apply in the case of Richard:

1. Richard will learn alternative social problem solving skills that he may use when he feels confronted or challenged.
2. Richard will develop relationships with a new set of positive role models or mentors.

Goal 1 emphasizes a direct reduction in the risk factor B, whereas goal 2 emphasizes the relationship of A with B by developing compensatory protective factors. Depending on case information not presented here, these goals may be sufficient to reduce his hostility. However, other goals focused on the context, X, may be helpful or necessary. For instance, Richard's teachers and/or parents might utilize less confrontational approaches when setting limits, or Richard might develop a way to avoid situations in which he feels confronted.

Of primary importance at this stage is to establish intervention goals that are grounded in case-based hypotheses about priority risk and protective factors. If this is the case, then goal attainment should imply a measurable reduction of risk on the risk assessment. To evaluate the sufficiency of the intervention goals, forensic social workers should answer the following question: Assuming that the intervention goal is achieved, will this lead to a reduction in measured risk on the risk assessment instrument? If answered in the negative, the goals should be reevaluated; it may be that the goals need to be more explicitly directed toward measurable risk and protective factors.

Develop Intervention Plans

Intervention plans build directly from intervention goals and describe the specific actions to be taken by youths, family members, the forensic social worker, and other relevant parties. Expert recommendations on the development of intervention plans emphasize two complementary themes: use of evidence-based interventions and use of informal community supports.

Support for the use of evidence-based interventions has grown since the "nothing works" era of the 1970s (Cullen, 2005). At that time, the results of more than one evaluation study into the effectiveness of psychosocial interventions in the criminal and juvenile justice systems cast a dim light on interventions generally. But since then, research has demonstrated the increasing effectiveness of carefully designed and carefully implemented psychosocial interventions. Brand-name interventions like multisystemic therapy for delinquent youths (Henggeler et al., 1998), aggression replacement therapy for violent youths (Goldstein, Glick, & Gibbs, 1998), and multidimensional family therapy for substance-abusing youths (Liddle, 2004) have all undergone rigorous empirical scrutiny. Unfortunately, brand-name evidence-based interventions are not available everywhere, nor have these interventions been extended to all potential priority risk and protective factors. However, it may be possible to construct interventions that approximate core characteristics of these evidence-based interventions. Lipsey and colleagues have conducted several large-scale meta-analyses that document the effectiveness of interventions generally and the characteristics of interventions associated with greater effectiveness more specifically (Landenberger & Lipsey, 2005; Lipsey & Wilson, 1998). Of particular interest are findings that certain intervention characteristics are consistently associated with greater intervention effectiveness. First, more effective interventions are implemented with fidelity; that is, intervention modifications are minimal, implementation across cases is consistent, and active efforts are undertaken to maximize youth involvement throughout the intervention. Second, longer interventions (longer than 6 months) tend to be more effective than shorter interventions. Third, many effective interventions are grounded in cognitive-behavioral principles that emphasize anger control or interpersonal problem solving. Other intervention types with strong records of success include programs that utilize volunteer counselors/mentors in conjunction with other intervention modalities and family-based interventions that target specific risk and protective processes.

In conjunction with the evidence-based practice movement, support for interventions grounded in positive youth development principles is gaining interest among forensic practitioners as well (Butts, Mayer, & Ruth, 2005; Torbet & Thomas, 2005). Positive youth development principles emphasize the connections that youths have, or can develop, with informal community-based resources and adults. Positive youth development interventions seek to develop opportunities for youth involvement on the one hand and develop competencies for skillful engagement by youths on the other hand. The emphasis of many youth development interventions is on building assets and protective factors in addition to, or even rather than, risk reduction. Mentoring programs and after-school programs are two types of interventions commonly identified with the positive youth development movement. When designing youth development interventions, forensic social workers should take care to consider the four protective processes outlined by Fraser (2004) as a means toward goal attainment.

To be effective, interventions should be precisely targeted. In the context of the case planning procedures recommended here, planned interventions should be directly related to the goals developed during the preceding stage. For Richard, this means that his clinical care coordinator might arrange for Richard's participation in an evidence-based social skills program that helps him to perceive and interpret the meaning of social interactions more effectively and that increases his repertoire of skillful responses when he feels confronted. Moreover, Richard may be referred to a mentoring program. Both interventions relate directly to the goals established in the preceding section.

To complete the integration of the statistical and impressionistic approaches to judgment and planning, forensic social workers should trace the case planning process backward from the intervention planning stage to the case assessment stage. At the end of the case planning process, it should be clear that interventions should be developed that are realistically expected to achieve explicitly stated goals, which are grounded in explicit hypotheses, which describe relations involving explicitly identified priority risk and protective factors, which were derived from a comprehensive assessment of youth risk and protective factors. When successful, a case plan developed with these procedures will have a high likelihood of altering the profile of risk and protective factors and to reduce or eliminate the occurrence of aggression and violence.

CONCLUSION

This chapter has argued for the compatibility of risk assessment instruments on the one hand and impressionistic case planning approaches on the other. It reviewed the literature on risk and resilience that guides the development of evidence-based interventions and youth development approaches and demonstrated that clinically useful risk assessment instruments incorporate many of the same risk and protective factors. Finally, it outlined an approach to case planning that integrates risk assessment instruments, clinical judgment, and critical thinking exercises. When implemented, this approach will result in highly focused intervention plans that target precisely defined risk and protective processes for change.

REFERENCES

Ayers, C. D., Hawkins, J. D., Peterson, P. L., Catalano, R. F., & Abbott, R. D. (1999). Assessing correlates of onset, escalation, deescalation, and desistance of delinquent behavior. *Journal of Quantitative Criminology 15*, 277–305.

Baird, C. (1984). *Classification of juveniles in corrections: A model systems approach.* Madison, WI: National Council on Crime and Delinquency.

Blum, J., Ireland, M., & Blum, R. W. (2003). Gender differences in juvenile violence: A report from Add Health. *Journal of Adolescent Health, 32*, 234–240.

Bonta, J. (1996). Risk-needs: Assessment and treatment. In A. T. Harland (Ed.), *Choosing correctional options that work: Defining the demand and evaluating the supply* (pp. 18–32). Thousand Oaks, CA: Sage.

Burchinal, M. R., Roberts, J. E., Hooper, S., & Zeisel, S. A. (2000). Cumulative risk and early cognitive development: A comparison of statistical risk models. *Developmental Psychology, 36*, 793–807.

Butts, J., Mayer, S., & Ruth, G. (2005). *Focusing juvenile justice on positive youth development.* Chicago: Chapin Hall Center for Children.

Cottle, C. C., Lee, R. L., & Heilbrun, K. (2001). The prediction of criminal recidivism in juveniles: A meta-analysis. *Criminal Justice and Behavior, 34*, 367–394.

Cullen, F. T. (2005). The twelve people who saved rehabilitation: How the science of criminology made a difference—The American Society of Criminology 2004 presidential address. *Criminology, 43*(1), 1–42.

Dawes, R. M. (1999). A message from psychologists to economists: Mere predictability doesn't matter like it should (without a good story appended to it). *Journal of Economic Behavior & Organization, 39*(1), 29–40.

Dawes, R. M., Faust, D., & Meehl, P. E. (1989). Clinical vs. actuarial judgment. *Science, 243*, 1668–1674.

Franke, T. M. (2000). The role of attachment as a protective factor in adolescent violent behavior. *Adolescent & Family Health, 1*, 40–51.

Fraser, M. W. (Ed.). (2004). *Risk and resilience in childhood: An ecological perspective* (2nd ed.). Washington, DC: NASW Press.

Fraser, M. W., Kirby, L. D., & Smokowski, P. R. (2004). Risk and resilience in childhood. In M. W. Fraser (Ed.), *Risk and resilience in childhood: An ecological perspective* (pp. 13–66). Washington, DC: NASW Press.

Frick, P. J. (2004). Developmental pathways to conduct disorder: Implications for serving youth who show severe aggressive and antisocial behavior. *Psychology in the Schools, 41*, 823–834.

Garmezy, N. (1971). Vulnerability research and the issue of primary prevention. *American Journal of Orthopsychiatry, 41,* 101–116.

Goldstein, A. P., Glick, B., & Gibbs, J. C. (1998). *Aggression replacement training: A comprehensive intervention for aggressive youth.* Champaign, IL: Research Press.

Griffin, P., & Torbet, P. (2002). *Desktop guide to good juvenile probation practice.* Pittsburgh, PA: National Center for Juvenile Justice.

Grisso, T., Vincent, G., & Seagrave, D. (Eds.). (2005). *Mental health screening and assessment in juvenile justice.* New York: Guilford Press.

Grove, W. M., & Meehl, P. E. (1996). Comparative efficiency of informal (subjective, impressionistic) and formal (mechanical, algorithmic) prediction procedures: The clinical-statistical controversy. *Psychology, Public Policy, and Law, 2,* 293–323.

Harachi, T. W., Fleming, C. B., White, H. R., Ensminger, M. E., Abbott, R. D., Catalano, R. F., et al. (2006). Aggressive behavior among girls and boys during middle childhood: Predictors and sequelae of trajectory group membership. *Aggressive Behavior, 32,* 279–293.

Healy, W. (1927). *The individual delinquent: A text-book of diagnosis and prognosis for all concerned in understanding offenders.* Boston: Little, Brown.

Henggeler, S. W., Borduin, C. M., Schoenwald, S. K., Rowland, M. D., & Cunningham, P. B. (1998). *Multisystemic treatment of antisocial behavior in children and adolescents.* New York: Guilford Press.

Herrenkohl, T. I., Huang, B., Tajima, E. A., & Whitney, S. D. (2003). Examining the link between child abuse and youth violence: An analysis of mediating mechanisms. *Journal of Interpersonal Violence, 18,* 1189–1208.

Herrenkohl, T. I., Tajima, E. A., Whitney, S. D., & Huang, B. (2005). Protection against antisocial behavior in children exposed to physically abusive discipline. *Journal of Adolescent Health, 36,* 457–465.

Hilton, N. Z., & Simmons, J. L. (2001). The influence of actuarial risk assessment in clinical judgments and tribunal decisions about mentally disordered offenders in maximum security. *Law and Human Behavior, 25*(4), 393–408.

Hoge, R. D. (2002). Standardized instruments for assessing risk and need in youthful offenders. *Criminal Justice and Behavior, 29,* 380–396.

Hoge, R. D., & Andrews, D. A. (2003). *The Youth Level of Service/Case Management Inventory (YCS/CMI): Intake manual and item scoring key.* Ottawa, Canada: Carleton University.

Howell, J. C. (1995). *Guide for implementing the comprehensive strategy for serious, violent, and chronic juvenile offenders.* Washington, DC: Office of Juvenile Justice and Delinquency Prevention.

Howell, J. C. (2003). *Preventing & reducing juvenile delinquency: A comprehensive framework.* Thousand Oaks, CA: Sage.

Jang, S. J., & Smith, C. A. (1997). A test of reciprocal causal relationships among parental supervision, affective ties, and delinquency. *Journal of Research in Crime and Delinquency, 34,* 307–336.

Klein, G. A. (1998). *Sources of power: How people make decisions.* Cambridge, MA: MIT Press.

Knoester, C., Haynie, D. L., & Stephens, C. M. (2006). Parenting practices and adolescents' friendship networks. *Journal of Marriage and Family, 68,* 1247–1260.

Krysik, J., & LeCroy, C. W. (2002). The empirical validation of an instrument to predict risk of recidivism among juvenile offenders. *Research on Social Work Practice, 12*, 71–81.

Landenberger, N. A., & Lipsey, M. W. (2005). The positive effects of cognitive-behavioral programs for offenders: A meta-analysis of factors associated with effective treatment. *Journal of Experimental Criminology, 1*, 451–476.

Liddle, H. A. (2004). Family-based therapies for adolescent alcohol and drug use: Research contributions and future research needs. *Addiction, 99*(Suppl. 2), 76–92.

Lipsey, M. W., & Derzon, J. H. (1998). Predictors of violent or serious delinquency in adolescence and early adulthood. In R. Loeber & D. P. Farrington (Eds.), *Serious & violent juvenile offenders* (pp. 86–105). Thousand Oaks, CA: Sage.

Lipsey, M. W., & Wilson, D. B. (1998). Effective intervention for serious juvenile offenders. In R. Loeber & D. P. Farrington (Eds.), *Serious & violent juvenile offenders* (pp. 313–345). Thousand Oaks, CA: Sage.

Lipshitz, R., Klein, G. A., Orasanu, J., & Salas, E. (2001). Focus article: Taking stock of naturalistic decision making. *Journal of Behavioral Decision Making, 14*(5), 331–352.

Lyle, C. G., & Graham, E. (2000). Looks can be deceiving: Using a risk assessment instrument to evaluate the outcomes of child protection services. *Children and Youth Services Review, 22*, 935–949.

MacKinnon-Lewis, C., Kaufman, M. C., & Frabutt, J. M. (2002). Juvenile justice and mental health: Youth and families in the middle. *Aggression and Violent Behavior, 7*, 353–363.

Masten, A. S., & Coatsworth, J. D. (1998). The development of competence in favorable and unfavorable environments: Lessons from research on successful children. *American Psychologist, 53*, 205–220.

Masten, A. S., Hubbard, J. J., Gest, S. D., Tellegen, A., Garmezy, N., & Ramirez, M. (1999). Competence in the context of adversity: Pathways to resilience and maladaptation from childhood to late adolescence. *Development and Psychopathology, 11*, 143–169.

Mears, D. P., Ploeger, M., & Warr, M. (1998). Explaining the gender gap in delinquency: Peer influence and moral evaluations of behavior. *Journal of Research in Crime and Delinquency, 35*(3), 251–266.

Meehl, P. E. (1954). *Clinical versus statistical prediction: A theoretical analysis and a review of the evidence.* Minneapolis: University of Minnesota Press.

Moffitt, T. E., Caspi, A., Harrington, H., & Milne, B. J. (2002). Males on the life-course persistent and adolescence-limited antisocial pathways: Follow-up at age 26 years. *Development and Psychopathology, 14*, 179–207.

Moffitt, T. E., Caspi, A. Rutter, M., & Silva, P. A. (2001). *Sex differences in antisocial behavior.* New York: Cambridge University Press.

Pollard, J. A., Hawkins, J. D., & Arthur, M. W. (1999). Risk and protection: Are both necessary to understand diverse behavioral outcomes in adolescence? *Social Work Research, 23*, 143–158.

Rhodes, J. E., Grossman, J. B., & Resch, N. L. (2000). Agents of change: Pathways through which mentoring relationships influence adolescents' academic adjustment. *Child Development, 71*, 1662–1671.

Rutter, M. (1979). Protective factors in children's responses to stress and disadvantage. In J. S. Bruner & A. Garten (Eds.), *Primary prevention of psychopathology* (pp. 49–74). Hanover, NH: University Press of New England.

Rutter, M. (2005). Environmentally mediated risks for psychopathology: Research strategies and findings. *Journal of the American Academy of Child and Adolescent Psychiatry, 44,* 3–18.

Sameroff, A. J., Peck, S. C., & Eccles, J. (2004). Changing ecological determinants of conduct problems from early adolescence to early adulthood. *Development and Psychopathology, 16,* 873–896.

Schwalbe, C. S. (2004). Re-visioning risk assessment for human service decision making. *Children and Youth Services Review, 26,* 561–576.

Schwalbe, C. S. (2007). A meta analysis of juvenile justice risk assessment predictive validity. *Law and Human Behavior, 31,* 449–462.

Schwalbe, C. S., Fraser, M. W., & Day, S. H. (2007). Predictive validity of the Joint Risk Matrix with juvenile offenders: A focus on gender and race/ethnicity. *Criminal Justice and Behavior, 34,* 348–361.

Shlonsky, A., & Wagner, D. (2005). The next step: Integrating actuarial risk assessment and clinical judgment into an evidence-based practice framework in CPS case management. *Child and Youth Service Review, 27,* 409–427.

Silverthorn, P., Frick, P. J., & Reynolds, R. (2001). Timing of onset and correlates of severe conduct problems in adjudicated girls and boys. *Journal of Psychopathology and Behavioral Assessment, 23,* 171–181.

Simons, R. L., Chao, W., Conger, R. D., & Elder, G. H. (2001). Quality of parenting as mediator of the effect of childhood defiance on adolescent friendship choices and delinquency: A growth curve analysis. *Journal of Marriage and Family, 63,* 63–79.

Simons, R. L., Simons, L. G., Burt, C. H., Brody, G. H., & Cutrona, C. (2005). Collective efficacy, authoritative parenting and delinquency: A longitudinal test of a model integrating community- and family-level processes. *Criminology, 43,* 989–1029.

Simourd, L., & Andrews, D. A. (1994). Correlates of delinquency: A look at gender differences. *Forum on Corrections Research, 6,* 26–31.

Stern, S. B., & Smith, C. A. (1998). Reciprocal relationships between antisocial behavior and parenting: Implications for delinquency intervention. *Families in Society, 80,* 169–181.

Stouthamer-Loeber, M., Loeber, R., Homish, D. L., & Wei, E. (2001). Maltreatment of boys and the development of disruptive and delinquent behavior. *Development and Psychopathology, 13,* 941–955.

Thornberry, T. P., Lizotte, A. J., Krohn, M. D., Farnworth, M., & Jang, S. J. (1991). Testing interactional theory: An examination of reciprocal causal relationships among family, school, and delinquency. *Journal of Criminal Law and Criminology, 82,* 3–35.

Torbet, P., & Thomas, D. (2005). *Advancing competency development: A white paper for Pennsylvania.* Pittsburgh, PA: National Center for Juvenile Justice.

Tversky, A., & Kahneman, D. (1974). Judgment under uncertainty: Heuristics and biases. *Science, 185,* 1124–1131.

Tversky, A., & Kahneman, D. (2002). Extensional vs. intuitive reasoning: The conjunction fallacy in probabilistic judgment. In T. Gilovich, D. Griffin, & D. Kahneman (Eds.), *Heuristics and biases: The psychology of intuitive judgment* (pp. 19–48). New York: Cambridge University Press.

Werner, E. E., & Smith, R. S. (1982). *Vulnerable but invincible: A study of resilient children.* New York: McGraw-Hill.

14

Contextualizing Girls' Violence: Assessment and Treatment Decisions

JUDITH A. RYDER, CINDY GORDON, AND JESSICA BULGER

Girls are rarely central to justice-related research, policy, or practice (Bloom, 2003). Indeed, it has only been in the past 30 years or so that female involvement in crime has become a topic of serious consideration in mainstream criminological literature. Even the more recent studies of gender and crime, however, have focused primarily on adult women, not girls (Zahn, 2006). In the juvenile justice literature, research on female delinquency continues to be overshadowed by that of males, who commit a disproportionate share of delinquent offenses and account for approximately 82% of all violent crimes (Snyder, 2006). Empirical data specific to violence among girls are limited, and, thus, the corresponding knowledge of appropriate treatment is fragmentary (Giordano, Cernkovich, & Lowery, 2004; Lanctôt, Émond, & Le Blanc, 2004). As a result, explanations of girls' violence have too often been left to sensationalized media stereotypes that have contributed to ineffective interventions and a proliferation of punitive social policies (Brown, Chesney-Lind, & Stein, 2007; Steffensmeier, Schwartz, Zhong, & Ackerman, 2005). Fortunately, new research has begun to investigate distinct gender pathways to crime (including variations in risks and strengths), and gender-responsive praxis have provided a more holistic understanding of appropriate treatment interventions.

Regardless of age, justice-involved females share many commonalities. Developmental differences, however, caution against the indiscriminate application of adult-based research findings to the lives of girls (Odgers, Reppucci, & Moretti, 2005; Vincent & Grisso, 2005). The purpose of this chapter is to provide practitioners with a general overview of what is currently known about violent behavior among females under the age of 18.[1] This includes a discussion of changing definitions and emerging theoretical perspectives and an examination of contributing risk factors. The chapter reviews violence risk assessment and discusses possible measurement issues for risk prediction, as well as treatment approaches that are both gender responsive and age appropriate for girls. Case examples, primarily from residential treatment centers, are used to enhance understanding of gender-responsive interventions. Although most reported female delinquency does not include physical violence and the number of girls arrested and detained for violent offending remains much smaller than the number of boys (Baum, 2005; Chesney-Lind & Belknap, 2004), it is important that practitioners and researchers alike become knowledgeable about the nature and extent of girls' violence and seek to develop gender-sensitive assessment tools and effective treatment responses.

DEFINITIONS, MEASURES, AND POLICY IMPLICATIONS

An increase in official incidence rates and widespread media coverage of violence enacted by girls has heightened the public's interest as well as its fears (Chesney-Lind & Eliason, 2006). On the one hand, an escalation in the number of person offense cases involving girls might suggest the need for more gender-responsive interventions. Unfortunately, misconceptions about the empirical data have instead contributed to advocacy and political actions that have had harsh consequences for girls (Luke, 2008; Simkins & Katz, 2002). It is therefore critical that those working with and for girls seek to understand their use of violence, beginning with how violence is variously defined and measured and the context in which behaviors occur.

Research consistently demonstrates that "estimating the rates for youth violence and gender is complicated by the definition of what is considered violent" (Leschied, Cummings, Van Brunschot, Cunningham, & Saunders, 2001, p. 202). Indeed, much of the debate regarding a putative escalation in violence by girls continues because of differing definitions. The *Oxford English Dictionary* distinguishes violence by its physicality. While aggression is defined as "an unprovoked attack; the first attack in a quarrel; an assault, an inroad," violence is more narrowly characterized as the "exercise of physical force so as to inflict injury on, or cause damage to, persons or property" (Simpson & Weiner, 1989a, 1989b).

The literature on boys' violence generally focuses on overt physical acts based on delinquent or criminal offenses (Farrington, 1998; Hawkins et al., 1998). Pollock and Davis (2005) note, however, that contemporary studies of girls often use aggression as a synonym for violence, thereby expanding the number and types of acts that may be counted. Making aggression synonymous with violence also minimizes the fact that aggression can be manifested in malicious words and nonphysical acts, and physical violence used in self-defense may be reactive, not aggressive (2005, p. 17). Different definitions and measures of violence inhibit meaningful comparisons across studies and programs and may contribute directly to ineffective or even harmful policies for girls. As history demonstrates, the way in which appropriate female behavior is defined has broad social and political consequences for how girls are treated and how their problems are addressed (Godfrey, 2004; Norton, 2002; Odem & Schlossman, 1991). To sort out some of the definitional variation, we begin with a review of national data sources and measures most often used to assess girls' violence.

Official Record Data

Official statistics describe offenses that come to the attention of the justice system. The two primary official data sources are the Uniform Crime Report (UCR) and the National Crime Victimization Survey (NCVS), each of which includes national, longitudinal data. The UCR consists of arrest data compiled by the FBI and provides annual information on sex- and age-specific arrests, categorized by offense. The NCVS is sponsored by the U.S. Department of Justice and the U.S. Census Bureau to collect data on crimes against persons from a nationally representative household sample.

The UCR's Violent Crime Index is the sum of four offenses that are also individually measured: murder and nonnegligent manslaughter, forcible rape, robbery, and aggravated assault. According to the index, juvenile violent crime arrests generally escalated in the late 1980s, peaked in 1994, and then dropped dramatically in the ensuing decade. In 2004, for all Violent Crime Index offenses combined, the number of juvenile arrests was the lowest since 1987 (Snyder, 2006, p. 4). Given the much larger number of boys represented in these law enforcement arrest data, however, the drop in juvenile violent crime was actually a drop in male offending.

For girls, there is variation in this narrative of decreasing crime. According to UCR data, between 1980 and 2004 juvenile female arrest rates grew more than those of males for the following offenses: simple assault (290% vs. 106%), weapons law violations (160% vs. 22%), and aggravated assault (93% vs. 11%) (Snyder, 2006, p. 8). These are large increases, but given that the base number of female offenders is so small, slight numerical changes can generate significant changes in the reported percentages.

A more telling indicator than percentage increase is the female proportion of juvenile arrests. For example, for all Violent Crime Index offenses combined, the female proportion of juvenile arrests steadily increased from 10% in 1980 to 19% in 2004 (Snyder, 2006, p. 3). This gradual rise over nearly a quarter of a century was primarily because of a significant increase in the female proportion of arrests for aggravated assault (Snyder & Sickmund, 2006, p. 128). During the decade in which overall juvenile violence decreased 22% (1995–2004), violent crime arrest rates for females decreased only 11%, while violent crime arrest rates for males decreased 35% (Snyder, 2006, p. 8). Although the female numbers remain relatively small, the UCR data provide statistical evidence of a rise in some violent offending by girls. This increase must be addressed in terms of theory, treatment, and policy.[2]

The other primary source of official data, the National Crime Victimization Survey, is helpful in understanding the volume and nature of crimes against juveniles ages 12 to 17, as well as trends in these offenses (Snyder & Sickmund, 2006, p. 27).[3] The NCVS gathers information on household victimizations (burglary, larceny, vehicle theft) and interpersonal violence victimization. It provides an estimate of offending rates for person offenses (other than murder) based on victims' reports of offender characteristics, including sex and age. The indices for violent crimes are comparable to those used in the UCR (Steffensmeier et al., 2005, p. 368).

When compared with UCR arrest data, NCVS victimization data indicate that, between 1980 and 2000, serious violent offenses by girls increased less sharply and decreased more steeply than those by boys (Stahl, 2004). In a decade of generally decreasing juvenile violent crime

(1993–2003), NCVS data also indicate that, of all nonfatal violent victimizations in which victims perceived offenders to be juveniles, three-fourths were attributed to male offenders (Baum, 2005, p.7).[4] Analyses of NCVS 1980–2003 data reveal very little change "or a lack of convergence in the gender gap for assault crimes and the Violent Crime Index over the past one to two decades" (Steffensmeier et al., 2005, p. 379).

Self-Report Studies

Self-report studies ask juvenile respondents to anonymously recount their own offenses. Two other widely cited sources for examining national trends in female juvenile crime are the ongoing Monitoring the Future (MTF) survey of high school seniors and the National Youth Risk Behavior Survey. These surveys are independent of criminal justice selection biases and consistently find stable gender differences in delinquency, including violent offending (Steffensmeier & Schwartz, 2004, p. 102). Evidence from these national self-report studies indicates that female adolescents do engage in violent behavior but at lower rates than their male counterparts (Elliott, 1994). Also, incidence and prevalence of violent behaviors tend to decline as girls age through adolescence (Ageton, 1983). Using National Youth Survey data to examine changes in the distribution, incidence, and prevalence of female delinquency, categorizing by race, social class, and place of residence, Ageton found that significantly higher proportions of Black and lower-class girls were involved in assaultive behaviors. Ageton and others suggest that, in the United States, race and class may be better predictors of violent crime than gender (Kruttschnitt, 1994; Laub & McDermott, 1985; Pollock & Davis, 2005).

In a major study of trends in girls' violence from 1980 to 2003, Steffensmeier et al. (2005) underscored the sensitivity of arrest statistics to criminal justice selection bias and the importance of analyzing additional and multiple data sources. The researchers used advanced time-series techniques to compare arrest data from the UCR with victimization data from the NCVS and nationally representative self-report data from the Monitoring the Future and National Youth Risk Behavior Surveys. Increases in juvenile female violence as reported in the UCR were not borne out in the other longitudinal, nonarrest sources. The other sources indicated little overall change in girls' level of violence (as measured by simple and aggravated assaults and the Violent Crime Index) over the past 20 years and little change in the female-to-male percentage of violent offending. The research concludes that any rise in juvenile female violence is "more a social construction than an empirical reality" (Steffensmeier et al., 2005, p. 397).

The Social Construction of Violence

Perhaps as critical as empirical data on girls' violence is the meaning that is attributed to the evidence (Cullen et al., 1998). The lens through which researchers, practitioners, and the public interpret official law enforcement statistics will determine positions on what those statistics represent (Luke, 2008). In an effort to understand the public's concern with rising violence among girls despite evidence of a decrease in percentages, Steffensmeier et al. (2005) linked assessment of the empirical data to normative and constructionist theories of crime and law. A normative perspective sees criminal law as being enforced in reaction to criminal acts. Girls, in this view, *are* becoming more violent; the official arrest statistics reflect reality. The purported increase in female juvenile violence is attributed to a number of causes, including strain and violence in society generally (Garbarino, 2006; Prothrow-Stith & Spivak, 2005; Schaffner, 2004); shifting gender role expectations (Pipher, 1994); greater risk of victimization (Brown & Gilligan, 1992); and increasing poverty and disenfranchisement among marginalized populations (Heimer, 2000; Jones, 2004; Ness, 2004).

A constructionist perspective, on the other hand, tends to see less change in girls' behaviors and more in the behavior of the state. For example, official categories of assault are broad and require subjective evaluations of intent and bodily harm. Law enforcement agencies are likely to differ in how and under what circumstances they make those determinations. Fueled by growing intolerance for social disorder and cultural anxiety "over shifting norms of gender and race" (Luke, 2008, p. 44), tough law-and-order policies have made girls likely subjects of increased sanctioning (Benekos & Merlo, 2008; Reitsma-Street, 2004).

For example, more girls are being referred to juvenile court under the auspices of school zero-tolerance policies, which often involve police arrests on campus for actions that previously were addressed by school administrators (Brown et al., 2007; Stein, 2001). In certain contexts, particularly in low-income and minority schools and communities, girls' disorderly conduct and verbal aggression are now more likely to be labeled simple assaults, and simple assaults are likely to be "upcharged" to aggravated assaults. In this fashion, behaviors previously considered nondelinquent (and dealt with unofficially) are relabeled as serious criminal acts (Chesney-Lind, 2004).

There is evidence too, that proarrest domestic violence statutes have brought more girls into the justice system, criminalizing, for example, girls defending a mother against a batterer (American Bar Association & National Bar Association, 2001; Chesney-Lind, 2002). These same laws have been used to arrest children fighting with parents. One study found that daughters were arrested in 92% of the cases, "whereas arrest occurred in 75 percent of incidents in which a son assaulted a parent" (Buzawa & Hotaling, 2006).

Constructionists have argued that stakeholders' (i.e., parents, schools, media, victim advocates, researchers) efforts to prevent, intervene, or otherwise manage girls' behaviors have actually contributed to "more elastic definitions of violence," increased criminalization of acts, and rising juvenile female arrests (Feld, 1998). This perspective contends that, while girls' actual behaviors may fluctuate somewhat, criminal justice practices have shifted significantly—reflecting changes in how society defines, and the extent to which it tolerates, female violence.

Aggression and Relational Violence

Overall, female rates of violent offending remain lower than male rates in virtually all times and places (Kruttschnitt, 2001). There is little debate that, among juveniles, girls engage in fewer and less serious forms of violence than do boys (Martino, Ellickson, Klein, McCaffrey, & Edelen, 2008; U.S. Department of Health and Human Services, 2001). When definitions of violence and aggression are broadened beyond physical actions, however, girls may be represented in quite a different manner. For example, one study found that girls had lower rates of school violence compared to boys when violence was defined as overt aggression, but girls were "proportionately more likely to appear in the data when verbal threats and intimidation" were included (Everett & Price, 1995). Björkqvist and Niemla (1992) also employ a broad definition of violence, arguing that it includes not only physical acts, but also intentions. The conceptualization of aggression in the psychological literature has recently shifted to include both direct (physical) and indirect (relational) forms, but the distinctions remain blurred (Odgers & Moretti, 2002). An analysis by Little, Henrich, Jones, and Hawley (2003) does, however, provide an outline of the general forms and specific functions of aggressive behavior.

Regardless of the label (e.g., indirect, covert, relational, social), girls' behaviors are being reexamined in the context of this more hidden form of aggression, with important ramifications for how girls are perceived, sanctioned, and treated (Chesney-Lind, Morash, & Irwin, 2007). Relational violence or aggression tends not to involve direct confrontation, but instead is a form of social manipulation (Björkqvist, 2001) that relies on hostile exploitation of relationships and the use of threats to dominate others and to inflict emotional harm (Crick & Grotpeter, 1995). Tactics are far-ranging and may include spreading rumors and lies, rolling eyes, excluding peers from group activities, withdrawing attention and affection, and using others to attack a victim (Björkqvist, Osterman, & Kaukiainen, 1992).

Björkqvist (2001) cautions against calling indirect aggression female because of the "enormous individual variation" and because types of aggression overlap. A number of studies, however, contend that, while girls are as aggressive as boys, that expression is gendered: female aggression tends to be expressed indirectly through the disruption of relationship, while male aggression tends to be manifested physically (Björkqvist & Niemla, 1992; Björkqvist et al., 1992; Crick & Grotpeter, 1995). Leschied and colleagues' (2001) extensive literature review on aggression in adolescent girls suggests that adolescent and younger girls use indirect, relational aggression more than physical aggression, especially when compared to boys—with the exception of verbal aggression, which boys tend to use more (Lindeman, Harakka, & Keltikangas-Javinen, 1997). These findings, however, are inconclusive. McMaster, Connolly, Pepler, and Craig (2002) found girls and boys engage in relational aggression to the same extent, while others found boys to be (moderately) more relationally aggressive (Little et al., 2003; Wolke, Woods, Bloomfield, & Karstadt, 2000).

What does seem to be clear is that, among girls, without comparisons to boys, covert, relational aggression is more common than is overt, physical aggression (Crick & Bigbee, 1998; Crick et al., 1999). Also, among victims, covert aggression is "particularly distressing for girls independent of whether such acts occur in conjunction with overt aggression" (Odgers & Moretti, 2002, p. 105). Awareness of both of these aspects is important for assessment and treatment planning, given that girls involved in the justice system are likely to have difficulties with relational aggression. Often related to prior victimizations, depression, and peer rejection, girls' aggression and hostility are likely to be manifested toward other similarly situated girls, as well as practitioners working within the system (Chesney-Lind & Belknap, 2004; Okamoto, 2002).

Conceptualizing aggression too broadly has the potential of exerting even greater social control over girls. Relabeling gossip, breaking of confidences, criticism of appearance, and name calling, for example, may simply encourage more surveillance of and intervention with girls' nondelinquent behaviors. The result may be the disproportionate processing and placement of lower-risk aggressive girls (Chesney-Lind, Morash, & Irwin, 2007; Leschied et al., 2001). Practitioners must be made aware of this likelihood and realize that the official criminal justice label is insufficient for assessing the nature of a girl's behavior or for determining appropriate treatment.

On the other hand, conceptualizing aggression as relational "has the potential for capturing better the developmental issues of adolescent girls" (Leschied et al., 2001, p. 208), who are socialized to value and define themselves in relation with others (Gilligan, Lyons, & Hammer, 1990; Miller, 1976; Surrey, 1991). Although the evidence is inconclusive, high levels of relational aggression may be a marker for overt forms of aggression (Odgers & Moretti, 2002). Overt and relational aggression appear to be distinct yet highly correlated, and it is possible that they derive from similar processes (Herrenkohl et al., 2007). Thus, addressing relational issues is an important aspect of assessing and treating aggression in girls.

GIRLS AND VIOLENT OFFENDING

In 2003, girls accounted for 14% (or 12,626) of all delinquent offenders in custody: 18% of all detained and 12% of all those committed.[5] Although these custodial numbers are low, they reflect an increase of 96% between 1991 and 2003 (Snyder & Sickmund, 2006, p. 206). Generally, juvenile female offenders in custody are young women of color. The peak age for girls in residential placement in 2003 was 16, with those age 15 and younger accounting for 46% of the residential population. The 2003 minority proportion of female juvenile offenders in custody was 55% (Snyder & Sickmund, 2006, p. 209). Minority overrepresentation in secure facilities is of concern, but such overrepresentation is often the result of decisions made much earlier, increasing at each stage of the justice system process (Poe-Yamagata & Jones, 2000).

Of all female delinquents held in custody in 2003, approximately 30% were held for person (violent) offenses, mostly for assaultive behaviors: homicide, 1%; sexual assault, 1%; robbery, 2%; aggravated assault, 8%;

simple assault, 14%; and other person offenses, 4% (Snyder & Sickmund, 2006, p. 210). Reflective perhaps of community racial and economic oppression (Miller, 1998), among girls in detention, Blacks had a higher proportion of person offenses (41%) than did Whites (31%) or girls of other races (27%) (Snyder & Sickmund, 2006, p. 170).

Homicide

Beyond basic demographic information, our understanding of violent offending among girls is limited, partially because of low incidence rates. For example, between 1984 and 2002, the largest number of juvenile female offenders involved in the most serious offense of homicide was 173 (compared to 2,952 males) (Snyder & Sickmund, 2006, p. 68). Loper and Cornell's (1996) analysis of FBI Supplemental Homicide Reports discerned that the pattern of homicide committed by 121 girls was "essentially distinct" from those of boys and women: homicides by girls were more likely to involve interpersonal and interfamilial conflict, a knife, and victims under the age of 13 years.

Another study of 29 adolescent female homicide offenders found, however, that the most frequently reported circumstance for the homicide was the commission of another crime, primarily assault and robbery (Roe-Sepowitz, 2007). The primary weapon was a car, followed by guns and knives. Although these homicide offenders knew their victims, they were not family members. In addition, these girls were more likely than those involved in interpersonal conflict to have had several prior delinquency referrals and a history of substance use.

Sexual Assault

Based on an international literature review, Hendriks and Bijleveld (2006) suggest that the best estimate for the female proportion of the total adolescent sex offender population is between 5% and 10%. Most studies conclude that girls begin sexual offending at a younger age than boys (Cavanaugh Johnson, 1989; Ray & English, 1995); tend to be between 12 and 15 years of age; and victimize children of primary school age (almost always a family member or acquaintance). Offenders tend to abuse two to three victims. In line with other studies, Hendriks and Bijleveld's own research in the Netherlands found that female offenders generally came from dysfunctional and chaotic family backgrounds that were "much more negative" than those of male offenders. Unlike some other studies (Fehrenbach & Monastersky, 1988), Hendriks and Bijleveld found that the majority of the girls did not offend alone but in the presence of one or more co-offenders.

Robbery

In a study of robbers, most of whom were in their late teens and early 20s, Miller (1998) found that men and women were motivated to rob for similar reasons, but the methods and strategies used were gendered. Making practical choices in the context of gender-stratified street settings, female robbers used various stereotypical perceptions of women to their advantage and thereby gained status, recognition, as well as money and goods. Most of the girls adjudicated for robbery in Ryder's study (2003) reported chaotic family situations and lived in violent, economically marginalized communities. Few robberies were financially motivated and little was gained; girls acted out of retaliation and revenge, using the robbery to maintain a modicum of control over others in a hostile world. Victims were generally female, both adults and juveniles. Other research indicates that most juvenile robberies are impulsive, unplanned events. Female robberies do not usually involve serious physical violence but may include physical contact such as "hitting, shoving, and fighting with the victim" (Chesney-Lind & Sheldon, 2004, p. 60).

Assault

Assaults account for most of the violent arrests of girls. Of all juvenile arrests for aggravated assault in 2004, nearly one-fourth were female, as were one-third of all juvenile arrests for other assaults (Snyder, 2006). Victims were primarily peers and family members. In a study that included young women convicted of violent crimes, serious assaults were generally alcohol- or drug-related and committed in conjunction with a robbery (Batchelor, 2005).

Ness (2004) argues that street fighting among girls has been underestimated and represents the majority of violent behavior in some impoverished neighborhoods. She illustrates how some girls take pleasure in physically dominating others, while noting the instrumental function it offers, including security, status, and self-esteem. Other research has found assaultive behaviors to be a source of protection and monetary gain (Brotherton, 1996; Campbell, 1984). In many situations such behaviors also serve as a coping or survival strategy, and fighting may be the most reliable social resource for young women in distressed communities (Jones, 2004). In her analysis of girl-on-girl assaults, Artz (1998) suggests that they represent a horizontal violence similar to the actions of other powerless groups; girls mimic the oppressor (males) and beat up similarly situated females.

RELATIONAL THEORY AND THE PATHWAYS PERSPECTIVE

Emerging research demonstrates that all violent offending by girls and young women is not the same, nor does it always conform to male patterns (Heimer & De Coster, 1999; Messerschmidt, 1986; Miller, 1998; White & Kowalski, 1992). While cautioning against lumping all females into a single group, feminist scholars have sought to tease out the gendered nature of violent offending and to determine the pathways girls take toward delinquency and crime (Belknap & Holsinger, 1998; Potter, 2006). Knowledge of these patterns is critical for practitioners engaged in assessing girls' violence and the design and implementation of treatment programs.

An increased understanding of gender differences has contributed to two developments important to the study of girls' violence. The first pertains to differences in how females and males mature psychologically. In contrast to traditional psychological theories that consider human development a progression from dependence to a self-sufficient, autonomous self, a relational model of women's psychology holds that females' path to maturity is through a sense of connection with others. Disconnections in relationships may be the source of many women's psychological problems (Covington, 2002; Miller, 1976).

Relational theory is important for making sense of the recurring themes of disconnection, violation, and victimization in the lives of female juvenile offenders. For example, while girls may be socialized to be more empathic than boys (Gilligan et al., 1990), much of the delinquency research indicates that girls in custody are often enmeshed in nonempathic relationships, with histories of loss, neglect, and abuse and, thus, may lack empathy for themselves or others or both (Covington, 2002). To better understand and address girls' violent offending, practitioners need to acknowledge these histories and help girls to experience new relationships that do not mirror the old (Robinson, 2007).

In a parallel vein, feminist pathway research recognizes that gendered differences in the lives of females and males help to shape patterns of criminal offending (Belknap & Holsinger, 1998; Steffensmeier & Allen, 1998). In particular, research examining childhood experiences that may place girls at risk for delinquency and violent offending consistently implicate early victimizations (Arnold, 1995; Chesney-Lind & Shelden, 2004; Siegel & Williams, 2003). Gender comparisons of childhood abuse and neglect indicate that both are more common, start earlier, and last longer for girls (e.g., Browne & Finklehor, 1986; Dembo, Williams, Wothke, Schmeidler, & Brown, 1992; McClellan, Farabee, & Crouch, 1997). One feminist argument theorizes a pathway beginning with victimization in the home, followed by running away (which is itself often criminalized), and the commission of crimes in order to survive (Belknap & Holsinger, 1998; Gilfus, 1992). Involvement in the illegal drug market may serve as a means to generate money and as a form of self-medication (Ireland & Widom, 1994; Krystal & Raskin 1970).

The profile that emerges of girls involved in violence presents three areas of concern: trauma, substance abuse, and mental health. Often closely entwined, each is a significant factor contributing to the possibility of delinquency and violent offending.

Traumatic Experiences

Traumatic events are deeply upsetting and substantially change how one thinks and feels about the world (Herman, 1997). Although defined and measured in a variety of ways (see Ryder, Langley, & Brownstein, 2008), traumatic events traditionally have been considered an extreme subset of stressful life events that break through internal protective defenses and overwhelm normal coping mechanisms (Dise-Lewis, 1988). Compared to their male counterparts, girls in custody are at greater risk for trauma exposure overall and to certain types of trauma in particular, and they are highly vulnerable to its comorbid effects (Brosky & Lally, 2004; Dixon, Howie, & Starling, 2005). The incarceration experience itself can be traumatic, and offenders with trauma histories are likely to have additional difficulties adjusting to confinement (Sherman, 2005).

Institutionalized girls report higher rates than boys for all types of abuse, particularly sexual abuse, and are significantly more likely than boys to report the belief that their abuse was related to their subsequent delinquency (Belknap & Holsinger, 2006). Seeking to explicate the mechanisms by which adjudicated girls' victimization contributed to their violent offending, Ryder (2007) found that multiple traumatic events disrupted primary relational bonds in early childhood, leaving them vulnerable to additional victimization and losses. A Canadian review of female offenders indicated that from 45% to 75% of incarcerated girls had been sexually abused (Corrado, Roesch, Hart, & Gierowski, 2002). In a qualitative study of non-justice-involved adolescent girls (Artz, 1998), those who had used violence reported significantly greater rates of sexual and physical victimization than their nonviolent female counterparts. A fifth of adolescent female homicide offenders reported prior sexual abuse (Roe-Sepowitz, 2007), and female sex offenders in the Netherlands reported that "neglect, abuse and sexual abuse (by family members) were the rule rather than the exception" (Hendriks & Bijleveld, 2006, p. 39). Similarly, girls bound over and sentenced to the adult criminal justice system reported themes of "sexual and physical abuse, neglect and disorder in the family" (Gaarder & Belknap, 2002, p. 509).

Considering the effects of victimization and other traumatic events on adult women, English, Widom, and Brandford (2001) note that abused and neglected females were nearly four times more likely than a matched control group to be arrested as a juvenile, twice as likely to be arrested as an adult, and nearly seven times more likely to be arrested as an adult for a violent crime. A longitudinal study of 127 females indicates that, although physical and sexual abuse during childhood and adolescence did not predict adolescent delinquency, such abuses were "potent predictors of adult criminality" (Cernkovich, Lanctôt, & Giordano, 2008, p. 3).

Substance Abuse

Drug and alcohol use is often "an attempt at self-help" (Krystal & Raskin 1970, p. 11) and may serve as a psychological escape—a strategy for coping with feelings of anxiety, anger, and depression (Belknap & Holsinger, 1998; Herman 1997; Ireland & Widom, 1994). There is much evidence to suggest that experiencing physical and sexual abuse, neglect, and other traumas increases the likelihood of using alcohol and drugs (Dembo, Williams, Lavoie, & Berry, 1989; Dembo, et al., 1990; Harlow, 1999; Ireland & Widom, 1994; Kingery, Pruitt & Hurley 1992; Smith & Thornberry, 1995). Furthermore, female abuse victims are more likely than males to develop drug problems and to be involved in drug-related crime (Harlow, 1999; Widom, Ireland, & Glynn, 1995). Anderson (1994) found that girls who used drugs were more likely to engage in fighting and gang membership, while other research reports that negative outcomes related to drug and alcohol use may be more severe for girls, particularly minority girls (Amaro, Blake, Schwartz, Flinchbaugh, 2001; Belenko, Sprott, & Peterson, 2004).

Mental Health

Among all youth exposed to trauma, girls are more likely than boys to develop mental health problems (Breslau, Davis, Andreski, & Peterson, 1991; Dembo, Schmeidler, Guida, & Rahman, 1998; Horowitz, Weine, & Jekel, 1995). Among youth in the juvenile justice system, approximately one-half meet criteria for at least two mental health disorders (Marsteller et al., 1997; Teplin, Abram, McClelland, Dulcan, & Mericle, 2002). Acoca (1999) found that, of the girls surveyed in California's juvenile justice system, more than half said that they needed psychological services, 24% had seriously considered suicide, and 21% had been hospitalized in a psychiatric facility. An Australian study of incarcerated girls suggests that, for some girls, both "trauma and PTSD may be predisposing factors for the development of other psychopathology" (Dixon et al., 2005, p. 803).

Girls may have a distinct profile of familial risk factors (Silverthorn & Frick, 1999), and there may be significant differences in how mental health is manifested in female and male adolescents (Alemagno, Shaffer-King, & Hammel, 2006; Hoyt & Scherer, 1998). Much research documents the tendency of girls to turn their emotional pain inward, where it is manifested in depression, substance abuse, and self-mutilation, before (in some cases) it is expressed physically (see, e.g., Artz, 1998; Campbell, 1994). Examining the relationship between clinical depression and antisocial behavior, Obeidallah and Earls (1999) determined that moderately depressed girls were more likely to be aggressive and to commit property crimes and crimes against other people than girls who were not depressed. Their research found that 82% of mildly to moderately depressed girls engaged in crimes against other persons, compared with 42% of girls who were not depressed. In addition, 57% of the mildly to moderately depressed girls engaged in higher levels of aggressive behavior, compared with 13% of those who were not depressed.

Given the substantial body of research linking trauma to subsequent internalizing and externalizing problem behaviors including aggression and violence, the need for intervention is particularly compelling. Treatment services, however, are hampered because detailed information about girls' trauma histories are not routinely collected, nor are gender-sensitive violence risk assessment tools readily available in juvenile justice settings (Lewis, 2006; Simkins & Katz, 2002).

VIOLENCE RISK ASSESSMENT

Clinicians learn early in training that, in order to provide optimal services for clients, a comprehensive clinical assessment must be conducted. This is the process of gathering information about the client for the purpose of gaining insight into the problems for which the individual is seeking treatment. The assessment includes family, developmental, educational, medical, social, and mental health histories and behavioral observations. These data inform the treatment plan, treatment strategy, and prognosis. Specifically, the assessment helps to identify variables that contribute to the current functioning of the girl. Once these are identified, the clinician and young woman work to eliminate, stabilize, or manage various factors so that the girl is in a better position to change behaviors, manage more effectively, and regain stability.

The paucity of empirical data on the developmental course of disruptive behavior problems and violence among girls, however, has frustrated clinicians, researchers, and policymakers alike. Most research has focused on boys, yet early identification and intervention is critical for young girls displaying disruptive behaviors who may be equally at risk for subsequent violence (Bierman et al., 2004, p. 137). Unfortunately, interventions developed for boys' behavior problems are frequently applied to girls, despite evidence of a female-specific set of risk factors (Hipwell & Loeber, 2006). The following section briefly reviews the existing literature on girls' violence and risk assessment, discusses the challenges of conducting risk assessments with girls, and presents some gender-responsive violence risk assessment tools.

Conducting a systematic and comprehensive assessment is essential for determining violence risk in girls and is the foundation of any effective treatment intervention (Borum, 2003; Grisso, 2005a). Violence risk assessments are often conducted at key decision-making points within the justice system, including at the initial detention decision, disposition and commitment to a secure facility, and transfer to adult court. Risk assessments help determine the level of risk that a girl poses to herself and others and assist in determining the level, type, and mix of program and supervision needs. The assessment can be accomplished through the use of early screening processes and tools, structured interviews, validated assessment instruments, and the gathering of data from other relevant resources.

Risk and protective factors are generally categorized according to individual, family, school, peer group, and community domains (Miller, Trapani, Fejes-Mendoza, Eggleston, & Dwiggins, 1995). Protective factors encourage positive behaviors, including healthy connections with family, peers, and schools; positive gender identification and self-concept; spirituality; and social supports. Risk factors are those that increase the individual's propensity of engaging in risky and delinquent behaviors, including violence. Several risk factors, such as age, gender, race, exposure to violence, and early criminal behavior, are static—that is, they cannot be changed in treatment. Others are dynamic and are directly related to an individual's delinquent behavior, such as attitudes, cognitions, and behavior regarding employment, education, peers, authority, substance abuse, and interpersonal relationships. To be effective, rehabilitative efforts must focus on factors that are both dynamic—amenable to change—and associated with the violent behaviors.

Violence risk assessments are most appropriate for prevention and intervention purposes rather than for prediction. Risk factors for youth violence are generally developmental and do change with time, and, thus, dangerousness is best thought of as existing on a continuum and varying with context (Borum & Verhaagen, 2006). There is no single factor that can predict future aggression, violence, or antisocial behavior, but it is possible for a single factor to disproportionately affect a particular girl's overall level of risk or for a combination of factors to significantly alter the risk level (Augimeri, Koegl, Levene, & Webster, 2005, p. 299).

Gender-Related Violence Risk Factors

Gender is one of the best predictors of delinquency, and patterns of delinquency are affected by gender. We know little, however, about what places girls at risk for aggressive behavior or what protects them. Violence risk assessments generally overlook gender and how events perceived as risk factors for violence (such as family experiences) may be gendered. This omission can "threaten the appropriateness of systemic interventions with and treatment responses to girls" (Belknap & Holsinger, 2006, p. 48).

While many risk factors for violence may apply similarly to males and females, girls have different developmental experiences and challenges, and, thus, it is also likely that some risk factors will vary. For example, studies of girls and violence report some unique concerns, including intrapersonal conflict "as reflected in a comorbidity of self-harm and suicide ideation with physical aggression" and the association between aggression and girls' victimization by family members (Leschied et al., 2001, p. 207). Furthermore, girls and boys differ in sensitivity and rate of exposure to common factors (Levene, Walsh, Augimieri, & Pepler, 2004; Moretti, Catchpole, & Odgers, 2005; Odgers, Schmidt, & Repucci, 2004).

Adolescent girls tend to have more serious problems than adolescent boys with self-image, sexual attitudes, family relations, and vocational and educational goals. Girls' self-esteem tends to diminish over the course of adolescence, and girls experience more episodes of depression, demonstrate lower levels of resilience, and attempt suicide more often than do adolescent boys (Miller et al., 1995). Studies report higher rates of eating disorders among girls and indicate that girls also may be more susceptible to psychological dysfunction as a response to traumatic events (Meichenbaum, 2006). Summarizing emerging research, Moretti, Catchpole, and Odgers (2005) indicate that factors that increase the risk for violence for girls include maltreatment, victimization, and trauma; family fragmentation and insecure attachment; peer relationships and early sexual maturation; and genetics (see Jaffee, Caspi, Moffitt, & Taylor, 2004; Rhee & Waldman, 2002). Additional gender-sensitive risk factors may include substance use and poor academic performance (Zahn, 2005). Girls tend to have multiple factors related to their delinquency, all of which need to be taken into account when assessing risks and needs (Loper, 2000).

Girls frequently enter the justice system for less serious offenses than boys, and, as a result, they are often pigeonholed into programs designed to provide higher surveillance and security measures than are needed (Chesney-Lind, 2000). Furthermore, when girls do engage in violent offending, it is often in the context of interpersonal relationships. Thus, gender-responsive assessment tools and practices are especially critical when first selecting girls to participate in programming that focuses on violent offending and for planning appropriate treatment.

Violence Risk Assessment Tools and Strategies for Girls

As previously noted, girls now account for nearly one-fifth of all juvenile arrests for violent crime, primarily because of a significant increase in the female proportion of arrests for aggravated assault (Snyder & Sickmund, 2006, p. 128). As a result, there is a growing need for practitioners to be able to better identify variation among girls who have engaged in violent behavior and to provide gender-responsive interventions. Most risk assessment instruments, however, are based on male data—just as treatment and policies governing service delivery have been gendered. One cannot assume that data obtained with such assessment tools will have the same meaning for both girls and boys or will provide an accurate assessment of gender-specific concerns and needs (Augimeri et al., 2005; Grisso, 2005b). One study utilizing separate risk assessment instruments for classifying male and female delinquents determined that not only did female risk factors differ substantially, but that separate instruments improved classifications for reoffending, especially for girls (Funk, 1999).

Adolescent girls present unique challenges for violence risk assessments, particularly because they are a decidedly marginalized and victimized population that often presents a complicated clinical profile. The high prevalence of mental disorders, victimization, and racial bias among the female juvenile justice population can make building initial rapport and conducting an assessment difficult. Addressing these factors, however, is essential even as it is important to recognize that abused and marginalized girls may be "less of a risk for future instrumental violence" because their actions often represent their attempt to "survive in extraordinary conditions as opposed to being motivated by thrill seeking or hedonistic goals" (Odgers et al., 2004, p. 20). Utilizing risk assessment data, treatment can be designed to assist in the "formation of healthy relationships and adaptive parenting skills—both of which form the context for the majority of violence that is committed by adult women" (Odgers et al., 2004, p. 202). Meichenbaum (2006) suggests that a gender-responsive assessment should evaluate for all forms of relational aggression, for strengths and signs of resilience, and should build in procedures to evaluate the effectiveness of intervention programs.

Structured Interviews and Risk Assessment

The assessment process can be viewed on a continuum including screenings, structured clinical interviews, third-party historical information, and validated actuarial tools. Individualized assessments need to use multimodal means to discover and address the history and the details of offenses as well as the life circumstances that moved girls into the juvenile justice system. A careful examination of this history should be brought to bear on decisions determining risk and security levels, as well as counseling and treatment responses.

Structured interviews have a specific format and address particular issues. Standardization ensures that all clients are asked the same questions, for the same specific purpose, and are assessed in a consistent manner. Structured violent risk assessments enable clinicians to objectively obtain information that will assist in determining factors that contribute to certain behaviors. When consistently applied, they can "increase case management efficacy and produce predictions of future violence that surpass those of unstructured clinical judgments" (Odgers et al., 2004, p. 195). Generally, formal assessment procedures offer greater validity, structure, and consistency to risk classification and help to match the most intensive interventions to youth with the greatest needs (Howell, 1995).

Although female-specific assessments are not widely available, some advances have been made. One risk assessment tool that has been validated for girls is the Early Assessment Risk List for Girls. A number of tools also have been assessed in terms of gender performance (gender analyzed) (Walters, 2008). These include the Youth Level of Service Case Management Inventory and the Global Risk Assessment Device. Individual states have also developed gender-analyzed tools—with mixed results (Walters, Winterfield, & Brumbaugh, 2007).

Early Assessment Risk List for Girls

The Child Development Institute (formerly the Earlscourt Child and Family Centre) in Toronto, Canada, is a treatment center for children under the age of 12 exhibiting serious aggressive and antisocial behaviors. The institute has developed gender-specific initiatives, including risk assessment tools, to augment and improve understanding of the developmental pathways of aggression. After developing a risk assessment tool for boys, the institute created a consultation version of the tool for use with girls—the Early Assessment Risk List for Girls (EARL-21G). These two instruments were modeled on an adult violence risk instrument commonly used in forensic and correctional settings (the HCR-20) and are among the first structured instruments developed for assessing violence risk in young children (Augimeri et al., 2005). The EARL-21G combines empirically supported risk factors applicable to behaviorally troubled girls with three gender-specific factors from a qualitative study conducted by the developers: social aggression, attention deficit hyperactivity disorder, and early sexual development (Levene et al., 2004).

The EARL-21G is designed to provide a platform for increasing clinicians' and researchers' understanding of girls' risk factors for violence and antisocial behaviors and to assist in the creation of effective clinical treatment plans of high-risk girls (Augimeri et al., 2005). It is a practical instrument/checklist with 21 items that are scored on a scale from 0 to 2. The items are intended to highlight a girl's strengths and weaknesses and to elicit thoughts about possible interventions. The instrument is divided into three sections. *Family items* are concerned with the extent to which the child has been supported, nurtured, disciplined, supervised, and encouraged. The *child items* address the child's ability to behave responsibly and sensibly, and the focus of the *responsivity* section is the ability of the girl and her family to engage in treatment and benefit from interventions.

A retrospective and prospective file study found interrater reliability and correlations between scores and subsequent youth and adult court convictions to be statistically significant. An evaluation of the Earlscourt Girls Connection, a gender-specific program for young girls exhibiting aggressive and antisocial behaviors that uses the EARL-21G, analyzed behavioral change according to primary caregivers' ratings. A comparison of admission scores with 6-month and 12-month follow-up found that, at follow-up, girls rated lower on the total score for externalizing behaviors and higher on prosocial behaviors (Walsh, Pepler, & Levene, 2002).

Youth Level of Service/Case Management Inventory

The Youth Level of Service/Case Management Inventory (YLS/CMI) is a standardized inventory designed to aid professionals in assessing adolescent offenders. The inventory assesses factors associated with recidivism risk and need and has been found to be predictive of factors pertaining to girls (Hoge, 2005). The tool is composed of seven parts and includes a 42-item checklist that produces a detailed survey of youth risk and needs factors to be used in formulating a case plan. The YLS/CMI is based on two assumptions. The first is that the causes of an adolescent's criminal activity are a complex network of interacting variables reflective of the adolescent's circumstances and characteristics. The second assumption is that interventions with high-risk adolescents can be effective in reducing the chances of future antisocial activity. To be effective, however, the interventions must be targeted to the criminogenic needs of the individual adolescent and delivered in an appropriate manner (Hoge, 2005).

Global Risk Assessment Device

The Global Risk Assessment Device (GRAD) is an Internet-based tool that was developed out of a need for standardized information about justice-involved youth and their families. It assesses potential threats to adolescents' developmental needs in 11 domains of risk/needs: prior offenses, family/parenting issues, deviant peer relationships, substance abuse, mental health issues, psychopathy, sexual activity and other health-related risks, leisure activities, accountability, education/work issues, and traumatic events (Gavazzi et al., 2003). Originally similar in content to several other assessment tools, the GRAD was expanded to address the unique risks to which girls are exposed. Thus, the GRAD includes the more gender-sensitive domains of traumatic events and sexual activity and other health-related risks. Also, the original domains were augmented with items that reflect female-specific manifestations of problem behavior (e.g., the peers domain includes items to assess relational aggression) (Gavazzi, Yarcheck, & Chesney-Lind, 2006).

Evidence suggests that the GRAD has excellent psychometric properties, but its gender-sensitivity nature was only recently considered. In a study including 305 male and female adolescent detainees, Gavazzi, Yarcheck, and Chesney-Lind (2006) found significant gender differences in risk/need scores. Girls scored significantly higher than boys on items related to traumatic events, family and parenting issues, mental health, and health issues and exhibited more risk for psychopathy. The reasons for being detained were also gendered. Girls were more likely to be held for incorrigible/unruly behavior and domestic violence (offenses including more family-related phenomena), while boys were more likely to be detained for property and violent offenses. Girls also reported significantly higher peer relationship risks, suggesting that girls fled family situations and engaged with delinquent peers on the streets. Findings support the need for "the development of gender-sensitive assessment instruments for use with juvenile offenders" (p. 605) as well as gender-responsive programming for girls and boys.

The development of comprehensive violence risk assessment procedures and tools is a work in progress. Although the risks and needs of girls and boys are often aligned along a common continuum, research has begun to identify important gender-based differences in the development and expression of aggression and violence. Thus, reliance on tools that only capture risks to which boys are traditionally exposed may suffice for some girls but will overlook risks such as traumatic events and mental health that are much more likely to predict future difficulties for many girls (Gavazzi et al., 2006).

GENDER-RESPONSIVE TREATMENT

Initiating treatment with girls who have used violence can be difficult. Girls often have complex clinical profiles and present to their clinicians as guarded and resistant. The violent behavior for which a girl has been referred may not (particularly in her opinion) warrant the prescribed punishment. Her violence may have served as a means to an end, enabling her to leave a violent home, meet a new peer group, increase her social status, or break free from imposed gender roles. It is also likely that she has an extensive history of abuse and neglect and struggles with substance abuse and mental health issues (Brosky & Lally, 2004; Browne & Finklehor, 1986; Chesney-Lind & Shelden, 2004; Dixon et al., 2005; Siegel & Williams, 2003). Her pathway to violence is often complicated, and her treatment must be comprehensive and sensitive to her unique needs.

The purpose of this section is to present gender-responsive principles for use in treatment with girls who have acted violently. Although a complete understanding of the treatment needs of girls who have used violence is still evolving, as are corresponding treatment interventions, a gender-responsive framework provides practitioners with guidelines with which to design appropriate treatment approaches. Gender responsiveness for girls has been defined as:

> intentionally allowing gender to affect and guide services in areas such as site selection, program development, content, and material to create an environment that reflects an understanding of the realities of girls' lives, and is responsive to issues and needs of the girls and young women being served. (Morgan & Patton, 2002, p. 58)

Placing the unique needs and concerns of girls in the forefront of all programming and treatment decisions is essential to this approach, particularly when seeking to intervene therapeutically in the lives of girls who have come to the attention of social services and the justice system because of violent behaviors. Although a violent offense is what led them through the door, the girls tend to bring into treatment a myriad of intertwined, complicated issues and concerns, including histories of traumatic events, conflicted relationships, losses, mental health issues, and struggles with gender norms and stereotypes. Together, these issues form an intricate web from which the clinician seeks to discern and selectively disentangle patterns of behavior in order to assist in girls' healthy development. Treatment interventions must also address public safety and protection concerns, and both relapse prevention and recidivism reduction depend in large part on mobilizing resources for girls that were not present when the offense occurred. Thus, a comprehensive approach to treatment moves beyond the individual girl to include services for and alliances with family and community supports—as appropriate.

A comprehensive approach addresses girls' behaviors in context and provides a continuum of services along three levels of care: primary, secondary, and tertiary prevention (Greene, Peters & Associates, 1998). The goal of primary prevention is to eliminate or minimize risk factors of female violence. Secondary prevention (or early intervention) is intended to provide early detection and treatment of initial problems caused by risky behaviors, and to prevent the development of future violence. The tertiary level in this continuum provides treatment and aftercare in an effort to "arrest the progression of problems caused by risky behaviors" (Greene, Peters & Associates, 1998, p. 41). Treatment in residential and secure settings may serve to interrupt violent behavior patterns and help girls develop perspective, consider responsibilities, and learn skills to address normal developmental tasks. Aftercare services and sanctions are included in the treatment model and are designed to prevent recidivism and provide alternative resources (Altschuler & Armstrong, 2001). The following section considers this third level in the continuum. It focuses on six key elements of gender-responsive treatment, largely based on the work of Covington and Bloom (2006) and Bloom, Owen, and Covington (2003). Case examples (using pseudonyms) from a clinical setting demonstrate the application of the gender-responsive principles.

Creating a Therapeutic Environment

Given the prevalence of trauma in the lives of many girls, and acknowledging the long-term consequences of unresolved traumatic experiences, a sense of safety must be the foundation of a gender-responsive therapeutic environment. Covington (2002) has noted the importance of the therapeutic milieu model, in which a carefully arranged environment is designed to reverse the effects of exposure to interpersonal violence. The therapeutic culture contains five fundamental and complementary elements, each of which can be incorporated into both institutional and community settings (Haigh, 1999). The elements are a culture of belonging (attachment); of safety (containment); of openness (communication); of participation and citizenship (involvement); and of empowerment (agency). Similarly, Patton and Morgan (2002) specify three environmental components essential to programs designed for girls: physical safety, emotional safety, and surroundings that place value on females.

Physical safety specifically refers to an environment void of "violence, physical and sexual abuse, verbal harassment, bullying, teasing, and stalking" (Patton & Morgan, 2002, p. 31). An environment's physical safety can be improved by ensuring that girls have private areas for hygiene practices and the physical checks associated with intake and security measures (Patton & Morgan, 2002; Zavlek & Maniglia, 2007). Meetings and group sessions should be in private and contained spaces. Within these spaces, comfortable chairs (such as beanbags and pillows) arranged in a circle can help girls feel physically protected. If the program does not provide a sense of physical safety, treatment effectiveness will be impeded.

Emotional safety is an especially critical component of the treatment environment. Research indicates a high rate of prior trauma among girls entering the justice system, and the juvenile justice experience itself frequently adds to girls' traumatic experiences. Residential placement can trigger painful memories and reactions, increase feelings of loss of control, and result in retraumatization. Adjustments in the physical environment, however, can help to minimize these reactions and promote a sense of emotional safety. Colors, lighting, and decorations should be selected to facilitate a calm environment, thereby decreasing feelings of anxiety and internal chaos that so often characterize girls involved in violent behaviors (Valentine Foundation & Women's Way, 1990).

It is important that girls are also protected from emotional harm from one another, and, thus, staff need to encourage girls to communicate and share their feelings, free of "negative or coercive behaviors, bias, racism, and sexism" (Patton & Morgan, 2002, p. 2; Valentine Foundation & Women's Way, 1990). Staff need to be attuned to the use of covert, relational aggression (e.g., insults, gossip, manipulation of relationships). A low staff-to-participant ratio makes it easier to discern and intervene in such behaviors, while simultaneously facilitating the development of trusting relationships between girls and program staff and among the girls themselves. Girls are often socialized to compete against each other, and they benefit from opportunities where they feel safe from such competition and are encouraged to relate to peers in a supportive manner.

Finally, the treatment environment should physically express the high value it places on females. A female-centered environment is designed to "enhance a girl's understanding of female development, honor and respect the female perspective, respond to girls' diverse heritages and life experiences, and empower young women to reach their full potential" (Patton & Morgan, 2002, p. 34). The physical environment can promote female empowerment through the prominent display and use of books, posters, pictures, magazines, videos, activities, inspirational messages, and guest speakers. Creating such an environment introduces girls to a range of new possibilities and opportunities, bolstering feelings of strength, achievement, and pride.

Female Role Models and Mentors

Girls in treatment for violent behaviors frequently lack positive female role models, and, thus, building effective relationships is an essential part of working with these girls. This is especially important work because incarcerated girls are likely to be on guard, watching and waiting for a false step, a reenactment of prior damaging relationships, or a broken promise. It is critical that staff separate the girl from her violent offense and take the time to listen to her. When girls feel heard and respected, they will slowly invite others to come closer and to learn about their world. Gilligan (1982) contends that relationships are the key to giving girls a sense of connection, and that attachment and interdependence are the groundwork of female identity development. Disruption of attachments and other losses, however, are likely to be significant factors in the violence that girls display (Ryder, 2007). Thus, during treatment, girls' relational issues need to be addressed, whether they are positive or negative in nature. Being genuine and consistent facilitates the development of a rich and enduring therapeutic relationship, which is critical to a girl's treatment success.

Mentors, either program staff or external individuals, can provide girls with nurturance and consistency, teach the skills needed to build and maintain healthy relationships, and model survival and growth (Morgan & Patton, 2002, p. 62). Specific attention should be paid to the relationship between girls and male treatment providers. Staff need to be aware of how prior male sexual abuse may contribute to incarcerated girls' sexualized behaviors and anger toward male staff, as well an increased sense of vulnerability. Although initially the therapeutic relationship with male staff may be particularly contentious, it can prove to be transformative. Establishing a relationship with an "emotionally supportive and caring male appears to be an extremely powerful intervention in itself" (Okamoto, 2002, p. 265).

Clinical Example

Jill was neglected and sexually abused within her birth family. After connecting and then terminating with several foster families, she was finally adopted. Shortly thereafter, however, Jill was sexually abused by her adoptive father. Jill subsequently began to threaten and physically assault people. Therapy placed Jill in a vulnerable position; her retaliation was in her strong, abrasive, and threatening words and her unkempt presentation. Over the course of treatment, Jill developed a push-and-pull relationship, exemplifying her relational worldview. She first presented with a tough attitude and poor hygiene, which she believed provided the greatest chance at protection from hurtful relationships. There were times when her yearning for connection would creep in and she was able to drop her guard slightly and present in a calm and engaging manner. As she experienced her therapist getting closer, however, Jill's sense of vulnerability escalated again, and she retreated back to her defensive, protective stance. This dialectic continued for several months and was also created in the milieu, particularly with one female staff member.

Gradually, within a physically and emotionally safe environment, and with two female adults helping to meet Jill's emotional need for empathy and compassion, Jill's threats and aggression decreased. Through the use of dialectical behavior therapy (DBT) (Miller, Rathus, & Linehan, 2007), Jill also learned to regulate her emotions and she began to regularly present with a calm and engaging manner. These supportive relationships and DBT helped Jill to begin to experience true growth and to recognize her own positive characteristics, rather than only the negative traits and behaviors that had often brought her attention.

A Focus on Female Competencies and Strengths

A positive self-concept is a critical protective factor for girls, and movement toward this—with a focus on eliciting and building upon strengths, talents, and goals—is to be encouraged (Belknap & Holsinger, 2006; Bloom, Owen, Deschenes, & Rosenbaum, 2002). To do so, clinicians need to learn what a girl believes she is good at and what she enjoys doing. Providing girls with the opportunity to engage in these activities is important for shifting their identity from that of a violent offender to a competent, strong individual. For example, for a girl who dreams of being a famous singer, staff are encouraged to find a way for her to participate with others in a choral group or talent show or to take lessons. Such actions demonstrate belief in the girl, support her goals, and allow her the opportunity to build competency in a prosocial manner.

Girls' competencies and strengths may be intertwined with their use of violence. For example, a girl struggling to manage relationships may use violence to achieve her relational goal. Rather than seeing her only as a violent, manipulative person, a gender-responsive approach sees her as someone who craves and values relationships. Some have suggested, for example, that engagement in indirect aggression can be a sign of social intelligence wherein a girl is able to "analyze social relations and manipulate them" for her own purposes. Encouraging a girl to redirect these same skills and use her social intelligence empathetically can build and strengthen her conflict resolution skills (Björkqvist, 2001, p. 273).

Girls need opportunities to view themselves as survivors rather than victims and to see the connections between their past traumas and their current violent behaviors. For example, recognizing that a girl ran away to escape an abusive situation and then assaulted others when angry may indicate violent combativeness, but it may also indicate resilience and agency and can serve as a foundation for learning healthy coping skills. It is important that girls be provided opportunities to discuss both their personal responsibility and accountability and that of others. Where appropriate, they may work toward making amends to those they hurt, which can be the most powerful part of treatment. Girls can then begin to learn and practice healthy boundaries and healthy relationships (Gaarder & Belknap, 2002; Leschied et al., 2001). Developing strengths based on existing competencies can help to improve girls' self-esteem, control, and prosocial behaviors while bolstering their sense of competence and worth (Greene, Peters & Associates, 1998; Morgan & Patton, 2002).

Case Example

Anna was 11 years old when she entered treatment for sexual aggression. In her short lifetime, Anna and her brother had sustained chronic and sadistic sexual abuse, which had continued undetected for years. Anna was overwhelmed with confusing sexual thoughts and feelings and could not discern whether her experiences were "normal." What was understood, however, was that she could not manage her sexual urges and she began to engage in sexually aggressive behaviors with her brother. Mimicking the behaviors of her abuser, she assumed a threatening demeanor and she exerted physical force to gain control over others. Anna also began to engage in self-injurious behaviors and to lie.

When Anna entered treatment, the shame surrounding her own abuse, in addition to the shame of sexually harming others, had destroyed any sense of self-worth. Anna was unable to believe that she was worthy of love and life, and certainly could not imagine why others would invest hope in her development process. It was initially unclear whether anything could alleviate such powerful shame.

The main treatment goal was to focus on Anna's strengths and competencies. Rather than viewing her as a child who engaged in horrific sexual behaviors, those working with Anna in the treatment community saw her sense of humor and her dramatic talents and consistently acknowledged these and other strengths. The treatment also sought to bring out Anna's sense of empathy, because she had steadfastly avoided accountability for her actions. Externally, she presented as one who did not understand the importance of being accountable for her behavior and did not care about those she hurt. Internally, she feared that verbalizing what she had done would equate her with the person who had abused her. Gradually, in a supportive environment, Anna was able to better understand that her hurtful behaviors were related to her own traumatic experiences, that she was not comfortable with them, and that she wanted to change. Bringing forth newly recognized competencies, including a sense of empathy for others, Anna began to take responsibility for her behaviors. As her strengths and competencies grew, Anna realized that accountability could be healing rather than shaming.

Individualized Treatment Planning

Treatment plans need to acknowledge that all girls are different despite the commonalities of gender and a violent offense (Zavlek & Maniglia, 2007). In 2003, for example, girls of racial and ethnic minority backgrounds constituted 55% of female offenders in residential custody (Snyder & Sickmund, 2006); clearly, those entering treatment represent a continuum of ethnic, racial, sexual, and religious cultures and identities as well as familial structures (see, e.g., Robinson, 2007). Moreover, each may engage in differing behaviors based on past and present worldviews and experiences.

Individualized treatment planning is determined by information gathered from the offender and all of the systems pertaining to her and her family. The nature of the offense helps to determine the level of treatment and the type and mix of services. Depending on individual needs, girls may require information and support around issues pertaining to physical as well as emotional and mental health, including the links among aggression, depression, posttraumatic stress disorder (PTSD), and substance abuse (Messer & Gross, 1994; Sherman, 2005). All such services must be delivered in a culturally competent and gender-sensitive manner.

Clinical Example

Jane, a 15-year-old African American girl, was severely traumatized during her childhood by ongoing neglect, physical and sexual abuse, and witnessing her father beat her mother. Clinical providers questioned treatment effectiveness and success after Jane perpetrated several assaults on caregivers. Simultaneously, Jane questioned how she could be successful in a clinical relationship in which she felt threatened by the emotional intimacy. Her fear of relational harm and need for self-protection provoked her physical aggression.

Interestingly, Jane began talking about wanting to help people, and the treatment team responded by scheduling a formal meeting with Jane to discuss her ideas. In the meeting, Jane talked about feeling better about herself when she was helping others and reported that this feeling never occurred in other activities or environments. She specifically mentioned wanting to help children in Africa. The treatment team determined that this would become the focus of treatment, because it was the first time that Jane demonstrated conviction about something and was willing to let adults into her life. Also, as a young Black woman, Jane was expressing a desire for a connection with her cultural heritage. A treatment plan was developed that included community service work in individual therapy, in milieu therapy, and with her mentor.

Jane conducted several community service projects, including recycling and selling artwork, with proceeds going to a charity organized to help children in Africa. Her mentor worked to educate Jane about the culture of different African countries and helped her to develop projects and goals. Jane's therapist worked to tie this all together by relating community service to Jane's past violent offenses. Community service is an option that enables girls to develop social capital and repair social connections. It also serves as a link between the treatment process and community integration.

Homogeneous Group Treatment

Homogeneous, female-centered group treatment is critical for girls, particularly in the beginning stages of treatment. Underlying all of the multiple issues is frequently a thick layer of shame that girls struggle to talk about or even acknowledge. Shame and anger surrounding past traumatic events may have motivated a girl's self-harm and violence toward others. Then, because the use of violence by girls is perceived as shameful both internally and externally, the girl is further shamed. A treatment group composed of only violent female offenders can decrease the shame each individual carries with her and can help to build a sense of community and individual self-worth. It is important for girls to be provided time to talk with one another in a safe, relational context (Leschied et al., 2001). Small groups held in contained settings help to ensure the physical and emotional safety of members. If possible, group meetings should be scheduled at different times than those of boys to provide more privacy.

Clinical Example

Fourteen-year-old Jasmine walked into group, her head down, her glance turned inward. Her shame and embarrassment were powerful. Her fear of having to share her story of violent behavior with other girls was paralyzing. She sat in a large chair that enveloped her body, hoping to shield herself from the girls around her. As the girls began sharing their personal stories, however, Jasmine began to increase her eye contact and sit up in her chair. She later reported that she had experienced a sense of calm run through her body.

Her reaction was unexpected; she was unsure how she could feel such calm in what she believed would be the worst experience of her life. What followed was even more alarming to her; she began speaking to the other girls in group about her own life story, sharing the horrific events that she had experienced, as well as the shameful ways that she treated others through her aggression. What Jasmine realized was that she didn't feel alone, despite sitting in a room of strangers. She felt supported by the similarities of the stories she heard, and she was comforted by the nodding heads as she shared her own narrative. Although she knew that she had a long road ahead of her, she had found a starting point where her efforts to change were supported, and she reported that, for the first time, she felt a piece of shame peel away.

Long-Term Community Support

Despite evidence that girls are most likely to succeed in the community when they have positive connections with individuals and a network of programs (Sherman, 2005), few aftercare structures exist to support girls' reentry into the community. One successful model is the intensive aftercare model developed by Altschuler and Armstrong (1994, 2001). Originally designed for male juveniles at high risk for reoffending, this model is compatible with best practices for female juvenile offenders, because it is based on comprehensive case management and "emphasizes individualized treatment plans and consistent relationships throughout the treatment process" (Ryder, 2008, p. 17). Continuity of care is stressed and a highly structured association of community-based resources can provide comprehensive services and help in creating social networks (Altschuler, 2008). The model encourages, for example, engaging women's organizations to provide speakers and or support; using community mentors who are representative of girls' culture as a female, or are ethnically/racially helpful to the girl's development; and providing girls with the opportunity to give back to the community or to individuals where trust has been compromised (Altschuler & Armstrong, 2001).

Another model is Boston's Female Focus Initiative (FFI). While in detention, girls are provided services through community-based programs, and these same programs work with the girls upon reentry into the community. The FFI connects girls with stable provider relationships, thus increasing their chances of success in the community and decreasing the possibility of recidivism (Sherman, 2005).

INTERVENTION OPTIONS

To address the needs of this population of girls, programs need to employ a range of interventions with behavioral, cognitive, relational, and systems perspectives (Covington & Bloom, 2006). Although many risk factors for girls' violence overlap with those of boys (Leschied et al., 2001), treatment plans also need to address girls' status in a gendered society, because their problems are often the result being female (i.e., sexual abuse, early pregnancy, male violence, occupational inequality). Gender-responsive programming as has been described in this chapter is built on a relational model (Gilligan, 1982; Miller, 1976), which also is complementary to interventions such as group therapy and a restorative justice perspective (Elis, 2005).

Other interventions include dialectical behavior therapy (Miller, Rathus, & Linehan, 2007), an evidenced-based practice designed to help manage dysregulated emotions that often stem from past abuse. Managing symptoms of trauma and allowing girls the opportunity to understand their past can be crucial elements of treatment. The therapy uses a combination of skills training, problem solving, and validation to help reduce self-destructive, impulsive, and aggressive behaviors (Trupin, Stewart, Beach, & Boesky, 2002; also see Pollack, 2005). Through DBT, girls focus on skill building in the areas of mindfulness, interpersonal effectiveness, emotion regulation, and distress tolerance. DBT skills training is most effective when it is taught in both individual and group therapy.

Several family therapy models are consistent with a gender-responsive model, including functional family therapy, multisystemic therapy, and brief strategic family therapy. Research demonstrates that family therapy improves family communications and relationships and controls imbalances. Family therapy can effect positive changes in the family, school, and community environment over the long term. Staff need to be aware, however, of interpersonal conflicts stemming from gender-related issues such as mother/daughter competition, abandonment and resentment, and familial relationships built on indirect and direct aggression. Girls and their families may need to be individually prepared ahead of time to work together, because family members may have contributed to a girl's offending or precipitated her involvement in the juvenile justice system (Altschuler & Armstrong, 2004). Preparatory meetings can help build safety and trust and model appropriate boundaries.

TARGET (Trauma Affect Regulation: Guide for Education and Treatment) is one educational and therapeutic approach to the prevention and treatment of PTSD that has been used effectively, although not exclusively, with girls (Ford, 2001). It is a strengths-based and sequential skill set that addresses the primary personal issues related to trauma. Most TARGET groups are single sex, making it possible to provide a safe place for those who may have experienced trauma perpetrated by members of the other gender and to help group members work on gender-specific issues in a sensitive manner.

Other curricula that are specific to girls that can be used in treatment of girls who have engaged in violence include *Voices: A Program of Self-Discovery and Empowerment* and *Girls Circle*. The *Voices* program draws upon various therapeutic approaches including psychoeducational, cognitive-behavioral, expressive arts, and relational theory. The curriculum is intended to guide girls through a journey of self-discovery by exploring topics of the self and connecting with others, healthy living, and the journey ahead (Covington, 2004). The workbook can be used in individual or group work and is accompanied by a facilitator's guide.

The *Girls Circle* curriculum is considered a "promising approach" by the Model Programs Guide of the Office of Juvenile Justice and Delinquency Prevention, and is based on relational theory, resiliency practices, and skills training. The structured support groups focus on "increasing positive connections, building empathic skills, and developing resiliency" and have resulted in significant increases in self-efficacy, body image, and social connection (Steese et al., 2006, p. 55).

CONCLUSION

Recent evidence of increasing numbers of girls charged and placed in custody for violent offenses has generated public concern. More importantly, perhaps, this evidence has spurred much-needed research that focuses exclusively on girls and the development of aggression and violent offending. This focus is critical for the development of prevention strategies, assessment tools, and treatment interventions that are effective and appropriate for girls. In addition to studies comparing violence between boys and girls, future research must consider within-group comparisons that examine contributions of particular variables to the development of aggression in girls and consider how girls differentially mediate their experiences in developing violent behaviors (Leschied et al., 2001). Causal explanations of girls' violence also require additional data pertaining to interpersonal and contextual factors that affect girls' lives.

We know a great deal about what girls need to live healthy lives. Additional research must be conducted, but it is imperative that we also address the gap between studies that document gender differences in the developmental course and risk factors for violence and the "implementation and formal evaluation of interventions that actually use this information" (Hipwell & Loeber, 2006, p. 249). Current knowledge must be used to inform and structure practices and policies that take girls seriously and that are committed to ameliorating the social and structural conditions that contribute to their distress.

NOTES

1. Generally, a state's juvenile court system has original jurisdiction over all youth charged with a law violation who were younger than age 18 at the time of the offense, arrest, or referral to court. Individual states, however, often have statutory exceptions to basic age criteria, including lower and upper age limitations (see Snyder & Sickmund, 2006, p. 103).
2. It is also important to remember the numerical differences between female and male arrests. In 2004, for example, girls represented 30% of all juvenile arrests—or 660,000, as compared to over 1.5 million male arrests. In that year, the female proportion of Violent Crime Index arrests was 19%, representing a total of 17,309 girls. Similarly, the female proportion of aggravated assaults grew to 24% in 2004; this totaled 14,508 females compared to 45,942 males (Snyder, 2006, p. 3).
3. A major limitation of the NCVS is that crimes against youth younger than age 12 are not collected.
4. Furthermore, most juvenile victims were female (Snyder & Sickmund, 2006, p. 31).
5. The female proportion of all juveniles held in custody varied by state. In Hawaii, Nebraska, North Dakota, South Dakota, and Wyoming, girls represented at least 25% of those in custody, whereas in Colorado, Maryland, New Jersey, and Rhode Island, girls represented no more than 10% of offenders in custody; Vermont held too few juveniles to calculate a reliable percentage (Snyder & Sickmund, 2006, p. 207).

REFERENCES

Acoca, L. (1999). Investing in girls: A 21st century strategy. *Juvenile Justice, 6*(1), 3–13.

Ageton, S. (1983). The dynamics of female delinquency, 1976–1980. *Criminology, 21*(4), 555–584.

Alemagno, S., Shaffer-King, E., & Hammel, R. (2006). Juveniles in detention. How do girls differ from boys? *Journal of Correctional Health Care, 12*(1), 45–53.

Altschuler, D. M. (2008). Rehabilitating and reintegrating youth offenders: Are residential and community aftercare colliding worlds and what can be done about it? *Justice Policy Journal, 5*(1). Retrieved November 23, 2008, from http://www.cjcj.org/justice_policy_journal

Altschuler, D. M., & Armstrong, T. L. (2001). Reintegrating high-risk juvenile offenders into the communities: Experiences and prospects. *Corrections Management Quarterly, 5*(3), 72–88.

Altschuler, D. M., & Armstrong, T. L. (2004). *Intensive juvenile aftercare reference guide.* Sacramento, CA: Juvenile Reintegration and Aftercare Center.

Amaro, H., Blake, S., Schwartz, P., & Flinchbaugh, L. (2001). Developing theory-based substance abuse prevention programs for young adolescent girls. *Journal of Early Adolescence, 21*(3), 256–293.

American Bar Association & National Bar Association. (2001). *Justice by gender: The lack of appropriate prevention, diversion and treatment alternatives for girls in the justice system*. Washington, DC: Author.

Anderson, N.L.R. (1994). Resolutions and risk taking in juvenile detention. *Clinical Nursing Research, 3*(4), 297–315.

Arnold, R. (1995). Processes of victimization and criminalization of Black women. In B. Price & N. Sokoloff (Eds.), *The criminal justice system and women: Offenders, victims and workers*. (pp. 136–146). New York: McGraw-Hill.

Artz, S. (1998). *Sex, power and the violent school girl*. Toronto, Canada: Trifolium Books.

Augimeri, L., Koegl, C., Levene, K., & Webster, C. (2005). Early assessment risk list for boys and girls. In T. Grisso, G. Vincent, & D. Seagrave, D. (Eds.), *Mental health screening and assessment in juvenile justice* (pp. 295–310). New York: Guilford Press.

Batchelor, S. (2005). Prove me the bam!: Victimization and agency in the lives of young women who commit violent offenses. *Probation Journal: The Journal of Community and Criminal Justice, 52*(4), 358–375.

Baum, K. (2005). *Juvenile victimization and offending, 1993–2003* (Bureau of Justice Statistics Special Report). Washington, DC: Bureau of Justice Statistics.

Belenko, S., Sprott, J., & Peterson, C. (2004). Drug and alcohol involvement among minority and female juvenile offenders: Treatment and policy issues. *Criminal Justice Policy Review, 15*(1), 3–36.

Belknap, J., & Holsinger, K. (1998). An overview of delinquent girls: How theory and practice have failed and the need for innovative changes. In R. Zaplin (Ed.), *Female offenders: Critical perspectives and effective interventions* (pp. 5–29). Gaithersburg, MD: Aspen.

Belknap, J., & Holsinger, K. (2006). The gendered nature of risk factors for delinquency. *Feminist Criminology, 1*(1), 48–71.

Benekos, P., & Merlo, A. (2008). Juvenile justice: The legacy of punitive policy. *Youth Violence and Juvenile Justice, 6*(1), 28–46.

Bierman, K., Bruschi, C., Domitrovich, C., Yan Fang, G., Miller-Johnson, S., & The Conduct Problems Prevention Research Group. (2004). Early disruptive behaviors associated with emerging antisocial behavior among girls. In M. Putallaz & K. Bierman (Eds.), *Aggression, antisocial behavior, and violence among girls* (pp. 137–161). New York: Guilford Press.

Björkqvist, K. (2001). Different names, same issues. *Social Development, 10*(2), 272–274.

Björkqvist, K., & Niemla, P. (1992). New trends in the study of female aggression. In K. Björkqvist & P. Niemla (Eds.), *Of mice and women: Aspects of female aggression* (pp. 3–16). San Diego, CA: Academic Press.

Björkqvist, K., Osterman, K., & Kaukiainen, A. (1992). The development of direct and indirect aggressive strategies in males and females. In K. Björkqvist & P. Niemla (Eds.), *Of mice and women: Aspects of female aggression* (pp. 51–64). San Diego, CA: Academic Press.

Bloom, B. (Ed.). (2003). *Gendered justice: Addressing female offenders*. Durham, NC: Carolina Academic Press.

Bloom, B., Owen, B., & Covington, S. (2003). *Gender-responsive strategies: Research, practice and guiding principles for women offenders*. Washington, DC: National Institute of Corrections.

Bloom, B., Owen, B., Deschenes, E., & Rosenbaum, J. (2002). Moving toward justice for female juvenile offenders in the new millennium: Modeling gender-specific policies and programs. *Journal of Contemporary Criminal Justice, 18*(1), 37–56.

Borum, R. (2003). Managing at-risk juvenile offenders in the community. *Journal of Contemporary Criminal Justice, 19*(1), 114–137.

Borum, R., & Verhaagen, D. (2006). *Assessing and managing violence risk in juveniles.* New York: Guilford Press.

Breslau, N., Davis, G., Andreski, P., & Peterson, E. (1991). Traumatic events and post-traumatic stress disorder in an urban population of young adults. *Archives of General Psychiatry, 48,* 216–222.

Brosky, B., & Lally, S. (2004). Prevalence of trauma, PTSD, and dissociation in court-referred adolescents. *Journal of Interpersonal Violence, 19*(7), 801–814.

Brotherton, D. (1996). Smartness, toughness and autonomy. *Journal of Drug Issues, 26*(1), 261–277.

Brown, L., Chesney-Lind, M., & Stein, N. (2007). Patriarchy matters: Toward a gendered theory of teen violence and victimization. *Violence Against Women, 13*(12), 1249–1273.

Brown, M., & Gilligan, C. (1992). *Meeting at the crossroads: Women's psychology and girls' development.* New York: Ballantine.

Browne, A., & Finkelhor, D. (1986). Impact of child sexual abuse: A review of the research. *Psychological Bulletin, 99,* 66–77.

Buzawa, E., & Hotaling, G. (2006). The impact of relationship status, gender, and minor status in the police response to domestic assaults. *Victims and Offenders, 1*(1), 1–38.

Campbell, A. (1984). *The girls in the gang.* New York: Blackwell.

Campbell, A. (1994). *Men, women, and aggression.* New York: Basic Books.

Cavanagh Johnson, T. (1989). Female child perpetrators: Children who molest other children. *Child Abuse and Neglect, 13*(4), 571–585.

Cernkovich, S., Lanctôt, N., & Giordano, P. (2008). Predicting adolescent and adult antisocial behavior among adjudicated delinquent females. *Crime & Delinquency, 54*(1), 3–33.

Chesney-Lind, M. (2000). What to do about girls. In M. McMahon (Ed.), *Assessment to assistance: Programs for women in community corrections* (pp. 139–170). Lantham, MD: American Correctional Association.

Chesney-Lind, M. (2002). Criminalizing victimization: The unintended consequences of pro-arrest policies for girls and women. *Criminology and Public Policy, 2*(1), 81–90.

Chesney-Lind, M. (2004, August). *Girls and violence: Is the gender gap closing?* VAWnet Applied Research Forum. Philadelphia: National Resource Center on Domestic Violence.

Chesney-Lind, M., & Belknap, J. (2004). Trends in delinquent girls' aggression and violent behavior: A review of the evidence. In M. Putallaz & K. Bierman (Eds.), *Aggression, antisocial behavior, and violence among girls: A developmental perspective* (pp. 203–220). New York: Guilford Press.

Chesney-Lind, M., & Eliason, M. (2006). From invisible to incorrigible: The demonization of marginalized women and girls. *Crime, Media, Culture, 2*(1), 29–47.

Chesney-Lind, M., Morash, M., & Irwin, K. (2007). Policing girlhood? Relational aggression and violence prevention. *Youth Violence and Juvenile Justice, 5*(3), 328–345.

Chesney-Lind, M., & Shelden, R. (2004). *Girls, delinquency and juvenile justice* (3rd ed.). Belmont, CA: Wadsworth.
Corrado, R., Roesch, R., Hart, S., & Gierowski, J. (2002). *Multi-problem violent youth: A foundation for comparative research on needs, interventions and outcomes.* Amsterdam: IOS Press.
Covington, S. (2002). A woman's journey home: Challenges for female offenders and their children. Paper for the Urban Institute "From Prison to Home" Conference. Retrieved February 2, 2008, from http://www.urban.org
Covington, S. (2004). *Voices: A program of self-discovery and empowerment for girls. Facilitators Guide.* Carson City, NV: Change Companies.
Covington, S., & Bloom, B. (2006). Gender-responsive treatment and services in correctional settings. *Women and Therapy, 29*(3/4), 9–33.
Crick, N., & Bigbee, M. (1998). Relational and overt forms of peer victimization: A multi-informant approach. *Journal of Consulting and Clinical Psychology, 66*(2), 337–347.
Crick, N., & Grotpeter, J. (1995). Relational aggression, gender and social-psychological adjustment. *Child Development, 66*(3), 710–722.
Crick, N., Werner, N., Casas, J., O'Brien, K., Nelson, D., Grotpeter, J., et al. (1999). Childhood aggression and gender: A new look at an old problem. In D. Bernstein (Ed.), *Nebraska symposium on motivation: Gender and motivation, 45,* 75–141. Lincoln: University of Nebraska Press.
Cullen, F., Wright, J., Brown, S., Moon, M., Blankenship, M., & Applegate, B. (1998). Public support for early intervention programs. *Criminal Justice and Behavior, 44*(2), 187–204.
Dembo, R., Schmeidler, J., Guida, J., & Rahman, A. (1998). A further study of gender differences in service needs among youths entering a juvenile assessment center. *Journal of Child and Adolescent Substance Abuse, 7*(4), 49–77.
Dembo, R., Williams, L., Lavoie, L., & Berry, E. (1989). Physical abuse, sexual victimization, and illicit drug use. *Violence and Victims, 4*(2), 121–138.
Dembo, R., Williams, L., Wothke, W., Schmeidler, J., & Brown, C. H. (1992). The role of family factors, physical abuse, and sexual victimization experiences in high-risk youths' alcohol and other drug use and delinquency: A longitudinal model. *Violence and Victims, 7*(3), 245–266.
Dembo, R., Williams, L., Wothke, W., Schmeidler, J., Getreu, A., Berry, E., et al. (1990). The relationship between cocaine use, drug sales and other delinquency among a cohort of high risk youths over time. In M. De La Rosa, E. Lambert, & B. Gropper (Eds.), *Drugs and violence: Causes, correlates, and consequences* (pp. 112–135). Research monograph No. 103. Rockville, MD: National Institute on Drug Abuse.
Dise-Lewis, J. (1988). The Life Events and Coping Inventory: An assessment of stress in children. *Psychosomatic Medicine, 50*(5), 484–499.
Dixon, A., Howie, P., & Starling, J. (2005). Trauma exposure, posttraumatic stress, and psychiatric comorbidity in female juvenile offenders. *Journal of the American Academy of Child & Adolescent Psychiatry, 44*(8), 798–806.
Elis, L. (2005). Restorative justice programs, gender, and recidivism. *Public Organization Review: A Global Journal, 5*(4), 375–389.
Elliott, D. (1994). Serious violent offenders: Onset, developmental course, and termination—The American Society of Criminology 1993 presidential address. *Criminology, 32*(1), 1–21.

English, D., Widom, C., & Brandford, C. (2001). *Childhood victimization and delinquency, adult criminality, and violent criminal behavior: A replication and extension.* Washington, DC: U.S. National Institute of Justice.

Everett, S., & Price, J. (1995). Student's perceptions of violence in the public schools. The Metlife survey. *Journal of Adolescent Health, 17*(6), 345–352.

Farrington, D. (1998). Predictors, causes and correlates of male youth violence. In M. Tonry & M. H. Moore (Eds.), *Crime and justice: A review of research* (Vol. 24, pp. 421–475). Chicago: University of Chicago Press.

Fehrenbach, P., & Monastersky, C. (1988). Characteristics of female adolescent sexual offenders. *American Journal of Orthopsychiatry, 58*(1), 148–151.

Feld, B. (1998). Juvenile and criminal justice systems' responses to youth violence. In M. Tonry and M. H. Moore (Eds.), *Crime and justice: A review of research* (Vol. 24, pp. 189–261). Chicago: University of Chicago Press.

Ford, J. (2001). *TARGET. Trauma affect regulation: Guide for education and treatment.* Farmington: University of Connecticut Health Center.

Funk, S. (1999). Risk assessment for juveniles on probation. *Criminal Justice and Behavior, 26*(1), 44–68.

Gaarder, E., & Belknap, J. (2002) Tenuous borders: Girls transferred to adult court. *Criminology, 40*(3), 481–517.

Garbarino, J. (2006). *See Jane hit: Why girls are growing more violent and what we can do about it.* New York: Penguin Press.

Gavazzi, S., Slade, D., Buettner, C., Partridge, C., Yarcheck, C., & Andrews, D. (2003). Toward conceptual development and empirical measurement of global risk indicators in the lives of court-involved youth. *Psychological Reports, 93,* 1239–1242.

Gavazzi, S., Yarcheck, C., & Chesney-Lind, M. (2006). Global risk indicators and the role of gender in a juvenile detention sample. *Criminal Justice and Behavior, 33*(5), 597–612.

Gilfus, M. (1992). From victims to survivors to offenders: Women's routes of entry and immersion in street crime. *Women and Criminal Justice, 4*(1), 63–89.

Gilligan, C. (1982). *In a different voice: Psychological theory and women's development:* Cambridge: MA: Harvard University Press.

Gilligan, C., Lyons, N., & Hammer, T. (Eds.). (1990). *Making connections: The relational worlds of adolescent girls at Emma Willard School.* Cambridge, MA: Harvard University Press.

Giordano, P., Cernkovich, S., & Lowery, A. (2004). A long-term follow-up of serious adolescent female offenders. In M. Putallaz & K. Bierman (Eds.), *Aggression, antisocial behavior, and violence among girls: A developmental perspective* (pp. 186–202). New York: Guilford Press.

Godfrey, B. (2004). Rough girls, 1880–1930: The "recent" history of violent young women. In C. Adler & A. Worrall (Eds.), *Girls' violence: Myths and realities* (pp. 21–39). Albany: State University of New York Press.

Greene, Peters & Associates. (1998). *Guiding principles for promising female programming: An inventory of best practices.* Washington, DC: U.S. Department of Justice, Office of Juvenile Justice and Delinquency Prevention.

Grisso, T. (2005a). Why we need mental health screening and assessment in juvenile justice programs. In T. Grisso, G. Vincent, & D. Seagrave (Eds.), *Mental health screening and assessment in juvenile justice* (pp. 3–21). New York: Guilford Press.

Grisso, T. (2005b). Evaluating the properties of instruments for screening and assessment. In T. Grisso, G. Vincent, & D. Seagrave (Eds.), *Mental health screening and assessment in juvenile justice* (pp. 71–93). New York: Guilford Press.

Haigh, R. 1999. The quintessence of a therapeutic environment: Five universal qualities. In P. Campling & R. Haigh (Eds.), *Therapeutic communities: Past, present and future* (pp. 246–247). London: Kingsley.

Harlow, C. (1999). *Prior abuse reported by inmates and probationers.* Washington, DC: U.S. Department of Justice, Office of Justice Programs.

Hawkins, J., Herrenkohl, T., Farrington, D., Brewer, D., Catalano, R., & Harachi, T. (1998). A review of predictors of youth violence. In R. Loeber & D. Farrington (Eds.), *Serious and violent juvenile offenders: Risk factors and successful interventions* (pp. 106–146). Thousand Oaks, CA: Sage.

Heimer, K. (2000). Changes in the gender gap in crime and women's economic marginalization. In G. LaFree (Ed.), *Criminal justice 2000: Vol. 1. Nature of crime. Continuity and change* (NCJ182408, pp. 427–483). Washington, DC: National Institute of Justice.

Heimer, K., & De Coster, S. (1999). The gendering of violent delinquency. *Criminology, 37*(2), 277–317.

Hendriks, J., & Bijleveld, C. (2006). Female adolescent sex offenders—An exploratory study. *Journal of Sexual Aggression, 12*(1), 31–41.

Herman, J. (1997). *Trauma and recovery.* New York: Basic Books.

Herrenkohl, T., McMorros, B., Catalono, R., Abbott, R., Hemphilll, S., & Toumbourou, J. (2007). Risk factors for violence and relational aggression in adolescence. *Journal of Interpersonal Violence, 22*(4), 386–405.

Hipwell, A., & Loeber, R. (2006). Do we know which interventions are effective for disruptive and delinquent girls? *Clinical Child and Family Psychology Review, 9*(3/4), 221–255.

Hoge, R. (2005). Youth Level of Service/Case Management Inventory. In T. Grisso, G. Vincent, & D. Seagrave (Eds.), *Mental health screening and assessment in juvenile justice* (pp. 283–294). New York: Guilford Press.

Horowitz, K., Wiene, S., & Jekel, J. (1995). PTSD symptoms in urban adolescent girls: Compounded community trauma. *Journal of American Academy of Adolescent Psychiatry, 34*(10), 1353–1361.

Howell, J. (1995). *Guide for implementing the comprehensive strategy for serious, violent and chronic juvenile offenders.* Washington, DC: U.S. Department of Justice.

Hoyt, S., & Scherer, D. (1998). Female juvenile delinquency: Misunderstood by the juvenile justice system, neglected by social science. *Law and Human Behavior, 22*(1), 81–107.

Ireland, T., & Widom, C. (1994). Childhood victimization and risk for alcohol and drug arrests. *International Journal of the Addictions, 29,* 235–274.

Jaffee, S., Caspi, A., Moffitt, T., & Taylor, A. (2004). Physical maltreatment victim to antisocial child. *Journal of Abnormal Psychology, 113,* 44–55.

Jones, N. (2004). "It's not where you live, it's how you live": How young women negotiate conflict and violence in the inner city. *Annals of the American Academy of Political and Social Science, 595,* 49–62.

Kingery, P., Pruitt, B., & Hurley, R. (1992). Violence and illegal drug use among adolescents: Evidence from the U.S. national adolescent student health survey. *International Journal of the Addictions, 27*(12), 1445–1464.

Kruttschnitt, C. (1994). Gender and interpersonal violence. In A. Reiss & J. Roth (Eds.), *Understanding and preventing violence: Vol. 3. Social influences* (pp. 293–376). Committee on Law and Justice, National Research Council. Washington, DC: National Academy Press.

Kruttschnitt, C. (2001). Gender and violence. In C. Renzetti & L. Goodstein (Eds.), *Women, crime and criminal justice: Original feminist readings* (pp. 77–92). Los Angeles: Roxbury.

Krystal, H., & Raskin, H. (1970). *Drug dependence: Aspects of ego function.* Detroit: Wayne State University Press.

Lanctôt, N., Émond, C., & Le Blanc, M. (2004). Adjudicated females' participation in violence from adolescence to adulthood. Results from a longitudinal study. In M. Moretti, C. Odgers, & M. Jackson (Eds.), *Girls and aggression: Contributing factors and intervention principles* (pp. 75–84). New York: Kluwer Academic.

Laub, J., & McDermott, M. (1985). An analysis of serious crime by young Black women. *Criminology, 23*(1), 81–98.

Leschied, A., Cummings, A., Van Brunschot, M., Cunningham, A., & Saunders, A. (2001). Aggression in adolescent girls: Implications for policy, prevention and treatment. *Canadian Psychology, 42*(3), 200–215.

Levene, K., Walsh, M., Augimieri, L., & Pepler, D. (2004). Linking identification and treatment of early risk factors for female delinquency. In M. Moretti, C. Odgers, & M. Jackson (Eds.), *Girls and aggression: Contributing factors and intervention principles* (pp. 147–164). New York: Kluwer Academic.

Lewis, M. (2006). *Custody and control: Conditions of confinement in New York's juvenile prisons for girls.* New York: Human Rights Watch/American Civil Liberties Association.

Lindeman, M., Harakka, T., & Keltikangas-Javinen, L. (1997). Age and gender differences in adolescents' reactions to conflict situations: Aggression, prosociality, and withdrawal. *Journal of Youth and Adolescence, 26*(3), 339–351.

Little, T., Henrich, C., Jones, S., & Hawley, P. (2003). Disentangling the "whys" from the "whats" of aggressive behavior. *International Journal of Behavioral Development, 27*(2), 122–133.

Loper, A. B. (2000). Female juvenile delinquency: Risk factors and promising interventions. *Juvenile Justice Fact Sheet.* Charlottesville: Institute of Law, Psychiatry & Public Policy, University of Virginia.

Loper, A., & Cornell, D. (1996). Homicide by juvenile girls. *Journal of Child and Family Studies, 5*(3), 323–336.

Luke, K. P. (2008). Are girls really becoming more violent? A critical analysis. *Affilia, 23*(1), 38–50.

Marsteller, F., Brogan, D., Smith, I., Ash, P., Daniels, D., Rolka, D., et al. (1997). *The prevalence of substance use disorders among juveniles admitted to regional youth detention centers operated by the Georgia Department of Children and Youth Services.* Center for Substance Abuse Treatment Final Report. Retrieved November 24, 2008, from http://www.behav.com/projects/CSATFinalReport.html

Martino, S., Ellickson, P., Klein, D., McCaffrey, D., & Edelen, M. (2008). Multiple trajectories of physical aggression among adolescent boys and girls. *Aggressive Behavior, 34*(1), 61–75.

McClellan, D. S., Farabee, D., & Crouch, B. M. (1997). Early victimization, drug use and criminality: A comparison of male and female prisoners. *Criminal Justice and Behavior, 24*(4), 455–476.

McMaster, L., Connolly, J., Pepler, D., & Craig, W. (2002). Peer to peer sexual harassment in early adolescence: A developmental perspective. *Development & Psychopathology, 14*(1), 91–105.

Meichenbaum, D. (2006.) *Comparison of aggression in boys and girls: A case for gender-specific interventions.* Miami, FL: Melissa Institute for Violence Prevention and Treatment. Retrieved January 30, 2008, from www.melissainstitute.org/articles

Messer, S. C., & Gross, A. M. (1994). Childhood depression and aggression: A covariance structure analysis. *Behaviour Research and Therapy, 32*(6), 663–677.

Messerschmidt, J. W. (1986). *Capitalism, patriarchy and crime: Toward a socialist feminist criminology.* Totowa, NJ: Rowman and Littlefield.

Miller, A., Rathus, J., & Linehan, M. (2007). *Dialectical behavior therapy with suicidal adolescents.* New York: Guilford Press.

Miller, D., Trapani, C., Fejes-Mendoza, K., Eggleston, C., & Dwiggins, D. (1995). Adolescent female offenders: Unique considerations. *Adolescence, 30*(118), 429–435.

Miller, J. (1998). Up it up. Gender and accomplishment of street robbery. *Criminology, 36*(1), 37–66.

Miller, J. B. (1976). *Toward a new psychology of women.* Boston: Beacon Press.

Moretti, M., Catchpole, R., & Odgers, C. (2005). The dark side of girlhood: Recent trends, risk factors and trajectories to aggression and violence. *Canadian Child and Adolescent Psychiatry Review, 14*(1), 21–25.

Morgan, M., & Patton, P. (2002). Gender-responsiveness programming in the justice system: Oregon's guidelines for effective programming for girls. *Federal Probation, 66*(2), 57–65.

Ness, C. (2004). Why girls fight: Female youth violence in the inner city. *Annals of the American Academy of Political and Social Science, 595,* 32–48.

Norton, M. (2002). *In the devil's snare. The Salem witchcraft crisis of 1692.* New York: Vintage.

Obeidallah, D., & Earls, F. (1999). *Adolescent girls: The role of depression in the development of delinquency.* Washington, DC: U.S. Department of Justice, National Institute of Justice.

Odem, M., & Schlossman, S. (1991). Guardians of virtue: The juvenile court and female delinquency in early 20th century Los Angeles. *Crime and Delinquency, 37*(2), 186–203.

Odgers, C., & Moretti, M. (2002). Aggressive and antisocial girls: Research update and challenges. *International Journal of Forensic Mental Health, 1*(2), 103–119.

Odgers, C., Reppucci, N., & Moretti, M. (2005). Nipping psychopathy in the bud: An examination of the convergent, predictive, and the theoretical utility of the PCL-YV among adolescent girls. *Behavioral Sciences and the Law, 23*(6), 743–763.

Odgers, C., Schmidt, M., & Repucci, N. (2004). Reframing violence risk assessment for female juvenile offenders. In M. Moretti, C. Odgers, & M. Jackson (Eds.), *Girls and aggression: Contributing factors and intervention principles* (pp. 195–210). New York: Kluwer Academic.

Okamoto, S. (2002). The challenges of male practitioners working with female youth clients. *Child & Youth Care Forum, 31*(4), 257–268.

Patton, P., & Morgan, M. (2002). *How to implement Oregon's guidelines for effective gender-responsive programming for girls: Report to the Oregon Criminal Justice Commission and the Oregon Commission on Children and Families*. Washington, DC: Office of Juvenile Justice and Delinquency Prevention, Office of Justice Programs.

Pipher, M. (1994). *Reviving Ophelia: Saving the selves of adolescent girls*. New York: Ballantine.

Poe-Yamagata, E., & Jones, M. (2000). *And justice for some*. National Council on Crime and Delinquency and Building Blocks for Youth. Retrieved November 23, 2008, from www.buildingblocksforyouth.org

Pollack, S. (2005). Taming the shrew: Regulating prisoners through women-centered mental health programming. *Critical Criminology, 13*(1), 71–87.

Pollock, J., & Davis, S. (2005). The continuing myth of the violent female offender. *Criminal Justice Review, 30*(1), 5–29.

Potter, H. (2006). An argument for Black feminist criminology: Understanding African American women's experiences with intimate partner abuse using an integrated approach. *Feminist Criminology, 1*(2), 106–124.

Prothrow-Stith, D., & Spivak, H. R. (2005). *Sugar and spice and no longer nice: How we can stop girls' violence*. San Francisco: Jossey-Bass.

Ray, J. A., & English, D. (1995). Comparison of female and male children with sexual behavior problems. *Journal of Youth and Adolescence, 24*(4), 439–451.

Reitsma-Street, M. (2004). Connecting policies, girls and violence. In M. Moretti, C. Odgers, & M. Jackson (Eds.), *Girls and aggression: Contributing factors and intervention principles* (pp. 115–130). New York: Kluwer Academic.

Rhee, S., & Waldman, I. (2002). Genetic and environmental influences on antisocial behavior. *Psychological Bulletin, 128*, 490–529.

Robinson, R. (2007). "It's not easy to know who I am": Gender salience and cultural place in the treatment of a "delinquent" adolescent mother. *Feminist Criminology, 2*(1), 31–56.

Roe-Sepowitz, D. (2007). Adolescent female murderers: Characteristics and treatment implications. *American Psychological Association, 77*(3), 489–496.

Ryder, J. (2003). *Antecedents of violent behavior: Early childhood trauma in the lives of adolescent female offenders*. Unpublished doctoral dissertation, City University of New York.

Ryder, J. (2007). "I wasn't really bonded with my family": Attachment, loss and violence among adolescent female offenders. *Critical Criminology, 15*(1), 19–40.

Ryder, J. (2008). Revamping the Altschuler and Armstrong Intensive Aftercare Program for use with girls in the juvenile justice system. *Women, Girls & Criminal Justice, 9*(2), 17, 18, 22, 26, 27, 32.

Ryder, J., Langley, S., & Brownstein, H. (2009). "I've been around and around and around": Measuring traumatic events in the lives of incarcerated girls. In R. Gido & L. Dalley (Eds.), *Women and mental health issues across the criminal justice system* (pp. 45–70). Upper Saddle River, NJ: Prentice Hall.

Schaffner, L. (2004). Capturing girls' experiences of "community violence" in the United States. In C. Alder & A. Worrall (Eds.), *Girls' violence: Myths and realities* (pp. 105–128). New York: State University of New York Press.

Sherman, F. (2005). *Thirteen pathways to juvenile detention reform: Detention reform and girls*. Baltimore: Annie E. Casey Foundation.

Siegel, J., & Williams, L. (2003). The relationship between child sexual abuse and female delinquency and crime: A prospective study. *Journal of Research in Crime and Delinquency, 40*(1), 71–94.

Silverthorn, P., & Frick, P. (1999). Developmental pathways to antisocial behavior: The delayed-onset pathway in girls. *Development and Psychopathology, 11*(1), 101–126.

Simkins, S., & Katz, S. (2002). Criminalizing abused girls. *Violence Against Women, 8*(12), 1474–1499.

Simpson, J., & Weiner, E. (Eds.) (1989a). Aggression. In *The Oxford English Dictionary* (2nd ed.). Oxford, England: Oxford University Press. Retrieved November 21, 2008, from http://dictionary.oed.com/cgi/entry/ 50004419

Simpson, J., & Weiner, E. (Eds.) (1989b). Violence. In *The Oxford English Dictionary* (2nd ed.). Oxford, England: Oxford University Press. Retrieved November 21, 2008, from http://dictionary.oed.com/cgi/entry/50277881

Smith, C., & Thornberry, T. (1995). The relationship between childhood maltreatment and adolescent involvement in delinquency. *Criminology, 33*(4), 451–477.

Snyder, H. (2006). Juvenile arrests 2004. *OJJDP Bulletin*. Washington, DC: U.S. Department of Justice, Office of Juvenile Justice and Delinquency Prevention.

Snyder, H., & Sickmund, M. (2006). *Juvenile offenders and victims: 2006 national report*. Washington, DC: U.S. Department of Justice, Office of Juvenile Justice and Delinquency Prevention.

Stahl, A. (2004). *A profile of females in the juvenile justice system*. Power Point presentation. Pittsburgh, PA: National Center for Juvenile Justice.

Steese, S., Dollette, M., Philips, W., Hossfeld, E., Matthews, G., & Taorimina, G. (2006). Understanding Girls Circle as an intervention on perceived social support, body image, self-efficacy, locus of control, and self-esteem. *Adolescence, 41*(161), 55–74.

Steffemeier, D., & Allen, E. (1998). The nature of female offending: Patterns and explanations. In R. Zaplin (Ed.), *Female offenders: Critical perspectives and effective intervention* (pp. 5–29). Gaithersburg, MD: Aspen.

Steffensmeier, D., & Schwartz, J. (2004). Trends in female criminality: Is crime still a man's world? In B. Price & N. Sokoloff (Eds.), *The criminal justice system and women: Offenders, prisoners, victims & workers* (3rd ed., pp. 95–111). New York: McGraw-Hill.

Steffensmeier, D., Schwartz, J., Zhong, H., & Ackerman, J. (2005). An assessment of recent trends in girls' violence using diverse longitudinal sources: Is the gender gap closing? *Criminology, 43*(2), 355–405.

Stein, N. (2001). Sexual harassment meets zero tolerance: Life in K-12 schools. In W. Ayers, B. Dohrn, & R. Ayers (Eds.), *Zero tolerance: Resisting the drive for punishment in our schools* (pp. 130–137). New York: New Press.

Surrey, J. (1991). The "self-in-relation": A theory of women's development. In J. Jordan, A. Kaplan, J. Miller, I. Striver, & J. Surrey (Eds.), *Women's growth in connection: Writings from the Stone Center* (pp. 51–66). New York: Guilford Press.

Teplin, L., Abram, K., McClelland, G., Dulcan, M., & Mericle, A. (2002). Psychiatric disorders in youth in juvenile detention. *Archives of General Psychiatry, 59*, 1133–1143.

Trupin, E., Stewart, D., Beach, B., & Boesky, L. (2002). Effectiveness of a dialectical behaviour therapy program for incarcerated female juvenile offenders. *Child and Adolescent Mental Health, 7*(3), 121–127.

U.S. Department of Health and Human Services. (2001). *Youth violence: A report of the Surgeon General*. Rockville, MD: U.S. Government Printing Office.

Valentine Foundation & Women's Way. (1990). *A conversation about girls*. Philadelphia: Authors.

Vincent, G., & Grisso, T. (2005). A developmental perspective on adolescent personality, psychopathology, and delinquency. In T. Grisso, G. Vincent, & D. Seagrave (Eds.), *Mental health screening and assessment in juvenile justice* (pp. 22–43). New York: Guilford Press.

Walsh, M., Pepler, D., & Levene, K. (2002). A model intervention for girls with disruptive behaviour problems: The Earlscourt Girls Connection. *Canadian Journal of Counseling, 36*(4), 297–311.

Walters, J. H. (February, 2008). Girls Study Group, personal correspondence.

Walters, J. H., Winterfield, L., & Brumbaugh, S. (2007). *Girls Study Group screening and assessment instrument review*. Presentation. Retrieved November 23, 2008, from http://girlsstudygroup.rti.org

White, J., & Kowalski, R. (1992). Deconstructing the myth of the nonaggressive woman: A feminist analysis. *Psychology of Women Quarterly, 18*(4), 487–508.

Widom, C., Ireland, T., & Glynn, P. J. (1995). Alcohol abuse in abused and neglected children followed-up: Are they at increased risk? *Journal of Studies on Alcohol, 56*(2), 207–217.

Wolke, D., Woods, S., Bloomfield, L., & Karstadt, L. (2000). The association between direct and relational bullying and behavior problems among primary school children. *Journal of Child Psychology and Psychiatry, 41*(8), 989–1002.

Zahn, M. (2005, November 16). *Causes and correlates of girls' delinquency*. Presentation at the American Society of Criminology conference, Toronto, Canada. Retrieved February 1, 2008, from http://girlsstudygroup.rti.org/docs/2005_ASC_C&C.ppt.pdf

Zahn, M. (2006). The Girls Study Group: Its creation and achievements. *The Criminologist, 31*(5), 1, 3–6.

Zavlek, S., & Maniglia, R. (2007). Developing correctional facilities for female juvenile offenders: Design and programmatic considerations. *Corrections Today, 69*(4), 58–63.

15 Identifying and Responding to Criminogenic Risk and Mental Health Treatment Needs of Crossover Youth

DENISE C. HERZ, SHARON HARADA,
GREGORY LECKLITNER, MICHAEL RAUSO,
AND JOSEPH P. RYAN

Despite growing recognition of and concern about the relationship between child maltreatment and delinquency, very little is known about the youth who cross into delinquency while under the care of child protective services. Research that does address this issue, however, indicates that these "crossover" youth need comprehensive services that account for different risk levels while simultaneously addressing behavioral health and social intervention needs. Unfortunately, these youth rarely receive coordinated care from both the child welfare and delinquency systems; rather, they often fall into the cracks that separate the two systems. This chapter examines the demographic and social backgrounds as well as the risk and treatment need levels of crossover youth charged with violent and nonviolent offenses in Los Angeles County. The implications of these results for building a comprehensive system of care across probation, child protective services, and the mental health care system are then discussed in relationship to current efforts to improve system collaboration in Los Angeles County.

CRIMINOGENIC RISK AND MENTAL HEALTH TREATMENT NEEDS OF CROSSOVER YOUTH WHO COMMIT VIOLENT OFFENSES

The advent of the juvenile court in 1899 established two systems to address the needs of children: the child welfare system for children who were victims of abuse and/or neglect and the delinquency system for children who committed criminal acts. Although these systems were intended to serve the needs of both sets of children, there was little recognition that some children would be both victims and offenders. Consequently, many youth who enter child protective services and subsequently commit a crime rarely receive coordinated care from both the child welfare and delinquency systems.

Youth who penetrate both the child welfare and delinquency systems are commonly referred to as crossover or dual-jurisdiction youth.[1] A youth enters both systems in one of three ways. The most frequent pathway occurs when a youth enters the child welfare system and later commits a crime while under the care and custody of child protective services. A second pathway involves a youth with prior, but not current, contact with child protective services who commits a crime and enters the delinquency system. A third possible pathway occurs when a youth with no prior child welfare system contact enters the delinquency system, and probation refers the case to child protective services for further investigation of abuse/neglect.

The prevalence of crossing over is difficult to estimate, because these youth are typically subsumed in agency-specific information systems that are rarely, if ever, integrated. Research on the relationship between child maltreatment and delinquency, however, estimates that between 9% and 29% of dependent children engage in delinquent behavior. Although the percentage of juvenile probationers with a history of abuse/neglect is even more difficult to measure, a recent study conducted by Halemba, Seigel, Lord, and Zawacki (2004) reported that 42% of youth in probation placements had current or prior involvement in the child welfare system.

These estimates are particularly meaningful when national statistics are considered. In 2003, there were 523,000 children in foster care (Snyder & Sickmund, 2006). If from 9% to 29% of foster care youth crossed over into delinquency, then between 47,070 and 151,670 youth under the care and custody of child protective services would be found in national juvenile arrest data. Similarly, juvenile custody data show that 96,655 juvenile offenders were housed in an out-of-home setting in 2003. Using the estimates from Halemba et al. (2004), at least 20,298 of these offenders would be crossover youth. Unfortunately, it is impossible to determine the full extent to which crossover youth are represented in the national delinquency statistics, because juvenile arrest statistics include multiple arrests for the same person and are often inflated due to the nature of juvenile offending (e.g., groups of youth are arrested for one offense). Juvenile custody data are also limited because they only capture youth placed in correctional institutions or residential placements, and not all juvenile offenders are placed in an out-of-home setting. Thus, the estimates most likely underestimate the true number of crossover youth in the United States.

Despite the ambiguous nature of prevalence estimates, the relationship between maltreatment and delinquency is well established. Yet we know surprisingly little about crossover youth beyond their history of maltreatment. Little to nothing is known, for example, about the demographic and background characteristics of these youth and their offending patterns, risk levels, treatment needs, treatment histories, and patterns of recidivism. The purpose of this chapter is to examine these characteristics and to compare them across crossover youth who were charged with violent offenses to those who were charged with nonviolent offenses. In particular, the following questions will be explored:

1. What are the demographic and background characteristics of crossover youth, and do these characteristics differ across nonviolent and violent?
2. What are the risk and treatment need levels for violent crossover youth, and do these levels differ across violent and nonviolent crossover youth?
3. To what extent was the treatment need for mental health problems met with the provision of treatment services? Do these relationships differ across nonviolent and violent?
4. How do risk levels, treatment need, and treatment history impact recidivism? Do these relationships vary across nonviolent and violent?

It is important to understand who crossover youth are and how their risk and treatment need levels impact services and recidivism, because such information holds significant potential to improve multisystem responses for not only crossover youth but for all juveniles handled in the delinquency system.

LITERATURE REVIEW

The Link Between Maltreatment and Delinquency

Victims of physical abuse and neglect are at an increased risk of engaging in delinquent behavior. Dependent youth are also arrested more often and begin offending at an earlier age relative to nondependent youth (Kelley, Thornberry, & Smith, 1997; Ryan & Testa, 2005; Stewart, Dennison, & Waterson, 2002; Widom, 1994; Widom & Maxfield, 1996; Zingraff, Leiter, Myers, & Johnsen, 1993). Dependent youth are also three times as likely as non-maltreated youth to be arrested for a violent offense (English, Widom, & Branford, 2002).

Little is known about the processing of crossover youth after they commit an offense. Although limited, some studies have examined the experiences of dependent youth who subsequently commit delinquent acts and found that the dependency status negatively influences decision making. Researchers at the Vera Institute of Justice examined 13,000 juvenile preadjudication detention decisions in New York City between 1997 and 1999 (Conger & Ross, 2001). The authors concluded that foster youth without prior involvement in juvenile corrections were more likely to be detained compared to nondependent delinquent youth.

In addition to the reports produced by the Vera Institute, researchers at Children's Rights in New York City completed a qualitative study focused on crossover youth. Morris and Freundlich (2004) interviewed a variety of stakeholders (e.g., foster parents, young adults, judges, and child welfare administrators) about foster youth experiences in the juvenile justice system. The authors concluded that the offenses associated with dependent youth entering the juvenile justice system were less serious compared to nondependent delinquents and that many stakeholders believed crossover youth were treated differently than their delinquency-only counterparts. Finally, Ryan et al. (2007) compared disposition outcomes between 2002 and 2005 across first-time offenders with an open child welfare case to first-time offenders without a child welfare case in Los Angeles County. Results showed that crossover youth were less likely to receive home on probation as a disposition outcome and were more likely to receive suitable placement dispositions (e.g., out-of-home placement in a probation group home) than offenders without a child welfare case.

The limited evidence that crossover youth receive harsher outcomes in juvenile justice processing raises the question of whether crossover youth are higher risk and have higher treatment needs than general population delinquent youth. To date, there are no published studies that examine the risk and treatment need levels of crossover youth or compare those levels to general population delinquents. Besides clarifying the impact of a youth's crossover status on harsher outcomes in juvenile justice processing, knowing their risk and treatment need levels is critical because it (1) provides guidance on identifying appropriate supervision plans for offenders and (2) helps build case plans to simultaneously reduce offenders' risk while improving their psychosocial functioning. For crossover youth, the identification of risk and treatment needs is particularly important, because it stresses the need for comprehensive, integrated responses for youth who penetrate and are failed by multiple systems.

Risk, Criminogenic Need, and Strengths

Andrews and Bonta (2006) as well as others have demonstrated that certain factors are empirically better at predicting recidivism than others. Factors or characteristics that increase the likelihood of recidivism are called risk factors, while characteristics that show a reduction in offending are considered strengths or protective factors. Risk factors are further distinguished into two types: static and dynamic. Static risk factors refer to characteristics that cannot be changed. For example, age at first arrest is a static risk factor because it increases the chance of offending (when the child is younger than 12 years old), and it cannot be changed regardless of the types of interventions available to the offender. Dynamic risk factors, on the other hand, are amenable to change. Poor academic performance, for instance, can be improved with the appropriate type and level of intervention. Dynamic risk factors are also known as criminogenic need. An offender's risk level can be assessed by quantitatively considering the static risks, criminogenic need, and strengths exhibited in his or her life. This information, in turn, provides the information needed to build an individualized case plan aimed at reducing an offender's risk level (i.e., providing intervention for criminogenic risk) and increasing his or her strengths (i.e., supporting and encouraging current and new strengths). By assessing risk, criminogenic needs, and strengths in this way, the appropriate targets for and levels of service can be identified, and methods to enhance personal strengths can be developed. Risk and need assessments offer the opportunity to generate case plans that integrate accountability and treatment, which has been shown repeatedly to have the most impact on reducing recidivism (see Andrews & Bonta, 2006, for further discussion of this issue).

To determine which criminogenic factors were most relevant in the assessment and case planning process, Andrews and Bonta (2006) summarized results from a number of studies and meta-analyses (pp. 63–70). The consistency of findings across studies is instructive to the use of risk assessment for offenders. Although a number of factors were related to recidivism, there were eight factors—referred to as the "central eight" risk/need factors—that were the strongest predictors of future offending. These central eight factors include having: a history of antisocial behavior (i.e., involvement in antisocial activities), an antisocial personality pattern (e.g., impulsiveness), antisocial cognition (i.e., attitudes, beliefs, etc., favorable to crime), antisocial associates (e.g., delinquent peers), poor-quality family relationships, poor school performance, low levels of involvement in prosocial leisure and recreational activities, and substance abuse. Mental illness was not a strong predictor of offending, but there is some evidence that it can moderate, or amplify, the impact of other risk/need factors. Thus, it is important that case plans address both risk/need factors and mental illness simultaneously.

Building comprehensive case plans from risk and need assessments has particular implications for the handling of crossover youth, because this population arguably presents a complex array of issues that require a wide variety of intervention strategies (Cocozza & Shufelt, 2007; Petro, 2006, 2007; Wiig & Tuell, 2004; Wiig, Widom, & Tuell, 2004). For instance, the family situation associated with child protection cases often requires an alternative placement option beyond the home and the use of innovative, evidenced-based programs that can engage and motivate the youth and family members to change; their mental health and substance abuse problems require accessing co-occurring treatment programs when available; and the presence of additional criminogenic need factors (e.g., antisocial beliefs, self-regulation) call for additional psychosocial interventions. To further investigate the need for comprehensive responses to crossover youth, we turn next to analysis of data from Los Angeles County.

THE JOINT ASSESSMENT PROCESS IN LOS ANGELES COUNTY

In the state of California, a youth may not be under formal, legal supervision of both the child welfare and delinquency systems simultaneously. California Welfare and Institutions Code (WIC) 241.1 outlines a process for determining whether a crossover youth will remain under the supervision of the Department of Children and Family Services (DCFS) or will be referred to the delinquency court once a youth is arrested and charged with a criminal offense. The Los Angeles County Juvenile

Court, in turn, created protocol to further define the 241.1 WIC process. The key aspect of this protocol is the requirement of a joint assessment report, including a joint recommendation submitted to the delinquency court by probation and the DCFS. This report is submitted to the court and all related parties for consideration in the outcome of the 241.1 WIC hearing. Outcomes in the 241.1 WIC hearing process include: (1) dismissal of the case; (2) retention of the case in the dependency court with informal probation ordered by the delinquency court; or (3) termination of the dependency case and formal probation ordered by the court. In Los Angeles County, all youth under the care of the DCFS who are charged with a crime receive a 241.1 WIC hearing except cases that are found unfit for juvenile court and filed in adult court or those cases waived to the adult court for criminal processing (direct file cases). For fitness cases, the 241.1 WIC hearing is suspended until a fitness hearing is held to determine whether the youth is fit to remain in juvenile court.

Two units in Los Angeles County are responsible for the completion of a 241.1 WIC joint assessment report: the DCFS 241.1 WIC unit and the probation 241.1 WIC or special investigations unit. Staff from both units are required to work collaboratively to produce a report that includes the following information: the elements/circumstances of the offense; victim information; dependency history; delinquency history; residence status/information; evidence of gang activity; evidence of alcohol/substance use; health/mental health information; school information; family information; minor's statement; parents' statement; interested parties statement; and joint analysis/evaluation of data to determine the joint recommendation and case plan. In addition, a psychological evaluation may be completed by the Department of Mental Health if the youth's defense attorney provides consent. The 241.1 WIC joint assessment reports are densely populated with information about the offender and the case; hence, they represent excellent and unique social artifacts from which to gather data.

Sample

The current study draws a sample of all first-time offenders ($N = 226$) from data previously collected from all 241.1 WIC joint assessment reports completed between April 1, 2004, and December 31, 2004 ($N = 581$). The sample was limited to first-time offenders in order to create equivalent groups with regard to prior offenses. This was particularly important given the study's focus on risk assessment. Offenders with different histories are arguably different with regard to risk and need, which would potentially confound the results of the current study. To explore the differences between nonviolent and violent offenders, the sample was distinguished by their most serious current, charged offense. Youth charged with offenses that involved the threat of or actual harm to others were coded as violent offenders, and all other youth were categorized as nonviolent offenders. These data present an exceptional opportunity to explore the prevalence and nature of risk and treatment need among crossover youth, because the joint assessment report followed a standard template, and completion of all sections was required by the court. Thus, there were little missing data.

Measures

Several measures were used to capture the demographics and current social situation, family characteristics, DCFS and juvenile justice experiences, risk levels, treatment need levels, and outcomes of crossover youth in Los Angeles County. A brief description of all the measures in each category is provided below:

Demographics and current social situation: The youth characteristics captured in this category include gender (male/female), race/ethnicity (Black, Latino, White, and other), age (in years), current living situation (home, relative, foster care, group home, residential treatment placement), and school status (not enrolled, enrolled).

Family characteristics: The characteristics in this category measured family history of criminal behavior, substance abuse, and/or mental health problems and whether youth currently received support (i.e., care, concern, and intention to contribute to youth's well-being) and/or stability (i.e., ability to consistently provide for youth's emotional and economic needs) from family member or other significant adult.

DCFS and juvenile justice experiences: DCFS experiences captured length of time in DCFS care, placement history, and treatment history. Because this sample of offenders did not have a history of prior offenses (only first-time offenders were selected for the current study), the only juvenile justice experience measured in this study was whether the youth was detained in juvenile hall at the time of the arrest.

Treatment need and concordance with treatment: Treatment need was measured by the prevalence of a mental health problem or substance abuse problem. Problems refer to diagnoses for a mental health or substance disorder as well as signs and symptoms of a mental health and/or substance abuse disorder. The range of problems include: none, mental health only, substance abuse only, and both mental health and substance abuse. Once the presence of a mental health problem was established, an additional variable was created to capture whether a youth with a mental health problem received treatment at some point in his or her time in DCFS care. Two outcomes were possible: no match (i.e., presence of mental health problem but no previous mental health treatment) and full match (i.e., presence of a mental health problem and previously received mental health treatment). Substance abuse was excluded from consideration, because the prevalence of substance abuse treatment was too small to be meaningful. This concordance measure has at least two limitations. First, it is not clear that the mental health problem was present before the treatment, and, second, there is no way to determine whether the treatment received was matched specifically to the individual needs of the youth. Nonetheless, this measure provides some insight into whether youth with mental health problems are receiving some intervention and whether that intervention reduces the likelihood of recidivism.

Risk and intervention need levels: Since the 241.1 WIC data were collected, the Los Angeles County Probation Department commissioned a validity study on its risk/need assessment tool, the Los Angeles Risk and Resiliency Checkup (LARRC; Yoo & Sosna, 2007). The LARRC was adapted from the San Diego County Probation Department's tool by the Los Angeles County Probation Department, and it is used throughout the county to assess risk levels among the juvenile population.

Yoo and Sosna's (2007) study utilized LARRC results from all first-time offenders processed by the Los Angeles County Probation Department between March and December 2005 ($N = 2,043$) and subsequently tracked these offenders for 2 years to measure recidivism. Using the LARRC results and recidivism data, the authors used factor analysis to assess which items were related to one another and to determine which scales were the strongest predictors of recidivism. The results of this study yielded nine scales: delinquent behavior; delinquent affiliations; delinquent orientation; substance abuse; family interactions; interpersonal relations; social isolation; academic engagement; and self-regulation. Four of these nine scales were the most predictive of recidivism. Thus, Yoo and Sosna recommended that the first four (delinquent behavior, delinquent affiliations, delinquent orientation, and substance abuse) be summed to assess individual risk levels. They further recommended that all nine scales be used to guide the development of a case plan, because each one was potentially indicative of key areas for intervention (Sosna & Yoo, 2007).

To guide the use of these scales for case planning, Sosna and Yoo (2007) identified thresholds to identify areas for behavioral and social intervention as part of a youth's case plan. Separate thresholds were identified for low-, moderate-, and high-risk offenders by Sosna and Yoo (2007). These threshold scores were then used in the current study to assess youths' need for intervention.[2] For example, a youth who scored high risk in family interactions should receive some type of family therapy; a youth who scored high risk in self-regulation should receive cognitive-behavioral intervention; and so on. The advantage of using the LARRC in this way is twofold. First, it provides an objective basis from which to assess a youth's needs and identify appropriate interventions, and, second, these scales can be directly linked to evidenced-based programming. The utility of this approach is impressive because it restructures the way in which risk is perceived and, as a result, holds the potential to significantly impact the way in which risk is addressed through supervision and programming.

Unfortunately, the LARRC was not completed on the cases in the 241.1 WIC study, but the data from this study were comprehensive enough to make an application of the LARRC scoring possible. Although not perfectly aligned, measures for all items listed in the LARRC could be identified and used to calculate scores for all the LARRC scales in the current study (see Appendix A at the end of this chapter for a list of measures for each scale). Nonetheless, applying the LARRC in this way is instructive in assessing offender risk as well as treatment needs.

Risk and treatment need: Using the prevalence of mental health problems and the LARRC assessment of risk level, a combined risk and treatment need measure was computed. The resulting categories include low risk/no mental health problem; low risk/mental health problem; moderate risk/no mental health problem; moderate risk/mental health problem; high risk/no mental health problem; and high risk/mental health problem.

Recidivism: The primary outcome measure used in this study is recidivism, which is measured by a new arrest between the youth's 241.1 WIC arrest documented in the study and December 31, 2005. It is important to note that a new arrest does not necessarily translate to a sustained petition, because our data did not cover a time span long enough to capture such information.

Procedures

Descriptive statistics were used to analyze the measures described above. Tests for significant differences between nonviolent and violent offenders were accomplished using chi-square tests or t tests for independent samples when appropriate.

Results

1. What are the demographic and background characteristics of crossover youth, and do these characteristics differ across nonviolent and violent offenders?

As shown in Table 15.1, two-thirds of nonviolent and violent offenders were boys, and over 80% of youth in both groups were living in an

Table 15.1

SUMMARY OF DEMOGRAPHICS AND BACKGROUND CHARACTERISTICS ACROSS NONVIOLENT AND VIOLENT OFFENDERS

CHARACTERISTIC	NONVIOLENT OFFENDERS (N = 123)		VIOLENT OFFENDERS (N = 103)	
	N	%	N	%
Gender				
Male	79	64.2	66	64.1
Female	44	35.8	37	35.9
Race/Ethnicity				
Black*	65	52.8	73	70.9
Hispanic*	44	35.8	21	20.4
White	13	10.6	7	6.8
Asian American	1	1.0	2	2.0
Living situation at time of arrest				
Home	19	15.4	17	16.5
Relative	34	27.6	21	20.4
Foster care	28	22.8	24	23.3
Group home	41	33.3	40	38.8
Actively attending school[1]	90	80.5	92	89.3

*$p < .05$; [1]$p < .10$

out-of-home placement at the time of their arrest. The most common placement for these youth was a group home (33.3% for nonviolent offenders and 38.8% for violent offenders). Violent offenders, however, were more likely than nonviolent offenders to be Black (70.9% compared to 52.8%) and slightly less likely to be Latino (20.4% compared to 25.8%). Violent offenders were also more likely than nonviolent offenders to attend (i.e., be enrolled in) school, but this difference was only marginally significant ($p < .10$).

The average length of time spent in DCFS care was 7.14 years (see Table 15.2). During this time, placement in out-of-home care was neither uncommon nor limited among nonviolent or violent offenders. Ninety-six percent of nonviolent offenders and 99% of violent offenders were placed in at least one out-of-home setting, and, on average, they had an average of 5.66 placements during their time in DCFS care. The type of placements youth received varied but was not exclusive. For instance,

Table 15.2

SUMMARY OF PLACEMENT HISTORIES ACROSS NONVIOLENT AND VIOLENT OFFENDERS

	NONVIOLENT OFFENDERS ($N = 123$)			VIOLENT OFFENDERS ($N = 103$)		
	N	%	MEAN (SD)	N	%	MEAN (SD)
Length of Department of Children and Family Services care	123		7.60 (5.13)	103		7.14 (5.38)
None	5	4.1	—	1	1.0	
Relative	84	68.3	1.68 (1.70)	63	61.2	1.49 (1.33)
Foster care	84	68.3	3.50 (3.09)	73	70.9	3.50 (2.97)
Group home[a]	67	54.5	2.45 (2.27)	68	66.0	2.34 (2.35)
Residential Treatment Placement (RTP)	25	20.3	1.64 (1.22)	18	17.5	1.39 (1.29)
Total placements	123		5.66 (5.71)	103		5.95 (5.40)

[a] $p < .10$

approximately two-thirds of youth in both offending groups were placed in relative, foster care, and group home settings. The only marginally significant ($p < .10$) difference between nonviolent and violent offenders was placement in a group home: violent offenders were slightly ($p < .10$) more likely to be placed in group homes (66% compared to 54.4%).

The results presented in Table 15.3 demonstrate that these youth have troubled family backgrounds that have impacted the stability and support provided by the immediate family. Twenty-five percent of nonviolent offenders and 33% of violent offenders (marginally significant at $p < .10$) had mothers with a documented history of criminal behavior,

Table 15.3

SUMMARY OF FAMILY HISTORY AND EXPOSURE TO VIOLENCE ACROSS NONVIOLENT AND VIOLENT OFFENDERS

CHARACTERISTIC	NONVIOLENT OFFENDERS ($N = 123$)		VIOLENT OFFENDERS ($N = 103$)	
	N	%	N	%
Mother's history[a]				
None	31	25.2	34	33.0
Criminal behavior (CB)	2	1.6	3	2.9
Mental health (MH)	10	8.1	5	4.9
Substance abuse (SA)	57	46.3	37	35.9
CB + MH	2	1.6	0	0
CB + SA	13	10.6	16	15.5
MH + SA	4	3.3	8	7.8
CB, MH, and SA	4	3.3	0	0
Exposed to domestic violence	37	30.1	40	38.8
No family stability or support	56	45.5	54	52.4
Stability—mother, father, sibling	22	17.9	13	12.6
Stability—other	33	26.8	22	21.4
Support—mother, father, sibling	32	26.0	23	22.3
Support—other	36	29.3	25	24.3

[a] $p < .10$

substance abuse problems, mental health problems, or a combination of the three.[3] About one-third had been exposed to domestic violence in some way, and about half of these youth did not have stability or support from any significant adult. When stability and support were present in a youth's life, it was more likely to come from a relative outside the immediate family (e.g., grandparent, aunt/uncle) or nonrelative (e.g., foster parent) than from within the immediate family.

2. What are the risk and treatment need levels for violent crossover youth, and do these levels differ across violent and nonviolent crossover youth?

As described earlier, the recalibration of the Los Angeles Risk and Resiliency Checkup (Yoo & Sosna, 2007; Sosna & Yoo, 2007) provided the

Table 15.4

SUMMARY OF RISK LEVELS AND MENTAL HEALTH/SUBSTANCE ABUSE PROBLEMS ACROSS NONVIOLENT AND VIOLENT OFFENDERS

	NONVIOLENT OFFENDERS ($N = 123$)		VIOLENT OFFENDERS ($N = 103$)	
	N	%	N	%
Risk levels				
Low	64	52.0	52	50.5
Moderate	51	41.5	42	40.8
High	8	6.5	9	8.7
Behavioral/social intervention scales				
Delinquent behavior	34	27.6	34	33.0
Delinquent affiliations[a]	19	15.4	8	7.8
Delinquent orientation	37	31.7	39	37.9
Substance abuse	34	27.6	20	19.4
Family interactions	100	81.3	91	88.3
Interpersonal skills	19	15.4	21	20.4
Social isolation	37	30.1	28	27.2
Academic engagement	37	30.1	28	27.2
Self-regulation	26	21.1	28	28.2

[a] $p < .10$

opportunity to compare risk levels and need for behavioral/social interventions across violent and nonviolent crossover youth. With regard to risk (see Table 15.4), crossover youth were most likely to be low risk (52% of nonviolent offenders, 50.5% of violent offenders) followed closely by moderate risk (41.5% of nonviolent offenders, 40.8% of violent offenders). Less than 10% of youth scored as high risk (6.5% of nonviolent offenders, 8.7% of violent offenders). Although there was a very slight elevation in the percentage of high-risk offenders in the violent group, this difference was insignificant. Consistent with this finding, both nonviolent and violent offenders had the same level of need for behavioral/social interventions. The scale with the highest demand for intervention was family interactions (81.3% of nonviolent offenders, 88.3% of violent offenders). This finding is consistent with the results related to family stability and support shown in Table 15.4. The scales with the second highest demand for intervention were delinquent orientation, social isolation, and academic engagement. For all three scales, approximately one-third of the crossover youth needed intervention. Slightly more than a quarter of youth also needed intervention for delinquent behavior and substance abuse.

The need for behavioral/social intervention was compared across risk levels of all offenders. Consistent with predictions, a smaller proportion of low-risk offenders demonstrated a need for various interventions

Table 15.5

COMPARISON OF LARRC INTERVENTION NEED LEVELS BY RISK LEVELS

	LOW RISK (N = 116)	MODERATE RISK (N = 93)	HIGH RISK (N = 17)
Delinquent behavior*	12.9	46.2	58.8
Delinquent affiliations	13.8	11.8	0
Delinquent orientation*	9.5	58.1	76.5
Substance abuse*	3.4	41.9	64.7
Family interactions	82.8	87.1	82.4
Interpersonal skills[1]	12.1	22.6	29.4
Social isolation*	20.7	35.5	47.1
Academic engagement[1]	28.4	24.7	52.9
Self-regulation*	14.7	31.2	52.9

*$p < .05$; [1]$p < .10$

than moderate- and high-risk offenders, and a smaller proportion of moderate-risk offenders had a need for intervention than high-risk offenders (see Table 15.5). This was the finding for all scales except delinquent affiliations and family interactions. The need for intervention related to delinquent affiliations was small for all groups but smallest for high-risk offenders. This is an interesting finding in that delinquency peer affiliation is often a major issue for adolescents involved with the juvenile justice system. Perhaps high-risk crossover offenders are not associating with delinquent peers, or the data provided in case files were not thorough enough to register this in the computation of the scale. The findings are far more prominent when family interactions are considered. The need for family intervention was extremely high and nearly identical for low-, moderate-, and high-risk offenders (82.8%, 87.1%, and 82.4%, respectively).

Although the LARRC provides substantial insight into offender risk and need for behavioral/social intervention, it does not measure the prevalence of mental health, and its measures for substance abuse are somewhat limited. According to case file information presented in Table 15.6, over three-quarters of youth had problems with mental health, substance abuse, or both. The differences were not significant across nonviolent and violent offenders, but the pattern for mental health/substance abuse problems was slightly different across groups. Violent offenders were most likely to have mental health problems only (40.8%), whereas nonviolent offenders were equally as likely to have a mental health problem only or co-occurring problems (30.9%). The prevalence of substance abuse among nonviolent offenders was also noticeably higher than among violent offenders.

Table 15.6

SUMMARY OF MENTAL HEALTH AND SUBSTANCE ABUSE PROBLEMS ACROSS NONVIOLENT AND VIOLENT OFFENDERS

TYPE OF MENTAL HEALTH/ SUBSTANCE ABUSE PROBLEM	NONVIOLENT OFFENDERS ($N = 123$)		VIOLENT OFFENDERS ($N = 103$)	
	N	%	N	%
Neither	25	20.3	25	24.3
Mental health only (MH)	38	30.9	42	40.8
Substance abuse only (SA)	22	17.9	9	8.7
Both MH and SA	38	30.9	27	26.2

To determine how risk interacted with behavioral health treatment need, a continuum of risk and need was created using LARRC risk levels and the presence of a mental health problem.[4] Table 15.7 displays the results of this process. Again, there were no significant differences across groups. For both groups, approximately one-quarter of offenders fell into the low-risk/mental health and into the low-risk/no mental health problem categories. Differences were noticeable, however, when the prevalence of mental health problems was considered for moderate- and high-risk offenders. Less than 10% of offenders were classified in the moderate-risk/no mental health group, but approximately one-third of offenders were classified in the moderate-risk/mental health group. The same pattern was found among high-risk offenders. Only 1% ($n = 1$ in each group) of offenders were placed in the high-risk/no mental health category, whereas slightly less than 10% were found in the high-risk/mental health group.

3. To what extent was treatment need for mental health problems met with the provision of treatment services? Does this relationship differ across nonviolent and violent?

Results related to treatment history are presented in Table 15.8.

Table 15.7

SUMMARY OF RISK LEVELS BY MENTAL HEALTH PROBLEM ACROSS NONVIOLENT AND VIOLENT OFFENDERS

	NONVIOLENT OFFENDERS ($N = 123$)		VIOLENT OFFENDERS ($N = 103$)	
	N	%	N	%
Low risk/no mental health	34	27.6	27	26.2
Low risk/mental health problem	30	24.4	25	24.3
Moderate risk/no mental health problem	12	9.8	6	5.8
Moderate risk/mental health problem	39	31.7	36	35.0
High risk/no mental health problem	1	.8	1	1.0
High risk/mental health problem	7	5.7	8	7.8

Table 15.8
SUMMARY OF TREATMENT HISTORIES ACROSS NONVIOLENT AND VIOLENT OFFENDERS

	NONVIOLENT OFFENDERS (N = 123)		VIOLENT OFFENDERS (N = 103)	
	N	%	N	%
Type of treatment received				
None	32	26.0	22	21.4
Mental health	82	66.7	78	75.7
Substance abuse	1	1.0	1	1.0
Mental health and substance abuse	8	6.5	2	1.9
Concordance between need and mental health treatment				
No match	26	21.1	20	19.4
Full match	97	78.8	83	80.6

These findings indicate that the majority of nonviolent (66.7%) and violent (75.7%) offenders received some type of mental health treatment while under the care of DCFS. Approximately one-quarter of youth did not receive any treatment, and 7.5% of nonviolent offenders and 2.9% of violent offenders received substance abuse treatment. These results are limited, though, in that they do not consider whether the youth needed treatment and also received treatment. To address this issue, a concordance measure was created to explore treatment history relative to treatment need. Based on this measure, slightly more than three-quarters of the youth with a need for mental health treatment received some type of mental health treatment, and approximately 20% of youth had a need but did not receive treatment. None of these findings differed significantly across nonviolent and violent offenders.

  4. How do risk levels, treatment need, and treatment history impact recidivism? Do these relationships vary across nonviolent and violent?

A comparison of recidivism rates between nonviolent and violent offenders shows no difference between the groups (see Table 15.9). Approximately one-quarter of offenders in both groups recidivated during the follow-up period. Recidivism, on the other hand, significantly differed across risk categories. Low-risk offenders were the least likely group to recidivate (16.4%). Moderate-risk offenders were twice as likely as the low-risk offenders to recidivate (30.1%), and high-risk offenders were two and a half times as likely as the low-risk offenders to recidivate (41.2%).

When recidivism across the risk/need categories is compared in Table 15.10, recidivism follows the same general pattern, with one striking difference. Recidivism within each risk group is increased with the

Table 15.9
RECIDIVISM RATES ACROSS NONVIOLENT AND VIOLENT OFFENDERS

	RECIDIVISM RATE	
	N	%
Type of offense		
Nonviolent offenders ($n = 123$)	30	24.4
Violent offenders ($n = 103$)	24	23.3
Risk level		
Low ($n = 116$)	19	16.4
Moderate ($n = 93$)	28	30.1
High ($n = 17$)	7	41.2

Table 15.10
RECIDIVISM RATES BY LEVEL OF RISK AND MENTAL HEALTH TREATMENT NEED

RISK/NEED LEVEL[a]	NUMBER IN GROUP	NUMBER RECIDIVATED	% RECIDIVATED
Low risk/no mental health	61	8	13.1
Low risk/mental health problem	55	11	20.0
Moderate risk/no mental health problem	18	4	22.2
Moderate risk/mental health problem	75	24	32.0
High risk/mental health problem	15	6	40.0

[a]The *high risk/no mental health problem* category was excluded because only two cases fell into this category: one nonviolent offender and one violent offender.

Table 15.11

RECIDIVISM RATES BY TREATMENT MATCH GROUPS

TREATMENT MATCH GROUP	NUMBER IN GROUP	NUMBER RECIDIVATED	% RECIDIVATED
No match	44	8	18.2
Full match	180	46	25.5

presence of a mental health problem. A final comparison of recidivism rates was made for the mental health need/treatment match measure. According to Table 15.11, the match group (25.5%) has a slightly higher recidivism rate than the no match (18.2%) group, but this difference is not statistically significant.

Discussion

Taken together, these results improve our knowledge and understanding of crossover youth. First-time nonviolent and violent offenders appear to be more similar than different. Most crossover youth are boys, but girls are represented at a slightly higher rate than in the general delinquency population. Black youth are overrepresented among crossover youth; crossover youth are most likely to be living in a group home at the time of their placement; and most of these youth are enrolled in school, although they may not be attending regularly. Unstable family situations are the norm for this group. Fathers are often absent, and the ability of single mothers to provide positive and consistent parenting for their young infants and toddlers is compromised by substance abuse, mental health problems, criminal behavior, and domestic violence (see Marsh, Ryan, Choi, & Testa, 2006). Almost half their lives have been spent in the child welfare system. They have moved from a life with their birth family to living with relative caretakers, to foster homes, and, finally, into the most restrictive end of the child welfare system—group home care.

With regard to criminogenic risk and treatment need, these crossover youth are predominately low risk, but a substantial portion of them have mental health problems that may contribute to recidivism. Further, mental health problems seem to be more problematic as criminogenic risk increases. Not surprisingly, high-risk offenders have the greatest need for behavioral/social interventions followed by moderate-risk and low-risk offenders, respectively. The current study suggests that most crossover youth are in need of interventions related to family interactions and that many need interventions for social isolation, delinquent affiliations, academic engagement, and self-regulation. A significant number of youth were also shown to need interventions related to interpersonal skills. When considered in the context of the histories of these youth, a picture begins to emerge of significant needs for treatment related to child abuse/neglect, exposure to traumatic events (domestic and likely community violence), depression/anxiety, conduct problems, possible learning disabilities, impulse and attention problems, and substance abuse.

Interestingly, the majority of these youth had received some type of mental health service, and many had several episodes of treatment. Yet these interventions did not reduce the likelihood of recidivism, but rather correlated with an increase in delinquent behavior. This study does not provide information regarding the type or intensity of treatment but concludes only that the treatment offered was ineffective as an intervention to reduce the likelihood of recidivism, leading one to question whether the mental health services received were appropriate; in other words, were the mental health services matched to the individual levels of risk and need of these youth?

BUILDING A COMPREHENSIVE APPROACH

These results offer substantial insight into how crossover youth should be handled. They stress the need to build a juvenile justice system of care in which multiple systems work together to accomplish the following (Stroud & Friedman, 1986):

- Clear definitions and recognition of the mental health, substance abuse, and behavioral problems
- Acceptance and integration of accountability as a response to delinquent behavior
- Standardized screening and assessment to identify the problem as early in the process as possible
- Matching both risks and needs to appropriate interventions in a continuum of care that integrates accountability (e.g., graduated sanctions), social interventions, and treatment interventions
- Accessing appropriate levels of care in the least restrictive setting

- Involving and engaging the family in treatment planning and programming
- Utilizing a strength-based approach to assessment and service provision
- Ensuring that programming is culturally competent and gender specific
- Active and ongoing partnerships between juvenile justice and behavioral health systems to formalize information sharing and collaborative planning and programming
- Ongoing commitment and investment from key stakeholders, interested parties, supervisors, and line staff

Building a juvenile justice system of care requires an integration of systems that traditionally work in isolation from one another. Rather than viewing juvenile justice as one system that refers to and receives referrals from other systems, a juvenile justice system of care requires that these systems work together to plan more efficient responses for offenders and provide more effective services to offenders. Such systems include (but are not limited to) the child welfare system, the mental health system, the substance abuse system, and education systems.

To date, there has been limited success in partnering these systems to improve overall responses to children and families. Instead, they typically operate separately due to different philosophies, policies, and protocols. The result of this fragmentation is the growing number of crossover youth with mental health and substance abuse problems in the juvenile justice system; further penetration into the juvenile justice system for youth in the child welfare system; further alienation for family and significant adults; and increased school failure.

To illustrate what can be accomplished with regard to multisystem collaboration and coordination, descriptions of developments related to the handling and treatment of crossover youth in Los Angeles County are provided from the Los Angeles County Probation Department, the Department of Children and Family Services in Los Angeles County, and the Los Angeles Department of Mental Health.

Probation

Data analyzed for this study confirm the need for enhanced case management interventions across a continuum of care, including a more comprehensive assessment to be provided to the courts in order to appropriately address a youth's criminogenic needs and ultimately reduce the likelihood of recidivism. The County of Los Angeles has taken steps to enhance interagency cooperation through the implementation of a dual-status pilot project in May 2007. Built on the initial 241.1 WIC protocol implemented in 1997 and predicated on the passage of Assembly Bill (AB) 129, the Probation Department and the Department of Children and Family Services (Child Welfare), in consultation with the presiding judge of juvenile court, created a jointly written protocol to allow the departments to jointly assess and recommend that a youth be designated as dual status.

Development of this protocol was accomplished under the leadership of the juvenile presiding judge through a countywide, multiagency collaboration. Overarching strategies incorporated in the revised 241.1 WIC pilot protocol include:

- Utilization of a multidisciplinary team (colocated to include probation, DCFS, the Department of Mental Health, and an education liaison) approach to jointly develop recommendations to court in order to determine which status would best serve the interests of the youth, considering community safety and victim rights
- Leveraging resources with public-sector agencies through an enhanced, structured, cross-systems assessment, including, where allowable, a mental health resource evaluation and enhanced educational input
- Individualized case planning and treatment services planning and delivery (including available evidenced-based programs)
- Implementation oversight and monitoring
- Development and tracking of cross-systems outcomes
- Formalized evaluation process

Additionally, through team oversight of the postdisposition supervision and case management process, priority is placed on identifying the best service delivery plan for the youth, including, where applicable, identifying appropriate placements. Several evidenced-based programs are in the implementation process in the county, and consideration for access/enrollment, including service availability is considered at the predisposition phase to assist with transition to implementation postdisposition.

It is recommended that, while specific enhancements continue to be implemented through the original 241.1 WIC protocol, work with our partners through the AB 129 pilot continue in order to have sufficient data to enable a reliable program evaluation and recommendations for possible countywide implementation. This would provide the departments and our partners with substantive information to accomplish informed decision making, with the eye toward outcomes and accomplishment of the goals of this countywide initiative.

Child Protective Services

From the perspective of the Los Angeles DCFS, at least four findings from the current study underscore the need for interagency communication and collaboration. First, children of color were disproportionately represented in the study. Second, children in the study had multiple out-of-home placements and had an average of 7 years in DCFS. Third, children did not have a clear treatment plan that was developed from a multidisciplinary perspective (assessment), which missed creating individualized plans based on appropriate matches between risk, need, and treatment.

Fortunately, DCFS has already started implementing several strategies specifically designed to address these issues. For disproportionality, DCFS has been analyzing and sharing data with our staff and community to help us understand why there is a disproportionate number of Black children in DCFS (9% represented in the general population but 33% in DCFS) and to help us develop strategies to reduce the disproportionate number. One specific strategy is team decision making (TDM), which is a process of bringing a team together (including family, the DCFS case worker, community stakeholders, any current service providers, and any family supports) to discuss a potential removal or placement move. By bringing together a team at a critical decision point with the family and their supports, DCFS believes the decision reached and the subsequent created plan will result in better outcomes for the child and family, because the family voice is at the table and is used to create an individualized plan. TDM also addresses the issues of placement moves and length of time children stay in DCFS. If the team is able to identify relative caregivers at the TDM, the child may not need to enter out-of-home care in the first place; but, if the decision is to remove the child from the family, there is an open, "straight talk" conversation that fosters partnership and honesty with the family to support them in getting their child back home.

Although TDM has been very successful, there remains a gap in developing clear, individualized assessments around mental health and delinquency risk factors. As described above, DCFS is currently working closely with probation and mental health to implement the 241.1 Multidisciplinary Team Pilot Program and to develop a prevention program to stop the child's progression to a 241.1 status.

The role of DCFS within the TDM approach is to provide detailed information about the youth's child welfare history and services and to discuss the possible outcomes for the case with the team's probation officer, Department of Mental Health clinician, and education representative. Together, the team identifies the youth's needs and accesses appropriate programming, preferably best practice approaches, within their agencies. The collective nature of the team approach simultaneously capitalizes on the resources of multiple agencies for the best interest of the child.

DCFS, probation, mental health, and education recently joined forces to create the Interagency Delinquency Prevention Program (IDPP), which identifies DCFS children presenting predelinquent behavior as early as possible. IDPP will be attached to the TDM, which DCFS implemented in 1998. Using previous research conducted on crossover youths, the IDPP management team believed this was an ideal timing opportunity to review the youth's situation and identify any needs/risk factors. Mirroring the TDM model, a multiagency assessment will be conducted and linkages to appropriate services will be made. By connecting IDPP and TDM, DCFS believes they will be able to identify the youths who are at higher risk earlier and ultimately provide the youths and their families with supportive and effective interventions sooner. Examples of potential DCFS interventions the IDPP team may refer to are the Permanency Planning Program (P3) and Wraparound. The efforts related to P3, for example, are focused on finding as many family members as possible to widen the possibility of reunification and permanency for many crossover youth. Wraparound creates an ongoing Child and Family Team that develops a comprehensive plan based on the strengths and the needs of the child and his or her family. In Los Angeles County, Wraparound is reserved for children who present with the most complex and enduring needs.

The use of Wraparound, IDPP, and TDM are all based on the notion of forming a team of concerned people to ensure that better decisions and planning are happening to secure safety and permanency for all DCFS youth, including crossover youth. But more importantly, all decisions are formed *with* the family and honor the family as experts on their children. By providing the family with voice and choice and access to the case planning process, the plan is no longer a DCFS plan, but the family's plan that DCFS supports. The results of this study showed that family instability is one of the constant factors in and predictors of subsequent juvenile activity, and, by working with the family as a whole, the ability to extend services to the adults is greater because the individualized plan becomes more about the family than about the child. Thus, if the family sees itself as part of the solution, the chances are higher that the family will take an active part in the achievement of the goals.

Although DCFS is making progress in addressing the issues of disproportionality, reducing the number of children in group homes, and developing better assessments, the findings of the current study highlight the need for improvement. Ultimately, using data to evaluate where we are and where we came from is helpful in understanding where we want to go and how to get there. As the data showed, the only way we will be able to get there is with the collective support of DCFS, DMH, probation, youths, and their families.

Mental Health

The results of this study demonstrate the intricate relationships that exist between child abuse and neglect, delinquent behavior, domestic violence, substance abuse, and mental health problems. The prevalence of mental health problems among the crossover population and their families is quite high and appears to contribute to a variety of child and family problems as well as the likelihood of recidivism for youth in the crossover population. Furthermore, it appears that receiving mental health treatment has no impact on recidivism.

This result is not surprising if one considers the current public mental health system for children in Los Angeles County and in many parts of the nation. Publicly funded mental health care for children and adolescents is a patchwork of various clinical approaches, and studies that have examined the effectiveness of such "usual care" approaches have been disappointing. Weisz (2004) reviewed 14 such studies and concluded that typical treatments had no effect. The use of case management and the integration of various approaches reflecting the cross-systems involvement of many of these children and youth have been advocated as a more responsive approach (Stroud & Friedman, 1986). However, evaluations of this approach such as the Fort Bragg study (Bickman, 1996; Bickman et al., 1995; Hamner, Lambert, & Bickman, 1997) and the Stark County, Ohio, study (Bickman, Noser, & Summerfelt, 1999; Bickman, Summerfelt, & Firth, 1997) raise questions about the effectiveness of this model. Although these studies suggest systems benefits, such as reduction in residential placement, improved access to services, and greater parent satisfaction with services received, there were no significant differences found between control and treatment groups with respect to clinical outcomes.

There have been tremendous advances in the past 20 years regarding our understanding of the causes of juvenile violence and delinquency. A number of interventions have been developed and, through evaluation using randomized clinical trials, have been shown to be effective in preventing or reducing delinquency (Mihalic, Fagan, Irwin, Ballard, & Elliott, 2004). These evidence-based practices generally employ an ecological or systems approach that views the child's behavior through the context of the child's family and the community and provide a high level of service intensity through small case loads for therapists. Yet these evidence-based treatment models such as Functional Family Therapy (FFT; Alexander, Pugh, Parsons, & Sexton, 2000) and comprehensive approaches such as Multisystemic Therapy (MST; Henggeler, Mihalic, Rone, Thomas, & Timmons-Mitchell, 2001) and Multidimensional Treatment Foster Care (MTFC; Chamberlain, 2003) are seldom available to children in the child welfare system. In addition to demonstrated effectiveness in improving client and family functioning, including reductions in delinquent behavior, FFT, MST, and MTFC have the added benefit of reducing substance abuse, a common co-occurring problem for crossover youth as shown in this study. As a result, these approaches would appear to be ideally suited for crossover youth and to offer the greatest hope for reducing the likelihood that children in the child welfare system will transfer into the juvenile or criminal justice systems. Other intensive in-home approaches such as Wraparound or Children's System of Care are widely recognized as preferred models, especially for children with the highest level of emotional and behavioral needs, but these programs are often either nonexistent in the community or not available to the degree needed to meet the demand (Burns & Goldman, 1999). These services are child centered and family focused; rely on a whatever-it-takes approach using strengths-based interventions; leverage child, family, and community supports; and are available to the child and family on a 24/7 basis.

The development and expansion of these effective treatment approaches cannot be accomplished in isolation by the public mental health system. Services such as these, especially those that are evidence-based, require specialized training, adherence to model fidelity, and, in some cases, ongoing consultation. Implementation, particularly in large, diversely populated areas such as Los Angeles County, can be difficult, and sustaining the practices once implemented presents additional challenges. Initial costs are high, though cost savings achieved through reductions in crime, less need for out-of-home care, and reduced reliance on costly congregate care offer opportunities for overall cost savings (Aos, Lieb, Mayfield, & Pennucci, 2004). Thus, only through collaboration with partners in child welfare and juvenile justice can these models be properly implemented and sustained. For example, the Los Angeles County Department of Mental Health, working with the DCFS, the California Institute for Mental Health, and contract mental health providers, recently implemented several evidence-based programs targeted to youth in the child welfare system, including MTFC and FFT. Additionally, MST programs were implemented specifically for youth who are the subject of a 241.1 evaluation. Delinquency and dependency courts, along with the DCFS and probation staff assigned to the 241.1 process, will identify youth appropriate for this program and make the necessary referrals. Referrals to the program are also generated from the AB 129 pilot project and the Interagency Delinquency Prevention Program.

The department has also implemented full-service partnership programs that provide intensive in-home services for a variety of target populations. Children and youth in the child welfare system and those who are outgrowing the child welfare system are focal populations for these efforts. The department is also contemplating significant expansion of intensive in-home services, similar to the children's system of care approach, for children who are served by the county's child welfare system or at risk of entering that system.

The department is also an active participant with the court, DCFS, and the Probation Department in the AB 129 pilot project, using a multidisciplinary team approach to the assessment of risk and needs similar to the one described in this study, and it continues to work with those from child welfare, juvenile justice, the court, and attorneys to resolve the legal barriers to the inclusion of mental health information in the multidisciplinary assessment process. This project is but one of a number of initiatives where mental health, child welfare, and juvenile justice have partnered in recent years.

CONCLUSION

The transfer of youth in the child welfare system to the juvenile justice system is an indictment of the systems that have been established to serve these young people. Only through the use of more effective interventions, partnerships among child- and youth-serving institutions, and ongoing perseverance can we expect to meet our obligations to those most vulnerable among us.

Creating a juvenile justice system of care represents an opportunity for jurisdictions to overcome many interagency differences to create a seamless system of integrated case management and services that builds on the strengths of each system while addressing individual gaps. In doing so, the juvenile justice system of care will improve the quality of care that youth, families, and communities receive; system effectiveness; and the efficient use of resources.

NOTES

1. These terms will be used interchangeably throughout the chapter.
2. Coding was reverse coded. In other words, having a risk factor was coded 0, and not having a risk factor/having a strength was coded as a 2. As a result, low scores denote high risk, and high scores denote high strengths.
3. Similar statistics for fathers were not presented because 55% of fathers were classified in records as "whereabouts unknown," and, as a result, their profiles were incomplete.
4. Substance abuse was excluded from this process because it is accounted for in the LARRC assessment of risk.

REFERENCES

Alexander, J. F., Pugh, C., Parsons, B. V., and Sexton, T. L. (2000). Functional family therapy. In D. S. Elliott (Ed.), *Blueprints for violence prevention* (Book 3, 2nd ed.). Boulder: Center for the Study and Prevention of Violence, Institute of Behavioral Science, University of Colorado.

Andrews, D. A., & Bonta, J. (2006). *The psychology of criminal conduct* (4th ed.). Cincinnati, OH: Mathew Bender.

Aos, S., Lieb, R., Mayfield, M. M., & Pennucci, A. (2004). *Benefits and costs of prevention and early intervention programs for youth.* Olympia: Washington State Institute for Public Policy.

Bickman, L. (1996). A continuum of care: More is not always better. *American Psychologist, 51,* 689–701.

Bickman, L., Guthrie, P. R., Foster, E. M., Lambert, E. W., Summerfelt, W. T., Brea, C. S., & Heflinger, C. A. (1995). *Evaluating managed mental health services: The Fort Bragg experiment.* New York: Plenum Press.

Bickman, L., Noser, K., & Summerfelt, W. T. (1999). Long-term effects of a system of care on children and adolescents. *Journal of Behavioral Health Services Research, 26,* 185–202.

Bickman, L., Summerfelt, W. T., & Firth, J. M. (1997). The Stark County Evaluation Project: Baseline results of a randomized experiment. In C. T. Nixon & D. A.

Northrup (Eds.), *Evaluating mental health services: How do programs work in the real world?* (pp. 231–258). Thousand Oaks, CA: Sage.

Burns, B. J., & Goldman, S. K. (Eds.). (1999). *Promising practices in Wraparound for children with severe emotional disorders and their families. Systems of care: Promising practices in children's mental health, 1998 series* (Vol. 4). Washington, DC: Center for Effective Collaboration and Practice, American Institutes for Research.

Chamberlain, P. (2003). *Treating chronic juvenile offenders: Advances made through the Oregon multidimensional treatment foster care model.* Washington, DC: American Psychological Association.

Cocozza, J., & Shufelt, J. (2007). Mental health and juvenile justice: The initial models for change experience. *The LINK (Child Welfare League of America), 6*(1), 1–13.

Conger, D., & Ross, T. (2001). *Reducing the foster care bias in juvenile detention decisions: The impact of project confirm.* New York: Vera Institute of Justice.

English, D., Widom, C., & Branford, C. (2002). *Childhood victimization and delinquency, adult criminality, and violent criminal behavior: A replication and extension.* Washington, DC: National Institute of Justice.

Halemba, G. J., Siegel, G. C., Lord, R. C., & Zawacki, S. (2004). *Arizona dual jurisdiction study: Final report.* Pittsburgh, PA: National Council for Juvenile Justice.

Hamner, K., Lambert, E. W., & Bickman, L. (1997). Children's mental health in a continuum of care: Clinical outcomes at 18 months for the Ft. Bragg Demonstration. *Journal of Mental Health Administration, 24*(4), 664–670.

Henggeler, S. W., Mihalic, S. F., Rone, L., Thomas, C., & Timmons-Mitchell, J. (2001). Multisystemic therapy. In D. S. Elliott (Ed.), *Blueprints for violence prevention* (Book 6, pp. 27–28). Boulder: Center for the Study and Prevention of Violence, Institute of Behavioral Science, University of Colorado.

Kelley, B., Thornberry, T., & Smith, C. (1997). *In the wake of child maltreatment* (NCJ 165257). Washington, DC: U.S. Department of Justice, Office of Juvenile Justice and Delinquency Prevention.

Marsh, J. C., Ryan, J. P., Choi, S., & Testa, M. (2006). Integrated services for families with multiple problems: Obstacles to family reunification. *Children and Youth Services Review, 28,* 1074–1087.

Mihalic, S., Fagan, A., Irwin, K., Ballard, D., & Elliott, D. (2004). *Blueprints for violence prevention.* Washington, DC: Office of Juvenile Justice and Delinquency Prevention.

Morris, L., & Freundlich, M. (2004). *Youth involvement in the child welfare and juvenile justice systems.* Washington DC: CWLA Press.

Petro, J. (2006). *Juvenile justice and child welfare agencies: Collaborating to serve dual jurisdiction youth survey report.* Washington, DC: Child Welfare League of America.

Petro, J. (2007). *Increasing collaboration and coordination of the child welfare and juvenile justice systems to better serve dual jurisdiction youth: A literature review.* Washington, DC: Child Welfare League of America.

Ryan, J. P., Herz, D., Hernandez, P., & Marshall, J. (2007). Maltreatment and delinquency: Investigating child welfare bias in juvenile justice processing. *Children and Youth Services Review, 29,* 1035–1050.

Ryan, J. P., & Testa, M. F. (2005). Child maltreatment and juvenile delinquency: Investigating the role of placement and placement instability. *Children and Youth Services Review, 27,* 227–249.

Snyder, H., & Sickmund, M. (2006). *Juvenile offender and victims: A national report.* Washington, DC: Office of Juvenile Justice and Delinquency Prevention.

Sosna, T., & Yoo, J. (2007). *LARRC case planning categories.* Los Angeles: Probation Department.

Stewart, A., Dennison, S., & Waterson, E. (2002). *Pathways from child maltreatment to juvenile offending.* Criminology Research Council, Final Report, Australia. Retrieved January 23, 2009, from http://www.CriminologyResearchCouncil.gov.av/Reports/Stewart.html

Stroud, B. A., & Friedman, R. (1986). *A system of care for children and youth with severe emotional disturbances* (Rev. ed.). Washington, DC: Georgetown University Child Development Center, CASSP Technical Assistance Center.

Weisz, J. R. (2004). *Psychotherapy for children and adolescents: Evidence-based treatments and case examples.* Cambridge, England: Cambridge University Press.

Widom, C. (1994). The role of placement experiences in mediating the criminal consequences of early childhood victimization. *Child Welfare Research Review, 1,* 298–322.

Widom, C. S., & Maxfield, M. G. (1996, 20 September). A prospective examination of risk for violence among abused and neglected children. *Annals of New York Academy of Sciences, 794,* 224–237.

Wiig, J., & Tuell, J. (2004). *Guidebook for juvenile justice and child welfare system coordination and integration: Framework for improved outcomes.* Washington, DC: Child Welfare League of America.

Wiig, J., Widom, C., & Tuell, J. (2004). *Understanding child maltreatment and juvenile delinquency: From research to effective program, practice, and systemic solutions.* Washington, DC: Child Welfare League of America.

Yoo, J., & Sosna, T. (2007). *LARRC risk level categories: Rationale for cutoff scores.* Los Angeles: Probation Department.

Zingraff, M., Leiter, J., Myers, K., & Johnsen, M. (1993). Child maltreatment and youthful problem behavior. *Criminology, 31,* 173–202.

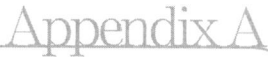

Appendix A

CORRESPONDENCE BETWEEN LARRC RISK/NEED SCALE SCORING AND 241.1 STUDY

SCALE	ITEM DESCRIPTION	CUT-POINT FOR INTERVENTION	RISK LEVEL THRESHOLDS
Delinquent behavior	Prior arrests Offenses committed under the influence Assaultive or fighting behavior Runaway Pattern of truancy in the past year Pattern of suspension or expelled from school Disruptive classroom/school behavior	Low risk ≤ 8 Moderate risk ≤ 7 High risk ≤ 4	*Males* Low ≥ 32 Moderate ≥ 19 and ≤ 31 High ≤ 18 *Females* Low ≥ 34 Moderate ≥ 20 and ≤ 33 High ≤ 19
Delinquent affiliations	Support/reinforcement in the community Significant crime in the neighborhood Presently not in an educational program Parental criminality or substance abuse Has gang affiliation or association Has delinquent friends	Low risk ≤ 7 Moderate risk ≤ 6 High risk ≤ 3	
Delinquent orientation	Delinquent orientation Supportive of delinquency Values honesty and integrity Values honesty and integrity Manipulative/deceitful	Low risk ≤ 4 Moderate risk ≤ 3 Low risk ≤ 1	
Substance abuse	Pattern of alcohol use Used mood-altering substance (not alcohol) Uses substances frequently Use interferes with daily functioning Early-onset substance abuse Sensation seeking	Low risk ≤ 7 Moderate risk ≤ 6 High risk ≤ 3	

(continued)

Appendix A

CORRESPONDENCE BETWEEN LARRC RISK/NEED SCALE SCORING AND 241.1 STUDY (*CONTINUED*)

SCALE	ITEM DESCRIPTION	CUT-POINT FOR INTERVENTION	RISK LEVEL THRESHOLDS
Family interaction	Extensive structured activities Participates in faith community Involved in community organization Communicates with family Constructive use of time at home Family activities Family support Unconditional regard from a parent Parental supervision deficiencies Chaotic family Parents model health moderation	Low risk ≤ 11 Moderate risk ≤ 9 High risk ≤ 6	
Interpersonal skills	Prosocial adult relations Poor relations with parents Positive peer relations Has at least one person to confide in Values dignity and the rights of others Ability to make friends Ability to communicate disagreements Self-efficiency in prosocial roles	Low risk ≤ 8 Moderate risk ≤ 6 High risk ≤ 4	
Social isolation	Socially isolated Very few prosocial acquaintances No meaningful relationship with any adult No prosocial interests	Low risk ≤ 4 Moderate risk ≤ 3 High risk ≤ 2	

(*continued*)

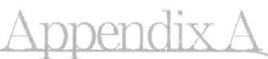

CORRESPONDENCE BETWEEN LARRC RISK/NEED SCALE SCORING AND 241.1 STUDY (*CONTINUED*)

SCALE	ITEM DESCRIPTION	CUT-POINT FOR INTERVENTION	RISK LEVEL THRESHOLDS
Academic Engagement	School engagement/bonds Attachments with academic achiever Positive interaction with teachers Educational aspirations Poor academic achievement		Low risk ≤ 5 Moderate risk ≤ 3 High risk ≤ 2
Self-regulation	Effectively manages peer pressure Youth is free of distressing habits Youth manages stress well Positive self-concept Self-control Problem-solving skills Plans, organizes, and completes tasks Anger management issues		Low risk ≤ 6 Moderate risk ≤ 4 High risk ≤ 2

Note: For all items, scoring for the LARRC is as follows: 0 = no indication of the characteristic; 1 = some indication of the characteristic; and 2 = indication of the characteristic.

16

Understanding Complexity in Sexually Abusive Youth

PHIL RICH

A STATISTICAL PICTURE OF JUVENILE SEXUAL CRIME

I know many people hate to read statistics, but bear with me while I provide an important picture about the incidence of general juvenile crime in the United States over the past decade and, in particular, sexual crimes during this same period.

Estimates show that juvenile participation in crime is a significant problem in the United States and, at the same time, indicate that, in recent years, juvenile participation in crime has decreased. The FBI Uniform Crime Report (U.S. Department of Justice, 2005), for instance, states that in 1996 approximately 20% of all arrests in the United States were of juveniles, but by 2005 this percentage had dropped to approximately 15.5%, or by about 4.3%. This is good news, but to put it into perspective, arrests for overall crime in the United States, and not just among juveniles, generally dropped during this same period by about 4.4%, so the reduction in juvenile arrests should be understood in the context of an overall drop in crime, as measured by arrests. That is, the drop in crimes for which adolescents were arrested was consistent with the overall drop in the crime rate, and not especially for juveniles.

Although there is a decrease in overall crime rates, including juvenile crime, there is not a clear decrease in overall arrest rates for juvenile sexual offending as a percentage of all arrests. In addition to the 4.4% decrease in the crime rate among the general U.S. population over the past decade, the 2005 FBI report (U.S. Department of Justice, 2005, Table 32) also notes a reduction of about 10.2% in sexual crimes among the general population. However, this is not the case with respect to juvenile sexual crime. Although there was a reduction of 4.3% in general juvenile arrests as a percentage of the total (for all crimes) over the decade, FBI figures show an overall *increase* of 0.7% in juvenile arrests for sexual crimes. Further, according to Table 32 of the FBI report, although the percentage of juvenile arrests for all crimes was 15.5%, the percentage of juvenile arrests for sexual crimes was higher and, in fact, has increased over the decade from 18.3% of all arrests for sexual crimes in 1996 to 19% of total sexual crime arrests in 2005. According to a recent bulletin by the Office for Juvenile Justice and Delinquency Prevention (Snyder, 2006), despite a decrease of 22% in overall juvenile arrests for all crimes in 2004, there was an increase of 12% in juvenile arrests for nonrape sexual offenses committed by juveniles.

Developing a picture of crime in the United States, including juvenile crime, is complicated, and Snyder (2006) warns that arrest rates are an inadequate means to fully assess crime rates. Frankly, it is difficult to clearly determine the percentage of crimes committed by juveniles, even when reading the annually published FBI reports, which tend to vary by table even within the same report. For instance, Table 32 of the 2005 FBI report shows that 15.5% of all crime arrests and 19% of all sexual crime arrests were of juveniles, but other tables in the same report show that juveniles accounted for 15.1% of all arrests in 2005 (Table 36) and either 17.6% or 20.2% of arrests for sexual crime arrests (Tables 36 and 38). According to data submitted to the National Incident-Based Reporting System between 1991 and 1996, juveniles were responsible for 23.2% of all sexual assaults (Snyder, 2000), although the FBI arrest report for 1996 shows that juveniles were responsible for 17.7% of these crimes (U.S. Department of Justice, 1996). Based on these figures, juvenile arrests for all crimes are somewhere between 15.1% and 15.5% for 2005, and for sexual crimes somewhere between 17.6% and 20.2%. In any case, we can see that juvenile sexual crime rates are higher than general juvenile arrests.

Not surprisingly, arrest statistics clearly indicate that most juvenile crimes, and particularly sexual crimes, are committed by males. 2003 arrest data reported by the National Center for Juvenile Justice (Snyder & Sickmund, 2006) show that boys accounted for 71% of all arrests and 92%

of juvenile sexual arrests, and Snyder (2000) reports that 96% of all sexual offenses in the United States between 1991 and 1996 were committed by males. In addition to being a male-dominated crime, FBI arrest statistics make it clear that juvenile sexual offenses are driven by adolescents rather than younger juveniles. In 2005, although juveniles younger than age 18 accounted for 17.6% of arrests for all sex crimes (Table 38), children age 12 and younger accounted for 2.7% of total arrests for sexual crimes; the remaining 14.9% of arrests were of adolescents age 13 to 17.

Breaking juvenile arrest statistics down further, relatively few juvenile sexual offenses involve forcible rape and are more often limited to less invasive sexual offenses. For instance, FBI statistics for 2005 (Table 32) show that nonrape sexual offenses are 336% more frequent than forcible rape among juvenile sexual offenders. Further, and of great significance, most juvenile sexual offenders victimize children. Data from the National Incident-Based Reporting System for 1991 to 1996 show that, although juveniles were responsible for 23% of all sexual assaults, they were responsible for 4% of sexual assaults against adults. And, whereas juvenile sexual offenders were responsible for 27% of sexual assaults against other adolescents, they were responsible for 39% of assaults against children age 6 to 11 and 40% of assaults against children younger than age 6 (Snyder, 2000). From another perspective, 58% of sexual crimes committed by juveniles were perpetrated against children younger than age 12, compared to 38% against adolescents and 6% against adults.

A PERSPECTIVE ON JUVENILE SEXUAL OFFENDERS

Accordingly, we can recognize juvenile sexual offenders as typically adolescent males most commonly engaging in nonforcible rape sexual offenses, and most typically against children age 12 or younger. Despite decreases in crime rates in the general population for all crimes and sexual crimes and decreases in general crime among juvenile offenders, it appears clear that we are not seeing a significant decrease in juvenile sexual crime. Although fluctuating, juvenile sexual crime has remained steady over the past decade, even increasing slightly (by 0.6%) as a percentage of total sexual crime arrests since 1996.

Given this simplistic statistical view of the juvenile sexual offender, we can nevertheless recognize sexually troubled behavior among adolescents as different than that of general adolescent conduct-disordered behavior. This is not only true in terms of the nature of the criminal behavior, but also in the consistent rate of such behavior (and even slight increase), as other juvenile and adult crime rates are dropping.

In fact, although many juvenile sexual offenders *do* have a history of nonsexual conduct-disordered behaviors (see, for instance, Efta-Breitbach & Freeman, 2004; O'Reilly & Carr, 2006; Worling & Långström, 2006) and are far more likely to get into future trouble for nonsexual rather than sexual behaviors, many juvenile sexual offenders do not meet the criteria for conduct disorder. In writing that approximately 50% of juvenile sexual offenders may be diagnosed with a conduct disorder, France and Hudson (1993) also imply that approximately half may *not* be conduct disordered. In their analysis of 24 studies that included over 1,600 juvenile sexual offenders and 8,000 nonsexual juvenile delinquents, Seto and Lalumière (2006) concluded that, although many juvenile sexual offenders are conduct disordered, they generally score lower in conduct-disordered behavioral problems than nonsexual juvenile delinquents. This was especially true of juvenile sexual offenders who assault children, who, as noted, appear to represent the majority of sexually aggressive juveniles; Seto and Lalumière suggest that it is in the *lack* or reduced level of conduct-disordered behavior that we see a substantial difference between juvenile sexual offenders and nonsexual juvenile delinquents.

In terms of recidivism, the literature repeatedly reports that juvenile sexual offenders are at far greater risk of recidivism for nonsexual offenses than they are for a new sexual offense and that recidivism rates for a sexual reoffense are relatively low for treated juvenile sexual offenders, often ranging between 7% and 15% in reported studies. For instance, in their meta-analysis of nine studies that included 2,986 juvenile sexual offenders, Reitzel and Carbonell (2006) showed recidivism rates of 12.5% for sexual crimes over an average 59-month follow-up period (compared to between 20.4% and 28.5% for different types of nonsexual recidivism). In their study of 636 juvenile sexual offenders, Epperson, Ralston, Fowers, Dewitt, and Gore (2006) found a 13.2% rate for sexual recidivism occurring prior to age 18, although they found a rate of 19.8% when they included juveniles who sexually reoffended after their 18th birthday. In their study of 156 juvenile sexual offenders, Parks and Bard (2006) found a 6.4% sexual offense rate compared to 30.1% for nonsexual recidivism over an average of 53 months postdischarge, although the authors note differences in the rate of recidivism for juvenile sexual offenders who molested children (4%), those who sexually abused peers and/or adults (9.8%), and those who had offenses against both groups of victims (6.5%).

Of note, the subject pool in Parks and Bard's study also showed the same sort of weighting toward juveniles who offended children, rather than juveniles offending peers or adults, with 45% more offenders of children than of peers. However, the authors selected age 10 or younger as the age at which victims were considered children, and victims age 11 and older as peers. Had they selected age 11 as the age at which victims were considered children (rather than peers), the number of child molesters in the study would have been greater, supporting the proposition that most juvenile sexual offenders select child victims.

Although we are learning about differences between juvenile sexual offenders and nonsexual juvenile offenders, as well as differences between juvenile sexual offenders who typically sexually abuse children and those who target peers or (with far less frequency) adults, juvenile sexually abusive behavior is not a cut-and-dried, well-understood phenomenon. It is not at all clear that juvenile sexual offenses are decreasing; they may be increasing or changing in character. In fact, although there is a clear and uniform overall decrease in the number of juveniles arrested for forcible rape over the 11 years spanning 1995 to 2005, there is a far smaller decrease in the number of juvenile arrests for other sexual offenses, and, in fact, for older adolescents, there is an increase in nonrape sexual offenses. The statistics are shown in Table 16.1. Essentially, despite an overall decrease of 31% in forcible rape arrests for all juveniles aged 17 and younger over this 11-year period, there is a 0.9% decrease in arrests for nonrape sexual offenses and an *increase* of 6.4% in nonrape sexual offenses for adolescents age 16 to 17.

As noted, juvenile arrest rates have generally decreased in conjunction with decreases in the arrest rate for the general population, so that juvenile decreases of 31.1% in arrests for forcible rapes closely matches the decrease of 29.2% in arrests of adults over the same period (1995–2005). However, for nonrape juvenile sexual offenses, there is a decrease of less than 1% in arrests and, for older adolescents, an increase in these crimes. So, based on arrest rates, it seems clear that, despite declining rates of juveniles (and others) engaging in rape, there is little change in the incidence of juvenile nonrape sexual offenses and an apparent increase for older adolescents.

To summarize, most juvenile sexual offenders are adolescent males more likely to engage in sexual crimes than nonsexual crimes and are less conduct disordered than nonsexual juvenile offenders. They typically

Table 16.1

PERCENTAGE CHANGE IN ARRESTS FOR SEXUAL OFFENSES COMMITTED BY JUVENILES, 1995 TO 2005

	ADULTS (AGE 18 AND OLDER)	ALL JUVENILES (YOUNGER THAN AGE 18)	JUVENILES (YOUNGER THAN AGE 12)	JUVENILES (AGES 13 TO 15)	JUVENILES (AGES 16 TO 17)
Forcible rape	−29.2	−31.1	−33.3	−32.5	−29.2
Nonrape sexual offense	−8.5	−0.9	−11.9	−1.4	+6.4

Note. Based on Table 38 of the 1995 and 2005 FBI Uniform Crime Reports, *Crime in the United States 2005*, by U.S. Department of Justice, Federal Bureau of Investigation, 2005. Washington, DC: U.S. Department of Justice.

engage in forms of sexual molestation other than forcible vaginal or anal rape, most often engage in sexually abusive behavior with prepubescent children, and, as a population group, are not significantly decreasing in numbers.

PATHWAYS AND CATALYSTS TO SEXUALLY ABUSIVE BEHAVIOR

Even though arrest rates for juvenile sexual offenses are not declining as rapidly as arrest rates for general crimes, and especially for nonrape sexual offenses (and may, in some case, be increasing), what *is* changing is our approach to recognizing, understanding, and treating juvenile sexual offending.

This includes recognizing characteristics that juvenile sexual offenders often have in common with one another and with nonsexual juvenile delinquents, as well as differences between juvenile sexual offenders and juvenile delinquents and differences among juvenile sexual offenders. Although we continue to look for similarities within the group, we more fully recognize what is now becoming a truism in the assessment and treatment of both adult and juvenile sexual offenders—that these are not homogeneous groups. Rather than a single common pathway leading to sexually abusive behavior, different pathways lead and contribute to both the development and onset *and* the maintenance and continuation of sexually abusive behavior, although different pathways share many features.

These common features are of importance in understanding the etiology of juvenile sexual offending, and one may simply extend that into the etiology of adult sexual offending. Although people are too complex for simple one-size-fits-all answers and despite individualized pathways, we can nevertheless lay down a general pathway along which sexual offenders inevitably travel in their development. That is, we're not likely to find someone who engages in sexually abusive behavior who has not developmentally experienced at least some of the conditions found along this metaphorical path. However, the pathway tends to be very general for antisociality, criminal behavior, mental health disorders, and dysfunctionality in general. In other words, it's a pathway that has good predictive power for problems in general but is too broad to have predictive power for sexually abusive behavior in particular. This general path frequently includes elements of suboptimal childhood experiences, including family instability and unstable living conditions, domestic violence, personal histories of neglect or abuse, and other disruptions to what we imagine to be optimal child development. However, we continue to try to narrow down the path in order to understand the specifics that create the branch along which some individuals veer toward sexually abusive behavior. What are the signposts that take some children and adolescents off the path of general antisociality and troubled behavior and onto the specific branch that leads to sexual offending? We have no definite answers, but we are closer to understanding key factors now than we were 10 years ago, or even 5 years ago, partly because we've become informed by a broader set of ideas and theories as we've become more educated about the children and adolescents with whom we work and our work with them.

Although adult and juvenile sexual offenders may start out along the same path, there are significant developmental differences between juvenile and adult sexual offenders (described below more fully); adult pathways become richer and more fully developed with the passage of time and developmental changes in their life circumstances and psychological and social makeup. Nevertheless, despite concerns about the "trickle-down phenomenon" described by Longo and Prescott (2006), in which our understanding and treatment of juvenile sexual offenders has been historically influenced and shaped by research and work with adult sexual offenders, it is also important to recognize similarities in the developmental pathways of adult and juvenile sexual offenders, especially because adult sexual offenders were once adolescents and, in some cases, adolescent sexual offenders. As such, it is difficult to discuss or understand the development of sexually abusive behavior in juveniles without also paying attention to the development of sexually abusive behavior in adults.

Malamuth (2003) describes two pathways leading to sexually abusive behavior in adult men. His model proposes that when early abusive experiences (one pathway) are combined with the development of narcissistic hostility to women (or hostile masculinity) (the second pathway), they interact to produce sexually abusive behavior, when *catalyzed* by low empathy. That is, men with traits of hostile masculinity and/or impersonal and promiscuous sexuality do not engage in sexual aggression if they display high levels of compassion and concern for others (i.e., they experience empathy). It is neither negative childhood experience nor hostile masculinity alone that makes the difference, nor both factors combined, but rather deficits in empathy and social connectedness serve as significant catalysts, helping to transform early experience and the development of antisocial attitudes into sexually abusive behavior.

Knight and Sims-Knight (2003) propose a similar model, although adding callousness and unemotionality that results from early physical and emotional abuse as a third pathway. The role of callous unemotionality in contributing to the development of sexually abusive behavior in men is close in principle and action to the low empathy/lack of compassion factor described by Malamuth in that it catalyzes other factors to produce sexually abusive behavior. In both models, a lack of empathy and compassion (i.e., callous unemotionality) fuels and catalyzes other experiences and attitudes, which come together to produce sexual aggression, driven, according to Knight and Sims-Knight, by emotional detachment—also a key element in Hayslet-McCall and Bernard's (2002) theory of male antisocial behavior.

As noted, being male is of special significance when discussing adult and juvenile sexual offending, because somewhere between 93% and 96% of all sexual crimes are committed by males. In describing the relationship between attachment theory and male criminality, Hayslett-McCall and Bernard (2002) consider the masculine identity to always be of concern, in the United States at least. They suggest that being a male is itself a risk for antisocial behavior, which they consider mediated through detachment that they assert is an acquired state resulting from the environment in which males are typically raised. Although they recognize that male criminal offending cannot be explained by a single theory, Hayslett-McCall and Bernard believe that antisocial, aggressive, and lack of self-regulated behavior in boys is driven by the child-rearing environment. However, because not every boy grows up to be aggressive or emotionally detached, it is unlikely that the child-rearing environment alone is the cause of male aggression; it is more likely that the interaction of both temperament and social connection, driven by early attachment experiences, produces antisocial behavior in males, but only when amplified and catalyzed by other factors along the developmental path.

EMPATHY, MORALITY, AND SOCIAL CONNECTION

When it comes to empathy, Whittaker, Brown, Beckett, and Gerhold (2006) found that the juvenile sexual offenders of children showed less sexual knowledge and increased distortions in empathy when compared to nonoffending adolescents, and they concluded that this combination may be critical in understanding the development of sexual offending in juveniles who sexually abuse children (again, it appears that this group represents the majority of juvenile sexual offenders, in the United States, at least). It is important to note that Whittaker et al. are describing a combination of at least two factors, because it is not likely that a lack of empathy is in itself a sufficient factor to explain the capacity to engage in sexually abusive behavior. However, it is probably a mistake to not consider empathy a significant factor, even though it is not powerful enough to produce sexually abusive and other criminal behavior on its own.

Although diminished empathy or deficits in empathy seems key to the development of sexually abusive—and, quite probably, all criminal—behavior, there is little specific evidence to support the idea that sexual offenders in general are any more deficient in empathy than any other group (see, e.g., Hudson and Ward, 2000). When studied, sexual offenders are no less empathic than others, including nonsexual criminal offenders and the general public. However, it may be appropriate to describe *distortions* in empathy, described in the Whittaker study, because research has suggested that sexual offenders possess general global empathy but experience diminished empathy when it comes to their victims. With regard to differences between global and victim-specific empathy, Webster (2002) found a gap between general empathy and victim-specific empathy in his study of incarcerated adult sexual offenders, writing that "sexual offenders are devoid of empathy for their victims" (p. 281). This suggests that sexual offenders may suppress empathy or distort experience in order to maintain sexually abusive behavior, and this may reflect errors in thinking or perspective taking rather than an incapacity for empathy. Keenan and Ward (2000) suggest that problems with victim empathy may be the result of a lack of mentalization (or the ability to reflect upon and imagine one's own mental experiences and the experiences of others, also known as metacognition), rather than a lack of empathy per se.

With particular regard to adolescent sexual offenders, similar to studies with adult sexual offenders, D'Orazio (2002) found no difference in the level of empathy between sexual offenders and nonoffenders, but did find juveniles in general to be less empathic than adults. She concluded that empathy is developmentally related and that reduced capacity for empathy in adolescents is normative and not related to juvenile antisociality. Hence, it is a mistake to consider the nature of adolescent empathy in the same terms as adult empathy or to map ideas about empathy deficits in adults onto adolescents and children. Nevertheless, D'Orazio found that sexual offenders low in perspective taking engaged in the most severe sexually abusive behavior, and it may well be that the capacity for perspective taking and understanding and caring about the experience of another is a critical element in the enactment of sexually abusive behavior. "Empathic distress" (or sympathy for the other) is described by Hoffman (2000) as key to empathy, and Vetlesen (1994) asserts that empathy establishes a relationship between self and others and is the basic human emotional faculty at the heart of all emotional connection with others. Underdeveloped or poorly formed social understanding and connection, as well as a limited vision of the mental states of self and others, may inhibit the development of age-expected empathy, allow empathic distress to be switched off or ignored, or allow the obvious experience of harm to others to be distorted and go unrecognized. Despite this, if we think of and judge adolescent empathy in adult terms, we risk seeing a lack of empathy in adolescents as pathological rather than as an unfolding developmental process. Adolescent empathy is thus best understood in the context of cognitive and emotional development, partly driven or impeded by either social connection or social disconnection.

In fact, it may be more relevant to consider empathy in juvenile sexual offenders as not simply the capacity to recognize and care about emotion in others, which may be limited in all adolescents, but also to feel connected to others. Here, we might consider the development of empathy in adolescents as not simply a feature of cognitive and emotional development, but also a feature and measure of social connection and belonging. When potentiated by and melded with other factors, limited empathy in adolescents, perhaps a normative state for most adolescents, may be reflected in a sense of disconnection and unrelatedness to others, and perhaps normative social values as a whole.

Moving from the development of empathy to another critical component of social connection and social behavior—that of moral development—Ashkar and Kenny (2007) propose that juvenile sexual offenders are arrested in their moral development. However, they suggest that the level of moral reasoning is tied to the context in which decision making occurs, and, although juvenile sexual offenders may be capable of a higher level of moral decision making, they are most likely to use less developed moral reasoning in situations that involve their engagement in sexually abusive behavior. Similar to ideas about the capacity for empathy and the experience of empathic distress (i.e., feeling sorry for others), this suggests that juvenile sexual offenders either have not developed or are able to switch off a higher level of moral reasoning, allowing them the ability to be sexually abusive. Ideas about empathy and morality are inevitably connected and similar because the two constructs are developmentally and cognitively linked, with morality serving as the attitudinal and behavioral equivalent of empathy. To this end, Hoffman (2000) describes the cognitive aspect of empathy as controlling the emotional experience by which empathic concern for others translates into and becomes congruent with moral codes and behavior. Similarly, Vetlesen (1994) writes that empathy is a precondition for moral decision making and that perceptions of morality are built on the experience of empathy for others. These authors see empathy and morality merging, where empathy builds the groundwork from which morality and moral identity emerges. We can reasonably infer that our social experiences, interactions, and behaviors are significantly related to the way in which we experience and connect with others (i.e., empathy) and decisions we make about how to behave and what to do in social situations and relationships (moral decision making). Social connection, then, is a product of empathic and moral development and the sense of social relatedness that is intrinsically connected.

We move, then, from understanding empathy as a product of and requirement for social relatedness to recognizing it as a prerequisite for the moral development that will allow empathy to be embedded and experienced in the structure and principles of social rules.

ATTACHMENT AND SOCIAL CONNECTION

In recognizing that empathic experience and moral reasoning play a key role in inhibiting or allowing antisocial behavior, including sexually abusive behavior, Stilwell, Galvin, Kopta, and Padgett (1998) describe moral development incorporating social values as well as early attachment experiences and subsequent social relatedness. Stilwell et al.'s model involves the transformation of attachment and social experiences into the values, attitudes, and beliefs that underlie relationships and behaviors, resulting in a moral conscience. Stilwell and colleagues describe the process of developing a social conscience, or the acquisition of morality, as the "moralization of attachment." Here, social connectedness and relatedness is simply another way of describing attachment.

Attachment in this context relates directly to principles of attachment theory that assert that we learn and form mental beliefs and opinions about ourselves and others through very early experiences of attachment with caregivers. These experiences subsequently provide the foundation for all social relationships that follow and our behavior in those relationships and, of equal importance, our experience of ourselves in social interaction and relationships (i.e., self-in-society). As described by Eagle (2006), someone with an insecure pattern of attachment and its corresponding cognitive schema is, by definition, someone who has had difficulty in the past and continues to have difficulty in the present with important others. This leads to possible impairment in social relatedness because, as Eagle notes, that person then fails to experience important others (i.e., attachment figures) as a source of security, safety, and consistency. In addition to building the basis for security in social relationships, early attachment experiences also train our capacity for metacognition and self-regulation, both key elements in social relatedness and social interaction. Of note, in their general theory of crime, Gottfredson and Hirschi (1990) assert that an absence of self-regulation is central to the development of all criminality.

Although attachment experiences and the related experience of social connection in both juvenile and adult sexual offenders has recently been the subject of significant discussion in the sexual offender treatment literature, including my own work (Rich, 2006), little research has been undertaken to better understand the significance of attachment in juvenile sexual offenders. Of the few researchers examining this subject, Mike Miner has done the most complete work, although it still in its early stages.

In general, Miner concludes that, in many respects, juvenile sexual offenders are no different than nonsexual juvenile offenders, and in some respects not especially different than nonclinical youth (that is, youth with no sexual or nonsexual offending behaviors). He does not consider juvenile sexual offenders to be more rejecting of social relationships than nonsexual juvenile delinquents, just less competent, and he believes that there is a link between attachment, social isolation, and sexually abusive behavior. For instance, in one study, Miner and Crimmins (1997) concluded that, although juvenile sexual offenders did not differ significantly than nonsexual juvenile delinquents in either attitude or behavior, they were significantly more isolated from family than nondelinquent youth and more socially isolated from peers than violent delinquents. Miner asserts that juvenile sexual abuse appears to be driven by social isolation and normlessness rather than by aggression, at least in those who molest children; he reports that juvenile sexual offenders who molest children have fewer friends, feel more isolated, associate with younger children, and have more concerns about masculinity than other juvenile sexual offenders or nonsexual juvenile offenders (Miner & Swinburne-Romine, 2004). This mirrors the conjecture of Hudson and Ward (2000) that sexually abusive behavior among adults is often more connected to the need for social connection and the acquisition of social goals than deviant sexuality.

Miner points to the importance of peer relationships in healthy and well-adjusted adolescent behavior, the centrality of attachment difficulties in the development of sexually abusive behavior, and the possibility that juvenile sexual offenders who molest children expect adult and peer rejection. In comparing differences in attitudes, normlessness, and social isolation among juvenile sexual offenders, nonsexual juvenile delinquents, and nondelinquent adolescents, Miner and Munns (2005) found that juvenile sexual offenders experienced more social isolation in school and in their families than nonsexual delinquents. Although, consistent with other research, they found that sexual offenders are quite similar to nonsexual juvenile delinquents, they also concluded that juvenile sexual offenders feel more isolated from their peers than nonsexual juvenile delinquents, and experience a deeper level of social isolation than nonsexual juvenile delinquents and nonoffenders. Miner suggests that the inability to experience satisfaction in social relationships may turn some adolescents to younger children to meet sexual and social needs. Miner also expects to find evidence that a high level of *hostile masculinity* is linked to juvenile sexual offending of peers and adults, whereas low *masculine adequacy* will be linked to juveniles who sexually abuse children.

If Miner's assertion about masculine self-image is correct—in which masculine inadequacy is prevalent in juvenile sexual offenders who assault children, and most juvenile sexual offenders molest children—then most juvenile sexual offenders not only fail to experience social connection with others but additionally experience self-doubts about their masculinity (compared to their imagined ideas about what it means to be a male). On this note, Hayslett-McCall and Bernard (2002) conjecture that most men experience themselves as violating standards of masculinity with respect to gender role expectations. When we add early negative experience, general deficits in social competency, sexual preoccupation, and sexual drive to Miner's model of masculine self-image, as well as exposure to sexual ideas and content in the developmental environment, we evoke a clearer understanding of the interacting and catalyzing factors that can produce sexually aggressive behavior in juveniles.

As we discuss antisociality and social relatedness, Hirschi's (2002) comment that the "bond of affection" for others is a major deterrent to crime (p. 82) is particularly relevant. He notes that we are moral beings to the extent that we have internalized the norms of society and "that the essence of internalization of norms, conscience, or superego lies in the attachment of individuals to others" (p. 18). Here, we rest on the idea that early attachment and bonding experiences are important components in: (1) the establishment of social connection and relatedness; (2) the development of critical self-regulatory and other social skills; and (3) the formation of identity, self-image, and mental representations of others. Taken alone, each of these elements is important in understanding the development of juvenile sexual offending. Together, they represent critical and intermeshed aspects of personal development, driving the capacity for self-efficacy and success and satisfaction in the social environment. In this regard, the social environment in which the child is raised, resulting in his or her sense of connection and relatedness to others, is not just an important but passive backdrop to the development of attachment and moral behavior; it is an *active* ingredient in social development.

THE HETEROGENEITY OF SEXUAL OFFENDERS

By now, it is clear that we don't, by any stretch of the imagination, fully understand the dynamics of sexually abusive behavior, not only with respect to why some adolescents (or children) engage in the behavior in the first place but also why some adolescents desist whereas others continue their sexually abusive behavior as adults. We must recognize, then, different pathways and different trajectories along those pathways based on different life experiences, different personality characteristics that in large measure are shaped by life experiences, different cognitive and emotional characteristics that serve to act upon the world and interpret experience, and different environmental forces that act upon the individual and sometimes redefine the pathway along which that individual is developmentally traveling.

However, we do have some clues and more complete and complex ideas about the development of sexually abusive behavior in juveniles, some of which have already been outlined. These are far more complex than ideas involving simple behavioral cycles and the acquisition of thinking errors or ideas that we can correct adult and juvenile sexually abusive behavior through the correction of thinking errors that are thought to be connected to sexually abusive behavior and the development of a simple relapse prevention plan. Our ideas have evolved beyond these simplistic notions about sexually troubled behavior and its treatment, in the literature of both adult and juvenile sex offender treatment. Although harm reduction and containment models are still the norm in the treatment of adult sexual offenders, based on the view that the safest and perhaps most effective approach to dealing with sexual offending is risk management rather than personal change, this is not the case in the treatment of juvenile sexual offenders. In fact, this is also changing to a limited degree in work with adult populations. Minimally, our view of what makes adult sexual offenders tick is changing, and we are more cognizant than ever about the complexity of these individuals and their needs, described well by Ward, Polaschek, and Beech (2006).

We have also come to recognize juvenile offenders as developmentally quite different than their adult counterparts in many, and perhaps most, respects and, in turn, have come to recognize children with sexual behavior problems as different than their adolescent counterparts. This is healthy movement. We, practitioners and researchers alike, have talked for a number of years about recognizing that the population of juvenile sexual offenders is heterogeneous, and we are now starting to take our own words to heart, at least among these three groups of child, adolescent, and adult offenders.

We also have come to actively seek an understanding of distinctions within each of these three groups. In the assessment and treatment of adult sexual offenders, for instance, our thinking has expanded beyond a single pathway model that leads to and explains sexually abusive behavior. Ward, Hudson, and Marshall (1996), for instance, describe a more complex model involving five different pathways, each of which involves unique psychological mechanisms that lead to sexually abusive behavior among subtypes of adults who sexually assault children, and each of which is independent of the others (Drake & Ward, 2003; Ward et al., 2006). Building on the idea of multiple pathways, Ward et al. (2004) have proposed a multidimensional model by which to understand recidivism among adult sexual offenders, dispensing with the idea that there is a single course of development and action that leads to sexual reoffense, and at the same time recognizing and explicitly identifying four subgroups of adult sexual offenders. Work like this has furthered not only our understanding of sexual offenders, but also pointed to the idea that human behavior is far too complex to be pigeonholed into single categories or described and understood by a single mechanism common to everyone who engages in similar behavior.

This same, more comprehensive and critical thinking has come into play in work with juvenile sexual offenders and children. For example, the recent task force report on children with sexual behavior problems, published by the Association for the Treatment of Sexual Abusers (ASTA; Chaffin et al., 2006), explicitly recognizes that, although many sexually reactive children have a history of prior sexual victimization, the origins of their sexual behavior problems are multifaceted and involve individual, biological, social, and familial factors. This newly emerging, and long overdue, thinking recognizes that there is no distinct or single profile for sexually reactive children any more than there is for juvenile or adult sexual offenders; nor is there a pattern that can readily distinguish sexually reactive children from other groups of children.

Further, Carpentier, Silovsky, and Chaffin (2006b) note that both research and clinical experience reveal that sexually reactive children are qualitatively different from juvenile adolescent and adult sexual offenders. They note, for example, that, although adolescent and adult sex offenders are predominantly male, the population of children with sexual behavior problems often includes a substantial number of girls. Additionally, Chaffin, Letourneau, and Silovsky (2002) report the likelihood of multiple trajectories for sexual behavior problems in children, with persistent sexually abusive behaviors as the exception rather than the norm. Based substantially on the results of a 10-year follow-up study of children with a mean age of 8 (Carpentier, Silovsky, and Chaffin,

2006a), the ATSA task force report concludes that few children continue to demonstrate sexual behavior problems into late adolescence or early adulthood.

THE DEVELOPMENTAL AND CONTEXTUAL NATURE OF JUVENILE SEXUAL OFFENDING

In addition to recognizing the heterogeneity of the population, we must also recognize the complexity of each individual within the population of sexually abusive youth. Further, with respect to the developmental differences that I have several times mentioned, we understand that juvenile offenders are very different from their adult counterparts, not only at the psycho-socio-emotional level, but the neurological level as well. The emotions, relationships, attitudes and ideas, cognitive capacities, place and role in society, and, not least of all, behaviors of adolescents are driven and motivated by very different experiences, forces, and factors than those of adults.

Highlighting these differences in understanding, evaluating, and making decisions about adolescent antisocial behavior, Steinberg and Scott (2003) describe young offenders as "less guilty by reason of adolescence." They consider adolescents developmentally immature when compared to adults, in particular with respect to their decision-making capacity, increased vulnerability to social circumstances, and still-forming character and personality, as well as brain maturation and general psychological development. Related directly to neurological development, they describe adolescents as less planful, thoughtful, and self-controlled than adults. Additionally, Steinberg (2003) warns against the "adultification" of juvenile offenders, noting descriptions that sometimes label young offenders as "career criminals," "super predators," and "fledgling psychopaths." In a similar vein, in a strong criticism of the legal and treatment system surrounding juvenile sexual offenders, Zimring (2004) argues that social and legal policies regarding adult and juvenile sexual offenders are based on broad stereotypes and fail to take into account the developmental status of juvenile sexual offenders with respect to the moral significance of current behaviors, predictions of future behavior, and implications for treatment.

Thus, the process of evaluation and treatment for sexually abusive youth requires a developmental approach to understanding and interpreting information, not only about the sexually abusive behavior itself, but also the individual juvenile sexual offender, and furthermore understanding the youth in the context of his or her *whole* life, rather than just the circumstances of the sexually abusive behavior. Morrison (2006), Longo (2002), Rich (2003), Ryan (1999), and others have referred to this "holistic" level of treatment, and, although we don't have true evidence-based treatments for sexually abusive youth (although we sometimes talk as though we do), it is nonetheless clear to us that "good" treatment for our clients and their families includes an approach that treats the whole child and not simply his or her sexually abusive or inappropriate behavior. Accordingly, we increasingly recognize the need to provide treatment that is not only comprehensive and individualized, but also aimed at the cognitive, emotional, and social developmental level of the client, thus addressing and treating the whole person and not simply the child as "juvenile sexual offender."

Equally, in the assessment of risk we no longer adopt or adapt adult methods of assessment, but instead recognize the imperative for a different assessment process—one that takes into account the developmental, contextual, and experiential particulars of adolescents. We see and increasingly embrace the importance of providing comprehensive assessment as we seek to recognize the particular pathway that led to and/or has maintained sexually abusive behavior in the child or adolescent, and our need to formulate an understanding of the individual youth. To this end, in the literature of juvenile sex offender treatment, we now see the emergence of practice standards and guidelines for the assessment of juvenile sexual offenders as well as assessment instruments that are increasingly used and accepted as state of the art for evaluating risk in juveniles that will continue to be developed and refined over time.

With regard to the contextual nature of treatment, the nonforensic mental health field has long accepted that individuals and their behavior must be understood in the context of their lives or the larger social systems to which they belong and within which they operate. To a great degree, these systems influence and define identity, role, attitudes, and behavior. Just as we have seen changes creeping into our understanding of and work with juvenile sexual offenders in general, the field is also beginning to recognize and accept that sexually abusive youth and their behaviors are part of and influenced by these larger systems. This introduces an ecological approach to understanding sexually abusive youth in situ, in which we recognize that these children and adolescents interact with and are influenced by systems within systems and, to a great degree, are the products of these nested and mutually interacting systems.

Elliot, Williams, and Hamburg (1998) describe the ecological-developmental approach as a framework by which human development is recognized as not occurring in isolation, but in social contexts. These contexts are interactive, not just between people and larger systems, but between and across systems in which interactions at every level influence and shape behavior and, in turn, are influenced and shaped by individual behavior. In the ecological environment, individuals live within subsystems that are subsumed by and nested within larger subsystems, through which they communicate and interact with other individuals, organized agents of society, and society itself (Bronfenbrenner, 1979). From this perspective, without reference to the larger ecological system that surrounds the individual, it is impossible to fully understand human interaction and behavior. The ability to understand human development, including the interplay between attachment and behavior, thus requires an understanding of the individual affected by all levels of the ecological system. This is as true for sexually abusive behavior as for any other behavior, and it requires a more complex view of individuals than a linear view that sees the individual developing and passing through life affected only by his or her immediate social environment.

DIFFERENT TREATMENT FOR DIFFERENT CLIENTS

At its heart, sex offender–specific treatment involves attacking the problem of sexually abusive behavior in juveniles, and we certainly approach the task with certain standard tools and ideas that are applied consistently with all of the children and adolescents we treat. For instance, although there has recently been a reaction to and possible movement away from a psychoeducational and partially cognitive-behavioral approach to sex offender–specific treatment, cycle and relapse prevention work remains relevant to treatment. That is, it remains important to help youth learn about their patterns of emotional, cognitive, and behavioral responses to their environment and thus help them understand more about themselves and how they engage in transactions and interactions with the world around them. This embodies a very basic model of cognitive-behavioral therapy and is certainly useful in helping youth and their families learn a basic language and set of ideas for working through sexual behavior issues, including motivation for sexually inappropriate behavior and how to deal with emotional and behavioral cycles that are dysfunctional and possibly harmful to others. Thus, the psychoeducationally driven model of identifying thinking errors, recognizing dysfunctional behavioral cycles, and developing safety (or relapse prevention) plans remains useful and a core component of sex offender–specific treatment, although we now see (thankfully) that such a simplistic model may be useful but is not likely to "fix" the problem for most of our clients.

Clearly, heterogeneity in juvenile sexual offenders creates a wide array of differences. Hence, even when applying a psychoeducational treatment model, we must recognize differences in our clients, most of which are obvious and some of which require different approaches to the teaching and delivery of even basic treatment ideas. Just as there are significant developmental differences between adults and adolescents, there are significant differences (which are so obvious as to not require further description) between adolescents and children age 12 and younger, between average- to high-IQ offenders and sexual offenders whose IQs fall into the borderline or mentally retarded range of intellectual functioning, between clients with significant psychiatric impairments and those who are relatively well functioning by comparison, and between male sexual offenders and female sexual offenders, as well as perhaps more subtle differences based on cultural, subcultural, and socioeconomic background. These differences require different approaches to the development of treatment content and the delivery of treatment, based on an understanding of differences between and among "classes" of juvenile sexual offenders and based not so much on typological differences (i.e., different "types" of sexual offenders) as on idiosyncratic, developmental, biological, and cultural differences. That is, even though basic psychoeducational ideas may be useful for all sexually abusive youth regardless of subgroup, content and delivery must be appropriate for the individual client being served.

However, going beyond simply individualizing basic treatment ideas to best fit different individuals and different subgroups of sexually abusive youth, treatment must focus on the psychosocial and developmental histories and current treatment needs unique to each individual client. That is, as is true for any form of mental health treatment, treatment for sexually abusive youth must be comprehensive, individually driven, and based on case formulation. This certainly fits well with the idea of risk, responsivity, and needs proposed by Hoge and Andrews (1996) and now increasingly well accepted in treating both adult and juvenile offenders. This set of related ideas bases the type and intensity of treatment required by each individual upon the assessed level of *risk* for that client, in combination with that client's expected level of treatment *response* and the expected treatment *needs* of that client. Although the risk–responsivity–needs model is typically used to assess case management needs, including the level of required treatment, it nevertheless highlights the idea that treatment is not one-size-fits-all, but requires differential application on a case-by-case basis.

THE DEVELOPING TREATMENT PERSPECTIVE

Treatment of sexually abusive behavior is about rehabilitation rather than cure. Hence, the goal is to change direction and rehabilitate attitudes, ideas, and behaviors that may be generally ineffective or antisocial, self-destructive, or harmful to others. In treatment, we seek to understand the source and the basis of problematic interactions and behaviors and rehabilitate the mental maps and cognitive schema that underlie and are essentially responsible for such problems.

Nevertheless, for all the reasons stated, when we talk about treatment, we cannot presently discuss pinpoint, razor-sharp treatment that we know to work or know to work with all juvenile sexual offenders, despite the attractiveness of simplistic psychoeducational and limited cognitive-behavioral models. However, we are able to create and test treatment modalities and techniques that have the promise of being effective. Some of these have some mild empirical support, whereas others are judged to have face value on the basis that we and others (for instance, family members or probation officers) recognize differences in the attitudes, cognition, or behaviors of our clients. Ultimately, because many juvenile sexual offenders do not reoffend sexually, we may argue that treatment appears to largely work, although it may not be treatment per se that is working; it may be apprehension or monitoring that reduces sexual recidivism. It is unlikely, though, that apprehension and monitoring themselves have great significance, because these same two conditions don't appear to be effective in preventing nonsexual recidivism, whereas so many kids seem to desist, rather that persist, from further sexually abusive activity. Hence, although we believe that treatment works for some juvenile sexual offenders, we do not understand what it is that works well in treatment, and, despite rumors to the contrary, we have no empirically validated treatments for adolescents that we know work.

Promising to further enhance the treatment process is the recognition of the centrality of the therapeutic relationship and its treatment alliance, as well as the introduction of elements of positive psychology. Here, we recognize that people have strengths upon which they can build in making improvements in their life and are motivated not just to avoid recidivism (an "avoidance" goal), but to accomplish desired and valued outcomes ("approach" goals). Whereas avoidance goals have long been a central feature in the treatment of sexual offenders and involve avoiding a behavior, approach goals are more synchronous with achievement and improvement. These elements of therapeutic relationship and the pursuit of positive goals are not only emerging in our work with sexually abusive youth, but in work with adult sexual offenders as well. The Good Lives model, which is designed to work with adult sexual offenders (but is finding a place in work with sexually abusive youth as well), shifts the focus in treatment from a containment and control model to a model of positive psychology. In this model, treatment works toward recognizing the identity, values, and beliefs with which the offender identifies so that he or she can work toward personal fulfillment and the development of prosocial social skills. The focus is not solely on risk reduction, but also on enhancing the capacity of the offender to improve his or her life. Thakker, Ward, and Tidmarsh (2006) "propose that the key theoretical perspective that guides treatment should be that of human well-being (i.e., good lives), rather than risk management, or relapse prevention" (p. 324). They assert that the focus of treatment should be on identifying obstacles to accomplishing "human goods" and the acquisition of the capacities and competencies required to achieve human goods in ways that are socially acceptable and personally satisfying.

In this vein, Yates (2005) notes that the aim in treatment is not to change the goal of social success, but to target the means the individual uses to achieve this goal. Hence, Ward and Stewart (2003) assert that the focus on a "good life," rather than risk containment and harm reduction, will contribute to the reduction of risk and the protection of society. Further, the expectation is that a focus on the acquisition of social skills and a personally fulfilling life will increase the offender's motivation to engage in treatment and enhance the ability of clinician and offender to work together as partners, thus strengthening the treatment alliance.

THE ROLE OF THE CLINICIAN

Clinicians working with adult sexual offenders have historically maintained a distance from their clients, leading to a sterile treatment environment and nonrelationally based treatment roles in which clinicians were both judgmental of their clients and confrontive in their behaviors. Treatment was more about the content of treatment than the act of engaging in the therapeutic process. That is, treatment was defined by tasks to be completed in treatment by the offender, rather than being focused on tasks and changes that might be accomplished through the therapeutic relationship.

The development of this model of adult sexual offender treatment is easy to recognize. These clinicians usually worked with their clients in prison or other forensic settings and adopted a hands-off approach to treatment that is not unusual, and even the norm, in such settings. Without special tools to work with sexual offenders, the simplistic and decidedly psychoeducational and nontherapeutic relapse prevention plan model crept in from the field of substance abuse treatment, and sex offender specific work also became heavily influenced by the criminal thinking errors model proposed by Yochelson and Samenow (1976). Treatment became further sterile and manualized, and only recently has this work been clearly recognized as ineffective (Marques, Wiederanders, Day, Nelson, & van Ommeren, 2005). Nevertheless, perhaps at the extreme end of the spectrum, it was even proposed that treatment methods were so sufficiently well specified that they could be taught to "intelligent laypeople" who could then presumably provide the treatment without clinicians (Quinsey, Harris, Rice, & Cormier, 1998, p. 72).

As more juvenile sexual offenders were identified in need of treatment, the trickle-down effect introduced a similar approach into their treatment. The same model of sterile, confrontive, and nonrelationally based treatment became the norm, driven by the accompanying simplistic, one-size-fits-all, psychoeducational and relapse prevention–driven model. Happily, as more clinicians recognized the complex needs of their clients and applied critical thinking to their work, unidimensional models that consider treatment to be essentially psychoeducational have been replaced by more clinically savvy models that recognize the wholeness and complexity of clients and their needs and the need for multidimensional treatment. As Longo and Prescott (2006) write, "our new century finds growing support for (this) holistic/integrated model of treatment" (p. 37).

Which takes us back to the centrality of the therapeutic relationship. A manualized approach to treatment emphasizes treatment technique over treatment approach and treatment content over treatment process and hence approaches treatment as technical, but even in the treatment of adult sexual offenders, we have seen recent changes. For instance, Marshall (2006) writes that manualized treatment in work with adult sexual offenders doesn't allow for necessary flexibility in clinical style or the development of the therapeutic alliance. He notes that rigid adherence to a manual reduces, if not eliminates, clinical flexibility and restricts the expression of therapist features that he writes have repeatedly been shown to be central to treatment in both general clinical treatment and sexual offender–specific treatment literature. Similarly, Marques et al. (2005) recognize that manualized treatments limit the ability to plan or implement treatment interventions based on individual case formulations, as well as the creativity and freedom of the clinician.

In recognizing the severe limitations of manual-driven treatment, the field is increasingly pulled toward treatment driven by individual case formulation, the skill of the clinician, and the therapeutic relationship. Moving away from reliance on and adherence to manualized treatment, we also realize the need to change our approach to treatment. For example, in work with adult sexual offenders, Beech and Hamilton-Giachritsis (2005) note a change in treatment technique from a direct and confrontational style, which they write is likely to lead to increased resistance rather than change, to the development of a supportive and emotionally responsive treatment relationship. In work with youth sexual offenders, the same is true, and Longo and Prescott (2006) write that hostile, confrontational, and harsh treatment styles are ineffective with sexually abusive youth; instead they stress the value of a warm, empathic, and rewarding approach in working with offenders. These relatively new ideas in sexual offender treatment—that we need to build therapeutic alliances with clients, help instill hope in them, and help them grow, rather than simply confront, challenge, and judge them—are welcome, and bring the treatment of juvenile and adult sexual offenders closer to therapeutic principles and processes already found in mainstream psychotherapy.

The conclusion of Marshall et al. (2003) that the behavior of the clinician in sexual offender treatment influences whether clients benefit from treatment is hardly a surprise, and has been recognized in the general field of counseling and psychotherapy for years. Marshall et al. (2003) and Marshall (2005) further note that the attributes and behaviors that therapists bring to treatment influence greater behavior change than those induced by manualized treatment procedures, and they recommend that clinicians adopt an empathic, warm, and rewarding style. There is a new awakening in the field of sexual offender treatment, in recognizing the importance of the clinician's role and the therapeutic relationship in the treatment process. In fact, this represents the increasing recognition in sex offender–specific treatment that the techniques and content of treatment are inadequate on their own and that treatment ideas and tasks are delivered and worked on most effectively through the therapeutic interaction between clinician and client.

In describing treatment in general, the principles of which are no different in work with sexual offenders, Lambert (1992) notes that 70% of treatment outcome involves the highly interpersonal factors introduced by the therapist and the client together, embodied in the therapeutic alliance that forms between them and through which the work of treatment is accomplished. He asserts that only 15% of the variance in treatment outcome is related to treatment technique. These ideas, and the idea that there are common factors found in all forms of effective treatment, are more recently supported by the findings of the American Psychological Association's Task Force on Empirically Based Principles of Therapeutic Change (Castonguay & Beutler, 2006). Briefly, out of 61 principles of therapeutic change, the task force reported the importance of client investment and participation in treatment, noting that effective treatments do not induce resistance in the client and that treatment outcome is enhanced if the client is willing to engage in the treatment process. With respect to the clinician, treatment effectiveness is likely to be enhanced if the therapist demonstrates open-mindedness and flexibility, is patient and able to tolerate any negative feelings he or she may experience about the client, and is comfortable with an emotionally connected treatment relationship. Further, treatment is likely to be beneficial if the therapist is able to facilitate a high degree of collaboration with the client and if a therapeutic alliance is established and maintained in which clinicians both experience empathy for their clients and are experienced by their clients as authentic in the relationship.

All of this speaks to the need for clinicians to engage clients in the treatment process and build a working relationship so that the client is an active participant in, and not simply the object of, the treatment process. Here, the client—in our case, sexually abusive youth—feels valued by and experiences empathy and warmth from the clinician, engages in a working alliance with the clinician, and experiences a genuine relationship with a genuine person rather than sterile treatment with a treatment technician. This, then, is the heart of the therapeutic relationship, as true for work with juvenile sexual offenders as any other population.

TREATMENT THROUGH SOCIAL CONNECTION AND THE DEVELOPMENT OF SOCIAL SKILLS

Given the presence of so many risks in the environment in which impressionable and still developing children and adolescents are raised, it is of note that, on the whole, relatively few youth engage in sexually abusive or inappropriate behavior. Accordingly, an important question is why so many children raised under adverse conditions and exposed to many inappropriate family and/or social messages don't become antisocial or criminal in their behavior or why they don't become juvenile sexual offenders when also exposed to highly sexualized environments, messages, or experiences.

The fact that most children raised under adverse conditions don't become seriously antisocial makes it clear that there are many factors that influence developmental pathways, probably too individualized for us to ever fully recognize or understand. One of these factors, however, is likely to be personal connection to an important attachment or other adult security figure. For instance, in their long-term study of high-risk children, Werner and Smith (1992, 2001) found that the presence of even one supportive person in the child's life throughout childhood and adolescence increased the chances of personal success despite high-risk life circumstances. Their findings reflect the balance that exists at each developmental stage, from childhood through adolescence, between stressful life events and risk factors that exacerbate vulnerability and protective factors that enhance resilience. In fact, it may be that the element of early attachment and its development into social relatedness not only provides a foundation for future relationships, but also serves as a mediating influence that acts upon and coalesces various other shaping forces, which, in some cases of suboptimal or insecure attachment, produces general antisocial behaviors and, in other instances, sexually abusive behavior.

Returning for a minute to the discussion at the beginning of this chapter, we can see that sexually abusive behavior is a different crime than others committed by adolescents, based purely on the fact that, while adult and juvenile crime rates are dropping, crimes involving juvenile sexual abuse are not, and in some cases are increasing. We also have good reason to hypothesize that social experiences and a sense of social connection have some influence in the motivations of sexually abusive adolescents to engage in sexual behaviors with children and, in fact, that most juvenile sexual offenders target children, rather than peers or adults.

Accordingly, in our treatment of sexually abusive youth, attachment experiences and related social relatedness and social competency should be targets for assessment and treatment. In terms of treatment, the focus is on rehabilitating the mental model (i.e., emotional and cognitive schema) that results from the accumulation of poor attachment experiences and their impact on a developing sense of self, others, and self-efficacy, as well as the capacity to engage in meaningful and satisfying social interactions and relationships (the "human goods" described by Thakker, Ward, and Tidmarsh, 2006). The goal of teaching sexually abusive youth psychoeducational concepts, such as dysfunctional behavioral cycles and thinking errors that contribute, or in some cases lead directly, to sexually abusive behavior, has been and remains an important element in sex offender–specific treatment. However, this work must be embedded in a larger and more complete treatment that also, and perhaps more significantly, addresses deficits in attachment, social relatedness, and social skills. These include a limited ability to form meaningful and satisfying relationships, experience empathy and concern for others, and engage in the behaviors, interactions, and relationships that are the backbone of appropriate social connection. These deficits further include a poorly developed capacity to recognize and understand one's mental state and the mental state of others (i.e., metacognition), an underdeveloped sense of moral decision making and behavior, and inadequate self-regulation, or the ability to recognize and manage one's own emotional state.

At the conclusion of this journey, then, from the incidence and nature of juvenile sexual offending through etiological factors, we arrive at a model of treatment that builds basic and important psychoeducational ideas and cognitive-behavioral principles into a larger integrated model of treatment that recognizes the uniqueness of individual developmental pathways that lead to sexually abusive behavior and the individuality of each sexually abusive youth who enters treatment. This model, however, not only recognizes the wholeness of the client, but also the holistic nature of treatment itself, incorporating and knitting together different elements into a larger multifaceted, multidimensional, and integrated whole. It also recognizes the central role of the clinician, including the attributes and approach of the clinician and the nature of the therapeutic relationship. This model goes far beyond single-minded and less complex models of treatment and beyond the ideas of manualized treatment; it is a far more complex, demanding, and intensive treatment process, requiring more skills from the clinician, as well as the clinician's ability to recognize, value, and empathize with the client, regardless of the behaviors that brought the client into treatment.

REFERENCES

Ashkar, P. J., & Kenny, D. T. (2007). Moral reasoning of adolescent male offenders: Comparison of sexual and nonsexual offenders. *Criminal Justice and Behavior, 34,* 108–118.

Beech, A. R., & Hamilton-Giachritsis, C. E. (2005). Relationship between therapeutic climate and treatment outcome in group-based sex offender treatment programs. *Sexual Abuse: A Journal of Research and Treatment, 17,* 127–140.

Bronfenbrenner, U. (1979). *The ecology of human development: Experiments in human behavior.* Cambridge, MA: Harvard University Press.

Carpentier, M. Y., Silovsky, J., & Chaffin, M. (2006a). Randomized trial of treatment for children with sexual behavior problems: Ten-year follow-up. *Journal of Consulting & Clinical Psychology, 72,* 482–488.

Carpentier, M., Silovsky, J., & Chaffin, M. (2006b). Treating children: Results from a 10-year follow-up. *The Forum, 18,* 4.

Castonguay, L. G., & Beutler, L. E. (2006). *Principles of therapeutic change that work.* New York: Oxford University Press.

Chaffin, M., Berliner, L., Block, R., Johnson, T. C., Friedrich, W., Louis, D., et al. (2006). *Association for the Treatment of Sexual Abusers task force report on children with sexual behavior problems.* Beaverton, OR: Association for the Treatment of Sexual Abusers.

Chaffin, M., Letourneau, E., & Silovsky, J. F. (2002). Adults, adolescents, and children who sexually abuse children: A developmental perspective. In J.E.B. Myers & L. Berliner (Eds.), *APSAC handbook on child maltreatment* (2nd ed., pp. 205–232). Thousand Oaks, CA: Sage.

D'Orazio, D. (2002). *A comparative analysis of empathy in sexually offending and non-offending juvenile and adult males.* Unpublished doctoral dissertation, California School of Professional Psychology at Alliant University, Fresno.

Drake, C. R., & Ward, T. (2003). Treatment models for sexual offenders. In T. Ward, D. R. Laws, & S. M. Hudson (Eds.), *Sexual deviance: Issues and controversies* (pp. 226–243). Thousand Oaks, CA: Sage.

Eagle, M. N. (2006). Attachment, psychotherapy, and assessment: A commentary. *Journal of Counseling and Clinical Psychology, 74,* 1086–1097.

Efta-Breitbach, J., & Freeman, K. A. (2004). Recidivism, resilience, and treatment effectiveness for youth who sexually offend. In R. Geffner, K. C. Franey, T. G. Arnold, & R. Falconer (Eds.), *Identifying and treatment youth who sexually offend: Current approaches, techniques, and research* (pp. 257–279). Binghamton, NY: Haworth Press.

Elliot, D. S., Williams, K. R., & Hamburg, B. (1998). An integrated approach to violence prevention. In D. S. Elliot, B. A. Hamburg, & K. R. Williams (Eds.), *Violence in American schools: A new perspective* (pp. 379–386). Cambridge, England: Cambridge University Press.

Epperson, D. L., Ralston, C. A., Fowers, D., Dewitt, J., & Gore, K. S. (2006). Actuarial risk assessment with juveniles who sexually offend: Development of the Juvenile Sexual Offense Recidivism Risk Assessment Tool-II (JSORRAT-II-II). In D. S. Prescott (Ed.), *Risk assessment of youth who have sexually abused* (pp. 118–169). Oklahoma City, OK: Wood & Barnes.

France, K. G., & Hudson, S. M. (1993). The conduct disorders and the juvenile sexual offender. In H. E. Barbaree, W. L. Marshall, & S. M. Hudson (Eds.), *The juvenile sex offender* (pp. 225–234). New York: Guilford Press.

Gottfredson, M. R., & Hirschi, T. (1990). *A general theory of crime.* Stanford, CA: Stanford University Press.

Hayslett-McCall, K. L., & Bernard, T. J. (2002). Attachment, masculinity, and self-control: A theory of male crime rates. *Theoretical Criminology, 6,* 5–33.

Hirschi, T. (2002). *Causes of delinquency.* New Brunswick, NJ: Transaction.

Hoffman, M. L. (2000). *Empathy and moral development: Implications for caring and justice.* Cambridge, England: Cambridge University Press.

Hoge, R. D., & Andrews, D. A. (1996). *Assessing the youthful offender: Issues and techniques.* New York: Plenum Press.

Hudson, S. M., & Ward, T. (2000). Interpersonal competency in sex offenders. *Behavior Modification, 24,* 494–527.

Keenan, T., & Ward, T. (2000). A theory of mind perspective on cognitive, affective, and intimacy deficits in child sexual offenders. *Sexual Abuse: A Journal of Research and Treatment, 12,* 49–60.

Knight, R. A., & Sims-Knight, J. E. (2003). The developmental antecedents of sexual coercion against women: Testing alternative hypotheses with structural equation modeling. In R. A. Prentky, E. S. Janus., & M. C. Seto (Eds.), *Sexually coercive behavior: Understanding and management: Vol. 989. Annals of the New York Academy of Sciences* (pp. 72–85). New York: New York Academy of Sciences.

Lambert, M. J. (1992). Implications of outcome research for psychotherapy integration. In J. C. Norcross & M. R. Goldstein (Eds.), *Handbook of psychotherapy integration* (pp. 94–129). New York: Basic Books.

Longo, R. E. (2002). A holistic approach to treating young people who sexually abuse. In M. C. Calder (Ed.), *Young people who sexually abuse: Building the evidence base for your practice* (pp. 218–230). Dorset, England: Russell House.

Longo, R. E., & Prescott, D. S. (2006). *Current perspectives: Working with sexually aggressive youth and youth with sexual behavior problems.* Holyoke, MA: NEARI Press.

Malamuth, N. M. (2003). Criminal and noncriminal sexual aggressors: Integrating psychopathy into a hierarchical-mediational confluence model. In R. A. Prentky, E. S. Janus., & M. C. Seto (Eds.), *Sexually coercive behavior: Understanding and management: Vol. 989. Annals of the New York Academy of Sciences* (pp. 33–58). New York: New York Academy of Sciences.

Marques, J. K., Wiederanders, M., Day, D. M., Nelson, C., & van Ommeren, A. (2005). Effects of a relapse prevention program on sexual recidivism: Final results from California's Sex Offender Treatment and Evaluation Project (SOTEP). *Sexual Abuse: A Journal of Research and Treatment, 17,* 79–107.

Marshall, W. L. (2005). Therapist style in sexual offender treatment: Influence on indices of change. *Sexual Abuse: A Journal of Research and Treatment, 17,* 109–116.

Marshall, W. L. (2006). The random controlled trial: Is this the most appropriate approach to evaluating effectiveness in sexual offender treatment? *Nota News, 54,* 5–6.

Marshall, W. L., Serran, G. A., Fernandez, Y. M., Mulloy, R., Mann, R. E., & Thornton, D. (2003). Therapist characteristics in the treatment of sexual offenders: Tentative data on their relationship with indices of behaviour change. *Journal of Sexual Aggression, 9,* 25–30.

Miner, M. H., & Crimmins, C.L.S. (1997). Adolescent sex offenders: Issues of etiology and risk factors. In B. K. Schwartz & H. R. Cellini (Eds.), *The sex offender: Corrections, treatment and legal practice* (pp. 9.1–9.15). Kingston, NJ: Civic Research Institute.

Miner, M. H., & Munns, R. (2005). Isolation and normlessness: Attitudinal comparisons of adolescent sex offenders, juvenile offenders, and nondelinquents. *International Journal of Offender Therapy and Comparative Criminology, 49,* 491–504.

Miner, M. H., & Swinburne-Romine, J. (2004, October). *Understanding child molesting in adolescence: Testing attachment-based hypotheses.* Presentation at the 8th International Conference of the International Association for the Treatment of Sexual Offenders, Athens, Greece.

Morrison, T. (2006). Building a holistic approach in the treatment of young people who sexually abuse. In R. E. Longo & D. S. Prescott (Eds.), *Current perspectives: Working with sexually aggressive youth and youth with sexual behavior problems* (pp. 349–368). Holyoke, MA: NEARI Press.

O'Reilly, G., & Carr, A. (2006). Assessment and treatment of criminogenic needs. In H. E. Barbaree & W. L. Marshall (Eds.), *The juvenile sex offender* (2nd ed., pp. 189–218). New York: Guilford Press.

Parks, G. A., & Bard, D. E. (2006). Risk factors for adolescent sexual offender recidivism: Evaluation of predictive factors and comparison of three groups based on victim type. *Sexual Abuse: A Journal of Research and Treatment, 18,* 319–342.

Quinsey, V. L., Harris, G. T., Rice, M. E., & Cormier, C. A. (1998). *Violent offenders: Appraising and managing risk.* Washington, DC: American Psychological Association.

Reitzel, L. R., & Carbonell, J. L. (2006). The effectiveness of sexual offender treatment for juveniles as measured by recidivism: A meta-analysis. *Sexual Abuse: A Journal of Research and Treatment, 18,* 401–421.

Rich, P. (2003). *Understanding juvenile sexual offenders: Assessment, treatment, and rehabilitation.* Hoboken, NJ: Wiley.

Rich, P. (2006). *Attachment and sexual offending: Understanding and applying attachment theory to the treatment of juvenile sexual offenders.* Chichester, England: Wiley.

Ryan, G. (1999). Treatment of sexually abusive youth: The evolving consensus. *Journal of Interpersonal Violence, 14,* 422–436.

Seto, M. C., & Lalumière (2006). Conduct problems and juvenile sexual offending. In H. E. Barbaree & W. L. Marshall (Eds.), *The juvenile sex offender* (2nd ed., pp. 166–188). New York: Guilford Press.

Snyder, H. N. (2000). *Sexual assault of young children as reported to law enforcement: Victim, incident, and offender characteristics* (NCJ 182990). Washington, DC: Bureau of Justice Statistics.

Snyder, H. N. (2006). *OJJDP juvenile justice bulletin: Juvenile arrests 2004.* Washington, DC: U.S. Department of Justice, Office of Justice Programs.

Snyder, H. N., & Sickmund, M. (2006). *Juvenile offenders and victims: 2006 national report.* Washington, DC: U.S. Department of Justice, Office of Justice Programs, Office of Juvenile Justice and Delinquency Prevention.

Steinberg, L. (2003, April 26). *Less guilty by reason of adolescence: A developmental perspective on adolescence and the law.* Invited master lecture at the biennial meetings of the Society for Research in Child Development, Tampa, FL.

Steinberg, L., & Scott, E. S. (2003). Less guilty by reason of adolescence. *American Psychologist, 58,* 1009–1018.

Stilwell, B. M., Galvin, M. R., Kopta, S. M., & Padgett, R. J. (1998). Moral volition: The fifth and final domain leading to an integrated theory of conscience understanding. *Journal of the American Academy of Child and Adolescent Psychiatry, 37,* 202–210.

Thakker, J., Ward, T., & Tidmarsh, R. (2006). A reevalaution of relapse prevention with adolescents who sexually offend: A Good-Lives model. In H. E. Barbaree & W. L. Marshall (Eds.), *The juvenile sexual offender* (2nd ed., pp. 313–335). New York: Guilford Press.

U.S. Department of Justice, Federal Bureau of Investigation. (1995). *Uniform Crime Reports for the United States, 1995.* Washington, DC: U.S. Department of Justice.

U.S. Department of Justice, Federal Bureau of Investigation. (1996). *Uniform Crime Reports for the United States, 1996.* Washington, DC: U.S. Department of Justice.

U.S. Department of Justice, Federal Bureau of Investigation. (2005). *Crime in the United States 2005.* Washington, DC: U.S. Department of Justice.

Vetlesen, A. J. (1994). *Perception, empathy, and judgment: An inquiry into the preconditions of moral performance.* University Park: Pennsylvania University Press.

Ward, T., Bickley, J., Webster, S. D., Fisher, D., Beech, A., & Eldridge, H. (2004). *The self-regulation model of the offense and relapse process: A manual: Vol. 1. Assessment.* Victoria, Canada: Psychological Assessment Corporation.

Ward, T., Hudson, S. M., & Marshall, W. L. (1996). Attachment style in sex offenders: A preliminary study. *Journal of Sex Research 33,* 17–26.

Ward, T., Polaschek, D.L.L., & Beech, A. R. (2006). *Theories of sexual offending.* Chichester, England: Wiley.

Ward, T., & Stewart, C. A. (2003). The treatment of sexual offenders: Risk management and good lives. *Professional Psychology: Research and Practice, 34,* 353–360.

Webster, S. D. (2002). Assessing victim empathy in sexual offenders using the victim letter task. *Sexual Abuse: A Journal of Research and Treatment, 14,* 281–300.

Werner, E. E., & Smith, R. S. (1992). *Overcoming the odds: High risk children from birth to adulthood.* Ithaca, NY: Cornell University Press.

Werner, E. E., & Smith, R. S. (2001). *Journeys from childhood to midlife: Risk, resilience, and recovery.* Ithaca, NY: Cornell University Press.

Whittaker, M. K., Brown, J., Beckett., R., & Gerhold, C. (2006). Sexual knowledge and empathy: A comparison of adolescent child molesters and non-offending adolescents. *Journal of Sexual Aggression, 12,* 143–154.

Worling, J. R., & Långström, N. (2006). Risk of sexual recidivism in adolescents who offend sexually: Correlates and assessment. In H. E. Barbaree & W. L. Marshall (Eds.), *The juvenile sex offender* (2nd ed., pp. 219–247). New York: Guilford Press.

Yates, P. M. (2005, Summer). Pathways to the treatment of sexual offenders: Rethinking intervention. *The Forum, 17*(3), 1–9.

Yochelson, S., & Samenow. S. E. (1976). *The criminal personality: Vol. 1. A profile for change.* Northvale, NJ: Jason Aronson.

Zimring, F. E. (2004). *An American travesty: Legal responses to adolescent sexual offending.* Chicago: University of Chicago Press.

17

Juvenile Stalking: An Overview of Assessment and Management Issues

R. GREGG DWYER
AND DEBORAH L. LAUFERSWEILER-DWYER

This chapter provides an overview of the phenomenon of stalking behavior by juveniles. The focus is on assessment and management of related mental health issues. Evidence-based guidance is provided where possible. Unfortunately, there is a paucity of published empirical studies of this type of behavior (McCann, 2003), and what is available is relatively new. Much of what is found in the literature is extrapolated from the literature on adult stalking behavior.

This chapter reviews the limited literature to provide suggestions for practical application. A working definition of juvenile stalking is followed by a description of assessment and treatment issues relevant to juveniles engaged in stalking. Management concerns are addressed from the perspective of mental health providers, and the chapter concludes with a brief critique of the literature and suggestions for future efforts.

JUVENILE STALKING DEFINED

The types of behaviors routinely found among juvenile stalkers include phone calls, letters, and physical contact (McCann, 2003). Definitions of stalking in the literature are typically based on one of three models: behavioral, medical (specifically, psychiatric), and legal. These are not mutually exclusive, but each provides a unique perspective of stalking. Although developed to understand adult stalkers, the framework will form the basis for our definition of juvenile stalking. Although not exhaustive given the limits of a book chapter, what follows is a sampling of definitions from each of these fields.

Behavioral

The behavior model derives its definition from the quality of the exhibited behaviors. Meloy and Gothard (1995) proposed the term *obsessional follower*, which Meloy (1996) later defined as including persons who follow the victims of their attention and those who exhibit abnormal or long-standing histories of threatening or harassing behavior directed at their victims. To allow for cases in which actual following does not occur, others use the descriptor *obsessional harassment,* which can include contact via telephone or mail, among other impersonal methods, and captures the victim's view of the behavior (Rosenfeld, 2000). Meloy (2002) has also defined the behavior by focusing on the victims. Specifically, he divided them into public and private figures.

Cupach and Spitzberg (1998) define stalking as a reoccurring and obsessive intrusion by one into the privacy of another without mutual consent. Their definition includes a continuum of behavior from socially acceptable to problematic. It is obviously more inclusive.

Mohandie, Meloy, McGowan, and Williams (2006) developed the four-category typology known as RECON, which is based on a nonrandom sample of 1,005 persons identified as stalkers. Although most of the subjects were adults, juveniles were included in their study. The first category, *intimate,* is the least likely to have psychotic symptoms and the most likely to engage in violence. The *acquaintance* type is the most persistent and the one most desirous of a relationship with his or her stalking target. *Public figure* stalkers represent the largest group and the most likely to have a history of a psychiatric diagnosis. They are typically the oldest, the least likely to escalate in behavior, and the least likely to threaten. Stalkers in the final category, *private stranger,* have a high prevalence of mental illness and female victims. They do not frequently assault their victims but rather want to talk.

Medical (Psychiatric) Model

There is no specific diagnosis for stalking, but the behavioral characteristics can sometimes meet the criteria for a *Diagnostic and Statistical Manual of*

Mental Disorders, 4th edition, text revision *(DSM IV-TR)* (American Psychiatric Association, 2001), diagnosis of delusional disorder, erotomanic type. Specifically, delusional disorder requires that the behavior under review is not bizarre (meaning it is plausible); is maintained for a minimum of 1 month; does not meet the criteria for a diagnosis of schizophrenia; lacks prominent auditory or visual hallucinations; tactile or olfactory hallucinations, when experienced, are congruent with the delusion; social functioning must be intact, with the obvious exception of the delusion's specific impact; mood symptoms, when present, must be brief relative to the delusion's duration; and the symptoms cannot be secondary to substance use or a general medical diagnosis (American Psychiatric Association, 2001). The subtype erotomanic requires that the person suffering the illness believe that he or she is the object of someone else's love, which may be "romantic" or "spiritual." The other person is frequently someone of prominence or at least of higher social status. The person with the delusion does not always attempt to make contact with this other person, but when efforts are made to do so, legal authorities can become involved (American Psychiatric Association, 2001).

Legal

Typically, legal definitions focus on the preoffending relationship between the stalker and the stalker's victim. A representative example is that developed by Palarea, Zona, Lane, and Langhinrichsen-Rohling (1999) from their study of Los Angeles Police Department cases. Their model is composed of three categories: simple obsessional, erotomanic, and love obsessional. The simple obsessional stalkers have relationships with their victims prior to the offending behaviors (Palarea et al., 1999; Zona & Sharma, 1993) and bear the highest risk of violence (Kienlen, Birmingham, Solberg, O'Regan, & Meloy, 1999; Schwartz-Watts & Morgan, 1998). The erotomanic stalkers, who are frequently women, believe they are loved by their victims, who are generally older men with higher status (Nadkarni & Grubin, 2000). The love obsessional type has had no prior relationship with the victim, who is often a celebrity, and is the most likely to have a psychiatric disorder (Palarea et al., 1999; Zona & Sharma, 1993).

The legal models are based on what has become known as antistalking legislation and consequently require the presence of a threat and criminal intent. The threatening behavior can be in the form of harassing phone calls or mail; watching; trespassing; vandalism; brandishing a weapon; intimidation of the victim's family; or threats of physical violence (McAnaney, Curliss, & Abeyta-Price, 1993). In addition, a pattern of behavior is often required, as is a realistic potential of real harm. The element of intent requires that the perpetrator of the behavior was acting purposefully, willfully, and knowingly (National Institute of Justice, 1993).

In this chapter, the terms *stalking* and *stalker* will be used for the convenience of avoiding gender-specific pronouns. *Juvenile* refers in this chapter to a person younger than age 18 unless otherwise specified.

ASSESSMENT AND TREATMENT

A precise prevalence is unknown for stalking in general, and it is even less clear for juvenile stalkers (McCann, 2003). McCann's (2001) review of the research literature revealed that stalking among high school and college students is significant, but minimal empirical evidence is available.

Given that there is no specific diagnosis of stalking in the *DSM IV-TR*, assessment cannot be simply a check of diagnostic criteria. Regardless of the definition used, the assessment of stalking behaviors should include an evaluation for the presence of a mental illness and for risk of violence. The former will aid identification of treatable conditions and ideal treatment setting. The latter is historically a difficult and typically unsuccessful task. Nevertheless, attempts should be made. Specifics of violence risk assessment are beyond the scope of this chapter but are contained in other chapters in this volume (see chapters 1, 2, and 3).

Evaluation for the presence of a psychiatric diagnosis should follow the same strategies employed when assessing someone for mental illness, regardless of the reason or presenting signs or symptoms. The mechanics of such a basic diagnostic evaluation are those common to the repertoire of most mental health providers. The diagnoses often associated with stalking behavior include delusional disorder, mood disorders, psychotic disorders, substance use disorders, obsessive-compulsive disorders, and certain personality disorders (Rosenfeld, 2000). No special techniques are necessary for identifying these just because the client has engaged in stalking behaviors.

Although no unique methods need be used, there are some cautions to keep in mind. First, it is not uncommon for persons to minimize their stalking behaviors, thus necessitating collateral sources (Rosenfeld, 2000). The prevalence rates for stalking are not well established, with both inaccurate accusations of stalking along with underdiagnosed cases occurring with unknown frequency (Rosenfeld, 2000). The circumstances of the accusations must be thoroughly understood to distinguish among psychotic, personality, mood, and delusional disorders and even situationally acceptable behaviors (Rosenfeld, 2000). To follow are suggestions from the literature regarding treatment approaches based on the diagnoses identified.

The field lacks efficacy studies for the treatment of stalking behavior in part because there is no specific treatment protocol (Rosenfeld, 2000). Consequently, the focus is typically on the individual symptoms and the disorders that include behaviors defined as stalking. For example, the treatment of delusions is usually with antipsychotic medications (Rosenfeld, 2000). Rosenfeld's (2000) review of the literature on this treatment modality revealed that studies focused on nonforensic samples, and he speculated that forensic populations might be less compliant with medication use. His review of psychotherapeutic techniques was mixed with regard to success. Again, the study samples were not of persons who had engaged in stalking behavior, but rather other types of delusional activity, and thus the relevance is questionable.

Stalking behaviors have been linked to schizophrenia, schizoaffective disorder, and mood disorders, such as bipolar disorder. These illnesses should be treated in the traditional manner, but studies report mixed success in using such methods to eliminate stalking behaviors (Rosenfeld, 2000). Antipsychotic and mood stabilizing medications have been used with complete, partial, and no resolution of obsessional following behaviors being reported in various studies (Rosenfeld, 2000). Cognitive-behavioral therapy, behavioral techniques, and psychoeducational approaches have also been tried, with none showing significance as the definitive choice (Rosenfeld, 2000).

Personality disorders are known to be difficult to treat regardless of the behaviors at issue (Rosenfeld, 2000). There is not a scientific base for the treatment of stalking behaviors due to personality disorders. Rosenfeld (2000) compared stalking behavior to domestic violence, for which personality disorder treatment has had some success when the offender wanted to cease his or her behavior (Rosenfeld, 2000). By extrapolating, one can presume the same approaches would be beneficial. Treatment should be directed to address the juvenile offender's relationships with others when a dysfunctional personality is identified (McCann, 2001).

It has been suggested that the presence of substance abuse disorders along with stalking behavior increases the risk of a violent outcome (Rosenfeld, 2000). As result, treating the substance abuse is imperative.

There is no reason to believe that traditional treatment protocols would not be applicable just because stalking behaviors are present. It is obviously important to screen for substance use problems, although this should be a part of all mental health assessments.

It is possible that some obsessional stalking is a manifestation of an obsessive-compulsive disorder (Rosenfeld, 2000). Although no research foundation exists in such a case, it stands to reason that methods of treating the underlying disorder would be effective in reducing or eliminating the stalking. Cognitive-behavioral, purely behavioral, and pharmacological approaches are the mainstay of treating obsessive-compulsive symptoms. These same methods should be tried if there are indications of an obsessive-compulsive process.

CLINICAL EXAMPLE

Based in part on a compilation of facts from actual stalking cases described by McCann (2001), the following fictitious case is provided to illustrate the assessment, treatment, and management techniques described in this chapter.

Prior to his recent charge of stalking, Bob had a history of both mental health and juvenile justice interventions. Beginning at age 8, Bob began to have trouble in school both academically and behaviorally. His grades dropped from primarily As and Bs to Ds and Fs, and his participation in extracurricular activities including sports and social clubs tapered from routine to nonexistent. In addition, Bob withdrew from his circle of friends and began to only interact with others in an aggressive and antagonistic manner.

Initially, Bob's change in academic performance and social interactions was attributed to his home life, which was punctuated by an emotionally and physically abusive father, who, during Bob's early years, had spent most of the time away from home either working on offshore oil rigs for 6 to 8 months at a time or in several extended residential substance use treatment programs. Bob's mother worked two jobs and spent the remainder of her time with online gambling sites. Around the time of Bob's 8th birthday, Bob's father changed jobs to warehouse work in their local community, so his infrequent and short visits to the household suddenly changed. With the increased frequency of interactions with Bob's father, Bob became more withdrawn, sullen, and aggressive. His role in the household as the only consistent male was usurped with his father's presence. Bob was first evaluated by his pediatrician on the suggestion of the school counselor, who suspected substance abuse. The pediatrician diagnosed Bob with attention deficit hyperactivity disorder (ADHD) and prescribed a stimulant. Although Bob took the medication as prescribed for several weeks, his symptoms did not improve, and Bob eventually began saving the pills for later sale to classmates.

By age 10, Bob began sampling the alcohol kept hidden in the family home by his father. After being discovered at age 12 by his father and subsequently physically beaten for drinking from his father's alcohol, Bob began seeking alternative methods to obtain alcohol. He attempted to befriend classmates who had a reputation for drug use as a source for alcohol. This arrangement lasted for only about a year due to Bob's poor social skills even for the group of youths, who typically were under the influence of one substance or another.

By this time, Bob had been picked up by the police on several occasions for shoplifting and attempted break-ins to his school and several residences. Because of his mother's job as a file clerk at the sheriff's department, Bob's legal transgressions resulted in his being driven home with no reports filed. On those occasions when Bob's father was at home when Bob was delivered by the police, Bob was physically beaten by his father, sometimes resulting in injuries that should have been treated by a medical professional. At age 13, after Bob burglarized a business and was apprehended, his juvenile justice record officially began. His first charge resulted in probation and mandatory mental health center treatment for what at that point was diagnosed as oppositional defiant disorder (ODD).

When puberty began for Bob at age 13, his attention shifted from petty crimes to obtain money for alcohol to a consuming interest in an older teenage girl who lived down the block from him and attended the same school as Bob. Bob still consumed alcohol as frequently as possible. Initially, he would only take notice of his female neighbor when she came and left from her home. Over a period of several weeks, he began thinking about her, drawing pictures of her, and fantasizing of ways to engage her in conversation. After several months of watching her from his bedroom window, which afforded him a line of sight to the front of her house, he began sneaking out of his home when he saw her return to her home at night. He would try to watch her through her bedroom window from a tree in her neighbor's yard. At school, he sought every opportunity to sit in places in the cafeteria and in the school yard where he would have a clear view of her eating lunch and interacting with her friends. He would follow her after school, even waiting outside the homes of her friends until she left and headed home.

By age 14, Bob filled all his waking moments with thoughts of his female neighbor and sought every opportunity to catch a glimpse of her. He obtained her e-mail address from an online Web site used by many of the students at their school. After several weeks of drafting messages, Bob eventually sent her an e-mail detailing his love for her and what he believed were signs that she loved him as well. At first, she dismissed the note as a prank of one of her friends. Bob began sending daily e-mails with increasingly sexually graphic descriptions of what he wanted and planned to do with her when they were finally alone together. Although she had ignored the first few e-mails, when the content became sexually explicit, she began sending responses back to Bob telling him to stop or she would call the police, and once she wrote that her boyfriend would make Bob stop. The e-mail referencing a boyfriend enraged Bob, and his e-mails turned violent, with threats of harm to both the neighbor and her boyfriend. The neighbor finally told her parents of the e-mails, the police were called, and the local Internet crime task force was able to trace the e-mails back to Bob. Bob was apprehended and charged with stalking after his e-mails were reviewed and photographs of the neighbor in various locations around the city and in her home were confiscated from Bob's bedroom. Bob was referred for a mental health evaluation prior to adjudication.

An assessment of Bob's behavior should include a comprehensive psychosocial evaluation. Records from his previous evaluation by his pediatrician, incident reports from all of his criminal activity, adjudication reports from those offenses that lead to charges, and school records will need to be obtained and reviewed to help establish a time line and possible etiologies and to identify symptoms of psychopathology. Such data will facilitate determining a diagnosis, assessing risk of future violence, developing a treatment plan, and identifying the ideal treatment setting.

The evaluation for a mental illness will be no different for Bob than for other teenagers. The clinician evaluating Bob should consider all the various categories of illnesses but be especially aware of those most likely to lead to stalking behaviors, including delusional disorders, mood disorders, psychotic disorders, substance use disorders, obsessive-compulsive disorders, and certain personality disorders (Rosenfeld, 2000). Minimization is a common trait among those who engage in stalking, so the use of collateral information sources, such as those already noted, will be critical in obtaining an accurate understanding of Bob's history and current behaviors.

Treatment planning will require a thorough assessment and accurate working diagnosis with a differential diagnostic list. Specific treatment will be focused on the working diagnosis with interventions based on Bob's symptoms. Compliance with treatment modalities can be problematic for persons with stalking behavior histories, and, in Bob's case, we know he was not compliant with treatment for ADHD. Bob's treatment plan will need to address all of Bob's mental health issues and not just those directly relevant to his stalking behaviors, especially given that the role of each of his treatment targets in his stalking behaviors may never be clear. Bob's history is positive for a poor opportunity for attachment, physical abuse victimization, substance use, ADHD, and ODD. Treatment specific for Bob's obsessional behaviors may require psychological interventions such as cognitive-behavioral therapy, psychoeducation, interpersonal skills training, and coping skills development. Pharmacological intervention such as mood stabilizers and antipsychotics may also be required beyond that used for his various psychiatric diagnoses. Earlier sections of this chapter provide details for these interventions and the mixed findings regarding their efficacy.

Because Bob's behaviors have the potential to affect not only his quality of life but also that of others and may even result in harm to others, management of Bob behavior beyond just mental health treatment will be necessary. Ideally, a multidisciplinary team approach should be used that includes a mental health component, the criminal justice system, the school system, and Bob's parents. The criminal justice system can employ measures to encourage compliance with the mental health treatment plan, such as mandatory court-ordered treatment and reporting to the court and/or probation or other legal agency failure to comply with treatment. A protection order may be helpful to provide a means of addressing concerns of the victim, should Bob be allowed to receive treatment in an outpatient setting. Bob's parents will need to be active participants in Bob's mental health treatment plan, education, and legal compliance. Given their history, this may require mental health services for them as a couple and/or individually. If an assessment of Bob's risk for violence or his mental health diagnosis warrants, Bob may be sent to an inpatient or residential care facility rather than a community-based treatment program. Details on violence risk assessment are provided elsewhere in this book.

MANAGEMENT

Given the potential for physical harm and the existence of legal prohibitions, the management of stalking behavior requires a combination of the criminal justice and mental health fields. The use of a multidisciplinary team (McCann, 2001) is ideal for addressing treatment, legal penalties, and protection orders (Meloy, 1997; Mullen, Pathe, Purcell, & Stuart, 1999). Mental health, law enforcement agencies, school officials, and parents should all be included in the management plan (McCann, 2003).

As already noted, treatment compliance is an issue, so methods of ensuring that the elements of the treatment plan are being followed must be in place. Checking blood levels of medications when possible, contact with third parties such as family members, and contact with victims may be necessary to ensure compliance (Rosenfeld, 2000). Legal intervention may be necessary to compel some with stalking behaviors to follow their treatment plans. These can be criminal or civil remedies. Ideally in the case of juvenile offenders, the parents or guardians would be supportive and active participants in ensuring compliance with the treatment plan. This is not always the case, and, even with the best of intentions, they are not always successful.

Some states allow for mandated treatment as part of criminal case sentencing or a condition of probation (Rosenfeld, 2000). This, of course, does not guarantee compliance, but it can provide for a mechanism to track and take action when treatment recommendations are ignored. The success of this avenue is obviously contingent on the availability of resources for providing the treatment, monitoring compliance, and addressing noncompliance. McCann (2001) recommended the use of probation with the requirement of mental health treatment and involuntary commitment if necessary. Civil remedies include involuntary inpatient and outpatient commitment to mental health treatment programs (Rosenfeld, 2000). Some assessment of dangerousness is typically required along with the presence of a mental illness, thus limiting the application of this choice (Rosenfeld, 2000).

Mullen et al.'s (1999) study of 145 stalkers ranging from 15 to 75 years of age revealed themes regarding treatment success, based on stalking motivation, that inform management strategies (Mullen et al., 1999). Stalkers who are hoping for an intimate relationship will require psychiatric intervention regardless of legal system involvement, whereas those reacting to rejection will likely stop when faced with legal sanctions. The targets of incompetent stalkers are generally safe with little effort by authorities, but preventing a new target is required. When predatory behavior is discovered, mental health providers can address the presence of paraphilias, but the legal system typically has a major role. Those who are stalking because of resentment pose the greatest challenge to both legal and mental health intervention.

CONCLUSION

The volume of empirical data to inform our understanding of juvenile stalking is minimal. As a result, assessment and management methods are often extrapolated from the research literature focused on adults and from studies of similar juvenile behavior such as sexual offending and general violence. This is obviously not ideal but at least serves as a starting point.

Although the constraints of a single book chapter prevent a comprehensive treatment of every aspect of juvenile stalking, this effort provides a foundation for mental health professionals faced with assessment and management of juveniles exhibiting such behaviors. More research is needed to understand the etiology, treatment, and prevention of juvenile stalking behaviors. An evidence base is needed to guide clinicians working with youth to improve their quality of life and prevent the victimization of others.

REFERENCES

American Psychiatric Association. (2001). *Diagnostic and statistical manual of mental disorders* (4th ed., text revision). Washington, DC: Author.

Cupach, W. R., & Spitzberg, B. H. (1998). Obsessive relational intrusions and stalking. In B. H. Spitzberg & W. R. Cupach (Eds.), *The dark side of close relationships* (pp. 233–263). Mahwah, NJ: Lawrence Erlbaum.

Kienlen K. K., Birmingham, D. L., Solberg, K. B., O'Regan, J. T., & Meloy, J. R. (1999). A comparative study of psychotic and non-psychotic stalking. *Journal of the American Academy of Psychiatry and the Law, 25,* 317–334.

McAnaney, K. G., Curliss, L. A., & Abeyta-Price, C. E. (1993). From imprudence to crime: Anti-stalking laws. *Notre Dame Law Review, 68,* 819–909.

McCann, J. T. (2001). *Stalking in children and adolescents: The primitive bond.* Washington, DC: American Psychological Association.

McCann, J. T. (2003). Stalking and obsessional forms of harassment in children and adolescents. *Psychiatric Annals, 33*(1), 637–640.

Meloy, J. R. (2002). Stalking and violence. In J. Boon & L. Sheridan (Eds.), *Stalking and psychosexual obsession* (pp. 105–124). London: John Wiley.

Meloy, J. R. (1996). Stalking (obsessional following): A review of some preliminary studies. *Aggression and Violent Behavior, 1*, 147–162.

Meloy, J. R. (1997). The clinical risk management of stalking: "Someone is watching over me." *American Journal of Psychotherapy, 51*, 174–184.

Meloy, J. R., & Gothard, S. A. (1995). Demographic and clinical comparison of obsessional followers and offenders with mental disorders. *American Journal of Psychiatry, 152*, 258–263.

Mohandie, K., Meloy, J. R., McGowan, M. G., & Williams, J. (2006). The RECON typology of stalking: Reliability and validity based upon a large sample of North American stalkers. *Journal of Forensic Sciences, 51*(1), 147–155.

Mullen, P. E., Pathe, M., Purcell, R., & Stuart, G. W. (1999). Study of stalkers. *American Journal of Psychiatry, 156*, 1244–1249.

Nadkarni, R., & Grubin, D. (2000). Stalking: Why do people do it? *British Medical Journal, 320*, 1486–1487.

National Institute of Justice. (1993). *Project to develop a model anti-stalking code for states* (NIJ Publication No. NCJ 144477). Washington, DC: U.S. Government Printing Office.

Palarea, R. E., Zona, M. A., Lane, J. C., & Langhinrichsen-Rohling, J. (1999). The dangerous nature of intimate relationship stalking: threats, violence, and associated factors. *Behavioral Sciences & the Law, 17*(3), 269–283.

Rosenfeld, B. (2000). Assessment and treatment of obsessional harassment. *Aggression and Violent Behavior, 5*(6), 529–549.

Schwartz-Watts, D., & Morgan, D. W. (1998). Violent versus nonviolent stalkers. *Journal of the American Academy of Psychiatry and Law, 26*, 241–245.

Zona, M., & Sharma K. L. (1993). A comparative study of erotomanic and obsessional subjects in a forensic sample. *Journal of Forensic Sciences, 38*, 894–903.

18 Applying Skills Directed Therapy to Aggressive Children

TAMMIE RONEN AND MICHAEL ROSENBAUM

Childhood aggression is one of the most troublesome behavioral problems in Israel and in the United States and has become a major social problem. One significant change that occurred in the study of aggression during the past decade was the shift in focus from the aggressive act per se and the effect of exposure to aggressive models to the aggressive child. Instead of putting the emphasis on aggressive events and the situations that instigate them, the focus now lies on individual differences in cognitive-affective dispositions and in biological predispositions that are assumed to be related to the expression of aggression in social contexts. Researchers are now looking at individual differences based on developmental, cognitive, and other internal components characterizing the aggressive child. This chapter describes the phenomenon of aggression and the theories that explain its occurrence and then proposes a new model for reducing aggression based on skills acquisition.

APPLYING SKILLS DIRECTED THERAPY TO AGGRESSIVE CHILDREN

Childhood aggression is one of the most troublesome behavioral problems in Israel and the United States. Aggression may be defined as overt

---

The authors would like to express their appreciation to Dee B. Ankonina for her editorial assistance.

acts in which aversive physical and verbal events are delivered to others (Buss, 1961; Kazdin, Rodgers, Colbus, & Siegel, 1987). This phenomenon constitutes a major social problem and comprises one of the most frequent reasons behind children's referrals to therapy (Herbert, 2002; Kazdin, 2003; Warman & Cohen, 2000; Webster-Stratton & Reid, 2003). Estimates have indicated that children with behavioral disorders account for from one-third to one-half of all child and adolescent clinic referrals (Herbert, 1987, 2002; Webster-Stratton & Reid, 2003).

Although the frequency of aggression is very high, agreement among researchers regarding aggression is very low. Standard definitions are lacking; explanations for the phenomenon are inconsistent; and the links between theory, assessment, diagnosis, therapy, and evaluation for this problem are weak (Kazdin, 1998).

The problem of aggressive behavior in children is addressed in the *Diagnostic and Statistical Manual of Mental Disorders* (*DSM-IV*; American Psychiatric Association, 1994) under the general category of attention deficit hyperactive and disruptive disorders, which includes conduct disorder, oppositional defiant disorder, disruptive behavior, and attention deficit hyperactive disorder. The most frequently used definitions are conduct disorder and oppositional defiant disorder.

In trying to differentiate between these, conduct disorder is diagnosed when children engage in a persistent pattern of behavior that violates either the basic rights of others or major age-appropriate societal norms or rules (American Psychiatric Association, 1994). Oppositional defiant disorder (ODD) is considered a less severe disorder but one that might presage conduct disorder (Scotti, Mullen, & Hawkins, 1998). ODD involves a recurrent pattern of negativistic, defiant, disobedient, and hostile behavior toward authority figures. It should last at least 6 months, during which four or more of the following are present: often loses temper; often argues with adults; often actively defies or refuses to comply with adults' requests or rules; often deliberately annoys people; often blames others for his or her mistakes or misbehavior; is often touchy or easily annoyed by others; is often angry and resentful; and/or is often spiteful or vindictive (American Psychiatric Association, 1994). Other *DSM-IV* criteria include clinically significant impairment in social, academic, or occupational functioning that stems from the disturbance in behavior and the stipulation that the child's oppositional behavior does not occur exclusively during the course of a psychotic or mood disorder. Differential diagnosis of ODD requires that criteria should not be met for either conduct disorder (aggression toward people or animals, destruction of property, a pattern of theft or deceit) or antisocial personality disorder (over age 18).

The lines between disruptive, oppositional defiant, and conduct disorders are often blurry, with definitions and groupings used interchangeably. Inconsistent and different views exist regarding how to identify those children who should be diagnosed with each of the separate disorders. Part of the complexity in achieving coherent, distinct definitions may be rooted in the extremely broad range of acting-out, undercontrolled, and externalizing behaviors (Achenbach, 1985, 1993; Kazdin, 1987, 1998) displayed by such children. Their behaviors include high rates of noncompliance and defiance in response to teacher requests, aggressiveness, cruelty toward peers, destructive acts, smart talk, lying, stealing, running away, cheating, and many more. Usually, children with disruptive behavior disorders also present comorbidity with learning difficulties, hyperactive and impulsive disorders, anger, anxiety, and depression. It is notably difficult to determine the etiological interrelations between the different comorbid childhood behaviors.

Aggressive children, as well as their peers who are the victims of aggression, suffer from behavioral as well as emotional problems, such as a decrease in their school achievements; a higher risk for dropping out of school; the development of antisocial behavior; and juvenile delinquency (Campbell, 1990; Kazdin & Weisz, 2003; Loeber & Farrington, 2000; McGinnis & Goldstein, 1997; Pope & Bierman, 1999).

CLASSIFICATIONS OF AGGRESSION

Several means have been suggested for classifying aggression. One of the most well known is proactive versus reactive responding. Reactive children are those who respond aggressively to others' aggression toward them. This group has a better prognosis than the other group: proactive children who initiate aggression toward others (Crick & Dodge, 1996; Hubbard, Dodge, Cillessen, Coie, & Schwartz, 2001).

Another classification of aggression is based on the type of aggression: direct versus indirect and physical versus verbal (Bjoerkqvist et al., 2001; Yudovfsky, Silver, Jackson, Endicott, & Williams, 1986). Verbal aggression is generally conceived as less severe and more frequent and acceptable in society than physical aggression. However, children with a higher rate of verbal aggression are also more likely to develop physical aggression

(Miller-Johnson, Coie, Maumary-Gremaud, & Bierman, 2002; Yudofsky et al., 1986).

DEVELOPMENTAL CHARACTERISTICS RELATED TO AGGRESSION

The main developmental component regarding aggression is gender (Bjoerkqvist et al., 2001). Although studies have reported that girls' aggression is on the rise, boys' aggression is still more frequent (Coie, Lochman, Terry, & Hyman, 1992; Crick, 1997; Crick & Grotpeter, 1995). Boys' aggression tends to remain more stable than that of girls, and boys are less prosocial but also less withdrawn than girls (Keltikangas-Jarvinen & Pakaslahti, 1999; Pulkkinen & Pitkanen, 1993; Warman & Cohen, 2000). A higher frequency of direct aggression emerged among boys, whereas girls presented a higher frequency of indirect aggression (Osterman et al., 1999).

Another important component is age. Aggression increases at the point of entry to preschool but tends to decrease naturally as children grow older. Thus, a higher rate of aggression is expected among younger children, with the exception of the small percentage of older children who develop conduct and antisocial disorders (Broidy et al., 2003).

Although gender and age are the main developmental components influencing aggression, one cannot ignore situational influences, especially transitions, crises, and distress. Epidemiological studies show that children respond to change by developing behavioral and emotional problems (Lapouse & Monk, 1958). This is true for any kind of change but especially among children in distress, in crisis, or in transitional or traumatic situations (Ronen, Rahav, & Apple, 2003; Ronen, Rahav, & Rosenbaum, 2003). Especially prominent under such conditions are affect-related symptoms: negative emotions (anger), anxiety, stress, and loneliness (Cole, Michel, & O'Donnell-Teti, 1994; Pope & Bierman, 1999).

NEW DIRECTIONS IN STUDYING AGGRESSION

Petit and Dodge (2003) noted that, "in spite of enormous attention to the issue, clinical practice and public policy have not had a significant impact on reducing the childhood violence" (p. 187). Obviously, then, research and practice on childhood aggression must change directions and emphases.

One of the most significant changes that has occurred in the study of aggression during the past decade is the shift in focus from the aggressive act per se and the effect of exposure to aggressive models (Bandura & Walters, 1963) to the aggressive child himself or herself (Hartup, 2005). Instead of putting the emphasis on aggressive events and the situations that instigate them, the focus now is on individual differences in cognitive-affective dispositions and in biological predispositions that are assumed to be related to the expression of aggression in social contexts (Tremblay, Hartup, & Archer, 2005). Researchers are now looking at individual differences based on developmental, cognitive, and other internal components characterizing the aggressive child.

Representative examples of this fairly new approach to the study of aggression can be found in the theoretical models developed by Dodge and Pettit (2003) and by Anderson and Bushman (2002). In their biopsychosocial model, Dodge and Pettit posit that "biological dispositions and socio-cultural contexts place certain children at risk in early life but that life experience with parents, peers, and social institutions increment and mediate that risk" (p. 349). An important part of their model describes how these factors lead children and adolescents to develop idiosyncratic social knowledge about their world. This knowledge may guide the individual child to process social information in a way that prompts the child to act aggressively. For example, an aggressive child is more likely to attribute malicious intentions to others than a nonaggressive child. Dodge and his colleagues worked for over two decades to substantiate their claim that the processing of social information is important to understanding why children act aggressively (e.g., Crick & Dodge, 1994; Dodge, 1986). Nevertheless, Dodge and Pettit noted that the magnitude of prediction of social information processing factors "in most studies is fairly modest" (p. 362).

The major strengths of Dodge and Pettit's model are that it combines both biological predispositions and social factors in one model and that it attempts to describe how these factors lead children to process social information in ways that may or may not encourage aggressive behavior. Rather than relating to situational stimuli per se, the model emphasizes the internal factors within the aggressive children that prompt aggressive behavior—that is, the child's response to the situational stimuli. Dodge and his coauthors relate to personal dispositions (such as sensitivity to rejection, hostility, and sense of loneliness) and point out the way children use their social schemas, social knowledge, and acquired rules to process social information and respond aggressively to the stimuli.

Similarly, the main thrust of the general aggression model (GAM) proposed by Anderson and Bushman (2002) was directed toward situational variables rather than personality variables. Joireman, Anderson, and Strathman (2003) revised the original GAM by giving more prominence to personality variables. Specifically, they addressed the issue of the "aggression paradox" (Husermann & Eron, 1989): Why do certain individuals habitually engage in aggressive acts, despite the apparently negative consequences? The seemingly best solution to such a paradox attributes the apparent consistency of aggressive behavior to personality variables rather than situational variables. Personality dispositions may lead individuals to act aggressively even when such behavior leads to punishment. According to Joireman et al., personality variables and situational variables interact to influence individuals' current affects, cognitions, and behaviors. Thus, as Joireman et al. demonstrated, individuals who tend to seek sensations (as a personality disposition; Zuckerman, 1994) are most likely to be attracted to aggression-eliciting situations. Furthermore, their findings revealed that people who tend to have a hostile view of the world and tend to be easily angered (both considered "traits") are more likely to act aggressively in response to aggressive challenges. Joireman et al. did not find, as they hypothesized, that the sensation-seeking–aggression relationship is mediated by hostility. Yet they found that anger is a mediator between hostility and physical aggression (cf. Buss & Perry, 1992).

In contrast to the social learning models of aggression (e.g., Bandura, 1973), the aforementioned aggression models do not dwell on the issue of how aggressive behavior is acquired, but rather focus on the personal and environmental factors that predispose the individual to behave aggressively ("risk factors"; Orpinas & Horne, 2006). In fact, research evidence is accumulating in support of the view that aggressive behavior exists in the behavioral repertoire of every individual. Furthermore, recent twin studies have revealed that individual differences in physical aggression are in large part determined by genetic factors (Brendgen, Vitaro, Boivin, Dionne, & Perusse, 2006) and to a lesser extent by environmental factors at least up to the age of 6 years. Rhee and Waldman (2002), who reviewed studies on aggression and antisocial behavior, suggested that genetic effects diminish with age. "As such, it is possible that heritable factors may play a larger role initially in placing a child at risk for reactively or proactively aggressive behavior but that later socialization experiences determine whether the child overcomes this risk" (Brendgen et al., 2006, p. 1309).

Tremblay and Nagin (2005) summarized previous research on physical aggression trajectories from early childhood to adulthood and concluded that the peak in frequency of physical aggression for the large majority of humans is probably between the second and fourth year after birth. A small proportion of children (probably around 6% of all children) exhibit physical aggression that declines more slowly, with a possible brief increase during adolescence (Broidy et al., 2003). Based on these epidemiological findings, Tremblay and Nagin (2005) suggested that physical aggression is neither a behavior that is socially learned nor a drive that must be satisfied. Rather, it is an internal disposition. "Children do not need to learn how to be aggressive, but how to control their aggressive behavior" (pp. 99–100). This view upholds the notion that physical aggression is and will always be part of humans' behavioral repertoire, although it is under control most of the time by most people.

Orpinas and Horne (2006) noted that, during the past 50 years, studies on child and adolescent aggression have focused primarily on the risk factors that predispose a child to behave aggressively. Only recently have educators and researchers begun to study the protective factors or the developmental assets that have the "potential to improve the well being of youth and to reduce aggression" (p. 34).

PERSONALITY-BASED MODEL OF AGGRESSION

The studies presented in this chapter focus on personal dispositions that act as vulnerability factors for aggressive behavior and on personal dispositions that protect the individual from acting aggressively. We conceptualized these personal variables within the cognitive-affective processing system framework (Mischel & Shoda, 1995).

We developed a personality-based model of aggressive behavior that derives from Mischel and Shoda's (1995) cognitive-affective system theory of personality, in which "individuals differ in how they selectively focus on different features of situations, how they categorize and encode them cognitively and emotionally, and how those encodings activate and interact with other cognitions and affects in the personality system" (p. 252). In this framework, *person variables* are cognitive-affective dispositions or units that consist of mental representations, such as encoding, expectations, beliefs, and affects that influence overt behavior. "The theory accounts for individual differences in overall average levels of behavior and for stable *if . . . then . . .* profiles of behavior variability across situations, as essential expressions of the same underlying personality system" (p. 252). Mischel and Shoda list five types of cognitive-affective units in the personality-mediating system: encoding categories, expectancies and beliefs, affects and emotions, goals and values, and competencies and self-regulatory plans.

In the studies reported below, we identify a number of cognitive-affective dispositions (CADs) that represent the five types suggested by Mischel and Shoda (1995). These include three aggression-promoting dispositions and two aggression-buffering dispositions that may affect overt behavior:

1. *Dispositional expectations.* We focused our research of dispositional expectations mainly on "rejection sensitivity," which was conceptualized as "the cognitive-affective processing disposition to anxiously expect, readily perceive, and intensely react to rejection" (Ayduk et al., 2000, p. 777). These kinds of expectations were closely linked to aggressive behavior (Leary, Twenge, & Quinlivan, 2006).
2. *Dispositional cognitive encoding.* We focused on hostile thought as a major cognitive disposition for interpreting others' behaviors or intentions. In this disposition, one encodes others' actions as basically hostile and not fair to oneself, and one encodes others' good intentions as suspicious (Buss & Perry, 1992).
3. *Dispositional affects and emotions.* In investigating aggression, the natural choice for study was the affective disposition of anger as an emotional internal response to external or internal cues (Buss & Perry, 1992).
4. *Goals and values* were also viewed as basic aspects of a cognitive-affective disposition. In particular, we focused on the study of prosocial goals as a motivational force to restrain aggression. The wish to become part of society and the need to be involved serve as goals that reduce one's aggressive responding and turn it into socially desirable responding (Ludwig & Pittman, 1999).
5. *Self-control.* In almost all of our studies, we focused on one's ability for self-control. That is, the tendency to use cognitive means such as cognitive reframing, attentional distraction, problem solving, and planning to attain specific goals even when confronting various obstacles.

We conceptualized that these five CADs' organization and interactions would determine whether aggressive behavior would be produced under specific social situations. Some of these CADs may serve as mediators between other CADs, and some may have a moderating or a constraining function on aggression. Most importantly, together with prosocial values, self-control skills were conceptualized as the major force against aggression, enabling humans to act positively rather than aggressively. Prosocial goals and self-control skills are stable personal dispositions that moderate and constrain the effects of aggression-promoting CADs on aggressive behavior.

On the other hand, dispositional rejection-sensitive expectations, hostile cognitive encoding, and angry emotions would be expected to exacerbate the effects of aggression-promoting CADs on aggressive behavior. For example, an individual's disposition toward hostilely encoding various social cues may mediate the relations between his or her expectations or basic beliefs about the nature of an interpersonal relationship (e.g., "She is being nice to me because she wants to exploit me for her own interests") and that individual's overt aggressive behavior. Yet, when individuals have long-range prosocial life goals as well as the necessary self-control and self-regulatory competencies, they should be able to minimize the effects of hostile cognitions on their expression of aggressive behavior (e.g., "I don't know why she is being nice to me, but if I am nice to her as well, we might become friends").

Studies Relating to the CAD Model

We recently conducted a series of studies to examine the CAD model of aggression. As mentioned, the model proposes that self-control processes moderate the connection between personal vulnerabilities and aggressive behavior by modifying the cognitive-affective aspects of aggression.

The first study was conducted to test the hypothesis that the relationship between rejection sensitivity and aggressive behavior is mediated by a disposition toward hostile encoding (to be labeled here as *hostility*) and negative affect (i.e., anger).

The participants were 771 adolescents who studied in the seventh and eighth grades in 12 different middle schools in central Israel. Each adolescent completed a set of questionnaires that included Buss and Perry's (1992) Aggression Questionnaire, comprising three subscales: aggressive behavior, hostile cognitions, and angry feelings. In addition, they were asked to complete the Rejection Sensitivity Questionnaire

(Downey, Lebolt, Rincon, & Freitas, 1998). To establish the reliability of the children's self-reports, the teachers were asked to assess their students on their level of aggressive behavior, social skills, and rejection sensitivity on a scale developed by Coie and Dodge (1988). Once the children's self-reports were found to be reliable and valid, we used only the data from the children. Using structural equations modeling, we found, as predicted, that both hostility and anger mediated the relationship between rejection sensitivity and aggressive behavior. More specifically, we found that rejection sensitivity, as a cognitive-affective disposition, led to hostility that in turn led to anger, and anger led to aggressive behavior. Children who expected social rejection tended to suspect the good intentions of others and often viewed other people as potentially hostile toward them. Hostility was often translated into angry feelings and aggressive behavior.

The findings emphasized the importance of considering the cognitions and emotions underlying aggressive acts. Changing one's hostile view of the social world may reduce aggressive behavior (Ronen, Weisbord, & Rosenbaum, 2007).

In a second study, we tested the hypothesis that self-control skills would moderate the effects of rejection sensitivity on aggressive behavior via the mediation of hostile cognitions. Among individuals who were high on rejection sensitivity and who had a rich repertoire of self-control skills, we predicted less hostile cognitions (and, consequently, less aggressive behavior) in comparison to individuals who were high on rejection sensitivity but who had a poor repertoire of self-control skills.

The 283 seventh- and eighth-graders (169 boys and 115 girls) who participated in the study completed the Children's Self-Control Scale (Rosenbaum & Ronen, 1991) in addition to the Rejection Sensitivity Questionnaire (Downey et al., 1998) and Aggression Questionnaire (Buss & Perry, 1992). As expected, self-control skills moderated the relationship between rejection sensitivity and hostility but not the relationship between rejection sensitivity and anger or aggressive behavior. Adolescents scoring high on self-control skills did not develop hostility even at high levels of rejection sensitivity. In contrast, those who were high on rejection sensitivity but low on self-control skills reported higher levels of hostility. It should be noted that these findings were only among the adolescents who were high on rejection sensitivity. No gender effects were found.

These outcomes indicated the importance of self-control skills in the process of controlling aggressive behavior. They also emphasized the

Chapter 18 Applying Skills Directed Therapy to Aggressive Children

utility of studying the hostile cognitions that underlie aggressive behavior (Weisbord, Rosenbaum, & Ronen, 2007).

The third study was conducted to examine whether two major personal dispositions moderate the relationship between hostility/anger and aggressive behavior. These dispositions were self-control skills and identification with social values. We conceived of these factors as two independent personality dispositions that, in interaction with each other, help control aggressive behavior. One's social values determine the social goals one is motivated to pursue, whereas self-control skills enable one to attain these goals by behaving in a nonaggressive way. Specifically, the major hypothesis tested in this third study was that children who have hostile cognitions and angry feelings will not behave aggressively if they have prosocial goals and have high levels of self-control skills. Furthermore, we hypothesized that children who had high levels of self-control skills but were low in prosocial values were likely to behave aggressively if they had hostile cognitions and angry feelings. These children would not be motivated to use their self-control skills to control their aggressive behavior.

Participants here comprised 450 children age 9 to 11 years in the fourth, fifth, and sixth grades of two elementary schools in central Israel. The children completed four scales: the Aggression Questionnaire (Buss & Perry, 1992), which has four subscales assessing hostility, anger, physical aggression, and indirect aggression; a three-item scale assessing the child's physical and verbal aggression; the Children's Self-Control Scale (Rosenbaum & Ronen, 1991); and the Pro-Social Self-Regulation Questionnaire (Ryan & Connell, 1989). In addition, teachers assessed the frequency and intensity of each child's behavioral problems, including aggressive behavior, using the Eyberg Child Behavior Inventory (Robinson, Eyberg, & Ross, 1980).

Overall, the data confirmed that hostility and anger correlated highly with aggressive behavior only in children who were low in prosocial values and low in self-control skills but not in children who were high on these two factors. Furthermore, only among children who were low in prosocial values did we find no correlation between self-control skills and aggressive behavior, in contrast to children who were high on prosocial values. Clearly self-control skills reduced aggressive behavior only in children with high levels of prosocial values. Interestingly, only among children who were low in anger and in self-control skills were higher prosocial values related to less aggressive behavior. Our findings clearly indicate that, although a child may have hostile cognitions and angry feelings, the child may not show any aggressive behavior if and only if he or she has a rich repertoire of self-control skills and prosocial values. Thus, self-control skills alone are not enough for controlling aggressive behavior. They must be accompanied by a motivation to use them for prosocial purposes.

These outcomes are important both for theorizing about personal dispositions that lead to aggressive behavior and for designing effective intervention programs. Any program to reduce aggressive behavior must consist of training in self-control skills as well as in the acquisition of prosocial values. Our findings also reemphasized the importance of hostile cognitions and angry feelings in the development of aggressive behavior (Eppel, Ronen, & Rosenbaum, 2007).

APPLYING INTERVENTIONS TO AGGRESSIVE BEHAVIOR

Kazdin (1998) noted three kinds of promising intervention programs for children who evidence behavioral disturbances: functional family therapy, parent and teacher counseling, and cognitive problem-solving models. Most interventions relate to the child's environment as responsible for his or her behavior, and they expect that changes in education style and discipline methods will change the child's behavior. Family therapists view the family as responsible for its problematic communication style, roles, and negotiations. Family therapy aims to change the members' roles and teach them a better way to relate to one another (Howard & Kendall, 1996; Kazdin, 1998; Patterson, 1982; Webster-Stratton, 1993). Parent and teacher supervision relies on the tenet that behavioral disturbances produce positive outcomes for the child, such as a sense of being strong and capable of achieving one's goals. Through supervision, parents and teachers learn to change these secondary outcomes and thereby to change the child's behavior (Hughes, 1993; Kazdin, 1998; Webster-Stratton, 1993).

Individual or group therapy with children takes a different viewpoint. Rather than searching for various ways to ensure child compliance, these methods encourage the child to apply skills toward changing his or her own behavior. Such intervention is based on the view of the disorder as a result of lacking skills, requiring application of new skills. A range of deficient skills characterize aggressive children in the cognitive, emotional, and behavioral domains (Bailey, 1998; Crick & Dodge, 1994; Hughes, 1993; Kazdin & Weisz, 2003; Kendall & Chu, 2000). In the cognitive domain, aggressive children express high rates of hostile cues in social situations; they attend to few cues when interpreting the meaning of others' behavior; and they attribute the behavior of others to hostile intentions when in ambiguous situations. When they are in contact with other aggressive children, they tend to underestimate their own level of aggression. Studies of children with behavioral disorders have revealed difficulties among these children suggesting that aggressive children present difficulties in delaying gratification, overcoming temptation, planning, and establishing targets and criteria for their behavior (Kazdin & Weisz, 2003; Kendall & Chu, 2000).

In the emotional domain, these children evidence difficulties in skills related to expressing both positive and negative emotion (Scotti et al., 1998), identifying emotion, understanding and accepting emotion, and controlling emotion (Ronen, 2004). As for the behavioral domain, children with behavioral disorders have been shown to lack the social skills necessary for conducting adequate interpersonal relationships (Crick & Dodge, 1994; Kazdin, 1998; Ronen, 2004).

Studies have pinpointed the efficacy of cognitive therapy in changing disruptive, defiant behavior (Bailey, 1998; Durlak, Fuhrman, & Lampman, 1991; Kendall & Chu, 2000; Ronen, 2003). The most popular cognitive techniques for reducing aggressive behavior consist of cognitive problem skill training and social skills training. Teaching a child to refrain from aggressive cognitions and to emphasize alternative social cognitions appears to successfully decrease aggressive behavior. Such programs incorporate constant reinforcements of prosocial behavior and discussions of antisocial behavior (Bailey, 1998), with training to improve social relationships via role play, observation, modeling, practicing techniques, and application of self-control skills.

SELF-CONTROL MODEL FOR AGGRESSION

The next section describes the Empowering Children and Adolescents Project as a model for evidence-based practice with aggression. The project, which was established in 2000 and supported by the JDC (Jewish Federation) and the Pratt Foundation, operates in the Bob Shapell School of Social Work at Tel-Aviv University, Israel. The project was founded to establish a clinical research center for study and intervention targeting children with oppositional defiant disorders and aggressive behavior, incorporating professional training in this specialized area and implementation of the intervention in educational and therapeutic settings around the country.

First, we will describe the importance of skills acquisition in child therapy; then, we will present the self-control model we have developed; finally, we will address the outcomes of implementations of our model with children and adolescents.

Importance of Skills Acquisition in Child and Adolescent Treatments

Lacking certain skills was found to be linked to behavioral disorders in several studies. Osterman et al. (1999) reported a correlation between aggression, especially physical aggression, and poor internal self-control skills. Bandura and his colleagues proposed self-efficacy (as an important cognitive skill) to be a major predictor in preventing transgressive behavior among children (Bandura, Caprara, Barbaranelli, & Pastorelli, 2001). They claimed that children with low academic self-efficacy, low social self-efficacy, and low personal self-efficacy will exhibit aggression.

Rosenbaum (1993, 1998) emphasized self-control as a set of goal-directed skills that enable humans to act upon their aims; overcome difficulties relating to thoughts, emotions, and behaviors; delay gratification; and cope with distress. Studies have pinpointed a link between self-control skills and the ability to cope with various types of distress such as anxiety (Hamama, Ronen, & Feigin, 2000; Ronen & Rosenbaum, 2001). Imparting children with self-control skills in school has emerged as an effective tool for reducing aggressive behavior (Ronen, 2003).

Skills-Directed Therapy Model for Children's Behavioral Disorders

Skills-directed therapy (SDT) focuses on skills acquisition and is conducted as a goal-directed therapy to determine which of the child's goals direct his or her behavior, which skills are needed for the child to become able to act in the desired manner, and which skills the child lacks and needs to learn in order to overcome the specific disorder. The skills in SDT are rooted in developmental psychology and combine features from all areas of the child's life.

In relating to cognitive development, the model emphasizes the fact that, at different ages and stages, children hold unique cognitive levels of comprehension that affect how the children construct and construe a view of the self and of the world (Mash & Barkley, 1996; Mash & Dozois, 1996). It is therefore crucial to consider children's linguistic skills (Luria, 1961; Vygotzky, 1962), skills for self-talk (Mischel, 1973, 1974), and ability to process social information (Crick & Dodge, 1994; Dodge & Pettit, 2003). The SDT model thus accounts for children's cognitive development by advocating that therapists utilize simple language familiar to children, focus on the specific ways in which children process information, and relate therapeutic techniques to the specific child's age and cognitive stage. Intervention targeting aggression is designed as a training course in children's skills for behavior change. The manuals and techniques derive from appealing methods such as imagery, metaphors, exercises, drawing, sculpturing, illustrations, and demonstrations, which serve to adapt the intervention's contents to children's cognitive ability for understanding the treatment's concepts (e.g., self-control). The child learns about the links between behaviors, emotions, and thoughts; learns to use self-talk and change automatic thoughts using day-to-day examples; experiences demonstrations, concretizations, role playing, and rehearsal in the therapeutic setting; and applies the learned skills at home.

Beyond cognitive features, SDT also takes into account children's emotional and social development as well as parental roles and cultural norms and influences. Regarding emotional features, the ability to experience, express, and understand emotions changes over children's development and holds important implications for interventions that train children in needed skills. Emotions can also be viewed as a set of skills enabling children to socialize and adjust to the world (Ronen, 2003; Shirk & Russell, 1996; Thompson, 1989). SDT interventions for children who exhibit aggression underscore the acquisition of skills for emotional change by pinpointing these children's ability to express, identify, accept, understand, and control emotions. Therapists work directly toward these goals, teaching children and training them in the needed emotions and practicing the learned skills.

Regarding social features, social experiences and social interactions crucially influence children's ability to become an integral part of society and to develop self-concept, self-identity, and self-control (Harter, 1983; Ronen, 2003). A child's behavior with peers, the peers' responses to the child, and the child's thoughts about those responses all comprise central factors in determining the child's self-perceptions. As children develop, they advance in their capacity to differentiate between self and others, not only as separate entities, but as possessing different subjective ways of coping and feeling. Both of these evolving processes are prerequisites for establishing and maintaining meaningful relationships (Schaffer, 1990, 1996). SDT interventions for children with aggression relate to social development in a group setting, by forming homogeneous groups of children who can practice in vivo communication, social relations, and social skills.

The SDT model also accounts for the parents' roles. Whenever a child is concerned, the parents should be involved. Parents comprise the child's immediate and main support system (Ronen, 2003). Parents not only act as important change agents for the child, but also hold responsibility for the child's learning, normal development, and ability for change (Patterson, 1975, 1982; Webster-Stratton, 1993, 1994). Among all their other roles, parents play very important roles for the child's skills acquisition, specifically as role models and direct trainers. SDT interventions emphasize the family role by designing parent supervision groups. Parents of each of the involved children participate in a parent group and undergo a similar program, relating first to themselves and how they can acquire skills and then to their children and how to educate their children to use appropriate skills.

And last but not least are the cultural elements of SDT. Being part of society and understanding cultural norms and rules hold critical importance for adequate social adjustment, prosocial behavior, positive communication, and social skills. Involvement in society necessitates a set of skills for adjustment and adaptation with society. The SDT model accounts for cultural norms and influences by trying to impart the child with skills for identifying environmental cues, cultural thinking, and other persons' perspectives (Dorfman, Meyer, & Morgan, 2004). Children practice such skills by analyzing stories, interpreting pictures, and relating to information raised in their day-to-day environment.

In sum, all of the developmental features, family components, and cultural considerations described above are integrated into a unified intervention model of self-control.

Self-Control Intervention Modules

The self-control intervention model developed by Ronen and Rosenbaum (2001) provides an extension of the basic self-control intervention program developed by Ronen to treat various children's disorders (Ronen, 1993a, 1993b, 2003). This model aims to impart children with self-control skills for reducing aggressive behavior. The model contains four modules.

The first module is *cognitive restructuring*. The child learns that the problem is a behavior, that a behavior can be changed if the child learns how to change it, and that change depends on the child (Beck, 1963; Beck, Emery, & Greenberg, 1985; Beck, Freeman, & Associates, 1990). The child acquires skills to observe the problem, assess it, set goals and targets for change, and redefine it as behavior that depends on the child. The therapist elicits cognitive restructuring by increasing children's self-efficacy about their ability to achieve change (Bandura, 1997), as well as by utilizing redefinition, changing attributional styles, and reframing the child's present functioning (Beck et al., 1985; Kanfer & Schefft, 1988; Meichenbaum, 1985). The techniques used include Socratic questions and paradoxical examples.

The second module is *problem analysis*. The child practices the skills for observing the links between the brain, body, and final problematic behaviors. The child learns to notice the links between thoughts, emotions, and behaviors and to understand the link between cause and effect (Beck, 1963; Ronen, 2003). The therapist uses rational analysis of these processes, employs written materials and anatomical illustrations of the human body, and helps the child accept responsibility for behaviors by learning to change the brain's commands. The child practices identifying automatic thoughts and uses the skills of self-talk and self-recording to change unmediated thoughts into mediated ones.

The third module is *attentional focus*. The child practices the skills needed to increase awareness of behavior and internal stimuli, raises sensitivity to the body, and particularly learns to identify internal cues related to the specific problem (Bandura, 1997; Mahoney, 1991, 1995). The therapist uses relaxation, concentration, and self-monitoring to promote achievement of these targets.

The fourth module is *self-control practice*. The child practices self-control skills such as self-talk, self-evaluation, self-monitoring, thinking aloud, and problem-solving skills (Barrios & Hartman, 1988; Brigham, Hopper, Shaw, & Emery, 1979; Ronen, 2003).

Application of the Model in Group Sessions

Aggression is a social problem. We therefore proposed that treating aggression in groups would enable children to experience in vivo different ways of relating to one another and to practice skills. The Empowering Children and Adolescents Project's overall goals consisted of studying the problem of ODD and aggression, developing an effective intervention manual, and training university students as well as field professionals to apply an effective intervention for children with ODD.

Children had been referred to the university project by social workers, teachers, counselors, or parents. The parents and the teachers completed the Conners (1969) and Eyberg scales (Robinson et al., 1980). Children who were assessed as high on both scales (suffering from a high frequency of behavior disorders) were invited to participate in the intervention groups. Usually, the adult environment (parents, teachers) was very interested in having the referred child participate in intervention. However, very rarely did the children themselves demonstrate motivation to do so. We wrote up a contract with the children, promising them that if they chose to leave the group after the first three sessions, they could drop out then.

The dropout rate was very low, usually occurring only if children were sick and could not attend and then lost momentum. After the first two or three sessions, children realized that they could benefit from the group and were happy to participate.

Children's Group Design

Each child participated in a 12-session course with a group that was homogeneous in terms of age and problems. Each 75-minute session presented new knowledge and combined demonstrations, practice, discussion, and homework assignments.

Because some of the children were very aggressive, the supervisor sat outside the room during sessions, in the event that the group leaders (who were students) found it difficult to cope with the children and needed help. Several times, the group leaders took one of the children outside to sign a behavioral contract with the supervisors stating that they could only continue participating if they improved their behavior in the group.

Session Contents

During this course, children learned what a behavior is, how to look at their aggression as a behavior, how their behavior is connected to their thoughts and emotions, what kinds of techniques can help them change their behavior, and so on. They learned to assess, evaluate, and plan the change process; they established criteria and expectations for change; they learned to observe, evaluate, and reinforce themselves;

and they learned to identify their internal cues and to replace automatic thoughts with mediated ones. The 12 sessions incorporated the following contents:

1. Getting to know the group members, presenting the program, exploring initial expectations, generating motivation for change, and developing an initial contract.
2. Increasing familiarity, clarifying expectations, learning about the term *behavior*, identifying behaviors that people exhibit, practicing observation methods.
3. Defining the client as a scientist and the intervention as a research study focusing on the client's behavior and the homework as research assignments.
4. Understanding that the behavior is related to commands the brain gives the body, identifying autonomous commands, and understanding how they take place and how they contribute to the existing problem.
5. Learning how to distinguish between autonomous and mediated commands, identifying the link that exists between an event and the interpretation we give it, understanding how a negative interpretation can be turned into a positive one.
6. Reviewing the connection between the event, the autonomous negative interpretation, and the planned positive interpretation; practicing focus on physical sensations and understanding how to identify the location of the sensation, its intensity, and what it indicates.
7. Identifying feelings, drawing a connection between feelings and physical sensations, identifying the internal cues pinpointing specific sensations and emotions, and drawing a connection between the situation/event, the intensity of the feeling, and the physical sensations.
8. Identifying various feelings and drawing a connection between the event and the feeling it arouses.
9. Learning about the link that exists between thoughts, feelings, and behaviors; learning how to modify behavior by changing the interpretation we attach to the event.
10. Learning how to use self-speech and self-instructions and developing tools and skills for modifying behavior.
11. Testing progress and continuing practice.
12. Evaluation and summary.

The Model's Implementation Outcomes

As a first phase, we applied this model at our university research clinic. For 3 years, students supervised by us conducted 10 groups of children and parents each semester. The groups showed a very small percentage of dropouts. After proving its efficacy, we started training teachers, educators, and social workers to apply the model each year in the children's natural settings. For the last 3 years, the program has been implemented in 10 to 20 new schools annually.

To assess the intervention's efficacy outcomes, we compared parents', teachers', and children's baseline reports with their termination reports, and we compared child treatment groups to control groups that were matched on aggression scores. Parents and teachers completed the Eyberg Child Behavior Inventory (Robinson et al., 1980) and the Conners Rating Scale (Conners, 1969). Children completed the Children's Problematic Behavior Inventory (Ronen, Rahav, & Moldavsky, in press), Buss and Perry's (1992) scale measuring aggression, and the self-control scale (Rosenbaum & Ronen, 1991).

Teachers, fathers, and mothers reported a significant decrease in the severity of children's behavior problems (Eyberg inventory) at the end of the program, compared to their preintervention ratings. The extent of reported change (the difference between Eyberg termination and baseline ratings) was 12.3 according to teachers, 10.0 according to mothers, and 6.3 according to fathers. (The scale scores ranged from 36 to 180.) Likewise, teachers, fathers, and mothers reported a significant reduction in children's rate of impulsive and disruptive behavior (Conners scale). The extent of reported change (the difference between the Conners termination and baseline ratings) was 5.43 according to teachers, 3.89 according to mothers, and 2.08 according to fathers. (The scale scores ranged from 12 to 36.) Children's self-reported aggressiveness also revealed a significant reduction, from 23.50 before the intervention to 21.66 at termination, a difference of 1.83. (The scale scores ranged from 13 to 65.) All differences were significant ($p < .05$). No significant change was observed in any of the scales in the control group when comparing baseline to termination.

In sum, mothers, fathers, teachers, and the children all provided feedback about the project's effectiveness. Outcomes from the first 3 years of conducting the treatment course in small children's groups revealed a very high percentage of change. That is, children attending these groups significantly improved their self-control skills and significantly reduced their aggressive behavior according to children's, parents', and teachers' assessments. The treatment boasted a very low dropout rate and a very high rate of maintaining treatment outcomes at the 2-year follow-up.

CONCLUSION

Aggression poses a major problem to the basic fabric of any society. As our research has shown, people often act aggressively against other people when they are excluded from society or when they fearfully expect to be rejected by significant others. Aggressive behavior is in direct contrast with the universal human need to belong. This has been labeled as the "aggression paradox." Individuals hurt mostly those people with whom they want to be closest. Why? In our research, we are trying to solve the puzzle of human aggressive behavior.

Based on past research, we believe that people are born with the basic disposition to solve interpersonal problems by acting aggressively. However, to be a part of society and satisfy their need to belong, everyone must learn to restrain aggressive behavior. Every society develops a set of laws and regulations to curb aggressive acts among its members. Most people fear punishment and have acquired enough social values to control their aggressive behavior.

The main focus of our research at the Schwartz Laboratory, with the help of the JDC and the Pratt Foundation, was to pinpoint the cognitive-affective dispositions that help individuals (children and adults) restrain their aggressive behavior through the use of self-control skills and the acquisition of prosocial values. As our studies have demonstrated, people control their aggressive behaviors by self-controlling their hostile cognitions (that usually lead to anger, which is followed by aggressive conduct). Prosocial values provide the guiding force behind the application of self-control skills to control one's hostility. Whereas most past research on aggression has focused on the aggressive act itself, our research is focused on the study of the cognitive-affective processes that lead one to act or not to act aggressively. We are interested specifically in understanding the cognitive-affective dispositions that lead a person to act nonaggressively even when provoked and even when there are no explicit sanctions against aggressive behavior. Early results of these intervention programs we developed, based on those assumptions, showed very encouraging results.

REFERENCES

Achenbach, T. M. (1985). *Assessment and taxonomy of child and adolescent psychopathology.* Beverly Hills, CA: Sage.
Achenbach, T. M. (1993). Implications of multiaxial empirically based assessment for behavior therapy with children. *Behavior Therapy, 24,* 91–116.
American Psychiatric Association. (1994). *Diagnostic and statistical manual of mental disorders* (4th ed.). Washington, DC: Author.
Anderson, C. A., & Bushman, B. (2002). Human aggression. *Annual Review of Psychology, 53,* 27–51.
Ayduk, O., Mendonza-Denton, R., Mischel, W., Downey, G., Peake, P., & Rodriquez, M. (2000). Regulating the interpersonal self: Strategic self-regulation for coping with rejection sensitivity. *Journal of Personality and Social Psychology, 79,* 776–792.
Bailey, V. (1998). Conduct disorders in young children. In P. Graham (Ed.), *Cognitive behaviour therapy with children and families* (pp. 95–109). Cambridge, England: Cambridge University Press.
Bandura, A. (1973). *Aggression: A social learning analysis.* Englewood Cliffs, NJ: Prentice Hall.
Bandura, A. (1997). *Self-efficacy: The exercise of control.* New York: W. H. Freeman.
Bandura, A., Caprara, G. V., Barbaranelli, C., & Pastorelli, C. (2001). Sociocognitive self-regulatory mechanisms governing transgressive behavior. *Journal of Personality and Social Behavior, 80,* 125–135.
Bandura, A., & Walters, R. H. (1963). *Social learning and imitation.* New York: Holt, Rinehart, & Winston.
Barrios, B. A., & Hartman, D. P. (1988). Fears and anxieties. In E. J. Mash & L. G. Terdal (Eds.), *Behavioral assessment of childhood disorders* (2nd ed., pp. 196–262). New York: Guilford Press.
Beck, A. T. (1963). Thinking and depression. *Archives of General Psychiatry, 9,* 324–333.
Beck, A. T., Emery, G., & Greenberg, R. L. (1985). *Anxiety disorders and phobias.* New York: Basic Books.
Beck, A. T., Freeman, A., & Associates. (1990). *Cognitive therapy of personality disorders.* New York: Guilford Press.
Bjoerkqvist, K., Osterman, K., Lagerspetz-Kirsti, M. J., Landau, S. F., Carpara, G. V., & Fraczek, A. (2001). Aggression, victimization and sociometric status: Findings from Finland, Israel, Italy and Poland. In R. J. Martin & D. B. Richardson (Eds.), *Cross-cultural approaches to research on aggression and reconciliation* (pp. 111–119). Hunting, NY: Nova Science.
Brendgen, M., Vitaro, F., Boivin, M., Dionne, G., & Perusse, D. (2006). Examining genetic and environmental effects on reactive versus proactive aggression. *Developmental Psychology, 42,* 1299–1312.
Brigham, T. A., Hopper, A. J., Shaw, B. F., & Emery, G. (1979). *Cognitive therapy of depression.* New York: Guilford Press.
Broidy, L. M., Nagin, D. S., Tremblay, R. E., Bates, J. E., Brame, B., Dodge, K. A., et al. (2003). Developmental trajectories of childhood disruptive behaviors and adolescent delinquency: A six site, cross national study. *Developmental Psychology, 39,* 222–245.
Buss, A. H. (1961). *The psychology of aggression.* New York: Wiley.

Buss, A. H., & Perry, M. (1992). The aggression questionnaire. *Journal of Personality and Social Psychology, 63*, 452–459.

Campbell, S. B. (1990). *Behavior problems in preschool children: Clinical and development issues*. New York: Guilford Press.

Coie, J. D., & Dodge, K. A. (1988). Multiple sources of data on social behavior and social status in the school: A cross-age comparison. *Child Development, 59*, 815–829.

Coie, J. D., Lochman, J., Terry, R., & Hyman, C. (1992). Predicting early adolescent disorder from childhood aggression and peer rejection. *Journal of Consulting and Clinical Psychology, 60*, 783–792.

Cole, P. M., Michel, M. K., & O'Donnell-Teti, L. (1994). The development of emotion regulation and dis-regulation: A clinical perspective. In N. A. Fox (Ed.), *The development of emotion regulation. Monographs of the Society for Research in Child Development, 59*, 73–100.

Conners, C. K. (1969). A teacher rating scale for use in drug studies with children. *American Journal of Psychiatry, 126*, 884–888.

Crick, N. R. (1997). Engagement in gender normative versus non-normative forms of aggression: Links to social-psychological adjustment. *Developmental Psychology, 33*, 610–617.

Crick, N. R., & Dodge, K. A. (1994). A review and reformulation of social information processing mechanisms in children's social adjustment. *Psychological Bulletin, 115*, 74–101.

Crick, N. R., & Dodge, K. A. (1996). Social information processing mechanism in reactive and proactive aggression. *Child Development, 66*, 993–1002.

Crick, N. R., & Grotpeter, J. K. (1995). Relational aggression, gender, and social-psychological adjustment. *Child Development, 66*, 710–722.

Dodge, K. A. (1986). A social information processing model of social competence in children. In M. Perlmuter (Ed.), *Minnesota symposium on child psychology* (pp. 77–125). Hillsdale, NJ: Erlbaum.

Dodge, K. A., & Pettit, G. (2003). A biopsychosocial model of the development of chronic conduct problems in adolescence. *Developmental Psychology, 39*, 1–41.

Dorfman, R. A., Meyer, P., & Morgan, M. L. (2004). *Paradigms of clinical social work: Emphasis on diversity* (Vol. 3). New York: Brunner-Routledge.

Downey, G., Lebolt, A., Rincon, C., & Freitas, A. (1998). Rejection sensitivity and children's interpersonal difficulties. *Child Development, 69*, 1074–1091.

Durlak, J. A., Fuhrman, T., & Lampman, C. (1991). Effectiveness of cognitive-behavior therapy for maladaptive children: A meta-analysis. *Psychological Bulletin, 110*, 204–214.

Eppel, E., Ronen, E., & Rosenbaum, M. (2007). Aggressive behavior: The moderating roles of self-control skills and identification with social values. *The Schwartz Research Report 2007* (pp. 28–29). Tel-Aviv: William S. Schwartz Laboratory for Health Behavior Research, Tel-Aviv University.

Hamama, R., Ronen, T., & Feigin, R. (2000). Self-control, anxiety, and loneliness in siblings of children with cancer. *Social Work in Health Care, 31*, 63–83.

Harter, S. (1983). Developmental perspectives on the self-system. In P. H. Mussen (Series Ed.) & E. M. Hetherington (Vol. Ed.), *Handbook of child psychology: Vol. 4. Socialization, personality, and social development* (pp. 275–386). New York: Wiley.

Hartup, W. W. (2005). The development of aggression: Where do we stand? In R. E. Tremblay, W. W. Hartup, & J. Archer (Eds.), *Developmental origins of aggression* (pp. 3–22). New York: Guilford Press.

Herbert, M. (1987). *Conduct disorders of childhood and adolescence: A social learning perspective* (2nd ed.). Chichester, England: Wiley.

Herbert, M. (2002). The human life cycle. In M. Davies (Ed.), *The Blackwell companion to social work* (2nd ed., pp. 355–365). Oxford, England: Blackwell.

Howard, B. L., & Kendall, P. C. (1996). Cognitive-behavioral family therapy for anxiety-disordered children: A multiple-baseline evaluation. *Cognitive Therapy & Research, 20,* 423–443.

Hubbard, J. A., Dodge, K. A., Cillessen, A.H.N., Coie, J. D., & Schwartz, D. (2001). The dyadic nature of social information processing in boys' reactive and proactive aggression. *Journal of Personality and Social Psychology, 80,* 268–280.

Hughes, J. (1993). Behavior therapy. In T. R. Kratochwill & R. J. Morris (Eds.), *Handbook of psychotherapy with children and adolescents* (pp. 185–220). Boston: Allyn & Bacon.

Husermann, L. R., & Eron, L. D. (1989). Individual differences and the trait of aggression. *European Journal of Personality, 3,* 95–106.

Joireman, J., Anderson, J., & Strathman, A. (2003). The aggression paradox: Understanding links among aggression, sensation seeking and the consideration of future consequences. *Journal of Personality and Social Psychology, 84,* 1287–1302.

Kanfer, F. H., & Schefft, B. K. (1988). *Guiding the process of therapeutic change.* Champaign, IL: Research Press.

Kazdin, A. E. (1987). *Conduct disorders in childhood and adolescence.* Newbury Park, CA: Sage.

Kazdin, A. E. (1998). Psychosocial treatments for conduct disorder in children. In D. E. Nathan & J. M. Gorman (Eds.), *A guide to treatments that work* (pp. 65–89). New York: Oxford University Press.

Kazdin, A. (2003). Problem-solving skills training and parent management training for conduct disorder. In A. E. Kazdin & J. R. Weisz (Eds.), *Evidence-based psychotherapies for children and adolescents* (pp. 241–262). New York: Guilford Press.

Kazdin, A. E., Rodgers, A., Colbus, D., & Siegel, T. (1987). Children's hostility inventory: Measurement of aggression and hostility in psychiatric inpatient children. *Journal of Clinical Child Psychology, 16,* 320–328.

Kazdin, A., & Weisz, J. R. (Eds.). (2003). *Evidence-based psychotherapies for children and adolescents.* New York: Guilford Press.

Keltikangas-Jarvinen, L., & Pakaslahti, L. (1999). Development of social problem-solving strategies and changes in aggressive behavior: A 7-year follow-up from childhood to late adolescence. *Aggressive Behavior, 25,* 269–279.

Kendall, P. C., & Chu, B. C. (2000). Retrospective self-reports of therapist flexibility in a manual-based treatment for youths with anxiety disorders. *Journal of Clinical Child Psychology, 29,* 209–220.

Lapouse, R., & Monk, M. A. (1958). An epidemiologic study of behavior characteristics in children. *American Journal of Public Health, 48,* 1134–1144.

Leary, M. R., Twenge, J. M., & Quinlivan, E. (2006). Interpersonal rejection as a determinant of anger and aggression. *Personality and Social Psychology Review, 10,* 11–132.

Loeber, R., & Farrington, D. P. (2000). Young children who commit crime: Epidemiology, development origins, risk factors, early interventions, and policy implications. *Development and Psychopathology, 12,* 737–762.

Ludwig, K. B., & Pittman, J. F. (1999). Adolescent prosocial values and self-efficacy in relation to delinquency, risky sexual behavior, and drugs. *Youth and Society, 30*(4), 461–482.

Luria, A. R. (1961). *The role of speech in the regulation of normal behaviors.* New York: Liverwright.

Mahoney, M. J. (1991). *Human change processes.* New York: Basic Books.

Mahoney, M. J. (1995). Continuing evolution of the cognitive sciences and psychotherapies. In R. A. Neimeyer & M. J. Mahoney (Eds.), *Constructivism in psychotherapy* (pp. 39–67). Washington, DC: American Psychological Association.

Mash, E. J., & Barkley, R. A. (Eds.). (1996). *Child psychopathology.* New York: Guilford Press.

Mash, E. J., & Dozois, D.J.A. (1996). Child psychopathology: A developmental-systems perspective. In E. J. Mash & R. A. Barkley (Eds.), *Child psychopathology* (pp. 3–60). New York: Guilford Press.

McGinnis, E., & Goldstein, A. P. (1997). *Skill streaming the elementary school child: New strategies and perspectives for teaching prosocial skills.* Champaign, IL: Research Press.

Meichenbaum, D. H. (1985). *Stress inoculation training.* New York: Pergamon.

Miller-Johnson, S. M., Coie, J. D., Maumary-Gremaud, A., & Bierman, K. (2002). Peer rejection and aggression and early starter models of conduct disorder. *Journal of Abnormal Child Psychology, 30*(3), 217–230.

Mischel, W. (1973). Toward a cognitive social learning reconceptualization of personality. *Psychological Review, 80,* 252–283.

Mischel, W. (1974). Processes in delay of gratifications. In L. Berkowitz (Ed.), *Advances in experimental and social psychology.* New York: Academic Press.

Mischel, W., & Shoda, Y. (1995). A cognitive-affective system theory of personality: Reconceptualization situations, dispositions, dynamics, and invariance in personality structures. *Psychological Review, 102,* 246–268.

Orpinas, P., & Horne, A. M. (2006). *Bullying prevention: Creating a positive school climate and developing social competence.* Washington, DC: American Psychological Association.

Osterman, K., Bjorkqvist, K., Lagerspetz, K.M.J., Charpentier, S., Carpara, G. V., & Pastorelli, C. (1999). Locus of control and three types of aggression. *Aggressive Behavior, 25,* 61–65.

Patterson, G. R. (1975). *Families: Applications of social learning to family life.* Champaign, IL: Research Press.

Patterson, G. R. (1982). *Coercive family process: A social learning approach.* Eugene, OR: Castalia.

Pettit, S. G., & Dodge, K. A. (2003). Violent children: Bridging development, intervention, and public policy. *Developmental Psychology, 39,* 187–188.

Pope, A. W., & Bierman, K. L. (1999). Predicting adolescent peer problems and antisocial activities: The relative roles of aggression and disregulation. *Developmental Psychology, 35*(2), 335–346.

Pulkkinen, L., & Pitkanen, T. (1993). Continuities in aggressive behavior from childhood to adulthood. *Aggressive Behavior, 19,* 249–263.

Rhee, S., & Waldman, I. D. (2002). Genetic and environmental influences on antisocial behavior: A meta-analysis of twin and adoption studies. *Psychological Bulletin, 29,* 490–529.

Robinson, A. E., Eyberg, M. S., & Ross, A. W. (1980). Inventory of child problem behavior. *Journal of Clinical Child Psychology, 9,* 22–29.

Ronen, T. (1993a). Adapting treatment techniques to children's needs. *British Journal of Social Work, 23,* 581–596.

Ronen, T. (1993b). Decision making about children's therapy. *Child Psychiatry and Human Development, 23,* 259–272.

Ronen, T. (2003). *Cognitive constructivist psychotherapy with children and adolescents.* New York: Kluwer/Plenum.

Ronen, T. (2004). Imparting self-control skills to decrease aggressive behavior in a 12-year-old boy. *Journal of Social Work, 4,* 269–288.

Ronen, T., Rahav, G., & Apple, N. (2003). Adolescent stress response to acute and continuous external stress: Terrorist attack. *Journal of Loss and Trauma, 8,* 261–282.

Ronen, T., Rahav, G., & Moldavsky, A. (in press). Aggressive behavior among Israeli elementary school students and associated emotional/behavioral problems and self-control. *School Psychology Quarterly.*

Ronen, T., Rahav, G., & Rosenbaum, M. (2003). Children's reactions to war situation as a function of age and sex. *Anxiety, Stress and Coping, 16,* 59–69.

Ronen, T., & Rosenbaum, M. (2001). Helping children to help themselves: A case study of enuresis and nail biting. *Research in Social Work Practice, 11,* 338–356.

Ronen, T., Weisbord, W., & Rosenbaum, M. (2007). Self-control skills as moderating the relationship between rejection sensitivity and hostile cognitions. *The Schwartz Research Report 2007* (pp. 18–19). Tel-Aviv: William S. Schwartz Laboratory for Health Behavior Research, Tel-Aviv University.

Rosenbaum, M. (1993). The three functions of self-control behavior: Redressive, reformative and experiential. *Work & Stress, 7,* 33–46.

Rosenbaum, M. (1998). Learned resourcefulness, stress, and self-regulation. In S. Fisher & J. Reason (Eds.), *Handbook of life stress, cognition and health* (pp. 483–496). Chichester, England: Wiley.

Rosenbaum, M., & Ronen, T. (1991, November). *Development of a rating scale for assessment of children's self-control skills (CSC).* Paper presented at the annual meeting of the Association for the Advancement of Behavior Therapy, New York.

Ryan, R. M., & Connell, J. P. (1989). Perceived locus of causality and internalization: Examining reasons for acting in two domains. *Journal of Personality and Social Psychology, 57,* 749–761.

Schaffer, H. R. (1990). *Making decisions about children: Psychology questions and answers.* Oxford, England: Blackwell.

Schaffer, H. R. (1996). *Social development.* Oxford, England: Blackwell.

Scotti, J. R., Mullen, K. B., & Hawkins, R. P. (1998). Child conduct and developmental disabilities: From theory to practice in the treatment of excess behaviors. In J. J. Plaud & G. H. Eifert (Eds.), *From behavior theory to behavior therapy* (pp. 172–201). Boston: Allyn & Bacon.

Shirk, S. R., & Russell, R. L. (1996). *Change process in child psychotherapy.* New York: Guilford Press.

Thompson, R. A. (1989). Causal attributions and children's emotional understanding. In C. Saarni & P. L. Harris (Eds.), *Children's understanding of emotion* (pp. 117–150). New York: Cambridge University Press.

Tremblay, R. E., Hartup, W. W., & Archer, J. (Eds.). (2005). *Developmental origins of aggression.* New York: Guilford Press.

Tremblay, R. E., & Nagin, D. S. (2005). The developing origins of physical aggression in humans. In R. E. Tremblay, W. W. Hartup, & J. Archer (Eds.), *Developmental origins of aggression* (pp. 83–106). New York: Guilford Press.

Vygotsky, L. (1962). *Thought and language.* New York: Wiley.

Warman, D. M., & Cohen, R. (2000). Stability of aggressive behaviors and children's peer relationships. *Aggressive Behavior, 26,* 277–290.

Webster-Stratton, C. (1993). Strategies for helping early school-aged children with oppositional defiant and conduct disorders: The importance of home-school partnerships. *School Psychology Review, 22,* 437–457.

Webster-Stratton, C. (1994). *Trouble families—problem children. Working with parents: A collaborative process.* Chicester, England: Wiley.

Webster-Stratton, C., & Reid, M. J. (2003). The incredible years parents, teachers, and children training series: A multifaceted treatment approach for young children with conduct disorders. In A. E. Kazdin & J. R. Weisz (Eds.), *Evidence-based psychotherapies for children and adolescents* (pp. 224–240). New York: Guilford Press.

Weisbord, N., Rosenbaum, M., & Ronen, T. (2007). Rejection sensitivity as an aggression enhancing cognitive-affective disposition. *The Schwartz Research Report 2007* (pp. 16–17). Tel-Aviv: William S. Schwartz Laboratory for Health Behavior Research, Tel-Aviv University.

Yudofsky, S. C., Silver, J. M., Jackson, W., Endicott, J., & Williams, D. (1986). The overt aggression scale for the objective rating of verbal and physical aggression. *American Journal of Psychology, 143,* 35–39.

Zuckerman, M. (1994). *Behavioral expression and biosocial bases of sensation seeking.* New York: Cambridge University Press.

19 Ecological and Evidence-Based Family Intervention for Juvenile Justice Practitioners

SUSAN B. STERN, JEANINE A. WEBBER,
AND LEENA K. AUGIMERI

This chapter focuses on evidence-based family ecological intervention models for a child or youth with either current or risk for juvenile justice involvement. A substantial body of treatment research supports approaches directed at augmenting parenting skills and modifying coercive family interactions with evidence that multifaceted research-based family interventions are effective in preventing future antisocial behavior and are stronger and more durable than those focused solely on children (Farrington & Welsh, 2006; Kazdin & Weisz, 1998; Kumpfer, 1999; Sexton, Alexander, & Mease, 2004; Taylor & Biglan, 1998). In like manner, prevention research draws attention to the family's importance both in the development and the early control of childhood aggression and conduct problems (Webster-Stratton & Taylor, 2001).

For younger children, aggression and conduct problems[1] strongly predict adolescent antisocial behavior and delinquency along with violence, drug use, school failure, and depression (Conduct Problems Prevention Research Group, 1992; Dishion, Patterson, Stoolmiller, & Skinner, 1991; Kazdin, 1995; Loeber, 1990; Webster-Stratton & Taylor, 2001), underlining the importance of early intervention to prevent or divert the documented negative prognostic trajectory. Early and effective intervention with children who are persistently disruptive or already labeled child delinquents decreases the likelihood of chronic delinquency, even in the face of exposure to risk factors at adolescence (Burns et al., 2003). As such, we discuss behavioral parent training, which has the strongest empirical support in the case of younger children and preadolescents exhibiting aggression and conduct problems, and we present a case example for a child delinquent that integrates a risk assessment model with family-based ecological intervention. Complicating the picture for case planning, children with conduct disorder often have comorbid conditions such as attention deficit hyperactivity disorder (ADHD), anxiety disorders, mood disorders, and learning disorders (Angold, Cotello, & Erkanli, 1999; Fergusson, Lynskey, & Horwood, 1996; Kazdin & Weisz, 1998; Loeber & Keenan, 1994) as our case example demonstrates.

At adolescence, the evidence-based treatments for youth with antisocial and delinquent behavior are more family systems than parent training oriented although the development of parenting skills and competence are still integrated into the models. Among these, we highlight Functional Family Therapy (Alexander, Pugh, Parsons, & Sexton, 2000) and Multisystemic Therapy (Henggeler, Schoenwald, Borduin, Rowland, & Cunningham, 1998), each developed specifically to treat delinquency, although both now target a range of problems of at-risk youth and their families, plus Multidimensional Treatment Foster Care (Chamberlain & Mihalic, 1998), which addresses a similar group of youth requiring out-of-home placement.

As with child conduct problems, adolescent antisocial behavior also does not occur in isolation, with evidence for a syndrome of problem behaviors that includes delinquency, substance use, school dropout, risky sexual activity, and teen pregnancy (Allen, Leadbeater, & Aber, 1994; Ary, Duncan, Duncan, & Hops, 1999; Donovan, Jessor, & Costa, 1988). A particularly important observation is the high rate of multiple or comorbid disorders among young people in juvenile custody in the United States, indicating both the seriousness of comorbid diagnoses and the urgent need to respond to these youths' needs (Abram, Teplin, McClelland, & Dulcan, 2003). Given the co-occurrence of drug use and delinquency, two additional evidence-based family-centered and ecological intervention models—Multidimensional Family Therapy (Liddle, 2002) and Brief Strategic Family Therapy (Szapocznik, Hervis, & Schwartz, 2003)—have relevance for practitioners in the juvenile justice system and could have been included in this review; however, they specifically target youth with substance abuse problems, which is beyond the scope of this chapter. Lastly, we will discuss some of the mechanisms of change across models and highlight assessment and treatment implications for juvenile justice practice.

WHY ECOLOGICAL?

Contemporary juvenile justice research is increasingly informed by social ecology theory (Bronfenbrenner, 1979; Fraser, 1996), which recognizes the importance of social context in understanding both the initiation and progression of problem behaviors. Consistent with this theoretical perspective, an impressive body of knowledge from longitudinal and modeling studies shows that antisocial and delinquent behaviors are multiple, determined by the reciprocal interaction of individual youth characteristics and characteristics of key social systems (e.g., family, school, peers, neighborhood) in which youth are embedded, underscoring the need for prevention and intervention programs that likewise target these multiple systems and the interactions among them (Fraser, 1996; Henggeler, 1991; Loeber & Farrington, 2001; Moretti, Odgers, & Jackson, 2004; Smith & Stern, 1997; Stormshak & Dishion, 2002). Whether a child or youth develops aggressive or antisocial behavior rests on the interplay between risk and protective factors at all levels of the child's environment, and it is the accumulation and interaction of risk rather than any single factor that increases the likelihood of adverse youth outcomes (Catalano & Hawkins, 1996; Grizenko & Pawliuk, 1994; Mrazek & Haggerty, 1994; Rutter, Giller, & Hagell, 1998). To the ecological perspective, an added developmental component captures the dynamic relationship as children interact with their environment over time in a reciprocal pattern to influence development and social patterns (Webster-Stratton & Taylor, 2001).

Two pathways have been identified for delinquency illustrating the differences in risk factors across developmental stages (Moffit, 1997; Patterson, Forgatch, Yoeger, & Stoolmiller, 1998): an early onset pathway beginning before puberty when family factors have the greatest impact and is more persistent across the life course and a trajectory of adolescent late starters for whom peers and school may become more predominant and who tend to engage in less serious and violent behaviors for a shorter duration (Krohn, Thornberry, Rivera, & Le Blanc, 2001; Moffitt, 1997; Simons, Wu, Conger, & Lorenz, 1994).

WHY FAMILY?

Although multiple risk factors across systems shape and maintain antisocial behavior and delinquency, *family processes* play a key role influencing youth behavior both directly and indirectly through interaction with other system influences, most notably peer relations with association with deviant peers the final pathway to delinquency (Ary et al., 1999; Thornberry, Huizinga, & Loeber, 1995; U.S. Department of Health and Human Services, 1999). Poor parent–child relationships, family conflict, and ineffective parenting practices significantly increase risk for antisocial behavior and delinquency (Henggeler & Sheidow, 2003; Loeber & Stouthamer-Loeber, 1986; Patterson, Reid, & Dishion, 1992; Smith & Stern, 1997). In the *affective* realm, low attachment or bonding, rejection, and hostility, as well as lack of parents'[2] support and involvement in their child's life, consistently have been linked with delinquency (Krohn, Stern, Thornberry, & Jang, 1992; Loeber & Stouthamer-Loeber, 1986). In contrast, family closeness is protective, with ties of affection and warmth encouraging parent–child involvement and positive family interaction, which, in turn, decrease the likelihood of deviant behavior (Kumpfer & DeMarsh, 1986; Patterson et al., 1992) and protect against negative peer influences, either by preventing contact with deviant peers or countering their influence (Poole & Regoli, 1980; Warr, 1993).

Effective parenting encompasses both socialization practices that shape and reinforce socially desirable and competent behavior and the parenting skills needed to control undesirable behavior. The research on family management and parenting is theoretically driven by Patterson's seminal coercion theory (Patterson, 1982; Patterson et al., 1992), a social learning model of the development and progression of antisocial behavior that incorporates the primary risk factors across systems. Supporting evidence suggests that the beginnings of antisocial behavior are indeed learned in the family, where daily interaction shapes aggression in young children when less skilled or stressed parents unintentionally reinforce child behaviors such as whining, noncompliance, and tantrums by giving in and failing to provide appropriate discipline. In a reciprocal manner, parent behavior is negatively reinforced by cessation of aversive child behavior, thereby perpetuating cycles of inconsistent parenting that, in turn, contribute to further antisocial behavior (Dishion, Patterson, & Kavanagh, 1992; Granic & Patterson, 2006; Patterson, 1995, Patterson & Dishion, 1988).

At the same time that the young aggressive child is developing coercive behaviors, he or she fails to learn those necessary for successful relationships with peers and in school. Upon entering school, a child who behaves aggressively is rejected by prosocial peers and is more likely to turn to other rejected and disruptive children, who reinforce one another's negative behaviors. Lacking behavioral and social competencies, the aggressive child also is at risk for academic difficulties. Peer rejection and school failures predict association with a deviant peer group, leading eventually to delinquency (Patterson et al., 1992).

When antisocial children reach early adolescence, developmental transitions require shifts in parental monitoring practices. Poor monitoring increases drift into a deviant peer group as teens spend more unsupervised time with their peers and effective monitoring is particularly significant for preventing arrest risk (Ary et al., 1999; Patterson et al., 1992; Snyder, Dishion, & Patterson, 1986). As coercive interactions continue to escalate in multiple settings, the additional problems outside the family intensify caregiver stress and further erode family control and climate (Ambert, 1992; Stern & Smith, 1999). Protective parent behaviors that can moderate risk—such as seeking information and support, parent–school involvement, and youth advocacy—may become less likely as caregivers are confronted by the demands of parenting a difficult youth (Boyd-Franklin & Bry, 2000; Stern & Smith, 1999).

Ineffective parenting practices, especially coercive interactions and poor monitoring, continue to maintain antisocial behavior into adolescence, even when deviant peers and school influences are taken into account (Dishion, Patterson, & Reid, 1988; Dishion et al., 1991; Patterson, DeBaryshe, & Ramsey, 1989; Vuchinich, Bank, & Patterson, 1992). Changes in parenting practices appear to be instrumental in altering child behavior in studies of change processes, supporting coercion theory's theoretical tenets and reinforcing the empirical base for parent training and family intervention (Dishion et al., 1992; Gardner, Burton, & Klimes, 2006; Huey, Henggeler, Brondino, & Pickrel, 2000; Kazdin & Weisz, 1998; Patterson, 1982, 2005; Schmidt, Liddle, & Dakof, 1996; Schrepferman & Snyder, 2002).

High levels of *family conflict* and *family violence* additionally increase risk for delinquency and youth violence (Thornberry, 1994; Thornberry et al., 1995). Family conflict, as one would expect, lessens parent–adolescent involvement. Consequently, these troubled relationships and decreased involvement contribute to inadequate monitoring, which again increases antisocial behavior both directly and indirectly by promoting association with deviant peers (Ary et al., 1999). Negative communication and problem-solving skill deficits exacerbate family conflict and are associated with delinquency and other negative outcomes for youth (e.g., Alexander, 1973; Hops, Tildesley, Lichtenstein, Ary, & Sherman, 1990) but not as strongly as are other family processes (Forehand, Miller, Dutra, & Chance, 1997; Smith & Stern, 1997). Notwithstanding, family intervention that targets communication and problem solving diminishes antisocial behavior, thus supporting their inclusion in intervention (Alexander et al., 2000; Bry, Conboy, & Bisgay, 1986; DeGarmo & Forgatch, 2004). Antisocial youths' poor communication and problem-solving skills also may interact with individual risk factors, including a cognitive bias to attribute hostile intent to others and beliefs supporting the use of aggression as a legitimate means to deal with conflict (Dodge & Frame, 1982; Slaby & Guerra, 1988). Individual parent factors such as adult criminality, antisocial personality disorder, substance abuse, and mental health disorders as well as adverse family circumstances including poverty, stress, and social isolation can contribute to increased risk for antisocial and delinquent behavior (Kumpfer, 1999; Patterson et al., 1992; Smith & Stern, 1997; Stern, Smith, & Jang, 1999). Although there are undoubtedly multiple pathways by which these factors affect youth outcomes, including genetic and cognitive ones, there is strong evidence that many influence behavior at least partially by disrupting parenting and family relationships (Conger & Elder, 1994; Conger, Patterson, & Ge, 1995; Stern & Smith, 1995; Stern et al., 1999). Consistent with the ecological model, research shows that family processes are further linked with risk factors at the school system level, indirectly affecting delinquency through lack of school success (Thornberry, Lizotte, Krohn, Farnworth, & Jang, 1991), and at the community level, where neighborhoods with high crime, disorganization, and mobility and low support present barriers to effective parenting (Peebles & Loeber, 1994; Stern & Smith, 1995).

THE CONTEXT OF CULTURE AND GENDER

Research on family processes and culture, while still in its early stages, increasingly addresses the many ways in which families of aggressive and antisocial youth differ and, thus, how their intervention needs may differ. Not meant as a full review or inclusive of the many aspects of family diversity (e.g., family structure, socioeconomic class), we briefly note two important areas to inform case planning and program development: ethnicity and gender. Emerging research findings on the relationship between family processes and ethnicity suggest that there may be some differences across ethnic groups (e.g., Catalano et al., 1992; McCluskey, & Tovar, 2003), although the findings are not consistent, and findings from some studies suggest that the relationship between family processes and delinquency or other adverse youth outcomes holds up across ethnic groups (Boyd-Franklin & Bry, 2000; Forehand et al., 1997; Kumpfer, 1999). There are even contradictory findings across studies that examine the same family process. Illustrative of this, Smith and Krohn (1995) found that parent control—which included both monitoring and discipline—was not associated with decreased delinquency for Hispanic adolescents in contrast with Black and White adolescents, whereas other studies have found that parental monitoring similarly decreases deviant behavior for Hispanic and Black youths (Forehand et al., 1997; Gorman-Smith, Tolan, Zelli, & Huesmann, 1996; Lamborn, Dornbusch, & Steinberg, 1996). Given the current state of evidence, practitioners should be aware of and continue to follow the research on family processes in light of its significance for adolescent behavior and clinical planning. Cultural responsivity suggests the need to individualize assessment and intervention and monitor outcomes for each youth and family.

In similar fashion, only recently have we begun to address the gender differences in risk and protective factors, family processes, and intervention outcomes for children and youth with conduct disorder and aggressive and antisocial behavior (Dodge, 2004; Ehrensaft, 2005; Levene, Walsh, Augimeri, & Pepler, 2004; Moretti et al., 2004). Studies specifically of high-risk samples (versus the general population) show that early sexual development, strained mother–daughter relationships (Levene, Madsen, & Pepler, 2005), disruptions in caregiving (Corrado, Odgers, & Cohen, 2000), socioeconomic disadvantages, and marital conflict (Keenan, Stouthamer-Loeber, & Loeber, 2005) are associated with early-onset disruptive behavior disorders in girls, whereas neighborhood problems and parental substance abuse have been found to be risk factors for conduct disorder in boys but not in girls (Keenan et al., 2005).

Once young people become involved in the justice system, their profiles and intervention needs differ significantly on the basis of gender. For example, girls are more likely than boys to have a history of victimization, chaotic family lives, more mental health needs, and family members who have had contact with the criminal justice system (Antonishak, Reppucci, & Mulford, 2004; Chamberlin & Moore, 2002). These findings suggest that, in contrast to boys, girls who come in contact with the criminal justice system have experienced different or more severe conditions that have interrupted healthy development and, as a consequence, may require more comprehensive mental health services, especially when a girl has been victimized. Moreover, because the relationship between mothers and daughters often is particularly strained when a young girl is experiencing serious behavior problems, focusing on the mother–daughter relationship is a priority for intervention.

FAMILY-BASED ECOLOGICAL AND EVIDENCE-BASED INTERVENTIONS

Not surprisingly in light of the research on family risk and protective factors that encompass dynamic interactional family processes, treatment outcome research demonstrates that families are key change agents for antisocial and delinquent youth (Henggeler & Sheidow, 2003; Kumpfer, 1999; Stern, 2001). All of the models next described are responsive to our knowledge of risk and protective factors across a child's and family's ecology, build on family interaction therapy and research, and are part of a program of ongoing research that informs evolving model development as well as sheds critical light on what actually occurs during intervention and mechanisms of change. Each addresses the coercive family interactions maintaining aggressive or antisocial behavior. Each model also has been recognized by reviewers and diverse federal agencies alike as "evidence-based" programs for child conduct problems and/or adolescent antisocial and delinquent behavior (Center for Substance Abuse Prevention; Elliott, 1998; Eyberg, Nelson, & Boggs, 2008; Kazdin & Weisz, 1998; Kumpfer, 1999; McBride, VanderWaal, VanBuren, & Terry, 1997; Office of Juvenile Justice and Delinquency Prevention, n.d.; U.S. Department of Health and Human Services, 1999, 2001; United States White House, n.d.). Different agencies use different designations to endorse interventions with what they consider strong empirical evidence of effectiveness (e.g., "model," "exemplary") and use slightly different criteria intended to ensure that the selected interventions have a strong conceptual framework, have been implemented with a high degree of fidelity, and have been rigorously evaluated (e.g., experimental design) with consistent positive findings, including independent replications. Despite this, the strength of research support for approaches designated as "evidence-based" varies as reflected in the comments on systematic reviews and our discussion throughout this chapter. Systematic reviews are designed to minimize bias in evidence assessment. A systematic review provides a thorough appraisal and synthesis of available research on a given topic based on a comprehensive and transparent search followed by a rigorous analysis of methodology and findings across identified studies including a meta-analysis when sufficient studies meet the required criteria. To this end, the Campbell Collaboration is an independent and international organization that engages in the production of systematic reviews, including an extensive international search of both published and unpublished research literature, to synthesize evidence on the effectiveness of interventions and policies in social welfare, education, and criminology. In doing so, it also seeks to establish a coherent, easily accessible library of knowledge for evidence-based practice in these fields. The following reviews provide current snapshots of the selected models that we believe juvenile justice practitioners and policy makers should be familiar with rather than full descriptions or systematic research appraisals, with ongoing research continuing to update the changing evidence base.

Behavioral Parent Training

Behavioral parent training models, often along with child cognitive-behavioral and social skills training to address individual risk factors and their interaction with other systems influences, are designed to help families with young children with early onset of serious conduct problems and focus on strengthening parent–child relationships and helping parents to foster positive behaviors in their children and effectively manage both common child behavior problems and more serious conduct. The intent is to impede negative developmental outcomes by teaching caregivers more effective child management strategies that increase positive parent–child interactions and minimize those that are negatively coercive (Smith & Stern, 1997; Taylor & Biglan, 1998).

Behavioral parent training programs have demonstrated impressive evidence of efficacy with over several hundred studies and recent meta-analyses reporting improved parenting practices and/or child behavior (Barlow & Parsons, 2004; Bunting, 2004; Maughan, Christiansen, Jenson, Olympia, & Clark, 2005; Serketich & Dumas, 1996). The programs are increasingly being replicated in effectiveness studies and disseminated and adopted internationally (Hutchings et al., 2007; Ogden, Forgatch, Askeland, Patterson, & Bullock, 2005). The empirically supported parenting programs targeting prevention and early intervention with high-risk families with children with behavioral problems include the renowned Oregon Social Learning Center model, *Parent Management Training* (Forgatch, 1994; Forgatch, & Patterson, 2005), *The Incredible Years* (Webster-Stratton & Herbert, 1994), *Helping the Noncompliant Child* (Forehand & McMahon, 1981), *Triple P* (Sanders, Markie-Dadds, & Turner, 1998, 2000), *Parent-Child Interaction Treatment* (Eyberg, Boggs, & Algina, 1995), and, most recently, the *SNAP (Stop Now And Plan)* program (Augimeri, Kogel, & Goldberg, 2001).

These programs are similar in theoretical underpinnings and intervention strategies, although the structure, format, and specific materials may differ. Based on Patterson's (1982) social learning coercion theory and Bandura's (1977, 1982) modeling and self-efficacy theories, evidence-based parent training emphasizes experiential learning methods for producing behavioral change; videotape, live modeling, and role play, or bug-in-the-ear in vivo training, together with home activities, provide for performance rehearsal, discussion, and feedback. These programs also tend to use a collaborative rather than a didactic approach to learning and aim to empower parents and increase their parenting confidence and self-efficacy (Sanders, Markie-Dadds, & Turner, 2003; Webster-Stratton & Herbert, 1994).

Research on the process of behavioral parent training points to the importance of maintaining a nonjudgmental attitude and atmosphere of mutual collaboration when working with parents (Webster-Stratton & Herbert, 1993, 1994). Without helping families to feel that they are contributing to the solution and actively soliciting their input, behavioral family intervention may well be ineffective at breaking through the resistance that is so often encountered in this work. A focus on parenting skills can inadvertently communicate the message that parents are to blame for their child's difficulties, negatively impacting the therapeutic alliance (Liddle, 1995; Stern & Smith, 1999). Process research shows that parent resistance and stress increase during some phases of parent training (Chamberlain, Patterson, Reid, Forgatch, & Kavanagh, 1984; Webster-Stratton & Spitzer, 1996) with further teaching and confrontation escalating resistance, whereas therapist reframing and support decreases it (Chamberlain et al., 1984; Patterson & Forgatch, 1985).

Parent training may be delivered through individual family treatment sessions or in a group format with some models encompassing both formats as well as multiple levels from primary prevention to intensive intervention (e.g., Triple P; Sanders et al., 2003). Because it is known that the risks associated with family adversity and parent mental health status negatively affect treatment engagement and outcome (Dumas & Wahler,

1983; Kazdin, Mazurick, & Bass, 1993; Prinz & Miller, 1994; Reyno & McGrath, 2006; Webster-Stratton & Hammond, 1990), investigators have expanded their programs to address engagement and retention and to enhance skills in other areas such as coping with extrafamilial stressors, parent depression, and conflict management and couples' communication, with positive outcomes for both children and their parents (see, e.g., Dadds, Schwartz, & Sanders, 1987; Kazdin & Whitley, 2003; Miller & Prinz, 1990; Sanders & McFarland, 2000; Wahler, Cartor, Fleischman, & Lambert, 1993).

Stop Now and Plan (SNAP®) Programs

One of the few evidence-based ecological parent training plus child skills model developed specifically for child delinquency is the Stop Now and Plan (SNAP®) programs (Burns et al., 2003; Howell, 2001). The SNAP programs are gender-sensitive, manualized, multicomponent interventions that work with the children, their families, schools, and communities (Child Development Institute, 2008a, 2008b; Levene, 2003). The SNAP Under 12 Outreach Project (SNAP ORP) initially opened its doors for service in the city of Toronto in 1985 in response to the decriminalization of children under 12 years of age in Canada. In 1996 the model expanded to include a gender-sensitive approach with the introduction of the SNAP Girls Connection (SNAP GC). The SNAP programs are part of a comprehensive crime prevention model initiated by the Centre for Children Committing Offences, a branch of the Child Development Institute, which includes gender-sensitive risk assessment and a police-community referral protocol. This approach allows police officers and other professionals to make timely referrals to local children's mental health agencies when they become aware of children at risk (Koegl, Augimeri, Ferrante, Walsh, & Slater, 2008).

Consistent with the literature on male delinquency, the majority of referrals to the SNAP ORP (boys program) are from the police, while most referrals to the SNAP GC are from schools, child welfare agencies, and other mental health professionals. Research findings suggest the program is effective in reducing problematic behaviors in both boys and girls (Augimeri, Farrington, Koegl, & Day, 2007; Koegl, Farrington, Augimeri, & Day, 2008; Lipman et al., 2008; Pepler et al., 2008). An intervention plan, responsive to the family's ecology, is developed by clinical staff and discussed with the family upon completion of an in-depth assessment that includes interviews and administration of standardized measures and the EARL gender-sensitive risk assessment tool (EARL-20B [Augimeri, Koegl, Webster, & Levene, 2001]; EARL-21G [Levene et al., 2001]). The EARLs are particularly helpful to clinicians at both the case planning and monitoring stages, because they aid in identifying which of the empirically known child, family, peer, and community risk factors are present in the family to help direct the intervention plan, priorities, and progress (Augimeri, Enebrink, Walsh, & Jiang, in press; Enebrink, Långström & Gumpert, 2006).

The SNAP programs incorporate behavioral, social skills, problem-solving, and cognitive-behavioral strategies. In addition to assisting caregivers in developing alternative and effective behavioral management strategies for their children's problematic behaviors, the 12-week parenting group also assists them in identifying strategies to gain the most benefit from existing protective factors such as established relationships with extended family and community organizations. The concurrent 12-week children's group teaches children self-control, self-regulation, problem-solving skills, and assertive behaviors in a gender-sensitive, child-friendly, and developmentally appropriate environment. In addition, other service components may be provided based on level of risk and need such as academic tutoring, family counseling, individual befriending, and school and community advocacy. Clinicians make referrals to any other resources a family may require and will work in cooperation and often assume a case management role when other service providers are involved with the child or family. Unlike the other evidence-based programs, SNAP was developed and continuously evaluated and refined by a community-based agency using a scientist–practitioner model demonstrating the feasibility of integrating it into agencies providing direct services to children and their families.

SNAP Clinical Case Example

> Michau is an outgoing, attractive, likeable 9-year-old boy with a nice sense of humor of African Canadian descent. He met all his developmental milestones on time (i.e., walking, talking, and toilet training) and is in good health except for occasional asthma. He began having behavioral difficulties at age 4 (e.g., serious temper tantrums, aggression, swearing, hitting). His mother attributes this to him witnessing and experiencing family violence and the violent death of an uncle he was very close to who was involved in gang activity at the time of his death. Michau struggles academically and has been labeled as having a learning disability; currently, he is 2 years behind

in reading and math. His teacher and mother report he has difficulty concentrating and is constantly fidgeting. At this time, no formal assessment has been conducted to determine the cause(s). Socially, Michau is an active boy who enjoys playing baseball, basketball, and football and considers himself "a born athlete." His mother, however, is guarded about his participating in activities in the community, because she reports it being a "tough" neighborhood. In regard to peers, he has a history of having difficulty with other children. Currently, he has two close friends; however, his mother is concerned about him hanging out with these boys and thinks they may "have a negative influence on him."

Michau lives with his mother and baby brother in a nice apartment that meets their needs. His mother works full-time but reports that finances are "tight." The family has support from the maternal grandmother and brother. As well, they have a few good family friends they can rely on. Mom also is able to access structured after school programs and has sought assistance from a local children's mental health center to deal with her son's anger outbursts. Michau reports a very loving and positive relationship with his mother. She has been his primary caregiver. Michau's biological father left the home when Michau was 6 years old due to domestic violence that resulted in him being incarcerated, although he currently lives in the same neighborhood and sees Michau regularly. Michau's mother reports that she and Michau are very affectionate toward each other and feels she is a "good mom" but says she needs to be more consistent with Michau. She feels that she has to overcompensate for the harsh and punitive discipline Michau experienced by his father and their marital issues, which resulted in child welfare involvement. In addition, Michau has had to cope with the birth of a baby brother, and that has been difficult for him because he has been the only child for the past 9 years.

Michau was referred to the SNAP ORP by the school social worker for aggressive behavior in the classroom and playground that resulted in numerous school suspensions. He also has had police contact for stealing, running away, and vandalism. He rated within the clinical range on the conduct problem subscale of the Child Behavior Checklist (Achenbach & Rescorla, 2001), a standardized measure of behavioral and emotional issues. Although Michau is able to distinguish right from wrong and feels "badly" when he does something wrong, he is defiant and has a number of "thinking errors" or cognitive distortions (e.g., thinks that no one likes him, thinks it is okay to steal candy because the store has "lots of candy and taking one doesn't hurt anyone or matter"). Overall, Michau is able to function at home and school but is experiencing issues in both these settings. He gets highly anxious when he is away from his mom for extended periods of time and seems sad and withdrawn at times. When assessed for interest in seeking help for their problems, Michau's mother was very open and willing to get help for herself and her son. She is extremely committed to engaging in the therapeutic process and contacted the children's mental health center to expedite the process. Michau is willing to work on his "issues" and was able to identify a goal for being involved in the program: "to control my anger."

The Eco-Map shown in Figure 19.1 provides a "word picture" of the family, giving a snapshot of subsystems such as supports, activities, health, school, peers, employment/financial, and other related factors pertaining to the target child and his family. The completed EARL-20B Summary Sheet (see Figure 19.2) is used to structure all the information provided about the case at hand to assess level of risk and clinical need.

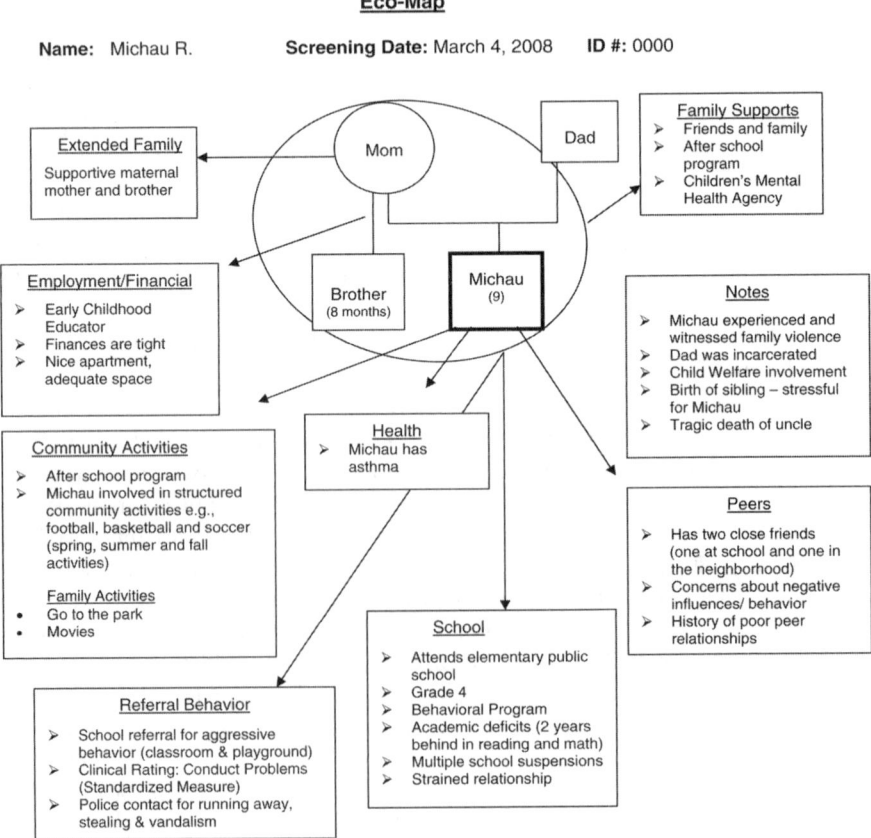

Figure 19.1 Eco-Map.

Chapter 19 Ecological and Evidence-Based Family Intervention

The EARL-20B Version 2 Summary Sheet
(To be used in association with the EARL-20B, Version 2 Manual)

Child's Name or ID#: Michau R. (First name SURNAME) Date: 2008 - 03 - 04 (YYYY-MM-DD)
Assessor: L.A. Child's DOB: 1999-02-15 (YYYY-MM-DD) Age: 9

Family Items			Rating (0-1-2)	Critical Risk
F1	Household Circumstances	mom employed, finances tight, adequate space, nice apartment	1	
F2	Caregiver Continuity	mom (primary), bio dad in and out, affectionate mom-child relationship	1	
F3	Supports	maternal mother & brother, friends, after school prog., children's mental health center	0	
F4	Stressors	strained school relationship, child welfare, M's asthma, birth of new baby, M's dad	2	√
F5	Parenting Style	mother – inconsistent, dad – harsh & punitive	2	√
F6	Antisocial Values and Conduct	dad - violent towards mom & M., incarceration	2	√

Child Items			Rating (0-1-2)	Critical Risk
C1	Developmental Problems	met all developmental milestones on time	0	
C2	Onset of Behavioral Difficulties	age 4 (serious temper tantrums & behaviour issues)	2	
C3	Abuse/Neglect/Trauma	witnessed & experienced family violence, death of uncle	2	√
C4	HIA (Hyperactivity/Impulsivity/Attention Deficits)	difficulty concentrating, fidgets, NO diagnosis	1	
C5	Likeability	attractive, nice sense of humor, polite, friendly, adults like him	0	
C6	Peer Socialization	2 close friends, concerns - negative influences, history of difficulty with peers	1	√
C7	Academic Performance	academic deficits, I.D.– 2 years behind in reading and math	2	
C8	Neighbourhood	"tough" but has access to structured community activities	1	
C9	Authority Contact	principals, teachers, police	2	
C10	Antisocial Attitudes	defiant, "thinking errors"/cognitive distortions, empathetic, knows right from wrong	1	
C11	Antisocial Behaviour	school suspensions, assault, aggression, vandalism, running away, swearing, stealing, bullying, CD clinical rating on standardized measure	2	√
C12	Coping Ability	issues at home/school, separation anxiety, over anxious, depressive symptoms	2	√

Responsivity Items			Rating (0-1-2)	Critical Risk
R1	Family Responsivity	mom willing to get help, active, committed (she contacted the agency)	0	
R2	Child Responsivity	wants to work on issues, able to identify a treatment goal	0	

Overall Clinical Judgment	LOW	MOD	HIGH √	TOTAL SCORE	24

Notes (Clinical Risk Management Plan): Major concerns pertain to C3 (Abuse, Neglect & Trauma), C12 (Coping Ability) and F6 (Antisocial Values and Conduct). Michau can be an explosive little boy who is engaging in a variety of antisocial behaviors. He is also struggling with the birth of his new baby brother (he was the only child up to this point). Based on the EARL risk summary (especially the critical risk factors) the following treatment considerations are recommended: (1) engage Michau in the SNAP® Children's Groups – learn self control and problem-solving strategies to help him control his anger, deal more effectively with his problems and cognitive distortions; (2) Mom to attend the SNAP® Parent Group – learn effective parent management strategies – in particular, how to be more consistent with her son; (3) Michau to receive some individual befriending with the SNAP® Group Leader and/or volunteer to work on his individual goals and work with the school regarding his academics and behavior issues; (4) further assessment required for Michau to investigate depression, anxiety, attention and abuse/trauma issues; (5) ensure positive mentors in Michau's life to buffer the possible impact of F6; (6) ensure Michau and mom have quality 1-to-1 time set aside to do something fun together; and (7) work out instrumental issues (e.g., transportation, babysitting) to ensure mom and Michau continue to be engaged in services.

Copyright © 2008 Child Development Institute

Figure 19.2 The EARL-20B Version 2 Summary Sheet.

This provides a one-page "transparent" summary of the case and the beginnings of a clinical risk management plan that is prescriptive in terms of interventions (see notes section).

As noted on the EARL-20B Summary Sheet, Michau received a total score of 24 and an overall clinical judgment of "high," indicating he is at high risk of engaging in future antisocial activities. Each EARL item is rated on a 3-point scale. A rating of 0 indicates that the characteristic or circumstance is not evident; a rating of 2 indicates that the characteristic or circumstance is present; and a rating of 1 indicates there is some, but not complete, evidence for the factor. The critical risk boxes are used to denote items that are of particularly high concern.

Based on Michau's EARL-20B risk summary, the notes section outlines a number of clinical services and strategies for identified areas of particular concern grounded in an ecological and social learning framework. The suggested plan targets both the child and parent and additional systems that may require assistance (e.g., school, community). In Michau's case, he is identified as an "explosive" boy who is engaging in antisocial activities. The suggested treatment plan is to engage him in the SNAP ORP, where he will have an opportunity to participate in the children's group and learn to control his anger and come up with appropriate solutions to his problems. In addition, this forum will also challenge any cognitive distortions and/or "thinking errors" such as "no one likes me" or "stealing is okay" in a supportive environment.

To ensure skill acquisition and generalization, the ORP child worker will work one-to-one with Michau on his individual treatment goal (i.e., control his anger) and ensure he is connected to structured neighborhood recreational activities where he will have an opportunity to develop positive peer relations and connections to community mentors (e.g., recreational coach). While Michau is engaged in his group, his mother will participate in the SNAP parenting group, where she will learn effective child management strategies and age-appropriate routines that she can implement at home with Michau. One of the areas of concern for Michau's mother was not being consistent with her parenting practices. This mostly pertained to the use of discipline. She indicated she had difficulty using discipline strategies consistently with her son because she felt "guilty" about the punitive discipline he experienced from his father. The parenting groups will teach her how to be more consistent with her parenting skills by introducing her to nonpunitive discipline strategies (e.g., removal of privileges and time out), addressing cognitions that interfere with discipline as needed, and helping her to coordinate special one-to-one time with Michau. This is especially important, because the two of them had spent a lot of time together before the birth of the baby.

In addition to the clinical risk management strategies, it is important for the treatment plan to address a number of other issues with particular concern in regard to items C3 (abuse, neglect, and trauma), C12 (coping ability), and F6 (antisocial values and conduct). Both Michau and his mother will need to be connected to a program that specializes in addressing the family violence trauma they experienced and their continued relationship with Michau's dad. This also may involve an assessment to investigate Michau's possible comorbid depression, anxiety, and attention issues. Lastly, it is imperative to ensure treatment compliance and success that instrumental factors such as transportation and child care are dealt with early on to ensure both Michau and his mother continue to be engaged in the treatment process.

Multidimensional Treatment Foster Care

The research evidence for parent training for adolescents is both more limited and more mixed than for younger children (Dishion & Andrews, 1995; Dishion & Patterson, 1992; Lundahl, Risser, & Lovejoy, 2006). The development of Multidimensional Treatment Foster Care (MTFC) speaks to both the difficulties of behavioral family intervention for adolescent delinquency in community settings (Dishion & Patterson, 1992) and the need for an alternative to the potentially ineffective practice of placing antisocial youth together in groups and living arrangements (Dishion, McCord, & Poulin, 1999; Dishion, Poulin, & Burraston, 2001; Hoagwood, Burns, Kiser, Ringeisen, & Schoenwald, 2001).

MTFC is an extension of Patterson's Parent Management Training to youth removed from their homes by authorities for chronic and severe antisocial behavior, emotional disturbances, and delinquency but considered safe to treat in the community. MTFC trains and supervises community families or experienced foster parents in family management to bring the adolescent's behavior under control while the youth's family receives parenting skills and family therapy and is supported toward reintegration and management of the adolescent. The youth is given skills training to get along with peers and in school, is closely supervised and cut off from delinquent peers, and participation in prosocial activities is facilitated. A case manager coordinates community contacts with parole or probation officers, the school, and others. MTFC significantly reduced incarceration compared with alternative residential care in two studies (Chamberlain, 1990; Chamberlain & Reid, 1998), with MTFC youth significantly less likely to have committed violent offenses at a 2-year follow-up of a randomized clinical trial (RCT) (Eddy, Whaley, & Chamberlain, 2004). In an extension of MTFC to girls referred by juvenile justice judges for chronic delinquency, intervention was modified by research on gender-specific processes related to social-relational aggression. Findings of an RCT and 2-year follow-up suggest beneficial decreases in delinquency-related outcomes as well as issues (e.g., high rate of mental health needs, the change process specific to girls) needing examination in future studies (Chamberlain, Leve, & DeGarmo, 2007; Leve, Chamberlain, & Reid, 2005). The conclusions of a recent systematic review substantiate the individual studies (Hahn et al., 2005), and the model also is reported to be a cost-effective alternative to residential treatment or incarceration (Chamberlain & Mihalic, 1998).

Functional Family Therapy

Functional Family Therapy (FFT) is a family systems model with a strong behavioral orientation that gives attention to the *function* of behavior in the family relational system and targets change in the maladaptive interactional patterns that maintain problem behaviors. It is a phase-oriented model in which FFT therapists initially concentrate on engagement and motivation by interrupting the family blaming process and developing a collaborative set.

FFT was one of the first models to address the difficulty of engaging in treatment youth and families in the juvenile justice system who often are angry, fearful, and disrespectful to one another and in many circumstances are likely to have failed at previous change attempts (Patterson et al., 1992; Stern & Smith, 1999). Engaging and motivating the family to set the stage for change occurs through building an alliance with all family members, reducing the negativity characteristic of many families, reframing the meaning of behavior and relationally defining problems, and developing an understanding of the problem behavior within the youth's and family's systemic context (Alexander et al., 2000). Once initially engaged, a culturally appropriate individualized plan that fits with the understanding of the function of the youth's behavior and the family's relational patterns is created during a behavior change phase that targets parenting skills (e.g., developmentally appropriate monitoring and supervision) and the establishment of positive communication and problem-solving interactions to manage conflict in a supportive family climate. A more multisystemic phase follows to help families generalize across situations, maintain change through relapse prevention, and support change by focusing on the family's relational needs and interactions with relevant systems in the youth's ecology (e.g., schools). Continuous monitoring and outcome accountability is an integral component of the model.

FFT is delivered either as a traditional clinic model or home-based service and has been offered in juvenile justice, mental health, and child welfare settings and, most recently, in school settings. Family members are all seen together, including younger siblings when appropriate. FFT researchers have examined in-session therapy process questions that have guided development of the model, most notably how to change negative, blaming family communication to better engage families and the effects of therapist characteristics and behavior on process and outcome (Alexander, Barton, Schiavo, & Parsons, 1976; Newberry, Alexander, & Turner, 1991; Robbins, Turner, Alexander, & Perez, 2003). Treatment outcome studies show that FFT decreases recidivism and out-of-home placement, improves family supportive relationships and climate, is cost-effective, and, of particular note, helps prevent younger siblings from entering the system (Alexander et al., 2000; Alexander & Parsons, 1973; Aos & Barnoski, 1998; Barton, Alexander, Waldron, Turner, & Warburton, 1985; Gordon, Arbuthnot, Gustafsond, & McGreen, 1988; Gordon, Graves, & Arbuthnot, 1995; Klein, Alexander, & Parsons, 1977). The model is being evaluated in a variety of dissemination and effectiveness contexts, including increasingly multicultural ones (Alexander et al., 2000), within statewide systems by community practitioners (e.g., Barnoski, 2004; Zazzali et al., 2007), and in international replications (Breuk et al., 2006). Most encouragingly, when the model is implemented with fidelity, lower recidivism rates and other related positive outcomes are being reported for this range of community settings and multiethnic participants (Sexton & Alexander, 2003). Currently, a Campbell Collaboration review of the effectiveness of FFT across studies is underway, an important development in light of its widespread use in the United States and increasing dissemination in other countries.

Multisystemic Therapy

Multisystemic Therapy (MST) was designed as an ecological model from its inception and has influenced the shift of other family intervention models in this direction. Based on Bronfenbrenner's (1979) theory of social ecology, MST has a consistency and coherence in integrating knowledge of risk and protective factors in a youth's and a family's ecology throughout its assessment and treatment procedures.

Services are provided using a family-preservation model in the youth's home and community, with extensive attention given to engagement as in the other approaches. Even though home-based treatment can facilitate engagement, it does not guarantee it, especially when engagement is viewed as an ongoing process signifying emotional investment and active participation and follow-through in intervention plans (Cunningham & Henggeler, 1999; Stern, 1999).

An ecological assessment of strengths and needs occurs across each of the systems that have been linked with antisocial behavior guided by the research on risk and protective factors. Protective factors provide clues or building blocks for how the youth and family can successfully make change, enhance change, or maintain changes. Because MST is a present-focused and future-oriented model, proximal causes are considered before distal ones when generating assessment hypotheses, although the latter are considered when they are linked with and impact current functioning (Henggeler et al., 1998).

Following assessment, treatment is individualized for each family, explicitly and systematically targeting the multiple domains in which the youth behavior is embedded using behavioral and cognitive-behavioral interventions with strong evidence of effectiveness as well as strategies from other empirically based or pragmatic problem-focused approaches such as structural and strategic family therapies. This does not necessarily mean that the worker intervenes in each system; rather, MST emphasizes empowering parents and other caregivers with the skills and support to develop and carry out change strategies across the key systems linked with adolescent problem behavior (Henggeler et al., 1998; Smith & Stern, 1997). Intervention strategies fall into five main categories, with interventions to modify parenting practices and strengthen family functioning at the core of the model. Other strategies target changing relationships with peers (specifically disengaging youth from deviant peers, fostering connection to prosocial peers and activities, and developing social competence and problem-solving skills); promoting academic and social competence in school and strengthening the family-school linkage (e.g., parent-teacher relationship); strengthening family linkages with community supports; and addressing individually oriented intervention when required.

The MST manual outlines guidelines for when to incorporate individual work into family treatment and details empirical interventions to address a range of difficulties such as caregiver substance abuse or psychiatric problems, youth cognitive and problem-solving deficits, and victimization sequelae (Henggeler et al., 1998). During MST engagement and intervention, therapists use an iterative process to identify obstacles to implementation, to test hypotheses about their role, and to generate solutions (Henggeler et al., 1998). Strategies for overcoming common barriers are described for each of the intervention areas.

Although MST treatment is individualized and highly flexible, enabling practitioners to build on each family's specific strengths and to be responsive to their cultural context, a set of nine principles provides a structured framework that guides MST case conceptualization and intervention. These include finding the fit between identified problems and the ecological context; targeting sequences of behavior within and between multiple systems (e.g., home, school) that maintain the problem; promoting the durability of treatment changes by empowering caregivers to similarly address family members' needs across ecological contexts; and continuous monitoring throughout treatment from multiple perspectives (e.g., father, grandmother, teacher, probation officer) to assess progress with providers (practitioner, supervisor, and support team) accountable for identifying and overcoming barriers to reaching treatment goals. Understanding how a family's culture contributes to problems and potential solutions is an important component of assessing the fit between identified problems and the broader systemic context (Brondino et al., 1997).

According to the remaining MST principles, interventions should target specific, well-defined problems, be present focused and action oriented, strengths based, developmentally appropriate for both youth and caregivers, require daily and weekly effort by everyone involved in carrying out tasks and working on achieving goals, and designed to promote responsible and decrease irresponsible behavior (Henggeler et al., 1998).

Individual studies report that MST has shown some significant positive results across settings in modifying family processes and in attenuating adolescents' serious antisocial behavior, including long-term reductions in delinquency recidivism, incarceration, and costs (Aos, Phipps, Barnoski, & Lieb, 2001; Sheidow, Henggeler, & Schoenwald, 2003). MST has reduced long-term rates of rearrest or out-of-home placement in three randomized trials with violent and chronic juvenile offenders (Borduin et al., 1995; Henggeler, Melton, Brondino, Scherer, & Hanley, 1997; Henggeler, Melton, & Smith, 1992; Henggeler, Melton, Smith, Schoenwald, & Hanley, 1993) and shown promising results in a small RCT with juvenile sex offenders (Borduin, Henggeler, Blaske, & Stein, 1990), although the latter findings should be viewed cautiously in light of a small sample size. In contrast, compared with usual community treatment, MST had limited effects in a study of substance abusing or dependent juvenile offenders with high rates of psychiatric comorbidity (Brown, Henggeler, Schoenwald, Brondino, & Pickrel, 1999; Henggeler, Clingempeel, Brondino, & Pickrel, 2002; Henggeler, Pickrel, & Brondino, 1999; Schoenwald, Ward, Henggeler, Pickrel, & Patel, 1996). As suggested by the researchers, poor treatment implementation fidelity and the need for enhancements to multisystemic therapy specific to a challenging population of drug-using offenders may have contributed to the disappointing outcomes. Additional studies focus on outcomes of MST for child abuse and serious emotional disorders (e.g., Brunk, Henggeler, & Whelan, 1987; Henggeler et al., 2003). Findings regarding changes in family functioning vary across studies, and two recent meta-analyses found no effects when individual study outcomes are pooled (Littell, 2005; Woolfenden, Williams, & Peat, 2003). Families in MST studies tend to be economically disadvantaged, and a high percentage are Black. In studies that have examined treatment differences, outcomes are reported to be equally effective for Black and White youth and families (Brondino et al., 1997). MST has been widely transported throughout the United States and internationally and has been examined in randomized trials in Canada and Norway (Leschied & Cunningham, 2002; Ogden & Amlund Hagen, 2006; Ogden & Halliday-Boykins, 2004; Schoenwald, Heiblum, Saldana, & Henggeler, 2008).

Despite encouraging findings from individual studies reported by MST investigators, recent findings from a large Canadian independent clinical trial of MST for serious young offenders (Leschied & Cunningham, 2002) and a Campbell Collaboration systematic review that included these findings (Littell, Popa, & Forsythe, 2005) raise issues about conclusions drawn previously. The meta-analysis findings were based on eight individual MST outcome studies that met scientific standards high enough to be included in a Campbell review. The Campbell review conclusion was that MST has not been shown to be more effective than alternative treatments (Littell, 2005), stimulating a spirited debate in the literature (Henggeler, Schoenwald, & Swenson, 2006; Littell, 2005, 2006, 2008). Although this finding is less favorable than those reported in individual studies and is at odds with previous reviewers' more positive assessment of the evidence base, evidence of no difference does not mean that MST does not work, only that it has not been shown to work better than the alternatives with which it was compared. We think that there are a number of reasons juvenile justice practitioners should be attentive to emerging MST findings given that MST is theoretically and empirically grounded, extensively studied with no evidence of harm (an important consideration) and there is no evidence suggesting an alternative more effective model (Littell et al., 2005; Stern, 2004).

It is possible that a Campbell review of any of the other models described in this chapter could raise issues similar to those identified for MST, because a systematic review and meta-analysis of outcomes from multiple studies may support a different conclusion than those drawn from the results of single studies or an unsystematic review. Littell's findings underscore the importance of rigorous and continuous research evaluations, culminating in well-executed systematic reviews in order to increase our certainty that a given intervention is effective. This is especially true as treatments deemed to be "evidence-based" are widely disseminated and extended to new populations and contexts (Stern, 2004), and such dissemination prior to a fairly high level of certainty should always be done cautiously and with continued evaluation.

LESSONS LEARNED FROM FAMILY RESEARCH: IMPLICATIONS FOR JUVENILE JUSTICE PRACTICE

As is evident in this overview of treatment outcome studies, the findings from family processes and family intervention research converge to underscore that families play a key role in and pose a frontline defense against childhood aggression and adolescent antisocial and delinquent behavior. Familiarity with these models provides the juvenile justice practitioner or program developer evidence-based methods to enhance practice. All the models reviewed offer systematic and planful, yet individualized and flexible, methods for working with the diversity of families seen in community practice. Though different, the approaches share several themes. Each acknowledges the multiple influences on youth development and the ecology of family life and incorporates these into its model in its own way. Each approach has evolved over years of (continuing) clinical research and has been modified in response to family needs, changing contexts, and research findings. Increasingly, investigators have turned to research on culture, gender, and comorbidity to further model development in the contemporary landscape. The existing research findings speak to the outcomes when intervention is delivered with fidelity—that is, in the manner validated and specified in program manuals and training. Effectiveness may be compromised when interventions previously found to be efficacious are not implemented with fidelity as some studies have shown (Elliott & Mihalic, 2004; Forgatch, Patterson, & DeGarmo, 2005; Henggeler et al., 1997; Huey et al., 2000; Sexton & Alexander, 2003; Stern, Alaggia, Watson, & Morton, 2008; Webster-Stratton, 2004) and/or are provided to clients whom the model was not intended to serve.

In addition to outcome studies of the effects of intervention, some program researchers have conducted process research to shed light on what actually transpires during sessions and critical mechanisms of change that lead to meaningful intervention implications (Liddle & Rowe, 2004; Sexton, Ridley, & Kleiner, 2004). Each approach targets parenting and family interactions, with shifts in parenting probably the most influential change mechanism identified in studies. All of the models reviewed give significant attention to culturally responsive engagement and the therapeutic alliance, with process studies across programs of family intervention research adding to our understanding of the complexity of therapeutic alliances in a family treatment context. Redefining the presenting problem by reducing blaming statements and reframing negative attributions, and decreasing within-session negativity, have emerged as key mechanisms for engagement and effective outcomes.

Regardless of whether one is in a setting that is implementing one of these models in its entirety, along with the training and supervision that are part of the dissemination packages for most evidence-based programs, the findings on change processes within and across models in conjunction with the evidence on effective outcomes speak directly to practitioners and program developers. As these models and processes are adopted in juvenile justice practice, ongoing monitoring and evaluation are needed to provide continuous quality assurance and to ensure that the evidence translates into effective outcomes for the children, youth, and families in our distinctive communities and that we do no harm.

NOTES

This chapter includes material previously published in "Evidence-Based Practice With Antisocial and Delinquent Youth: The Key Role of Family and Multisystemic Interventions," by S. B. Stern, 2004, in H. E. Briggs & T. Rzepnicki (Eds.), *Using Evidence for Social Work Practice* (pp. 104–127), Chicago: Lyceum Books, and is used with the consent of Lyceum Books.

1. See chapter 18 for a discussion of terms. We use aggression and conduct problems or conduct disorder to refer to both *DSM-IV* diagnosed (American Psychiatric Association, 2000) and undiagnosed disruptive/externalizing behavior problems in children.
2. The term *parent* is used for consistency but reflects the range of child caregiver arrangements.

REFERENCES

Abram, K. M., Teplin, L.A., McCelland, G. M., & Dulcan, M. K. (2003). Comorbid psychiatric disorders in youth in juvenile detention. *Archives of General Psychiatry, 60*, 1097–1108.

Achenbach, T. M., & Rescorla, L. A. (2001). *Manual for the ASEBA school age forms and profile*. Burlington: University of Vermont, Research Center for Children, Youth and Families.

Alexander, J. F. (1973). Defensive and supportive communication in normal and deviant families. *Journal of Consulting and Clinical Psychology, 40*, 223–231.

Alexander, J. F., Barton, C., Schiavo, R. S., & Parsons, B. V. (1976). Behavioral interventions with families of delinquents: Therapist characteristics and outcome. *Journal of Consulting and Clinical Psychology, 44*(4), 656–664.

Alexander, J. F., & Parsons, B. V. (1973). Short-term behavioral intervention with delinquent families: Impact on family processes and recidivism. *Journal of Abnormal Psychology, 81*, 219–225.

Alexander, J. F., Pugh, C., Parsons, B., & Sexton, T. (2000). Functional family therapy. In D. S. Elliott (Series Ed.), *Blueprints for violence prevention* (Book 3). Golden, CO: Venture Publishing.

Allen, J. P., Leadbeater, B. J., & Aber, J. L. (1994). The development of problem behavior syndromes in at-risk adolescents. *Development and Psychopathology, 6*, 323–342.

Ambert, A. M. (1992). *The effect of children on parents*. New York: Haworth Press.

American Psychiatric Association. (2000). *Diagnostic and statistical manual of mental disorders* (4th ed., text revision). Washington, DC: Author.

Angold, A., Costello, E. J., & Erkanli, A. (1999). Comorbidity. *Journal of Child Psychology and Psychiatry, 40*(1), 57–87.

Antonishak, J., Reppucci, N. D., & Mulford, C. F. (2004). Girls in the justice system: Treatment and intervention. In M. Moretti, C. Odgers, & M. Jackson (Eds.), *Girls and violence: Contributing factors and intervention principles*. Perspectives in Law and Psychology Series (pp. 165–181). New York: Kluwer Academic/Plenum Press.

Aos, S., & Barnoski, R. (1998). *Watching the bottom line: Cost-effective interventions for reducing crime in Washington*. Olympia: Washington State Institute for Public Policy, RCW13.40.500.

Aos, S., Phipps, P., Barnoski, R., & Leib, R. (2001). *The comparative costs and benefits of programs to reduce crime*. Olympia: Washington State Institute for Public Policy, Document 01-15-1201.

Ary, D. V., Duncan, T. E., Duncan, S. C., & Hops, H. (1999). Adolescent problem behavior: The influence of parents and peers. *Behaviour Research and Therapy, 37*, 217–230.

Augimeri, L. K., Enebrink, P., Walsh, M., & Jiang, D. (in press). Gender-specific childhood risk assessment tools: Early Assessment Risk List of Boys (EARL-20B) and Girls (EARL-21G). In R. K. Otto and K. Douglas (Eds.), *Handbook of violence risk assessment tools*. New York: Routledge.

Augimeri, L. K., Farrington, D. P., Koegl, C. J., & Day, D. M. (2007). The SNAP™ under 12 outreach project: Effects of a community based program for children with conduct problems. *Journal of Child and Family Studies, 16*, 799–807.

Augimeri, L. K., Koegl, C. J., & Goldberg, K. (2001). Children under 12 who commit offenses: Canadian legal and treatment approaches. In R. Loeber & D. Farrington

(Eds.), *Child delinquents: Development, intervention and service needs* (pp. 405–414). Thousand Oaks, CA: Sage.

Augimeri, L. K., Koegl, C. J., Webster, C. D., & Levene, K. S. (2001). *Early assessment risk list for boys* (Version 2). Toronto, Canada: Earlscourt Child and Family Centre.

Bandura, A. (1977). *Social learning theory.* Englewood Cliffs, NJ: Prentice Hall.

Bandura, A. (1982). Self-efficacy mechanisms in human agency. *American Psychologist, 84,* 191–215.

Barlow, J., & Parsons, J. (2004). Group-based parent-training programmes for improving emotional and behavioral adjustment in 0–3 year old children. *Cochrane Database of Systematic Reviews, 2,* 1–48.

Barnoski, R. (2004). *Outcome evaluation of Washington state's research-based programs for juvenile offenders: Appendix.* Olympia: Washington State Institute for Public Policy.

Barton, C., Alexander, J. F., Waldron, H., Turner, C. W., & Warburton, J. (1985). Generalizing treatment effects of functional family therapy: Three replications. *American Journal of Family Therapy, 13,* 16–26.

Borduin, C. M., Henggeler, S. W., Blaske, D. M., & Stein, R. (1990). Multisystemic treatment of adolescent sexual offenders. *International Journal of Offender Therapy and Comparative Criminology, 35,* 105–114.

Borduin, C. M., Mann, B. J., Cone, L. T., Henggeler, S. W., Fucci, B. R., Blaske, D. M., et al. (1995). Multisystemic treatment of serious juvenile offenders: Long term prevention of criminality and violence. *Journal of Consulting and Clinical Psychology, 63,* 569–578.

Boyd-Franklin, N., & Bry, B. H. (2000). *Reaching out in family therapy: Home-based, school, and community interventions.* New York: Guilford Press.

Breuk, R. E., Sexton, T. L., van Dam, A., Disse, C., Doreleijers, T., Slot, W. N., et al. (2006). The implementation and the cultural adjustment of functional family therapy in a Dutch psychiatric day-treatment center. *Journal of Marital and Family Therapy, 32*(4), 515–530.

Brondino, M. J., Henggeler, S. W., Rowland, M. D., Pickrel, S. G., Cunningham, P. B., & Schoenwald, S. K. (1997). Multisystemic therapy and the ethnic minority client: Culturally responsive and clinically effective. In D. K. Wilson, J. R. Rodrigue, & W. C. Taylor (Eds.), *Health-promoting and health-compromising behaviors among minority adolescents* (pp. 229–250). Washington, DC: American Psychological Association.

Bronfenbrenner, U. (1979). *The ecology of human development: Experiments by nature and design.* Cambridge, MA: Harvard University Press.

Brown, T. L., Henggeler, S. W., Schoenwald, S. K., Brondino, M. J., & Pickrel, S. G. (1999). Multisystemic treatment of substance abusing and dependent juvenile delinquents: Effects on school attendance at posttreatment and 6-month follow-up. *Children's Services: Social Policy, Research, & Practice, 2*(2), 81–93.

Brunk, M., Henggeler, S. W., & Whelan, J. P. (1987). A comparison of multisystemic therapy and parent training in the brief treatment of child abuse and neglect. *Journal of Consulting and Clinical Psychology, 55,* 311–318.

Bry, B. H., Conboy, C., & Bisgay, K. (1986). Decreasing adolescent drug use and school failure: Long-term effects of targeted family problem-solving training. *Child & Family Behavior Therapy, 8,* 43–59.

Bunting, L. (2004). Parenting programmes: The best available evidence. *Child Care in Practice, 10*(4), 327–343.

Burns, B. J., Howell, J. C., Wiig, J. K., Augimeri, L. K., Welsh, B. C., Loeber, R., et al. (2003). *Treatment, services, and intervention programs for child delinquents* (Juvenile Justice Bulletin, NCJ 193410). Washington, DC: Office of Juvenile Justice and Delinquency Prevention.

Catalano, R. F., & Hawkins, J. D. (1996). The social development model: A theory of antisocial behaviour. In J. D. Hawkins (Ed.), *Delinquency and crime: Current theories* (pp. 149–197). New York: Cambridge University Press.

Catalano, R. F., Morrison, D. M., Wells, E. A., Gillmore, M. R., Iritani, B., & Hawkins, J. D. (1992). Ethnic differences in family factors related to early drug initiation. *Journal of Studies on Alcohol, 53*(3), 208–217.

Chamberlain, P. (1990). Comparative evaluation of specialized foster care for seriously delinquent youths: A first step. *Community Alternatives: International Journal of Family Care, 2,* 21–36.

Chamberlain, P., Leve, L. D., & DeGarmo, D. S. (2007). Multidimensional treatment foster care for girls in the juvenile justice system: 2-year follow-up of a randomized clinical trial. *Journal of Consulting and Clinical Psychology, 75*(1), 187–193.

Chamberlain, P., & Mihalic, S. F. (1998). Multidimensional treatment foster care. In D. S. Elliott (Series Ed.), *Blueprints for violence prevention* (Book 8). University of Colorado, Center for the Study of and Prevention of Violence. Boulder, CO: Blueprints Publications.

Chamberlain, P., & Moore, K. J. (2002). Chaos and trauma in the lives of adolescent females with antisocial behaviour and delinquency. *Journal of Aggression, Maltreatment & Trauma, 6,* 79–108.

Chamberlain, P., Patterson, G.R., Reid, J. B., Forgatch, M. S., & Kavanagh, K. (1984). Observations of client resistance. *Behavior Therapy, 15,* 144–155.

Chamberlain, P., & Reid, J. B. (1998). Comparison of two community alternatives to incarceration for chronic juvenile offenders. *Journal of Consulting and Clinical Psychology, 66,* 624–633.

Child Development Institute. (2008a). *SNAP® children's group manual.* Toronto, Canada: Author.

Child Development Institute. (2008b). *SNAP® parent group manual.* Toronto, Canada: Author.

Conduct Problems Prevention Research Group. (1992). A developmental and clinical model for the prevention of conduct disorders: The FAST Track program. *Development and Psychopathology, 4,* 509–527.

Conger, R. D., & Elder, G. H. (1994). *Families in troubled times: Adapting to change in rural America.* New York: Aldine de Gruyter.

Conger, R. D., Patterson, G. R., & Ge, X. (1995). It takes two to replicate: A mediational model for the impact of parents' stress on adolescent adjustment. *Child Development, 65,* 541–561.

Corrado, R., Odgers, C., & Cohen I. (2000). The incarceration of female young offenders: Protection for whom? *Canadian Journal of Criminology, 4*(2), 189–207.

Cunningham, P. B., & Henggeler, S. W. (1999). Engaging multiproblem families in treatment: Lessons learned throughout the development of multisystemic therapy. *Family Process, 38*(3), 265–286.

Dadds, M. R., Schwartz, S., & Sanders, M. R. (1987). Marital discord and treatment outcome in behavioural family therapy for child conduct disorders. *Journal of Consulting and Clinical Psychology, 55,* 396–403.

DeGarmo, D. S., & Forgatch, M. S. (2004). Putting problem solving to the test: Replicating experimental interventions for preventing youngsters' problem behaviors. In R. D. Conger, F. O. Lorenz, & K.A.S. Wickrama (Eds.), *Continuity and change in family relations* (pp. 267–290). Mahwah, NJ: Erlbaum.

Dishion, T. J., & Andrews, D. W. (1995). Preventing escalation in problem behaviors with high-risk young adolescents: Immediate and one-year outcomes. *Journal of Consulting and Clinical Psychology, 63,* 538–548.

Dishion, T. J., McCord, J., & Poulin, F. (1999). When interventions harm: Peer groups and problem behaviour. *American Psychologist, 54,* 755–764.

Dishion, T. J., & Patterson, G. R. (1992). Age effects in parent training. *Behavior Therapy, 23,* 719–729.

Dishion, T. J., Patterson, G. R., & Kavanagh, K. A. (1992). An experimental test of the coercion model. In J. McCord & R. E. Tremblay (Eds.), *Preventing antisocial behavior: Interventions from birth through adolescence* (pp. 53–282). New York: Guilford Press.

Dishion, T. J., Patterson, G. R., & Reid, J. (1988). Parent and peer factors associated with early adolescent drug use: Implications for treatment. In E. Radhert & J. Grabowski (Eds.), *Adolescent drug abuse: Analysis of treatment research, NIDA research monograph* (Vol. 77, pp. 69–93). Washington DC: U.S. Government Printing Office.

Dishion, T. J., Patterson, G. R., Stoolmiller, M., & Skinner, M. I. (1991). Family, school, and behavioral antecedents to early adolescent involvement with antisocial peers. *Developmental Psychology, 27,* 172–180.

Dishion, T. J., Poulin, F., & Burraston, B. (2001). Peer group dynamics associated with iatrogenic effect in group interventions with high-risk young adolescents. *New Directions for Child and Adolescent Development, 91,* 79–92.

Dodge, K. A. (2004). Public policy and the "discovery" of girls' aggressive behaviour. In M. Putallaz & K. L. Bierman (Eds.), *Aggression, antisocial behavior, and violence among girls* (pp. 302–312). Duke Series in Child Development and Public Policy. New York: Guilford Press.

Dodge, K. A., & Frame, C. M. (1982). Social cognitive biases and deficits in aggressive boys. *Child Development, 53,* 620–635.

Donovan, J. E., Jessor, R., & Costa, F. M. (1988). Syndrome of problem behaviour in adolescence: A replication. *Journal of Consulting and Clinical Psychology, 56*(5), 762–765.

Dumas, J. E., & Wahler, R. G. (1983). Predictors of treatment outcome in parent training: Mother insularity and socioeconomic disadvantage. *Behavioral Assessment, 5,* 301–313.

Eddy, J. M., Whaley, R. B., & Chamberlain, P. (2004). The prevention of violent behaviour by chronic and serious male juvenile offenders: A 2-year follow-up of a randomized clinical trial. *Journal of Emotional and Behavioral Disorders, 12*(1), 2–8.

Ehrensaft, M. K. (2005). Interpersonal relationships and sex differences in the development of conduct problems. *Clinical Child and Family Psychology Review, 8*(1), 39–63.

Elliott, D. S. (Series Ed.). (1998). *Blueprints for violence prevention.* University of Colorado Center for the Study and Prevention of Violence. Boulder, CO: Blueprints Publications. Retrieved August 1, 2008, from http://www.colorado.edu/cspv/blueprints

Elliott, D. S., & Mihalic, S. (2004). Issues in disseminating and replicating effective prevention programs. *Prevention Science, 5*(1), 47–72.

Enebrink, P., Långström, N., & Gumpert, C. H. (2006). Predicting aggressive and disruptive behavior in referred 6- to 12-year-old boys: Prospective validation of the EARL-20B Risk/Needs Checklist. *Assessment, 13,* 356–367.

Eyberg, S. M., Boggs, S., & Algina, J. (1995). Parent-child interaction therapy: A psychosocial model for the treatment of young children with conduct problem behaviour and their families. *Psychopharmacology Bulletin, 31,* 83–91.

Eyberg, S. M., Nelson, M. N., & Boggs, S. R. (2008). Evidence-based psychosocial treatments for children and adolescents with disruptive behavior. *Journal of Clinical Child & Adolescent Psychology, 37,* 215–237.

Farrington, D. P., & Welsh, B. C. (2006). *Saving children from a life of crime: Early risk factors and effective interventions: Studies in crime and public policy.* New York: Oxford University Press.

Fergusson, D. M., Lynskey, M. T., & Horwood, L. J. (1996). Origins of comorbidity between conduct and affective disorders. *Journal of American Academy Child Adolescent Psychiatry, 35*(4), 451–460.

Forehand, R. L., & McMahon, R. J. (1981). *Helping the noncompliant child. A clinician's guide to parent training.* New York: Guilford Press.

Forehand, R., Miller, K. S., Dutra, R., & Chance, M. W. (1997). Role of parenting in adolescent deviant behavior: Replication across and within two ethnic groups. *Journal of Consulting and Clinical Psychology, 65*(6), 1036–1041.

Forgatch, M. S. (1994). *Parenting through change: A training manual.* Eugene: Oregon Social Learning Center.

Forgatch, M. S., & Patterson, G. R. (2005). *Parents and adolescents living together: Part 2. Family problem solving.* Champaign, IL: Research Press.

Forgatch, M. S., Patterson, G. R., & DeGarmo, D. S. (2005). Evaluating fidelity: Predictive validity for a measure of competent adherence to the Oregon model of parent management training. *Behavior Therapy, 36,* 3–13.

Fraser, M. W. (1996). Aggressive behaviour in childhood and early adolescence: An ecological-developmental perspective on youth violence. *Social Work, 41*(4), 347–361.

Gardner, F., Burton, J., & Klimes, I. (2006). Randomised controlled trial of a parenting intervention in the voluntary sector for reducing child conduct problems: Outcomes and mechanisms of change. *Journal of Child Psychology and Psychiatry, 4*(11), 1123–1132.

Gordon, D. A., Arbuthnot, J., Gustafsond, K. E., & McGreen, P. (1988). Home-based behavioral systems family therapy with disadvantaged juvenile delinquents. *American Journal of Family Therapy, 16,* 243–255.

Gordon, D. A., Graves, K., & Arbuthnot, J. (1995). The effect of functional family therapy for delinquents on adult criminal behavior. *Criminal Justice and Behavior, 22,* 60–73.

Gorman-Smith, D., Tolan, P. H., Zelli, A., & Huesmann, L. R. (1996). The relation of family functioning to violence among inner-city youths. *Journal of Family Psychology, 10,* 115–129.

Granic, I., & Patterson, G. R. (2006). Toward a comprehensive model of antisocial development: A dynamic systems approach. *Psychological Review, 113*(1), 101–131.

Grizenko, N., & Pawliuk, N. (1994). Risk and protective factors for disruptive behavior disorders in children. *American Journal Orthopsychiatry, 64*(4), 534–544.

Hahn, R. A., Bilukha, O., Lowy, J., Crosby, A., Fullilove, M. T., Liberman, A., et al. (2005). The effectiveness of therapeutic foster care for the prevention of violence: A systematic review. *American Journal of Preventive Medicine, 28*(2S1), 72–90.

Henggeler, S. W. (1991). Multidimensional causal models of delinquent behavior. In R. Cohen & A. Siegel (Eds.), *Context and development* (pp. 211–231). Hillsdale, NJ: Erlbaum.

Henggeler, S. W., & Borduin, C. M. (1990). *Family therapy and beyond: A multisystemic approach to treating the behavior problems of children and adolescents.* Pacific Grove, CA: Brooks/Cole.

Henggeler, S. W., Clingempeel, W. G., Brondino, M. J., & Pickrel, S. G. (2002). Four-year follow-up of multisystemic therapy with substance abusing and dependent juvenile offenders. *Journal of the American Academy of Child & Adolescent Psychiatry, 41*(7), 868–874.

Henggeler, S. W., Melton, G. B., Brondino, M. J., Scherer, D. G., & Hanley, J. H. (1997). Multisystemic therapy with violent and chronic juvenile offenders and their families: The role of treatment fidelity in successful dissemination. *Journal of Consulting and Clinical Psychology, 65,* 821–833.

Henggeler, S. W., Melton, G. B., & Smith, L. A. (1992). Family preservation using multisystemic family therapy: An effective alternative to incarcerating serious juvenile offenders. *Journal of Consulting and Clinical Psychology, 60,* 953–961.

Henggeler, S. W., Melton, G. B., Smith, L. A., Schoenwald, S. K., & Hanley, J. H. (1993). Family preservation using multisystemic treatment: Long-term follow-up to a clinical trial with serious juvenile offenders. *Journal of Child and Family Studies, 2,* 283–293.

Henggeler, S. W., Pickrel, S. G., & Brondino, M. J. (1999). Multisystemic treatment of substance abusing and dependent delinquents: Outcomes, treatment fidelity, and transportability. *Mental Health Services Research, 1,* 171–184.

Henggeler, S. W., Rowland, M. D., Halliday-Boykins, C., Sheidow, A. J., Ward, D. M., Randall, J., et al. (2003). One-year follow-up of multisystemic therapy as an alternative to the hospitalization of youths in psychiatric crisis. *Journal of the American Academy of Child and Adolescent Psychiatry, 42,* 543–551.

Henggeler, S. W., Schoenwald, S. K., Borduin, C. M., Rowland, M. D., & Cunningham, P. B. (1998). *Multisystemic treatment of antisocial behavior in children and adolescents.* New York: Guilford Press.

Henggeler, S. W., Schoenwald, S. K., & Swenson, C. C. (2006). Methodological critique and meta-analysis as Trojan horse. *Children and Youth Services Review, 28,* 447–457.

Henggler, S. W., & Sheidow, A. J. (2003). Conduct disorder and delinquency. *Journal of Marital and Family Therapy, 29*(4), 505–522.

Hoagwood, K., Burns, B. J., Kiser, L., Ringeisen, H., & Schoenwald, S. K. (2001). Evidence-based practice in child and adolescent mental health services. *Psychiatric Services, 52*(9), 1179–1189.

Hops, H., Tildesley, E., Lichtenstein, E., Ary, D., & Sherman, L. (1990). Parent–adolescent problem-solving interactions and drug use. *American Journal of Drug and Alcohol Abuse, 16,* 239–258.

Howell, J. C. (2001). Juvenile justice programs and strategies. In R. Loeber & D. Farrington (Eds.), *Child delinquents: Development, intervention and service needs* (pp. 305–321). Thousand Oaks, CA: Sage.

Huey, S. J., Henggeler, S. W., Brondino, M. J., & Pickrel, S. G. (2000). Mechanisms of change in multisystemic therapy: Reducing delinquent behavior through therapist adherence and improved family and peer functioning. *Journal of Consulting and Clinical Psychology, 68*, 451–467.

Hutchings, J., Bywater, T., Daley, D., Gardner, F., Whitaker, C., Jones, K., et al. (2007). Parenting intervention in sure start services for children at risk of developing conduct disorder: Pragmatic randomised controlled trial. *British Medical Journal, 334*, 678–682.

Kazdin, A. E. (1995). *Conduct disorders in childhood and adolescence.* Newbury Park, CA: Sage.

Kazdin A. E., Mazurick, J. L., & Bass, D. (1993). Risk for attrition in treatment of antisocial children and families. *Journal of Clinical Psychology, 22*, 2–16.

Kazdin, A. E., & Weisz, J. R. (1998). Identifying and developing empirically supported child and adolescent treatment. *Journal of Consulting and Clinical Psychology, 66*, 19–36.

Kazdin, A. E., & Whitley, M. K. (2003). Treatment of parental stress to enhance therapeutic change among children referred for aggressive and antisocial behavior. *Journal of Consulting and Clinical Psychology, 71*, 504–514.

Keenan, K., Stouthamer-Loeber, M., & Loeber, R. (2005). Studying conduct problems in girls. In D. J. Pepler, K. C. Madsen, C. Webster, & K. S. Levene (Eds.), *The development and treatment of girlhood aggression* (pp. 29–46). Mahwah, NJ: Erlbaum.

Klein, N. C., Alexander, J. F., & Parsons, B. V. (1977). Impact of family systems intervention on recidivism and sibling delinquency: A model of primary prevention and program evaluation. *Journal of Consulting and Clinical Psychology, 45*, 469–474.

Koegl, C. J., Augimeri, L. K., Ferrante, P., Walsh, M., & Slater, N. (2008). A Canadian programme for child delinquents. In R. Loeber, W. N. Slot, P. van der Laan, & M. Hoeve (Eds.), *Tomorrow's Criminals: The development of child delinquency and effective intervention* (pp. 285–300). Aldershot, The Netherlands: Ashgate.

Koegl, C. J., Farrington, D. P., Augimeri, L. K., & Day, D. M. (2008). Evaluation of a targeted cognitive-behavioural programme for children with conduct problems—The SNAP® Under 12 Outreach Project: Service intensity, age and gender effects on short- and long-term outcomes. *Clinical Child Psychology and Psychiatry, 13*(3), 419–434.

Krohn, M. D., Stern, S. B., Thornberry, T. P., & Jang, S. J. (1992). The measurement of family process variables: The effect of adolescent and parent perceptions of family life on delinquent behavior. *Journal of Quantitative Criminology, 8*, 287–315.

Krohn, M. D., Thornberry, T. P., Rivera, C., & Le Blanc, M. (2001). Later delinquency careers. In R. Loeber and D. P. Farrington (Eds.), *Child delinquents* (pp. 67–93). Thousand Oaks, CA: Sage.

Kumpfer, K. L. (1999). *Strengthening America's families: Exemplary parenting and family strategies for delinquency prevention.* U.S. Department of Justice. Retrieved June 5, 2001, from http: //www/strengtheningfamilies.org

Kumpfer, K. L., & DeMarsh, J. P. (1986). Family environmental and genetic influences on children's future chemical dependency. In S. Griswold-Ezekoye, K. L. Kumpfer, & W. Bukoski (Eds.), *Childhood and chemical abuse: Prevention and intervention* (pp. 49–91). New York: Haworth.

Lamborn, S. D., Dornbusch, S. M., & Steinberg, L. (1996). Ethnicity and community context as moderators of the relations between family decision making and adolescent adjustment. *Child Development, 67,* 283–301.

Leschied, A. W., & Cunningham, A. (2002). *Seeking effective interventions for serious young offenders: Interim results of a four-year randomized study of multisystemic therapy in Ontario, Canada.* London, Canada: Centre for Children and Families in the Justice System.

Leve, L. D., Chamberlain, P., & Reid, J. B. (2005). Intervention outcomes for girls referred from juvenile justice: Effects on delinquency. *Journal of Consulting and Clinical Psychology, 73*(6), 1181–1185.

Levene, K. S. (2003). *SNAP™ girls group manual: The girls club.* Toronto, Canada: Earlscourt Child and Family Centre.

Levene, K. S., Augimeri, L. K., Pepler, D., Walsh, M., Webster, C. D., & Koegl, C. J. (2001). *Early Assessment Risk List for girls—Version 1, Consultation edition (EARL-21G).* Toronto, Canada: Earlscourt Child and Family Centre.

Levene, K. S., Madsen, K. C., & Pepler, D. J. (2005). Girls growing up angry: A qualitative study. In D. J. Pepler, K. C. Madsen, C. Webster, & K. S. Levene (Eds.), *The development and treatment of girlhood aggression* (pp. 169–190). Mahwah, NJ: Erlbaum.

Levene, K. S., Walsh, M. M., Augimeri, L. K., & Pepler, D. J. (2004). Linking identification and treatment of early risk factors for female delinquency. In M. Moretti, C. Odgers, & M. Jackson (Eds.), *Girls and violence: Contributing factors and intervention principles* (pp. 131–146). Perspectives in Law and Psychology Series. New York: Kluwer Academic/Plenum Press.

Liddle, H. A. (1995). Conceptual and clinical dimensions of a multi-dimensional, multi-systems engagement strategy in family based adolescent treatment. *Psychotherapy, 32,* 39–54.

Liddle, H. A. (2002). Multidimensional family therapy for adolescent cannabis users. *Cannabis Youth Treatment Series,* Volume 5. Rockville, MD: Center for Substance Abuse Treatment, Substance Abuse and Mental Health Services Administration.

Liddle, H. A., & Rowe, C. L. (2004). Advances in family therapy research. In M. Nichols & R. Schwartz (Eds.), *Family therapy: Concepts and methods* (6th ed., pp. 395–435). Boston: Allyn & Bacon.

Lipman, E. L., Kenny, M., Sniderman, C., O'Grady, S., Augimeri, L., Khayutin, S., et al. (2008). Evaluation of a community-based program for young boys at risk of antisocial behaviour: Results and issues. *Journal of the Canadian Academy of Child and Adolescent Psychiatry, 17*(1), 12–19.

Littell, J. H. (2005). Lessons from a systematic review of effects of multisystemic therapy. *Children and Youth Services Review, 47,* 445–463.

Littell, J. H. (2006). The case for multisystemic therapy: Evidence or orthodoxy? *Children and Youth Services Review, 28,* 458–472.

Littell, J. H. (2008). Evidence-based or biased? The quality of published reviews of evidence-based practices. *Children and Youth Services Review, 30,* 1299–1317.

Littell, J. H., Popa, M., & Forsythe, B. (2005). Multisystemic therapy for social, emotional, and behavioural problems in youth aged 10–17 (Cochrane Review). *Cochrane Database of Systematic Reviews*, Issue 4. Chichester, England: Wiley.

Loeber, R. (1990). Development and risk factors of juvenile antisocial behaviour and delinquency. *Clinical Psychology Review, 10*, 1–41.

Loeber, R., & Farrington, D. P. (2001). *Child delinquents: Development, intervention, and service needs*. Thousand Oaks, CA: Sage.

Loeber, R., & Keenan, K. (1994). Interaction between conduct disorder and its comorbid conditions: Effects of age and gender. *Clinical Psychology Review, 14*(6), 497–525.

Loeber, R., & Stouthamer-Loeber, M. (1986). Family factors as correlates and predictors of juvenile conduct problems and delinquency. In M. Tonry & N. Morris (Eds.), *Crime and Justice: An Annual Review of Research, 7*, 29–149.

Lundahl, B., Risser, H. J., & Lovejoy, M. C. (2006). A meta-analysis of parent training moderators and follow up effects. *Clinical Psychology Review, 26*, 86–104.

Maughan, D. R., Christiansen, E., Jenson, W. R., Olympia, D., & Clark, E. (2005). Behavioral parent training as a treatment for externalizing behaviors and disruptive behaviour disorders: A meta-analysis. *School Psychology Review, 34*(3), 267–286.

McBride, D., VanderWaal, C., VanBuren, H., & Terry, Y. (1997). *Breaking the cycle of drug use among juvenile offenders*. Washington, DC: National Institute of Justice.

McCluskey C. P., & Tovar, S. (2003). Family processes and delinquency: The consistency of relationships by ethnicity and gender. *Journal of Ethnicity in Criminal Justice, 1*(1), 37–61.

Miller, G. E., & Prinz, R. J. (1990). Enhancement of social learning family interventions for child conduct disorder. *Psychological Bulletin, 108*, 291–307.

Moffitt, T. E. (1997). Adolescence-limited and life-course-persistent offending: A complementary pair of developmental theories. In T. P. Thornberry (Ed.), *Advances in criminological theory: Vol. 7. Developmental theories of crime and delinquency* (pp. 11–54). New Brunswick, NJ: Transaction Publishers.

Moretti, M. M., Odgers, C. L., & Jackson, M. A. (2004) Girls and aggression: A point of departure. In M. Moretti, C. Odgers, & M. Jackson (Eds.), *Girls and violence: Contributing factors and intervention principles* (pp. 147–163). Perspectives in Law and Psychology Series. New York: Kluwer Academic/Plenum Press.

Mrazek, P. J., & Haggerty, R. J. (Eds.). (1994). *Reducing risks for mental disorders: Frontiers for preventive intervention research*. Washington, DC: National Academy Press.

Newberry, A. M., Alexander, J. F., & Turner, C. W. (1991). Gender as a process variable in family therapy. *Journal of Family Psychology, 5*, 158–175.

Office of Juvenile Justice and Delinquency Prevention. (n.d.). *Model programs guide*. Retrieved July 29, 2008, from http://www.dsgonline.com/mpg2.5/mpg_index.htm

Ogden, T., & Amlund Hagen, K. (2006). Multisystemic treatment of serious behaviour problems in youth: Sustainability of effectiveness two years after intake. *Child and Adolescent Mental Health, 11*(3), 142–149.

Ogden, T., Forgatch, M. S., Askeland, E., Patterson, G. R., & Bullock, B. M. (2005). Implementation of parent management training at the national level: The case of Norway. *Journal of Social Work Practice, 19*, 317–329.

Ogden, T., & Halliday-Boykins, C. A. (2004). Multisystemic treatment of antisocial adolescents in Norway: Replication of clinical outcomes outside the US. *Child and Adolescent Mental Health, 9*, 77–83.

Patterson, G. R. (1982). *Coercive family process.* Eugene, OR: Castalia.

Patterson, G. R. (1995). Coercion as a basis for early age of onset for arrest. In J. McCord (Ed.), *Coercion and punishment in long term perspectives* (pp. 81–105). New York: Cambridge University Press.

Patterson, G. R. (2005). The next generation of PMTO models. *The Behavior Therapist, 28*(2), 25–32. Retreived December 14, 2007, from http://www.isii.net/website.isii/pdfarticles/new/The%Next%20Generation%20of%20PMTO%20models.pdf

Patterson, G. R., DeBaryshe, B. D., & Ramsey, E. (1989). A developmental perspective on antisocial behavior. *American Psychologist, 44*(2), 329–335.

Patterson, G. R., & Dishion, T. (1988). Multilevel family process models: Traits, interactions, and relationships. In R. A. Hinde & J. Stevenson-Hinde (Eds.), *Relationships within families: Mutual influences.* Oxford, England: Clarendon Press.

Patterson, G. R., & Forgatch, M. (1985). Therapist behavior as a determinant for client noncompliance: A paradox for the behavior modifier. *Journal of Consulting and Clinical Psychology, 53*, 846–851.

Patterson, G. R., Forgatch, M. S., Yoerger, K. L., & Stoolmiller, M. (1998). Variables that initiate and maintain an early-onset trajectory for juvenile offending. *Development and Psychopathology, 10*, 531–547.

Patterson, G. R., Reid, J. B., & Dishion, T. J. (1992). *Antisocial boys.* Eugene, OR: Castalia.

Peebles, F., & Loeber, R. (1994). Do individual factors and neighborhood context explain ethnic differences in juvenile delinquency? *Journal of Quantitative Criminology, 10*, 141–157.

Pepler, D., Walsh, M., Yuile, A., Levene, K., Vaughan, A., & Webber, J. (2008). *Bridging the gender gap: Interventions with aggressive girls and their parents.* Manuscript submitted for publication.

Poole, E. D., & Regoli, R. M. (1980). Parental support, delinquent friends, and delinquency: A test of interaction effects. *Journal of Criminal Law and Criminology, 70*(2), 188–193.

Prinz, R. J., Miller, G. E. (1994). Family-based treatment for childhood antisocial behaviour: Experimental influences on dropout and engagement. *Journal of Consulting and Clinical Psychology, 62*, 645–650.

Reyno, S. M., & McGrath, P. J. (2006). Predictors of parent training efficacy for child externalizing behaviour problems: A meta-analytic review. *Journal of Child Psychology and Psychiatry, 47*(1), 99–111.

Robbins, M. S., Turner, C. W., Alexander, J. F., & Perez, G. A. (2003). Alliance and dropout in family therapy for adolescents with behaviour problems: Individual and systemic effects. *Journal of Family Psychology, 17*(4), 534–544.

Rutter, M., Giller, H., & Hagell, A. (1998). *Antisocial behaviour by young people.* New York: Cambridge University Press.

Sanders, M. R., Markie-Dadds, C., & Turner, K.M.T. (1998). *Practitioner's manual for Enhanced Triple P.* Brisbane, Australia: Families International.

Sanders, M. R., Markie-Dadds, C., & Turner, K.M.T. (2000). *Practitioner's manual for Standard Triple P.* Brisbane, Australia: Families International.

Sanders, M. R., Markie-Dadds, C., & Turner, K.M.T. (2003). Theoretical, scientific and clinical foundations of the Triple P-Positive Parenting Program: A population approach to the promotion of parenting competence. *Parenting Research and Practice Monograph 1*, 1–24.

Sanders, M. R. & McFarland, M. (2000). The treatment of depressed mothers with disruptive children: A controlled evaluation of cognitive behavioral family intervention. *Behavior Therapy, 31*(1), 89–112.

Schmidt, S. E., Liddle, H. A. & Dakof, G. A. (1996). Changes in parenting practices and adolescent drug abuse during multidimensional family therapy. *Journal of Family Psychology, 10*, 12–27.

Schoenwald, S. K., Heiblum, N., Saldana, L., & Henggeler, S. W. (2008). The international implementation of multi-systemic therapy. *Evaluation and the Health Professions, 31*(2), 211–215.

Schoenwald, S. K., Ward, D. M., Henggeler, S. W., Pickrel, S. G., & Patel, H. (1996). MST treatment of substance abusing or dependent adolescent offenders: Costs of reducing incarceration, inpatient, and residential placement. *Journal of Child and Family Studies, 5*, 431–444.

Schrepferman, L., & Snyder, J. (2002). Coercion: The link between treatment mechanisms in behavioral parent training and risk reduction in child antisocial behavior. *Behavior Therapy, 33*, 339–359.

Serketich, W. J., & Dumas, J. E. (1996). The effectiveness of behavioral parent training to modify antisocial behavior in children: A meta-analysis. *Behavior Therapy, 27*, 171–186.

Sexton, T. L. & Alexander, J. F. (2003). Functional family therapy: A mature clinical model for working with at-risk adolescents and their families. In T. L. Sexton, G. R. Weeks, & M. S. Robbins (Eds.), *Handbook of family therapy* (pp. 323–348). New York: Taylor & Francis.

Sexton, T. L., Alexander, J. F., & Mease, A. L. (2004). Levels of evidence for the models and mechanisms of therapeutic change in couple and family therapy. In M. J. Lambert (Ed.), *Bergin and Garfield's handbook of psychotherapy and behaviour change* (5th ed., pp. 590–646). New York: Wiley.

Sexton, T. L., Ridley, C. R., & Kleiner, A. J. (2004). Beyond common factors: Multilevel-process models of therapeutic change in marriage and family therapy. *Journal of Marital and Family Therapy, 30*(2), 131–149.

Sheidow, A. J., Henggeler, S. W., & Schoenwald, S. K. (2003). Multisystemic therapy. In T. L. Sexton, G. R. Weeks, & M. S. Robbins (Eds.), *Handbook of family therapy* (pp. 303–322). New York: Taylor & Francis.

Simons, R. L., Wu, C., Conger, R. D., & Lorenz, F. O. (1994). Two routes to delinquency: differences between early and late starters in the impact of parenting and deviant peers. *Criminology, 32*, 247–275.

Slaby, R. G., & Guerra, N. G. (1988). Cognitive mediators of aggression in adolescent offenders: 1. Assessment. *Developmental Psychology, 24*, 580–588.

Smith, C. A., and Krohn, M. D. (1995). Delinquency and family life among male adolescents: The role of ethnicity. *Journal of Youth and Adolescence, 24*, 69–93.

Smith, C. A., & Stern, S. B. (1997). Delinquency and antisocial behaviour: A review of family processes and intervention research. *Social Service Review, 71*, 382–420.

Snyder, J., Dishion, T. J., & Patterson, G. R. (1986). Determinants and consequences of associating with deviant peers during preadolescence and adolescence. *Journal of Early Adolescence, 6,* 29–43.

Stern, S. B. (1999). Challenges to family engagement: What can multisystemic therapy teach family therapists? *Family Process, 38*(3), 281–285.

Stern, S. B. (2001). Outcomes research for children and adolescents: Implications for children's mental health and managed care. In N. W. Veeder & W. Peebles-Wilkins (Eds.), *Managed care services: Policy, programs and research* (pp. 187–212). New York: Oxford University Press.

Stern, S. B. (2004). Evidence-based practice with antisocial and delinquent youth: The key role of family and multisystemic interventions. In H. E. Briggs & T. Rzepnicki (Eds.), *Using evidence for social work practice* (pp. 104–127). Chicago: Lyceum Books.

Stern, S. B., Alaggia, R., Watson, K., & Morton, T. R. (2008). Implementing an evidence-based parenting program with adherence in the real world of community practice. *Research on Social Work Practice, 18*(6), 543–554.

Stern, S. B., & Smith, C. A. (1995). Family processes and delinquency in an ecological context. *Social Service Review, 69,* 703–731.

Stern, S. B., & Smith, C. A. (1999). Reciprocal relationships between antisocial behavior and parenting: Implications for delinquency intervention. *Families in Society, 80,* 169–181.

Stern, S. B., Smith, C. A., & Jang, S. J. (1999). Urban families and adolescent mental health. *Social Work Research, 23,* 15–27.

Stormshak, E. A., & Dishion, T. J. (2002). An ecological approach to child and family clinical and counselling psychology. *Clinical Child and Family Psychology Review, 5*(3), 197–215.

Szapocznik, J., Hervis, O., & Schwartz, S. (2003). Brief strategic family therapy for adolescent drug abuse. *Therapy Manuals for Drug Abuse Series,* Manual 5. Rockville, MD: National Institute on Drug Abuse.

Taylor, T. K., & Biglan, A. (1998). Behavioral family interventions for improving child-rearing: A review of the literature for clinicians and policy makers. *Clinical Child and Family Psychology Review, 1,* 41–59.

Thornberry, T. (1994). *Violent families and youth violence: Fact sheet #21.* Washington, DC: Office of Juvenile Justice and Delinquency Prevention.

Thornberry, T. P., Huizinga, D., & Loeber, R. (1995). The prevention of serious delinquency and violence: Implications from the program of research on the causes and correlates of delinquency. In J. C. Howell, B. Krisberg, J. D. Hawkins, & J. J. Wilson (Eds.), *A sourcebook: Serious, violent, and chronic juvenile offenders* (pp. 213–237). Newbury Park, CA: Sage.

Thornberry, T. P., Lizotte, A. J., Krohn, M. D., Farnworth, M., & Jang, S. (1991). Testing interactional theory: An examination of reciprocal causal relationships among family, school and delinquency. *Journal of Criminal Law and Criminology, 82,* 3–35.

U.S. Department of Health and Human Services. (1999). *Mental health: A report of the surgeon general.* Rockville, MD: U.S. Department of Health and Human Services, National Institutes of Health, National Institute of Mental Health.

U.S. Department of Health and Human Services. (2001). *Youth violence: A report of the surgeon general.* Rockville, MD: U.S. Department of Health and Human Services,

Centers for Disease Control and Prevention, National Center for Injury Prevention and Control; Substance Abuse and Mental Health Services Administration, Center for Mental Health Services; and National Institutes of Health, National Institute of Mental Health.

United States White House. (n.d.). *Community guide to helping America's youth.* Retrieved July 30, 2008, from http://helpingamericasyouth.gov/programtool-ap.cfm

Vuchinich, S., Bank, L., & Patterson, G. R. (1992). Parenting, peers, and the stability antisocial behavior in preadolescent boys. *Developmental Psychology, 28,* 510–521.

Wahler, R. G., Cartor, P. G., Fleischman, J., & Lambert, W. (1993). The impact of synthesis training and parent training with mothers of conduct-disordered children. *Journal of Abnormal Child Psychology, 21,* 425–440.

Warr, M. (1993). Parents, peers, & delinquency. *Social Forces, 72*(1), 247–264.

Webster-Stratton, C. (2004). *Quality training, supervision, ongoing monitoring, and agency support: Key ingredients to implementing the Incredible Years programs with fidelity.* Retrieved August 1, 2008, from www.incredibleyears.com/library

Webster-Stratton, C., & Hammond, M. (1990). Predictors of treatment outcome in parent training for families with conduct problem children. *Behavior Therapy, 21,* 319–337.

Webster-Stratton, C., & Herbert, M. (1993). What really happens in parent training? *Behaviour Modification, 17,* 405–456.

Webster-Stratton, C., & Herbert, M. (1994). *Troubled families—problem children: Working with parents: A collaborative process.* Chichester, England: Wiley.

Webster-Stratton, C., & Spitzer, A. (1996). Parenting a young child with conduct problems. New insights using qualitative methods. In T. H. Ollendick & R. J. Prinz (Eds.), *Advances in clinical child psychology* (pp. 1–62). New York: Plenum Press.

Webster-Stratton, C., & Taylor, T. (2001). Nipping early risk factors in the bud: Preventing substance abuse, delinquency, and violence in adolescence through interventions targeted at young children (0–8 years). *Prevention Science, 2*(3), 165–192.

Woolfenden, S. R., Williams, K., & Peat, J. K. (2003). Family and parenting interventions in children and adolescents with conduct disorder and delinquency aged 10–17. *Cochrane Database of Systematic Reviews, 2*(2001): CD003015.

Zazzali, J. L., Sherbourne, C., Hoagwood, K. E., Greene, D., Bigley, M. F., & Sexton, T. L. (2008). The adoption and implementation of an evidence based practice in child and family mental health services organizations: A pilot study of functional family therapy in New York state. *Administration Policy and Mental Health, 35,* 38–49.

Index

AB. *See* Assembly Bill (AB)
Absence seizures, 232
Abstinence violation effect (AVE), 187
Abuse, childhood, 127
Abuse Behavior Inventory, 165
Abusive tactics, 124
Accompanied offender, 202–203
Acquaintance typology, 562
ACT. *See* Assertive community treatment (ACT)
Action stage, 91
Actuarial assessment, 54
Actuarial decision making, 54, 381–382
Actuarial violence risk assessment tools, 132–133, 426
ACUTE. *See* Adolescent and Child Urgent Threat Evaluation (ACUTE)
Acute dynamic factors, 48
AD. *See* Alzheimer dementia (AD)
Addiction disorders, 127
ADHD. *See* Attention deficit hyperactivity disorder (ADHD)
Adjusted actuarial approach, 57–58
Admission criteria for psychopathy treatment, 270
Adolescent and Child Urgent Threat Evaluation (ACUTE), 411–412
Adolescent-limited offenders, case of, 365–368
Adolescent sex offenders, 204–205
Adoption and Safe Families Act, 130
Adult sexual offender clinicians, role of, 550–553
Adult trauma, 128–129
Affective responses, impaired, 318

Age, 18–19
Aggression
  case assessment of youth, 438–439
  classifications of, 575–576
  defined, 451
  developmental characteristics related to, 576
  indirect, 456
  interventions for, 584–585
  personality-based model of, 579–584
  relational violence and, 455–457
  risk factors for, 431–434
  self-control model for, 585–593
  skills directed therapy for, 573–575
  study of, 576–579
  verbal, 456
Aggression Questionnaire, 581–582
Aggressive behavior. *See* Aggression; Aggressive children
Aggressive children, 573–593
  See also Aggression
Alcohol hallucinosis, 226
Alcohol withdrawal, 226
Ali, Mohammed, 236
Alzheimer dementia (AD), 229
American Psychiatric Association (APA), 9, 247
American Psychological Association's Task Force on Empirically Based Principles of Therapeutic Change, 553
Amygdala, 225
Anamnestic assessment, 55
Anchoring bias, 46
Anger, 137
Anne E. Casey Foundation, 392

639

Antisocial offender development, 322
Antisocial personality disorder (ASPD), 147, 247–249
Anti stalking legislation, 563
APA. *See* American Psychiatric Association (APA)
Appraisal, risk, 67–70
Approach goals, 550
Area under the curve (AUC), 91
Arizona Risk/Needs Assessment Instrument (ARNA), 393
ARNA. *See* Arizona Risk/Needs Assessment Instrument (ARNA)
ASPD. *See* Antisocial personality disorder (ASPD)
Assault
 girls' violence, 459–460
 psychopathy, 284–285
Assembly Bill (AB), 517
Assertive community treatment (ACT), 293–294
Assessment
 of criminogenic need, 499–500
 for juvenile stalking, 564–566
 of psychopathy, 249–253
 tools for youthful populations, 377–378
 for victims of IPV, 164–166
Association for the Treatment of Sexual Abusers, 189
Assumption of psychological complexity, 332
Assumption of similarity, 333
Attachment theory, 536, 540–542
Attentional focus, 589
Attention deficit hyperactivity disorder (ADHD), 354, 355
Attribution biases, 299
Atypical anti psychotics, 237
AVE. *See* Abstinence violation effect (AVE)
Avoidance goals, 550
Avoidant-active relapse, 194

Back on Track, 396–398
Bandura, Alfred, 182
Barriers of psychopathy treatment, 287–288

Basal ganglia, 224, 236
Base rate data, 11, 47
Behavioral chain analysis, 144
Behavioral model of juvenile stalking, 562
Behavioral parent training, 609–612
Behavior Assessment System for Children Self-Report of Personality, 413
Below-average intellectual functioning, 287–288
Beyond Trauma: A Healing Journey for Women (Covington), 146
Biases
 anchoring, 46
 attribution, 299
 judgment errors and, 45–47
Bipolar disorder, 565
Bob Shapell School of Social Work, 585
Boundaries of practitioner/client, 259–262
Brain stem, 223
Brain tumors, 234–235
Brand-name interventions, 443
A Brief History of Behavioral and Cognitive Behavioral Approaches to Sexual Offenders (Marshall/Laws), 180
Bucy, Paul, 228
Bureau of Justice Statistics, 123, 226

CAD. *See* Clinical Assessment of Depression (CAD); Cognitive-affective dispositions (CAD) model
CAD model of aggression, 581–584
California Board of Corrections, 294
Callous unemotionality, 536
Cambridge Study of Delinquent Development, 384
Campbell Collaboration, 622–623
Case-based causal hypotheses, 440–441
Case management, defined, 292–293
Case management inventory, 469
Case planning process, 436–438
Castration, 184
Casual risk factor, 85–86
CBCL. *See* Child Behavior Checklist (CBCL)

CBT. *See* Cognitive-behavioral therapy (CBT)
CD. *See* Conduct disorder (CD)
CDI. *See* Children's Depression Inventory (CDI)
Centers for Disease Control, 157
"Central eight" risk/need factors, 500
Central nervous system (CNS), 223
Cerebellum, 223
Cerebrum, 223
Change
  process of, 142–144
  stages of, 91
  theory of, 188
Changeable risk factors. *See* Dynamic/static factors
Child Behavior Checklist (CBCL), 413
Child Development Institute, 468
Childhood abuse, 127
Child instruments, 469
Child molestation, 191–192, 197
Child protective services, 518–520
Children's Depression Inventory (CDI), 412
Children's Problematic Behavior Inventory, 592
Children's Self-control Scale, 582
Child's welfare system, 495–496
Classification of Violence Risk (COVR), 57
Cleckley, Hervey, 243
Clinical assessment, 54
  of psychopathy, 250–251
Clinical Assessment of Depression (CAD), 412, 580
Clinical interview, 61–67
Clinical items of HCR-20, 30–31
Clinical judgment, 45, 381
Clinical status variables, 87
CNS. *See* Central nervous system (CNS)
Cognitive-affective dispositions (CAD) model, 584–587
Cognitive-behavioral therapy (CBT), 94, 183–184
Cognitive restructuring, 589
Collateral informants, 60–61

Colorado Youthful Offender Level of Service Instrument, 392
Combining data, methods for, 54–58
Command hallucinations, 53
Communication, risk, 24–25
  report writing and, 70–76
Community reentry, 147–148
Community services, 166
Community support variables, 87
Compassion fatigue, 336–340
  prevention of, 340
  warning signs of, 339
Complex partial seizures (CPSs), 232–233
Comprehensive assessment, 464
Computer-based recidivism instruments, 407–411
Conceptual actuarial, 95
Conduct disorder (CD), 354, 355–356
Confirmatory factor analyses, 410
Confusional state, 225–226
Conners Rating Scale, 592
Consequences for rule-breaking behavior, 273–274
Contemplation, 91
Contemporary approaches to sex-offender-specific treatment, 189–211
  diversity, 201–208
  etiological theories, 197–201
  professional discretion, 208–211
  sex offender, defined, 190–197
Controversies of PCL-R, 315–319
Conversion disorder, 233
Convictions, criminal, 283
Co-occurring personality disorder, 83
Corpus callosum, 224
Correctional officers, 271
Correctional treatment, 88
Counseling for IPV, 166
Countertransference, defined, 329
Countertransference issues of MO, 329–336
  case vignette, 331–336
Court-referred batterer program, 128, 168
Covington, Stephanie, 146

COVR. *See* Classification of Violence Risk (COVR)
CPSs. *See* Complex partial seizures (CPSs)
Criminal attitude, 85–86
Criminal convictions, 283
Criminal history of high-risk offenders, 283–284
  criminal convictions, 283
  incarceration, history of, 283
  trial, 284
Criminality, 97
Criminal Sentiments Scale Modified (CSS-M), 300
Criminogenic factors of sex-offender-specific treatment, 198–201
Criminogenic need
  assessment of, 499–500
  defined, 23
  targeting, 298
Criminogenic need focus of treatment, 264–265
Criminogenic risk, 495–497
Crossover youth, 495–522
  criminogenic risk, 495–497
  joint assessment process, 500–515
  juvenile justice system of care, building, 515–522
  LARRC Risk/Need Scale, 526–528
  literature, 497–500
  mental health treatment, 495–497
  See also Youth violence
CSS-M. *See* Criminal Sentiments Scale Modified (CSS-M)

Daubert v. Merrell Dow Pharmaceuticals, 45
DBT. *See* Dialectical behavior therapy (DBT)
DCFS. *See* Department of Children and Family Services (DCFS)
Decision point, 379–380
Degeneracy, 356–357
Déjà vu, 232–233
Delinquency and maltreatment, link between, 497–499
Delirium, 225–226
Delirium tremens, 226

Delusions, 226
Dementia, 229–231
  frontotemporal, 229
Demographic risk factors of violent behavior, 18–20
Department of Children and Family Services (DCFS), 500–501, 517
Department of Mental Health, 517
Dependence, 127
Depression, 230
Depressive position, 322–323
Deprivation-violence connection, 313–314
Destabilizers, 32
Destructive envy, 322–323
Detachment, emotional, 536
Developmentally disabled sex offenders, 205–206
Deviance, sexual, 197
Deviance training, 369–370
Diagnostic and Statistical Manual of Mental Disorders (DSM), 49, 190, 247
Dialectical behavior therapy (DBT), 143, 147, 475, 481
Disabled sex offenders, developmentally, 205–206
Discharge planning, 147–148
Disconnection, 460
Discriminate function analyses, 410
Dispositional cognitive encoding, 580
Dispositional expectations, 580
Disruptive behavior disorders, 354–356
Distortion, 537
Diversity approach to sex-offender specific treatment, 201–208
  adolescent sex offenders, 204–205
  developmentally disabled sex offenders, 205–206
  female sex offenders, 201–204
  responsivity principle, 207–208
Domestic violence courts, 167–168
Domestic Violence Intake Center, 167
Donaldson, Kenneth, 7–8
Dopamine, 237
Dorsolateral prefrontal circuit, 225
Down's syndrome, 229

DSM. *See Diagnostic and Statistical Manual of Mental Disorders* (DSM)
Dual-jurisdiction youth. *See* Crossover youth
Dunedin Multidisciplinary Health and Development Study, 361
Dynamic risk profile, 92–93
Dynamic/static factors, 83–115
  dynamic variables, 98–100
  predictors, 109–115
  risk assessment tools, 86–88
  risk factors, static *vs.* dynamic, 84–86
  for sex offenders, 93–109
  of treatment program, 106–109
  VRS, 88–93
Dynamic variables
  dynamics of, 98–100
  sexual recidivism and, 94–95
  VRS-SO, 95–97
Dynamic *vs.* static risk factors, 84–86
  See also Dynamic/static factors

Earlscourt Child and Family Centre, 468
EARL-20B. *See* Early Assessment Risk List for Boys (EARL-20B)
EARL-20G. *See* Early Assessment Risk List for Girls (EARL-20G)
Early Assessment Risk List for Boys (EARL-20B), 400–401
Early Assessment Risk List for Girls (EARL-20G), 400–401, 468–469
Ecological and evidence-based family intervention, 608–623
  behavioral parent training, 609–612
  FFT, 618–619
  MST, 619–623
  MTFC, 617–618
  SNAP®, 612–617
Ecological intervention. *See* Ecological and evidence-based family intervention
Eco-Map, 614
Ecstasy, 227
Education, 20
EEG. *See* Electroencephalograph (EEG)

Effective parenting, 604
Electroencephalograph (EEG), 233
Emotional detachment, 536
Emotional regulation deficits, 128
Empathic questioning, 62
Empathy of juvenile sex offenders, 537–539
Empathy training, 262–263
Empirical actuarial approach, 94
Employment, 20
Empowering Children and Adolescents Project, 585
Encephalopathy, 225–226
Envy, destructive, 322–323
Epilepsy, 231–232
EPS. *See* Extrapyramidal symptoms (EPS)
"Escape theory" of suicide, 322
Estimate of Risk of Adolescent Sexual Offense Recidivism (ERASOR), 403–405
Etiological theories, 197–201
Evidence-based, concept of, 390
Evidence-based family intervention *See* Ecological and evidence-based family intervention
Evidence-based risk factors, 386–387
  mental disorder, 386–387
  self-harm, 387
Evil, defined, 319–321
Extrafamilial child molesters, 193
Extrapyramidal symptoms (EPS), 237
Eyberg Child Behavior Inventory, 583, 592

FACT. *See* Forensic assertive community treatment programs (FACT)
Factitious disorder, 233
Family-based intervention. *See* Ecological and evidence-based family intervention
Family conflict, 605
Family diversity, 606–608
Family instruments, 469
Family processes, 603–606
Family violence, 605
Federal Rule of Evidence 703, 61

Female delinquent offenders, 457–460
  assault, 459–460
  homicide, 458
  robbery, 459
  sexual assault, 458–459
  See also Girls violence; Women's violence
Female Focus Initiative (FFI), 480
FFI. *See* Female Focus Initiative (FFI)
FFT. *See* Functional Family Therapy (FFT)
Fixated child molester, 192
Forensic assertive community treatment programs (FACT), 293–294, 304–305
Forensic practitioners, 23
Forensic treatment issues, 139–148
  discharge planning, 147–148
  group interventions, 144–147
  therapeutic environment, 141–142
  therapeutic process, 142–144
  therapeutic relationship, 139–140
Fox, Michael J., 236
Frontal lobe, 223, 225
Frontal-subcortical circuit, 225
Frontotemporal dementia (FTD), 229–230
Frye v. United States, 45
FTD. *See* Frontotemporal dementia (FTD)
Functional Family Therapy (FFT), 113, 521, 618–619

Gage, Phineas, 228
GAM. *See* General aggression model (GAM)
Gangs, 110
Gender, 19
Gender-related risk factors of girl's violence, 465–466
Gender-responsive intervention, 135–139
Gender-responsive treatment for girl's violence, 471–480
  homogeneous group treatment, 479–480
  individualized treatment planning, 477–479
  long-term community support, 480
  role models/mentors, female, 474–475
  self-concept, female, 475–477
  therapeutic environment, 472–474
Gender-responsive violence risk assessment, 129–133
Gender-specific model of intergenerational transmission, 127
General aggression model (GAM), 578
Generalized tonic-clonic seizures (GMS), 232
General self-regulation, 99, 199–200
General Statistical Information for Recidivism, 86
Girls Circle, 482
Girl's violence, 449–482
  aggression, 455–457
  defined, 450–451
  gender-responsive treatment, 471–480
  interventions, 480–482
  measurements of, 450–451
  relational theory, 460–464
  self-report studies of, 453–454
  social construction of, 454–455
  statistics for, 451–452, 457–460
  violence risk assessment, 464–471
  See also Female delinquent offenders; Women's violence
Global Risk Assessment Device (GRAD), 468, 470–471
Global Risk Assessment Device (GRADcis™), 409–411
GMS. *See* Generalized tonic-clonic seizures (GMS); Grand mal seizure (GMS)
Good Lives model, 550
GRAD. *See* Global Risk Assessment Device (GRAD)
GRADcis™. *See* Global Risk Assessment Device (GRADcis™)
Grand mal seizure (GMS), 232
Group interventions, 144–147
Group sessions, 589–591
Guided clinical assessment, 55

Hallucinations, 226
Hare, Robert, 244–247

Harm, 43
HCR-20. *See* Historical, clinical, risk management-20 (HCR-20)
HCR-20 Violence Risk Management Companion Guide, 133
Health effects of IPV, 159–160
Healy, William, 431
Helping Women Recover (Covington), 146
Heterogeneity, 548
Heterosexual IPV, 129
Heterotypic continuity, 358
Heuristics, 437
High-risk offender issues, 283–284
 criminal history, 283–284
 psychopathy, 283
HIQ. *See* Hostile Interpretations Questionnaire (HIQ)
Historical, clinical, risk management-20 (HCR-20), 27–28
 clinical items contained in, 30–31
 historical items of, 28–30
 risk assessment research, 14–16
 risk management items contained in, 31–32
Historical foundations of sex offender-specific treatment, 180–187
 cognitive-behavioral therapy, 183–184
 early evolution, 180–183
 hormonal approaches, 184–186
 relapse prevention, 186–187
Historical items of HCR-20, 28–30
Homegrown risk tools, 392–393
Homicide, 458
Homogeneous group treatment, 479–480
Hormonal approach for sex offender-specific treatment, 184–186
Hostile Interpretations Questionnaire (HIQ), 300
Hostile masculinity, 541
Hostility, 137, 141, 581
Huntington disease, 236–237
Hypersensitivity, 319
Hypothalamus, 225

IDPP. *See* Interagency Delinquency Prevention Program (IDPP)
Immigrants, 163
Impressionistic approach, 437
Impulsivity, 128
Incarceration, 123–125, 283
Incentives, individualized, 287–288
Incentive systems, 263–264, 273
Incest, 193
Incidence rates of IPV, 158
Indirect aggression, 456
Individualized assessment of violent behavior, 58
 clinical interview, 61–67
 third-party information, 59–61
Individualized behavior cycle, 289–290
Individualized incentives, 287–288
Individualized treatment plan (ITP)
 girls' violence, 477–479
 psychopathy, 272–273, 283
Individual risk factors of violent behavior, 18
Institutional objectives, 276
Instruments, properties of, 389–391
Integrated treatment approach, 137–139
Interagency Delinquency Prevention Program (IDPP), 519
Internal metabolic derangement, 225–226
Internal placement issues, 266–267
International Classification of Diseases, 49
Interventions
 aggression, 584–585
 brand-name, 443
 gender-responsive, 135–139
 goals, 441–442
 group, 144–147
 for IPV, 164–168
 MCSTAR, 301–305
 perpetrators, 168–169
 plans, development of, 442–444
 social workers, 169–170
 types of, 480–482
Interview questions, violent behavior, 66
Intimacy deficits, 99, 199
Intimate partner violence, 128–129
Intimate partner violence (IPV), 157–170
 effects of, 159–160
 factors associated with, 161–163

IPV (*continued*)
  incidence rates, 158
  interventions for, 164–170
Intimate typology, 562
IPV. *See* Intimate partner violence (IPV)
ITP. *See* Individualized treatment plan (ITP)
It's Coming From the Tower (Clayton), 235

JAIS. *See* Juvenile Assessment and Intervention System (JAIS)
Jamais vu, 232–233
Jesness Inventory-Revised (JI-R), 401–402
Jewish Foundation, 585
JI-R. *See* Jesness Inventory-Revised (JI-R)
Joint assessment process in Los Angeles County, 500–515
  discussion, 514–515
  measures, 502–504
  procedures, 505
  results, 505–514
  sample, 501–502
Joint Risk Matrix, 426–427
J-SAT. *See* Justice System Assessment and Training (J-SAT)
J-SOAP-II. *See* Juvenile Sex Offender Assessment Protocol-II (J-SOAP-II)
J-SORRAT-II. *See* Juvenile Sexual Offense Recidivism Risk Assessment Tool-II (J-SORRAT-II)
Judgment, structured professional, 382–383
Judgment errors, 45–47
Justice System Assessment and Training (J-SAT), 402
Juvenile, defined, 564
Juvenile Assessment and Intervention System (JAIS), 407–408
Juvenile justice practitioners, 601–624
  family diversity, 606–608
  family processes, 603–606
  social ecology theory, 603

See also Ecological and evidence-based family intervention
Juvenile justice system of care, 515–522
Juvenile Sex Offender Assessment Protocol-II (J-SOAP-II), 405–406
Juvenile sex offenders
  complexity of, 545–547
  perspective on, 531–534
  risk assessments for, 403–407
  statistics, 529–531
  typologies of, 204
  See also Youth violence
Juvenile Sexual Offense Recidivism Risk Assessment Tool-II (J-SORRAT-II), 407
Juvenile stalking, 561–571
  assessment for, 564–566
  behavioral model, 562
  clinical example of, 566–569
  defined, 561–564
  legal model, 563–564
  management, 570–571
  medical model, 562–563
  psychiatric model, 562–563
  treatment for, 564–566
Juvenile violence offenders
  patterns of, 356–368
  treatment of, 368–372
  See also Youth violence

Kayser-Fleischer rings, 237
Kinsley, Alfred, 182
Klüver, Heinrich, 228
Kluver Bucy syndrome, 228
Knowledge, application of, 387–388

LARRC. *See* Los Angeles Risk and Resiliency Checkup (LARRC)
Legal-empirical-forensic model of forensic practice, 44–45
Legal model of juvenile stalking, 563–564
Lerner-Wren, Ginger, 294
Lesbian, gay, bisexual, and transgender (LGBT) community, 162
Leuprolide (Lupron), 184
Level of Service Inventory-Revised (LSI-R), 75–76, 111

Level of Services Inventory (LSI), 111
Lexico-semantic processing, abnormal, 318
LGBT. *See* Lesbian, gay, bisexual, and transgender (LGBT) community
Life-course persistent offending, 362–365
Likert scale, 89
Limbic system, 223, 225
Literature
  criminogenic risk, 497–500
  mental disorders and violence, 295–299
Location for psychopathy treatment, 270
Logistic regression analyses, 403
Long-term community support, 480
Los Angeles County joint assessment process, 500–515
Los Angeles Police Department, 563
Los Angeles Risk and Resiliency Checkup (LARRC), 526–528
Lover/teacher offender, 202–203
LSI. *See* Level of Services Inventory (LSI)
LSI-R. *See* Level of Service Inventory-Revised (LSI-R)
Lupron (leuprolide), 184

MacArthur Violence Risk Assessment Study, 16–18
Magnetic resonance imaging (MRI), 235
Maintenance stage, 91
Male-coerced offender, 202
Male criminality, 536
Malignant pseudoidentification, 322, 331
Malingering, 233
Maltreatment and delinquency, link between, 497–499
Maricopa County Adult Probation Department, 303
Marlatt, G. A., 186
Marshall, William, 183
Masculine adequacy, 542
"The Mask of Sanity" (Cleckley), 243, 315
Massachusetts Treatment Center (MTC), 192
Maternal depression, 127

MCSTAR. *See* Montgomery County Supervised Treatment After Release (MCSTAR) program
MDMA. *See* Methylene-dioxymethamphetamine (MDMA)
Measures of objectives, 276
Medical model of juvenile stalking, 562–563
Medroxyprogesterone (MPA), 184
Mental disorders, 128
  evidence-based risk factor, type of, 386–387
  literature concerning violence and, 295–299
  symptoms of, 52
Mental effects of IPV, 160
Mental health
  criminogenic risk, 520–522
  girls violence, 463–464
  treatment needs of crossover youth, 495–497
Mentally Ill Offender Crime Reduction grant program, 294
Mentally ill offenders, 291–305
  background of, 292–294
  literature concerning mental disorders and violence, 295–299
  MCSTAR program for, 299–305
Mentors, female, 474–475
Metacognition, 538
Methylene-dioxymethamphetamine (MDMA), 227
Mini-Mental State Exam (MMSE), 230–231
Minnesota Sex Offender Screening Tool-Revised, 94
Mississippi Delinquency Risk Assessment Scale, 392
MMSE. *See* Mini-Mental State Exam (MMSE)
MO. *See* Morally objectionable (MO)
Model Programs Guide, 482
Moffitt, Terrie, 357
Molestation, child, 191–192
Monahan, John, 9
Monitoring the Future (MTF) survey, 453

Montgomery County Supervised
    Treatment After Release
    (MCSTAR) program, 299–305
  intervention, 301–305
  measures of, 300
  outcomes of, 300–301
Mood disorders, 565
Moral development, 539
Moral insanity, 242
Morality of juvenile sex offenders,
    537–539
Morally objectionable (MO), 311–340
  compassion fatigue, 336–340
  countertransference issues, 329–336
  defined, 312
  deprivation-violence connection,
    313–314
  envy, 322–323
  evil, 319–321
  nihilism, 324–326
  persecution, 321–323
  psychopathic personality, 315–319
  substratum, 313–314
  treatment approaches, 326–328
Motivation goals, 257–258
Movement disorders, 236–238
MPA. *See* Medroxyprogesterone (MPA)
MRI. *See* Magnetic resonance imaging
    (MRI)
MST. *See* Multisystemic Therapy (MST)
MTC. *See* Massachusetts Treatment
    Center (MTC)
MTF. *See* Monitoring the Future (MTF)
    survey
MTFC. *See* Multidimensional Treatment
    Foster Care (MTFC)
Multidimensional family therapy, 443
Multidimensional Treatment Foster Care
    (MTFC), 521, 617–618
Multisystemic Therapy (MST), 370–371,
    619–623
Myelin, 223

National Council on Crime and
    Delinquency (NCCD), 393, 407
National Crime Victimization Survey
    (NCVS), 451, 453

National Institute of Corrections, 298
National Institute of Mental Health's
    Epidemiologic Catchment Area, 51
National Institute on Drug Abuse, 371
National Longitudinal Survey of Children
    and Youth, 110
National Youth Survey, 385
NCAR. *See* North Carolina Assessment of
    Risk (NCAR)
NCCD. *See* National Council on Crime
    and Delinquency (NCCD)
NCVS. *See* National Crime Victimization
    Survey (NCVS)
Need principle, 23, 88, 189
Neuroanatomy, 223–225
Neuroleptics, 237
Neuron, 223
Neuropsychiatric deficits
  in psychopathy, 318
Neuropsychiatry, 221–238
  delirium, 225–226
  movement disorders, 236–238
  neuroanatomy, 223–225
  substance abuse, 226–235
Nihilism, 324–326
Noncriminogenic needs, 75
Noncriminogenic variables, 207–208
North Carolina Assessment of Risk
    (NCAR), 393–394
North Carolina Department of Juvenile
    Justice, 393
North Dakota Risk Assessment
    Instrument, 392

Obsessional follower, 562
Obsessional harassment, 562
Occipital lobe, 223
O'Connor v. Donaldson, 7–8
ODD. *See* Oppositional defiant
    disorder (ODD)
Offense pathway distinctions, 193–194
Office of Juvenile Justice and
    Delinquency Prevention,
    351–352, 407
Oppositional defiant disorder (ODD),
    354–355, 574
Orbital frontal circuit, 225

Orchiectomy, 184
Orders of protection, 166–167
Oregon Social Learning Center, 610

PACT. *See* Positive Achievement Change Tool (PACT)
Paranoia, 137
Paranoid-schizoid position, 322
Paraphilic disorders, 190
Parenting, effective, 604
Parietal lobe, 223
Parkinson disease (PD), 236
Partner Violence Screen (PVS), 165
Pathways perspective and relational theory, 460–464
Pavlov, Ivan, 181
PCC. *See* Psychology of Criminal Conduct (PCC)
PCL-R. *See* Psychopathy Checklist-Revised (PCL-R)
PCL-SV. *See* Psychopathy Checklist-Screening Version (PCL-SV)
PD. *See* Parkinson disease (PD)
Perpetrators, interventions for, 168–169
Persecution, 321–323
Personal agency, 142–144
Personality-based model of aggression, 579–584
Personality disorder, 128, 565
Personality variables, 87
Personal support, 31
Person variables, 579
PET. *See* Positron emission tomography (PET)
Petit mal epilepsy, 232
PETRA. *See* Psychosocial Evaluation and Threat Risk Assessment (PETRA)
Phallometric method, 182
Phase system, 274–275
Pick's disease, 229, 230
PID. *See* Pride in Delinquency (PID) Scale
PIL. *See* Purpose-in-Life (PIL) Test
Pinel, Philippe, 242
Pituitary gland, 225
Poddar, Berkley, 7

Poddar, Prosenjit, 7
Policy implications, 450–451
Positive Achievement Change Tool (PACT), 397
Positron emission tomography (PET), 230
Posttraumatic stress disorder (PTSD), 122
Practitioners
  forensic, 23
  legal precedent, 6–8
  psychopathy, 256–264
Pratt Foundation, 585
Precontemplation, 91
Prediction of violence. *See* Violence risk assessment
Predictors of youth violence, static and dynamic, 109–115
Predisposed offender, 202
Pregnancy, 159
Premortem strategy, 440
Preparation stage, 91
Pride in Delinquency (PID) Scale, 300
Primary prevention, 472
Priority risk factors, 439–440
Private stranger typology, 562
Probability, 74
Probation, 516–518
Problem, theory of, 188
Problem analysis, 589
Procedures for psychopathy treatment, 269
Process variables, 207–208
Professional discretion principle, 189, 208–211
Program goals for psychopathy treatment, 269
Progressive supranuclear palsy, 237
Pro-Social Self-Regulation Questionnaire, 583
Protection, orders of, 166–167
Protective factors, 429, 431–434, 439–440
Pseudoseizures, 233
Pseydodementia, 230
Psychiatric Epidemiology Research Interview, 11
Psychiatric model of juvenile stalking, 562–563

Psychological complexity, assumption of, 332
Psychology of Criminal Conduct (PCC), 89
Psychometrics, properties of, 389–391
Psychopath, defined, 242
Psychopathia Sexualis (Psychopathy of Sex), 180
Psychopathic personality, 315–319
Psychopathy, 241–277
  assessment, 249–253
  checklist, 26–27, 244, 246
  high-risk offender issues, 283–284
  history of, 242–249
  individualized behavior cycle, 289–290
  individualized treatment plan, 283
  internal placement issues, 266–267
  neuropsychiatric deficits in, 318
  as a risk factor, 21–22
  staff, 269, 284
  target behavior, 284–286
  treatment and, relation between, 255–265
  See also Treatment, psychopathy
Psychopathy Checklist-Revised (PCL-R), 244–247
  psychopathic personality, 315–319
  Robert Hare, 244–247
Psychopathy Checklist-Screening Version (PCL-SV), 26–27, 246
Psychopathy of Sex *(Psychopathia Sexualis)*, 180
Psychopathy Treatment Program (PTP), 326–327
Psychosocial Evaluation and Threat Risk Assessment (PETRA), 412–413
Psycological escape, 462
PTP. *See* Psychopathy Treatment Program (PTP)
PTSD. *See* Posttraumatic stress disorder (PTSD)
Public figure typology, 562
Purpose-in-Life (PIL) Test, 324
Purposive Behavior in Animals and Men (Tollman), 182
PVS. *See* Partner Violence Screen (PVS)

RAI. *See* Risk assessment instruments (RAI)
Rape, 192
Rapid assessment instruments, 165
Rapid Risk Assessment for Sex Offender Recidivism, 23, 94
Rationality-within irrationality, 297
Rational model of treatment, 135–136
Receiver operating characteristics (ROC) curves, 91, 391
Recidivism
  measures of, 276–277
  risks for, evaluating, 388–391
  screening, risk for, 377–378
  sexual, 94–95
  See also Recidivism instruments
Recidivism instruments, 392–413
  for evaluation of risk of harm, 411–413
  risk assessments for juvenile sexual offenders, 403–407
  risk/needs assessment, 394–403
  screening tools, 392–394
  web/computer-based, 407–411
RECON, 562
Referral, methods of, 169
Rejection Sensitivity Questionnaire, 582
Relapse prevention (RP) theory, 94, 97, 186–187
Relational aggression, 141
Relational theory, 460–464
  mental health, 463–464
  and pathways perspective, 460–464
  substance abuse, 462–463
  traumatic events, 461–462
Relationship instability, 128
Reliability
  of VRS, 91–92
  of VRS-SO, 98
Reoffense, sexual, 194–195
Resilience, 428–431
Responsivity instruments, 469
Responsivity principle, 24, 88, 189, 207–208
Restraint, theory of, 142
Risk
  assessment of, concept for, 385
  criminogenic, 495–497

defined, 428–431
elements of, 43
youth violence, 112–113
Risk appraisal, 67–70
Risk assessment. *See* Violence risk assessment
Risk assessment evaluation. *See* Violence risk assessment evaluation
Risk assessment instruments (RAI), 392
Risk assessment research. *See* Violence risk assessment research
Risk assessment risk factors. *See* Violence risk assessment risk factors
Risk assessment tools. *See* Violence risk assessment tools
Risk communication, 24–25
  report writing and, 70–76
  transparent, 71
Risk factors
  defined, 499–500
  See also Violence risk assessment risk factors
Risk for Sexual Violence Protocol (RSVP), 95
Risk management, 23–24
  items contained in HCR-20, 31–32
Risk Matrix2000, 94
Risk-need-responsivity model, 23
Risk/needs assessment instruments for recidivism, 394–403
  EARL-20B, 400–401
  EARL-20G, 400–401
  JI-R, 401–402
  RRC, 402–403
  SAVRY, 398–400
  WSJCA, 396–398
  YLS/CMI, 394–396
Risk of harm, evaluation of, 411–413
  ACUTE, 411–412
  PETRA, 412–413
Risk principle, 23, 88, 189
Risk & Resiliency Checkup (RRC), 402–403
Risk status, 48
Robbery, 459
ROC. *See* Receiver operating characteristics (ROC) curves

Role models, female, 474–475
RP. *See* Relapse prevention (RP) theory
RRC. *See* Risk & Resiliency Checkup (RRC)
RSVP. *See* Risk for Sexual Violence Protocol (RSVP)
Rule-breaking behavior, 273–274

SAVRY. *See* Structured Assessment of Violence Risk of Youth (SAVRY)
Schizoaffective disorder, 565
Schizophrenia, 128, 565
Screening
  assessment *vs.*, 164–166, 388–389
  tools, 392–394
  for victims of IPV, 164–166
SDT. *See* Skills-directed therapy (SDT) model
Secondary prevention, 472
Seeking Safety (Najavits), 145
Seizures, 231–234
  stages of, 233
Selective serotonin reuptake inhibitors (SSRIs), 185
Self-concept of female, 475–477
Self-control intervention modules, 588–589
Self-control model for aggression, 585–593
  group sessions, 589–591
  outcomes of, 592–593
  results of, 592–593
  SDT model, 586–588
  self-control intervention modules, 588–589
  skills acquisition, importance of, 586
Self-control practice, 589
Self-harm, 137, 387
Self-initiated abuser, 202
Self-injurious behavior, 286
Self-regulation
  general, 99, 199–200
  sexual, 99, 200
Self-reported violence, 21
Self-report studies, 453–454
Serotonin, 237
Service management inventory, 469

Sex offender
  defined, 190–197
  developmentally disabled, 205–206
  dynamic and static factors for, 93–94, 93–109
  heterogeneity of, 542–545
  juvenile, 547–549
Sex offender attitudes, 99
Sex Offender Need Assessment Rating (SONAR), 95
  factors of, 99
Sex Offender Risk Appraisal Guide, 23
Sex offender-specific treatment, 179–211
  contemporary approaches to, 189–211
  current challenges of, 187–189
  historical foundations of, 180–187
Sex offender treatment, defined, 179
Sex Offender Treatment and Evaluation Project (SOTEP), 210
Sexual Abuse: A Journal of Research and Treatment (Miner), 210
Sexual arousal, 182, 184–185
Sexual assault, 458–459
The Sexual Behavior of Females (Kinsley), 182
The Sexual Behavior of Males (Kinsley), 182
Sexual deviance, 97, 197
Sexually abusive behavior, 534–537
Sexually abusive youth, 529–556
  attachment, 540–542
  characteristics of, recognizing, 534–537
  clinician, role of, 550–553
  empathy, 537–539
  heterogeneity of, 542–545
  morality, 537–539
  sex-offender-specific treatment, 547–549
  social connection, 537–542
  treatment of, 549–550
  See also Juvenile sex offenders
Sexual offender clinicians, 550–553
Sexual recidivism
  dynamic variables and, 94–95
  static variables and, 94
Sexual reoffense, 194–195
Sexual self-regulation, 99, 200

Sexual Violence Risk-20, 23, 95
SGFP. *See* Specialty Guidelines for Forensic Psychologists (SGFP)
Sheldon, William, 357
Shelter for victims of IPV, 166
Similarity, assumption of, 333
Single-photon emission computed tomography (SPECT), 230
SIQ. *See* Suicide Ideation Questionnaire (SIQ)
Skills acquisition, 586
Skills-directed therapy (SDT) model
  for aggression, 573–575
  for behavioral disorders, 586–588
Skinner, B. F., 181
SNAP®. *See* Stop Now and Plan (SNAP®) program
SNAP Girls Connection (SNAP GC), 611
SNAP Under 12 Outreach Project (SNAP ORP), 611
Social connection, 537–542
  social skills, development of, 554–556
  treatment through, 554–556
Social construction of violence, 454–455
Social ecology theory, 603
Social influences
  negative, 99
  significant, 199
Social potency, 384–385
Social skills, development of, 554–556
Social Work and Human Services Treatment Planner, 169
Social workers, intervention approaches for, 169–170
Socioeconomic status, 19, 127
SONAR. *See* Sex Offender Need Assessment Rating (SONAR)
SOTEP. *See* Sex Offender Treatment and Evaluation Project (SOTEP)
Specialty Guidelines for Forensic Psychologists (SGFP), 61, 71–72
SPECT. *See* Single-photon emission computed tomography (SPECT)
SPJ. *See* Structured professional judgment (SPJ)
SSRIs. *See* Selective serotonin reuptake inhibitors (SSRIs)

Stable dynamic factors, 48
STABLE-2007, 199
Staff, psychopathy
   assault, 284
   training, 269
Stages of Change model, 89
Stalker, defined, 564
State-based risk tools, 392–393
State Industrial School for Girls
      (Lancaster, Massachusetts), 356
Static-99, 23, 195
Static variables
   sexual recidivism and, 94–95
   VRS, 89–91
   VRS-SO, 95–97
Static *vs.* dynamic risk factors, 84–86
   See also Dynamic/static factors
Statistical approach, 437
Status epilepticus, 232
Stereotaxic neurosurgery, 184
Stockholm Project Metropolitan,
      295–296
Stop Now and Plan (SNAP®) program,
      612–617
Strength and criminogenic risk, 499–500
Strengths-based model of treatment,
      135–136
Stress, 32
Structured Assessment of Violence Risk
      of Youth (SAVRY), 112, 398–400
Structured interviews
   gender-responsive violence risk
      assessment, 130–132
   risk assessment and, 467–468
Structured professional judgment (SPJ),
      55, 382–383
Substance abuse, 226–235
   brain tumors, 234–235
   dementia, 229–231
   dependence, 127
   girls violence, 462–463
   seizures, 231–234
   traumatic brain injury, 227–229
Substantia nigra, 236
Substratum, 313–314
Suicidal ideation, 137
Suicide Ideation Questionnaire (SIQ), 412

Supervision, cooperation with, 200–201
Supervision of practitioners, 259
Supplemental Homicide Reports, 458
Support, personal, 31
Symptomatology, 223
Systematic assessment, 464

Tarasoff v. Regents of the University
      of California, 6–7
TARGET (Trauma Affect Regulation:
      Guide for Education and
      Treatment), 481
Target behaviors, 284–286
   assault, 284, 285
   self-injurious behavior, 286
Targets of treatment, 197–201
   criminogenic factors, 198–201
TCO. *See* Threat/control-overrise (TCO)
      symptoms
TDM. *See* Team decision making (TDM)
Teacher/lover offender, 202–203
Team decision making (TDM), 518
Temporal lobe, 223, 225
Temporal lobe epilepsy, 232–233
Tertiary prevention, 472
Therapeutic environment, 141–142
   creation of, 472–474
Therapeutic milieu model, 472
Therapeutic nihilism, 330–331
Therapeutic relationship, 139–140
Third-party information (TPI), 59–61
Thorndike, Edward L., 181
Threat/control-overrise (TCO) symptoms,
      10, 52
Tollman, E. C., 182
TPI. *See* Third-party information (TPI)
Training of practitioners, 259
Transparent risk communication, 71
Transtheoretical Model (TTM), 89,
      142–143
Trauma, childhood, 127
Trauma-informed interventions, 136–137
Traumatic brain injury, 227–229
Traumatic experiences, 461–462
Treatment
   approaches for MO, 326–328
   dynamic risk factors of, 106–109

Treatment (*continued*)
    for juvenile stalking, 564–566
    for juvenile violence offenders, 368–372
    for sex offender-specific treatment, 180–211
    strengths-based model of, 135–136
    through social connection, 554–556
    violence risk assessment to, linking, 133–134
    See also Treatment, psychopathy
Treatment, psychopathy, 255–265
    activities, 271–272
    admission criteria for, 270
    consequences of, 273–274
    correctional officers, 271
    criminogenic need focus of, 264–265
    implementing, 277
    incentive system for, 273
    individualized plan, 272–273
    location for, 270
    measures of objectives, 276
    objectives, 276
    outcomes of, 275–276
    overview of, 268–277
    phase system, 274–275
    practitioners, roles of, 256–264
    procedures for, 269
    program goals of, 269
    recidivism, 276–277
    staff training, 269
    treatment team, 270–271
Treatment activities for psychopathy, 271–272
Treatment goals, 257–258
Treatment modality, 258–259
Treatment of MO, guiding principles for, 328
Treatment perspective, 258–259
Treatment population
    defined, 190–197
    offense pathway distinctions, 193–194
    risk, classification based on, 194–197
    typologically, 191–193
Treatment responsivity, 97
Treatment targets, 85, 91
Treatment team, 270–271

Trial, 284
Trust, 139–140
TTM. *See* Transtheoretical Model (TTM)
Tumors, defined, 234
Typical antipsychotics, 237
Typological definitions, 191–193

UCR. *See* Uniform Crime Report (UCR)
Unaided clinical judgment, 55
Underrecognized populations, IPV in, 162–163
Uniform Crime Report (UCR), 353, 451
U.S. Census Bureau, 451
U.S. Department of Health and Human Services, 371
U.S. Department of Justice, 451
U.S., youth violence in, 351–356

Validity
    of VRS, 91–92
    of VRS-SO, 98
VASOR. *See* Vermont Assessment of Sex Offender Risk (VASOR)
Vera Institute of Justice, 498
Verbal aggression, 456
Vermont Assessment of Sex Offender Risk (VASOR), 95
Vicarious traumatization, 337–338
Violence, family, 605
Violence instruments, 392–413
Violence reduction program, 83, 327
Violence Reduction Program (VRP), 327–328
Violence Risk Appraisal Guide (VRAG), 12–14
Violence risk assessment, 3–32
    approaches/frameworks to, 381–383
    case vignette, 25–32
    concept of, 42–43
    defined, 4–5, 42–44, 378–383
    instruments, 434–444
    for juvenile sex offenders, 403–407
    objectives of, 43–44
    practitioners, role of, 6–8
    recidivism, instruments for, 394–403
    risk communication, 24–25
    risk management, 23–24

Index **655**

special considerations for, 383–391
specification of, 23
structured interviews and, 467–468
treatment, 23–24, 133–148
See also Violence risk assessment evaluation; Violence risk assessment research; Violence risk assessment risk factors
Violence risk assessment, case vignette, 25–32
HCR-20, 27–31
information, identification of, 26
psychopathy checklists, 26–27
risk assessment tools, 26
Violence risk assessment evaluation, 41–76
approaching the, 44–45
biases, 45–47
clinical interview, 66
combining data, methods for, 54–58
components of, 25
for girls violence, 464–471
individualized, 58–67
judgment errors, 45–47
parameters of, 5–6
report writing, 70–76
risk appraisal, 67–70
risk assessment, defined, 42–44
risk communication, 70–76
risk factors, 47–49
Violence risk assessment research, 8
first generation of, 9–11
HCR-20, 14–16
MacArthur Violence Risk Assessment Study, 16–18
second generation of, 11–14
third generation of, 14–18
VRAG, 12–14
Violence risk assessment risk factors
aggression, 431–434
classification based on, 194–197
demographic, 18–20
history as a, 20–21
individual, 18–22
key, 49–54
psychopathy, 21–22, 251–256
recidivism, 388–391

static *vs.* dynamic, 84–86
youth, 112–113
See also Women's violence, risk factors for
Violence risk assessment tools, 26
evolution of, 86–88
for girls violence, 466–471
knowledge, application of, 387–388
Violence Risk Scale (VRS), 88–93
dynamic risk profile, 92–93
reliability of, 91–92
static and dynamic variables of, 89–91
validity of, 91–92
Violence Risk Scale-Sexual Offender (VRS-SO)
conceptualization of, 105
dynamic/static factors, 93–94
dynamic variables of, 95–97
illustration of, 100–105
psychometric properties of, 98
reliability of, 98
sexual recidivism, 94–95
static variables of, 95–97
treatment program for, 106–109
validity of, 98
Violence Risk Scale-Youth Version (VRS-YV), 113–115
purpose of, 113
Violent behavior
history of, 20–21
interview questions, 66
social construction of, 454–455
of youth, 383–384
Violent Crime Index, 353
Voices: A Program of Self-discovery and Empowerment, 482
VRAG. *See* Violence Risk Appraisal Guide (VRAG)
VRP. *See* Violence Reduction Program (VRP)
VRS. *See* Violence Risk Scale (VRS)
VRS Manual, 89
VRS-SO. *See* Violence Risk Scale-Sexual Offender (VRS-SO)
VRS-SO Score Sheet©, 103
VRS-YV. *See* Violence Risk Scale-Youth Version (VRS-YV)

Washington State Institute for Public Policy, 397
Washington State Juvenile Court Assessment (WSJCA), 396–398
Watson, John B., 181
Web-based recidivism instruments, 407–411
Web/computer-based tools, 407–411
  GRADcis™, 409–411
  JAIS, 407–408
  Youth COMPAS, 408–409
Welfare and Institutions Code (WIC), 500–501
Wernicke-Korsakoff syndrome, 230
"What works" literature, 87–88
Whitman, Charles, 235
WIC. See Welfare and Institutions Code (WIC)
Wilson disease, 237
Women's violence, 121–148
  contextual issues, 122–125
  etiology of, 125–126
  forensic treatment issues, 139–148
  gender-responsive intervention, 135–139
  gender-responsive violence risk assessment, 129–134
  risk factors for, 126–129
  See also Female delinquent offenders; Girls violence; Women's violence, risk factors
Women's violence, risk factors, 126–129
  abuse, childhood, 127
  adult trauma, 128–129
  intimate partner violence, 128–129
  mental disorder, 128
  substance abuse and dependence, 127
  trauma, childhood, 127
Worcester Public Schools, 356
World Health Organization, 159
Wraparound approaches, 113

WSJCA. See Washington State Juvenile Court Assessment (WSJCA)

YASI. See Youth Assessment and Screening Institute (YASI)
YLS/CMI. See Youth Level of Service/Case Management Inventory (YLS/CMI)
Youth Assessment and Screening Institute (YASI), 397
Youth Correctional Officer Management Profiling for Alternative Sanctions Risk and Needs Assessment (Youth COMPAS), 408–409
Youthful populations
  assessment tools for, 377–378
  recidivism, 377–378, 392–413
  risk assessment, 378–383, 383–391
Youth Level of Service/Case Management Inventory (YLS/CMI), 111, 394–396, 468
Youth violence, 349–372
  adolescent-limited offenders, 365–368
  juvenile violence offenders, 356–372
  life-course persistent offenders, 362–365
  predictors of, 109–115
  risk assessment tools, 387–388
  risks, 112–113
  United States statistics, 351–356
  VRS-YV, 113–115
  See also Crossover youth; Juvenile sex offenders; Juvenile violence offenders; Youth violence and aggression
Youth violence and aggression, 425–444
  Joint Risk Matrix, 427
  protective factors, 431–434
  resilience, 428–431
  risk, 428–431
  risk assessment instruments, 434–444
  risk factors, 431–434